Contributions by

JOHNNYE AKIN, PH.D.
University of Denver, Denver, Colorado

SARA C. FINLEY, M.D.
University of Alabama in Birmingham School of Medicine

WAYNE H. FINLEY, PH.D., M.D.
University of Alabama in Birmingham School of Medicine

ROLAND R. HAWES, D.M.D., M.S.
Case Western Reserve University School of Dentistry, Cleveland, Ohio

H. PERRY HITCHCOCK, D.M.D., M.S.D.
University of Alabama in Birmingham School of Dentistry

STANLEY E. KELLER, D.M.D., M.S.
University of Alabama in Birmingham School of Dentistry

DAVID B. LAW, D.D.S., M.S.
University of Washington School of Dentistry

THOMPSON M. LEWIS, D.D.S., M.S.D.
University of Washington School of Dentistry

LINCOLN R. MANSON-HING, D.M.D., M.S.
University of Alabama in Birmingham School of Dentistry

CHARLES A. McCALLUM, JR., D.M.D., M.D.
University of Alabama in Birmingham School of Dentistry

PALMI MOLLER, D.M.D., M.S.
University of Alabama in Birmingham School of Dentistry

GILBERT J. PARFITT, F.D.S.R.C.S., M.R.C.S., L.R.C.P.,
   D.M.D., F.R.C.D.(C.)
Faculty of Dentistry, University of British Columbia

SATISH R. RAO, B.D.S., M.S.
Howard University College of Dentistry, Washington, D.C.

LOUIS W. RIPA, D.D.S., M.S.
Eastman Dental Center, Rochester, New York

DAVID L. RUSSELL, D.M.D., M.S.
University of Alabama in Birmingham School of Dentistry

JOSEPH M. SIM, D.D.S., M.S.D.
Southern Illinois University School of Dental Medicine

JOE P. THOMAS, D.D.S., M.S.D.
University of Alabama in Birmingham School of Dentistry

GWENYTH R. VAUGHN, PH.D.
University of Alabama in Birmingham School of Dentistry

JOSEPH F. VOLKER, D.D.S., M.S., PH.D.
University of Alabama in Birmingham

CLINICAL PEDODONTICS

4th edition

SIDNEY B. FINN, D.M.D., M.S.

Professor of Dentistry (Pedodontics), Senior Investigator,
Institute of Dental Research
University of Alabama in Birmingham School of Dentistry

illustrated with 354 figures

W. B. SAUNDERS COMPANY
Philadelphia, London, and Toronto

W. B. Saunders Company: West Washington Square
Philadelphia, Pa. 19105

12 Dyott Street
London, WC1A   1DB

833 Oxford Street
Toronto, Ontario M8Z 5T9, Canada

Clinical Pedodontics   ISBN   0-7216-3637-3

Print No.:   9   8   7   6   5   4   3

This book is dedicated to children,
in whose hands the future lies.

CONTRIBUTORS

SIDNEY B. FINN, D.M.D., M.S.

Professor of Dentistry, Senior Investigator, Dental Research Institute, University of Alabama in Birmingham

and

JOHNNYE AKIN, Ph.D.

Professor of Speech-Communication, Linguistics, University of Denver, Denver, Colorado

SARA C. FINLEY, M.D.

Associate Professor of Pediatrics; Assistant Professor of Physiology and Biophysics, University of Alabama in Birmingham. Affiliated with University of Alabama Hospitals and Clinics, and The Children's Hospital of Birmingham

WAYNE FINLEY, Ph.D., M.D.

Professor of Pediatrics; Assistant Professor of Biochemistry; Assistant Professor of Physiology and Biophysics, University of Alabama in Birmingham. Affiliated with University of Alabama Hospitals and Clinics, and The Children's Hospital of Birmingham

ROLAND R. HAWES, D.M.D., M.S.

Professor and Chairman, Pedodontics Department, Case Western Reserve University School of Dentistry, Cleveland, Ohio. Director of Pediatric Dentistry, Rainbow Babies and Children's Hospital, Cleveland, Ohio

H. PERRY HITCHCOCK, D.M.D., M.S.D.

Chairman, Department of Orthodontics, University of Alabama in Birmingham, School of Dentistry. Orthodontic Consultant, Birmingham Veterans Administration Hospital, Birmingham, Alabama

STANLEY E. KELLER, D.M.D., M.S.

Professor of Dentistry, University of Alabama School of Dentistry. Consultant, Veterans Administration Hospital, Birmingham, Alabama

DAVID B. LAW, D.D.S., B.S.D., M.S.

Professor and Chairman, Department of Pedodontics, University of Washington School of Dentistry. Consultant, University Hospital; Children's Orthopedic Hospital and Medical Center; U.S. Public Health Service Hospital, Seattle, Washington

THOMPSON M. LEWIS, D.D.S., M.S.D.

Professor of Pedodontics, University of Washington School of Dentistry. Attending Pedodontist, Children's Orthopedic Hospital; Consultant in Pedodontics, University of Washington, Seattle, Washington

LINCOLN R. MANSON-HING, D.M.D., M.S.

Professor of Dentistry and Chairman, Department of Dental Roentgenology, University of Alabama School of Dentistry

CHARLES A. McCALLUM, Jr., D.M.D., M.D.

Dean, School of Dentistry, University of Alabama in Birmingham, Birmingham, Alabama

PALMI MOLLER, D.M.D., M.S.

Professor of Dentistry, University of Alabama in Birmingham, School of Dentistry

GILBERT J. PARFITT, F.D.S., R.C.S., M.R.C.S., L.R.C.P., D.M.D., F.R.C.D.(C)

Professor and Head of Oral Medicine, Faculty of Dentistry, University of British Columbia, Vancouver, B.C.

SATISH R. RAO, B.D.S., M.S.

Assistant Professor of Dentistry, Department of Pedodontics, Howard University College of Dentistry, Washington, D.C.

LOUIS W. RIPA, D.D.S., M.S.

Chairman, Department of Pedodontics, School of Dentistry, State University, Stony Brook, New York

DAVID L. RUSSELL, D.M.D., M.S.

Associate Professor of Dentistry and Chairman, Department of Pedodontics, University of Alabama School of Dentistry. Chief of Dental Services, The Children's Hospital, Birmingham, Alabama

JOSEPH M. SIM, D.D.S., M.S.D.

Associate Professor and Chairman, Department of Pediatric Dentistry, Southern Illinois University School of Dentistry, Carbondale, Illinois

JOE PRICE THOMAS, D.D.S., M.S.D.

Associate Professor of Dentistry, University of Alabama School of Dentistry; Clinical Investigator, Institute of Dental Research; Director of Postgraduate Pedodontics. Staff, Birmingham Children's Hospital, Birmingham, Alabama

GWENYTH R. VAUGHN, Ph.D.

Associate Professor of Speech Pathology and Audiology, University of Alabama in Birmingham, Schools of Dentistry and Medicine; Chief, Audiology-Speech Pathology Service, Birmingham Veterans Administration Hospital, Birmingham, Alabama

JOSEPH F. VOLKER, D.D.S., M.S., Ph.D.

President, University of Alabama in Birmingham

PREFACE TO THE FOURTH EDITION

Dentistry for children can be divided conveniently into three broad categories: prevention, diagnosis, and correction. To treat disease by prevention is the most desirable and should occupy the pages at the beginning of this book. However, in a broad sense, whatever one does for the child can be construed as preventive; therefore, which chapters should come first remains debatable. Because certain aspects of prevention are frequently taught as separate courses the chapters have been arranged in sequence for introducing the student to clinical procedures.

Because pedodontic knowledge is expanding and encompassing wider areas of interest several new chapters have been added. These include chapters on chromosomal disorders, removable partial dentures and communicative disorders in children. Several chapters have been either deleted or combined with other text material. Many of the illustrations have been improved or are new.

The authors are indebted to individuals too numerous to mention separately; however, special credit is due Miss Catherine Sims and Dr. J. Barenie for critically reading many of the chapters, to Mrs. Wynell Wade for her assistance in assembling the material, and to Mrs. C. Mayhall for a number of the sketches.

SIDNEY B. FINN

PREFACE TO THE FIRST EDITION

This textbook on dentistry for children has been prepared for the teaching of undergraduate dental students and for the general practitioner who wishes to keep abreast of the newer concepts and techniques in this broad field. We have tried to present the material in a clear and easily readable style and to avoid dogmatism.

Every author has the desire to make the contents of his book as all-encompassing as possible. However, because of the enormous scope of pedodontics, it becomes necessary to strike a balance between the purely theoretical and the extremely practical. In this situation, the purpose for which the book is designed must determine how the balance is weighed. We have attempted to mix the theoretical with the practical, but have placed the emphasis on practicality.

Certain material pertinent to the practice of dentistry for children has received insufficient coverage elsewhere and has been made an integral part of this textbook; other theoretical material, which is fully covered elsewhere in the dental curriculum, has not been stressed. Among the subjects which have been included in this textbook are parent counseling, the problem of pain, oral diagnostic procedures, antimicrobial agents, extensive pulpal techniques, the handling of the handicapped child in the dental office, the construction of mouth protectors, the role of heredity, biopsy techniques and hospital admittance procedures.

As dentistry advances, greater emphasis is being placed upon prevention in order to maintain an ideal oral structure. To this end, the authors have devoted a large portion of this textbook. We have tried to make the chapters on preventive orthodontics and the prevention of dental caries unique in clarity and comprehensiveness.

The authors wish to express their appreciation for the cooperation given by all who participated in making this dream a reality. Our thanks go to William Bowen and Joseph Mineo, who prepared the photographs, and to John Desley, who prepared the drawings. A special citation is certainly due our neglected families, who have borne with infinite stoicism this necessary, but temporary, division of loyalty.

THE AUTHORS

CONTENTS

1

THE CHILDREN'S DENTIST, HIS PRACTICE, AND HIS COMMUNITY

by SIDNEY B. FINN

Dentistry for children is perhaps the most needed and yet the most neglected of all the services performed by the dentist. In spite of its extreme importance, some dentists are prone to discount its value because of an unawareness of, or indifference to, the newer concepts of present day pedodontics and the ultimate goals to be achieved. The value of this service cannot be exaggerated, for inadequate or unsatisfactory dental treatment during childhood may damage permanently the entire masticatory apparatus, leaving the individual with many of the dental problems so common in today's adult population.

When a dentist assumes the responsibility of working on children, he must expect the task to be somewhat difficult, for practicing exemplary dentistry for children is not easy. It requires the acquisition and utilization of a vast knowledge of dentistry, of which much is common to adult practice, but much is unique and pertinent to children alone. If the practitioner is willing to expend the additional effort required to master the subject, he will find that working on children becomes one of the most satisfying experiences in all dental practice.

Dentistry for children requires more than routine dental knowledge, for one is dealing with organisms that are in their formative years. Only in children does one find this rapid growth and development in which individuals are constantly changing. What is assumed to be a normal developmental pattern for any child is certainly not fixed and may be capable of modification. The pedodontist is in a position to alter the growth pattern and resistance to disease of the oral tissues in these patients to produce a more ideal oral structure from a metabolic, functional and esthetic viewpoint.

In dentistry for children, one is dealing mainly with prevention. There is virtually no important phase of this field that is not preventive in its broad context.

In this respect, pediatric dentistry is a truly dedicated service, for prevention is the ultimate goal of all medical science.

The dentist who works on children has three responsibilities: (1) to his patient; (2) to his community; (3) to himself. The dentist's responsibility to himself is here considered first, for by being conscientious about his own requirements he simultaneously serves his patient and his community better.

THE DENTIST'S RESPONSIBILITY TO HIMSELF

During his dental education, the student should acquire two desirable attributes which will help him throughout his career: ego and humility. Both will afford him stature in achieving success in his chosen field.

His ego should make him proud of his chosen profession, a profession that has contributed to the alleviation of pain and suffering and has materially fostered the elevation of health standards. Graduation from a recognized dental school implies that the basic education he has received is as adequate as is possible to obtain. He is as well equipped to practice his profession as are practitioners of other professions. Realization of these facts should give him the confidence so necessary to a professional career, which in turn should give him enough dignity to assume his rightful place in the community.

The dentist should have sufficient humility to realize that with increased ability comes increased responsibility. His responsibilities must never be taken lightly. Dentistry is an ever-growing profession, expanding in knowledge and technique. The dentist can never stop learning. His skill and knowledge either continue to improve and grow or he stagnates and becomes relatively less effective. He must continue and put into practice that which he continues to learn. This implies attending professional meetings, refresher courses, lectures, seminars, and conferences. The dentist should not only subscribe to but read professional journals, textbooks, and all literature that will increase his knowledge and ability. To all this, he must apply a critical appraisal to either accept or reject new information. A healthy skepticism is desirable but should not blind one to proved facts.

Finally, the dentist should have sufficient humility to be honest in his appraisal of himself and render the finest service of which he is capable. He must never be satisfied with inadequate judgment or inferior technique.

The dentist who enjoys practicing his profession has a responsibility to himself and his family to earn a comfortable livelihood from it. This may involve sage judgment in selecting, establishing and conducting a practice as well as the necessary ability and personality.

An effort should be made to establish oneself in the community in which he practices, and, if children are to constitute a part of this practice, good liaison should be established with public and private school teachers and administrators. An opening wedge in this direction can be volunteering your services in promoting oral hygiene among the children by speaking at Parent-Teacher Association meetings and school assemblies. The dentist may also assist those in charge of health teaching to establish oral health clubs, set up displays and promote home care among the students. Bringing dental health information to parents, teachers and students alike is one of the finest services offered by the dentist to his community as well as being an excellent practice builder.

OFFICE MANAGEMENT

Good business practices are as essential to a profession as they are to other enterprises. There is no reason why a dentist with personality and skill should find himself incompetent in practice management. The next few pages, therefore, are broadly concerned with the routine of office management.

Office Decoration

There are many factors that should be considered in locating an office for the type of practice you wish to establish, such as: the area's social and economic status, transportation and parking facilities, and easy access to schools and residential areas.

Once the location is selected, the type of office decoration must be considered. If one is to limit one's practice to children, the entire office from the reception room through the treatment rooms can have a definite motif. Decorations and accouterments depicting definite settings such as the circus, the West, outer space or nursery rhymes add to the warmth and fantasy of the office and tend to dispel fear. An aquarium is always a source of entertainment and may be placed either in the reception room or in the treatment room where it is visible to the child in the chair. Soothing, muffled music in the reception room has a comforting effect on both parent and patient and dispels the coldness often felt in a silent room. If adults are to bring children to the dental office, reading material should be available for adults as well as for children. Cookbooks afford busy mothers interesting reading. A pencil and pad bearing the inscription, "Copy a recipe and prepare a new dish for your child," can be placed alongside the cookbook for the mother to copy any recipe she may wish to take home. Thus an interesting and productive waiting period is provided the mother while the child is in the treatment room. The waiting room can also be used to present dental health material.

If the practice will not be limited to children, an area in the reception room should be set aside for children. (See Chapter 3, Child Management in the Dental Office.)

Ancillary Personnel

The dentist should realize the limitations of his allotted working time and, whenever possible, should employ personnel to permit him more time for those tasks that cannot be delegated to others. The selection of proper help, whether hygienist, assistant or secretary, is important and should be done with great care. Hiring should be on a trial basis only. Even with the highest qualifications, a hygienist or assistant is good only if she can fit satisfactorily into the regime of your office. The most competent personnel may have to be trained to do things as you want them done. This assumes greater importance with increasing expansion of duties for these individuals.

The efficient utilization of chairside assistants is extremely important in a pedodontic practice because (1) it decreases the length of the dental appointment, thus aiding in child management; (2) time and motion studies have shown that an assistant decreases the number of steps and movements necessary, resulting in less fatigue to the dentist; and (3) the dentist practices more efficiently and more rapidly, thereby becoming more productive, and increasing his income. The amount of work accomplished more than compensates for the expenditure of salary for the chairside assistant.

The following paragraphs depict the proper utilization of a chairside assistant. To get the most out of this type of arrangement, modern equipment is important. Contour chairs have been found most effective in a children's practice (Fig. 1–1). The patient rests in a supine position with his body parallel to the floor and feet slightly elevated. The assistant's arms are held slightly above the child's chest and afford a comforting feeling of security to him. There is no cuspidor available so he cannot use the diversionary tactic of frequent expectoration. Saliva is removed by suction.

The dentist operates in a sitting position on a comfortable, contoured stool. The assistant sits across the chair from him completely unencumbered by a dental unit. All equipment is conveniently located near the assistant. High and low speed handpieces, suction, air and water syringes are mounted on a bracket extending partially over the chair. Well integrated instruction makes it possible for these implements to be handed to the dentist as needed (Fig. 1–2).

The assistant has everything needed for any specific procedure within easy reach without leaving her chair. In a portable cabinet alongside her are the amalgamator and all needed general supplies and drugs (Figs. 1–3 and 1–4).

Each operation has its own tray (setup) of instruments which are selected from

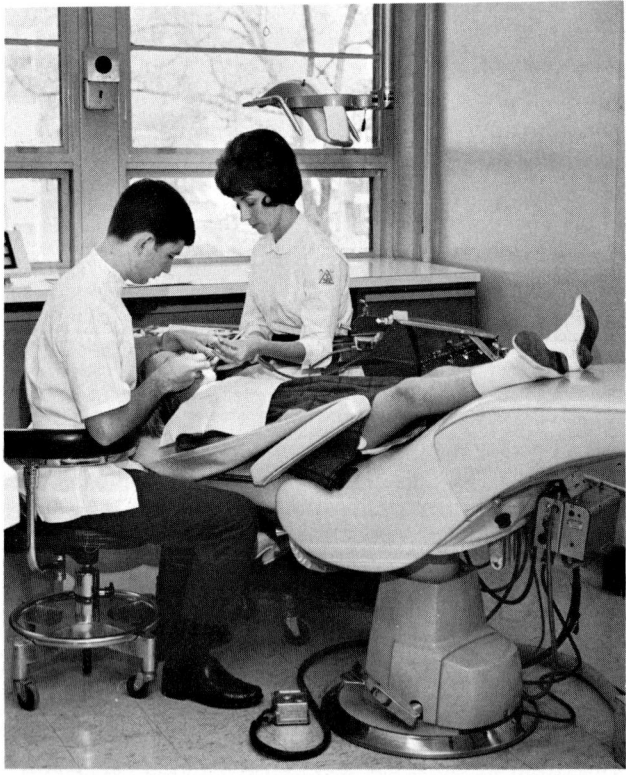

Figure 1–1   Notice the relaxed, comfortable position of the child, the dentist, and the assistant. The equipment projects from a bracket extending over the arm of the chair in close proximity to the assistant.

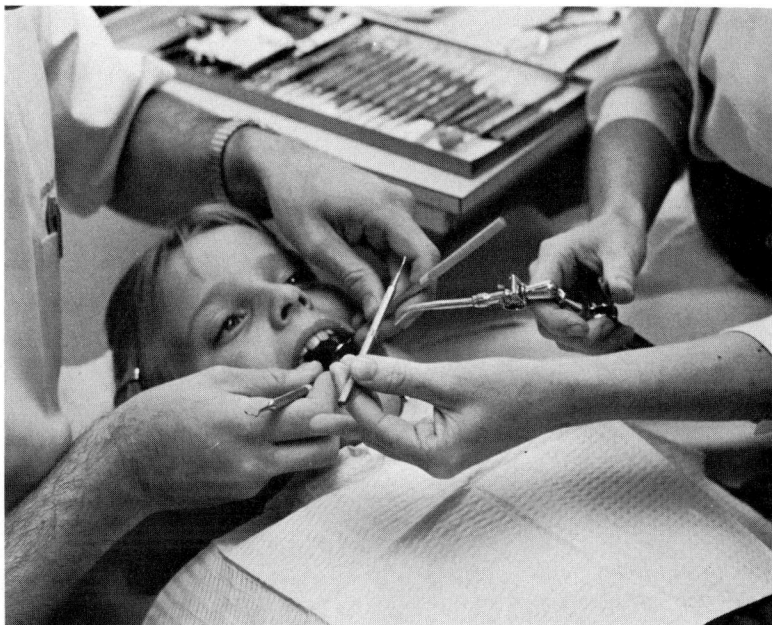

Figure 1–2 Through integrated training all four hands are being utilized; the assistant exchanges instruments as needed, using the fingers of one hand to give and remove instruments simultaneously.

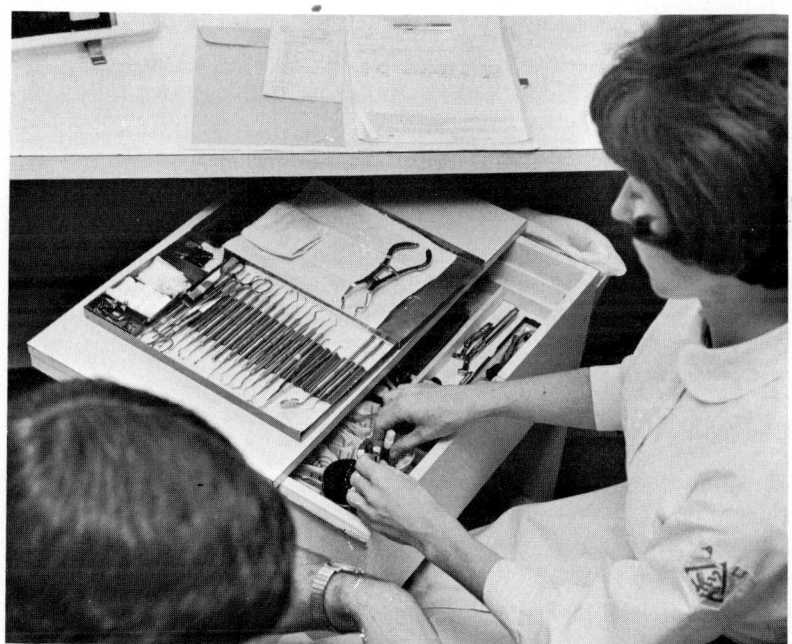

Figure 1–3 The portable cabinet with sliding top. In the front half are visible topical and local anesthetics, cotton supplies, handpieces, etc.

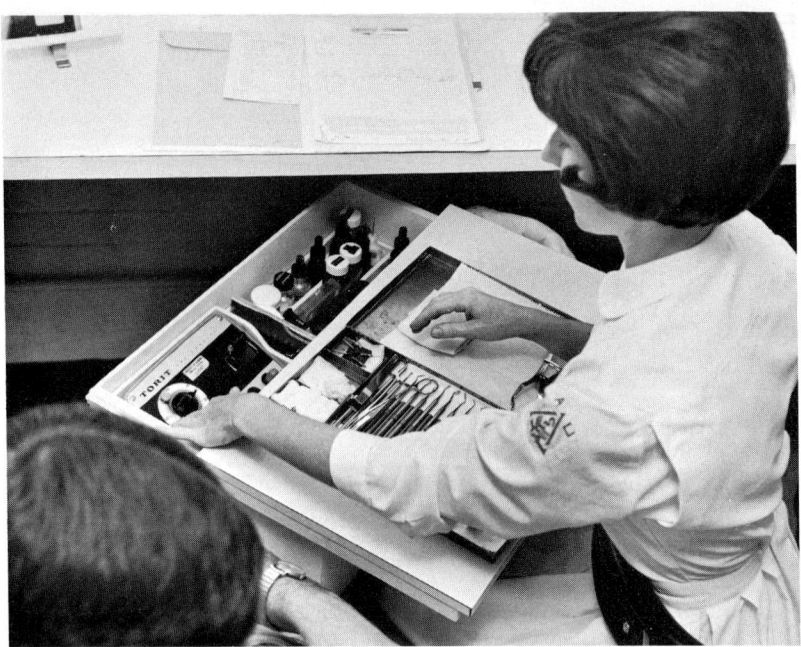

Figure 1-4   Under the back half of the sliding top are visible necessary drugs, filling materials, and mechanical amalgamator.

the cabinet drawers and placed on the top cover of the cabinet to meet the needs of the operation.

All instruments are handed to and removed from the dentist's hands by the assistant in what might be called a fluid exchange without need for the dentist to divert his attention (Fig. 1-5) while she continues to assist in other dental procedures such as operating the suction or using the air or water spray.

The concept of "four-handed dentistry" implies that the assistant's hands are constantly employed in the treatment of the child. It is not necessary for the dentist to divert his hands or his attention from the task he is performing, thus curtailing the amount of unnecessary motion while accomplishing a great deal more work. This concept is widely used in today's modern practice of dentistry for children.

Health Education Room

Space should be allocated in the dental office where the child and parent can be given proper instruction in preventive procedures. Although this information can be presented in any area of the dental office, a separate room away from possible areas of stress to the patient is most desirable. Instruction in oral hygiene procedures should be explained fully and participation by the child should be made mandatory until toothbrushing and flossing become an established habit pattern. This may require observing the patient go through the routine a number of times.

There are many adjuncts available, recently in kit form, to teach the children and attendant parents. Educating the parent is desirable to fortify and supervise the child while performing these duties at home. Slides, film strips, records, films, pamphlets, charts and models are available from a number of sources such as the American Dental Association. The justifiable emphasis presently being placed on plaque control, including its removal, must be an integral part of the educational program. Techniques such as plaque staining, and the phase-microscope (preferably for double viewing) to demonstrate viable microorganisms are valuable teaching aids to convince the patient and parent. A well illuminated mirror before which children can practice and perfect their toothbrushing and flossing technique will be of great benefit. Caries activity tests can also be used as an educational tool.

Introductory Information

The importance of obtaining complete identifying information and past history of the patient at the first visit cannot be emphasized too strongly. Generally the first visit of the child to the office is made in the company of a parent. The child may make subsequent visits alone and will be unable to offer the desired information. Printed forms should be on hand to facilitate recording these data, which should include the following items: the patient's full name and nickname; both parents' names, address, and telephone number; person responsible for payment of fees, his address, telephone number, occupation, and firm for which he works. One should also request and record the name of the person who referred the parent or patient to your office. It is a polite gesture to send this person a card of appreciation.

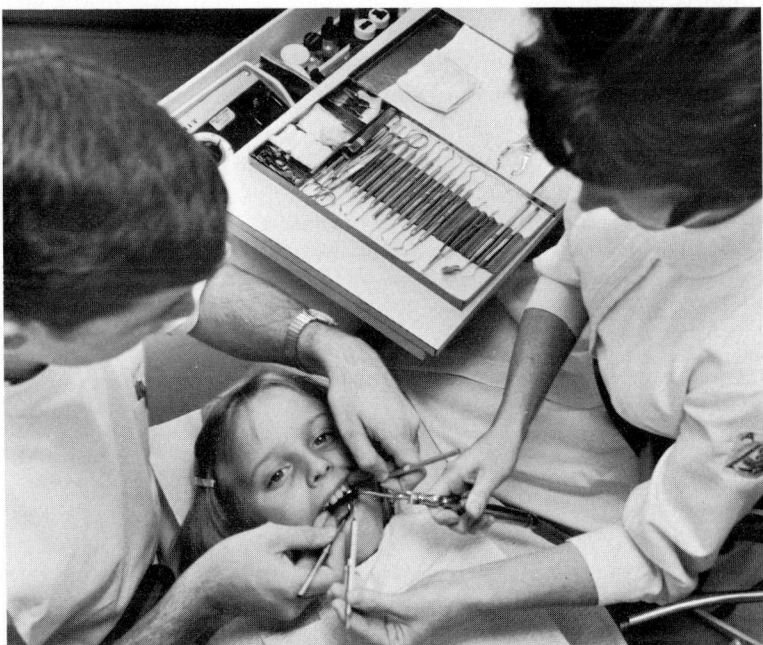

Figure 1–5 The illustrated tray is equipped for amalgam preparation and restoration. Trays are sterilized as a unit, then stored until needed.

Patient History

A thorough and revealing past history is essential if untoward difficulties are to be avoided during the course of dental treatment. The leading questions to be asked can be available on printed forms especially designed for the purpose. The dentist should take a complete past history and record the chief complaint. If the chief complaint is an emergency, the patient should receive treatment of a palliative or corrective nature during this visit.

The technique of appraising the patient and taking a complete history is described in Chapter 5.

Other information that should be obtained is whether the child receives regular physical examinations, and the name and address of the physician. If the child has been referred by a pediatrician, the latter should be consulted before treatment is started. A personal letter expressing your appreciation should be sent him. It is also helpful to learn if the child fears dental treatment and why. This information can be obtained from the parent. The record should be completed with the date and signature of the person giving the information and his relation to the patient.

Preliminary Examination and Consultation

After this preliminary information is obtained, the person taking the history escorts the patient and parent into the treatment room. The patient is seated in the chair, the identification and history cards are carefully studied and the oral cavity is thoroughly examined. A careful evaluation is made of the entire physical structure of the child. It should be suggested to the parent that at this visit the teeth should be cleaned, a topical fluoride applied to the teeth and tooth brushing instruction given. A full-mouth x-ray survey should be made and impressions taken for study models. After this information is assembled, a more accurate appraisal of the condition of the mouth, with suggested plans of treatment, can be made. Since this involves some time and study, another appointment is made for the parents at which time a complete diagnosis of the case is presented so the parents will be aware of the problems involved, along with the probable cost. Depending upon the financial condition of the family, alternate treatment plans may be suggested.

In quoting estimates, avoid giving exact figures or mentioning the exact number of cavities. If a definite number is quoted, the parent may be disappointed later on if another cavity is found or if more involved and complicated procedures are required than were originally anticipated. Never discuss fees with a minor. Always make sure that a parent or someone responsible for payment approves the estimate.

Audio-visual aids are of assistance in presenting the treatment plan to parents. A well diversified stock of models, charts and pictures assists in clarifying unfamiliar facts (Fig. 1–6).

Recalls

One of the fundamentals of a successful pedodontic practice is a good recall system. Parents appreciate being reminded that it is time for their child's re-examination. It indicates to them that you are earnestly endeavoring to prevent serious damage to the child's teeth.

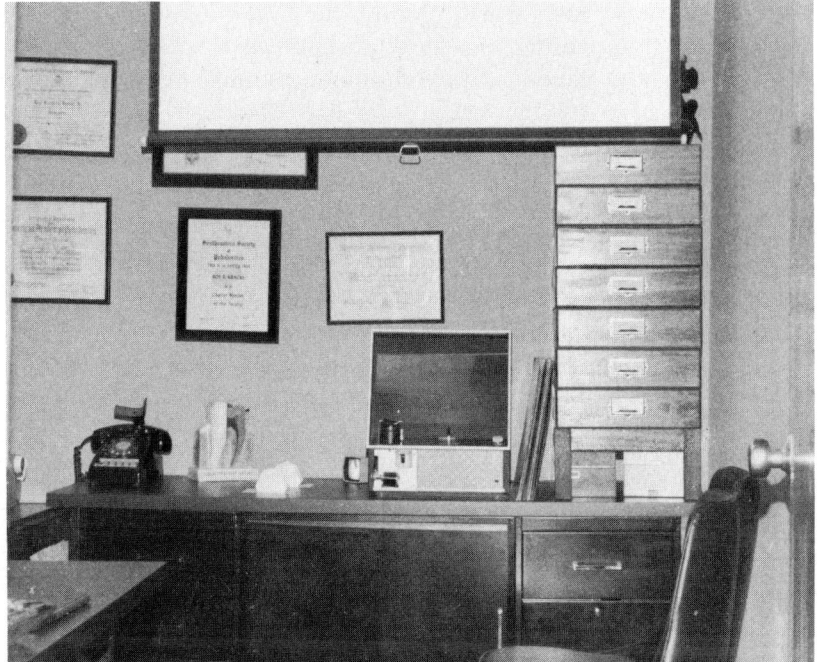

Figure 1–6   A health education room. Video material is projected from an adjoining room onto the screen. (Courtesy of Dr. Roy Kracke.)

After all necessary dental treatment has been completed, the hygienist, assistant or secretary should explain that periodic examinations are necessary if the child's teeth are to be maintained in as good a condition as they presently are. She can then suggest that she would be glad to call the parent when it is time for a re-examination.

The frequency of recall should be based on the caries susceptibility of the individual. Children with an active caries potential should be recalled at least every three months. Children with a low caries potential should be recalled approximately every six months.

An appointment book or appointment card file for recalls can be maintained to expedite notifying patients or parents. All notifications by telephone are made at least two weeks before the appointment time and followed up by an appointment card one week before this time.

THE DENTIST'S RESPONSIBILITY TO HIS PATIENT

The dentist's responsibility to his patient requires that he use good judgment in planning and executing treatment. This service must be performed to the best of his ability, and a fair and just fee should be charged for it. One of the first prerequisites for good office management is patient management. To fulfill his responsibility to his patient, the dentist must be able to handle children well. Inability to manage them may defeat all attempts to perform high quality dentistry. Emphasis must be placed on prevention, which requires not only a knowledge of preventive techniques but also the scientific knowledge of their functions. A competent dentist should be able to answer patient and parent inquiries intelligently with correct and factual knowledge.

Children's dentistry demands the use of diagnostic aids as well as a correct interpretation of the findings, both in emergency situations and in routine problems.

If the dentist can put into practice all of the aforementioned principles he is well on his way to discharging his responsibility to his patient. Beyond these, he must convey to patient and parent the value of good dentistry. He must convince them that good dentistry for children is an investment in future health. Good dentistry does not begin at the dental chair. It begins at home in proper oral hygiene, in an adequate diet, in carbohydrate restriction, in participation in community efforts for water fluoridation, in establishing dental programs for the indigent. Thus effective dentistry can be practiced without a dental chair. Its impact on the public may be as necessary as the effort expended at the dental chair. In other words, children's dentistry involes both education and service.

PROFESSIONAL RELATIONSHIPS

The dentist's responsibilities to his patients may require that he be a liaison between the parent and the physician or the parent and a hospital. The referral may be to a specialist in some branch of dentistry. These referrals should be executed with dispatch and as efficiently as possible. The parents should be informed of the need for consultation or hospitalization. If there is a risk involved, it must always be put in writing and the dentist should be sure that there is complete understanding by the parent.

Good rapport can be established with the pediatricians and general practitioners in town. Frequently the services of a pediatrician will prove of assistance in diagnostic problems. If a child patient appears ill, his temperature is taken and if elevated and no oral symptoms are present, the child should be referred to his pediatrician or general practitioner for diagnosis and treatment. A clinical oral thermometer should be available in every dental office. The pediatrician in turn will refer patients with oral problems to the dentist. Complete cooperation can exist between the allied professions. When the dentist first opens his office he should introduce himself to the pediatricians or general practitioners in the neighborhood or town. Such an association can build mutual respect.

THE DENTIST'S RESPONSIBILITY TO HIS COMMUNITY

The present day children's dentist is becoming more and more aware of his responsibilities to his community. These responsibilities transcend his duties as a chairside practitioner to make him a crusader for the elevation of the dental health standards of all children in the community. As a member of the healing profession, he assumes his rightful position alongside the pediatrician and the public health worker in bettering the general health of the community. The children's dentist can be the instigator and key worker in all community programs dealing with children's dental health, for no one knows better than he the communal needs. By fostering these programs, he instills in people a better appreciation of the value of dentistry, for a person cannot appreciate what he does not understand. Dental service is valued only if it comes to be regarded as a necessity; it becomes so regarded only when people learn that they should not and cannot do without it. This is the basis of all public health educational programs.

If the dentist displays no interest or desire to better the dental health of the community outside of his dental office, he has no right to complain if the public does not appreciate the value of early prevention and treatment of dental ills. The dentist must assume the role of dental educator. This is especially important in small cities and towns, where the number of professional public health educators is limited and where their varied duties in this large field may preclude giving sufficient attention to dental health.

The most satisfactory method of educating the people of a community is through public health dental programs. These may be quite varied and depend a great deal upon the needs of the community and the money available for such a program.

The most successful program is one that is continuous, whether it be preventive or corrective. People have a tendency to forget unless they are constantly reminded. Many persons, for instance, never visit a dentist until an aching tooth reminds them that aid is available; the public as a whole is apathetic.

Children's Dental Health Day (or Week) is celebrated once a year and it is effective to a certain degree. However, to have a definite and long-lasting impact on the community, dental health education must be brought before the public every day until it becomes an integral part of community life. It must be pressed with vigor until every member of the community is cognizant of his family's dental needs and is willing to participate by simply taking his own children to the dental office. If every parent assumes this responsibility, the community will have gone a long way in solving the problems of children's dental needs. To meet the needs of those who cannot afford private dentistry, programs must be established.

Community dental programs, to be complete, should embody two types of service: prevention and correction. The extent of these programs is dependent upon the available funds and available personnel.

PREVENTIVE PROGRAMS

Preventive programs should be educational as well as clinical. The educational aspects of a program stress the importance of preserving the teeth and periodontal tissues as well as limiting the possibility of malocclusion. In accomplishing this, one must present all aspects of the problem.

Emphasizing Needs

The needs of the community for dental care, as expressed by the prevalence of dental caries, periodontal disease, and malocclusion, must be presented to the community leaders and to the public in general for them to realize the magnitude of the problem. The sequelae of dental neglect must be emphasized to demonstrate the seriousness of public apathy. Once the responsible public is familiarized with the definite need for a dental program, community cooperation will be enlisted with less difficulty.

Teaching Preventive Methods

Assuming that the need has been well publicized, the next step is the development of an educational program on methods and techniques of preventing oral disease and malocclusion.

Oral Hygiene.   The importance of oral hygiene and home care, including the technique of proper tooth brushing, should receive considerable attention. Tooth brushing technique can be taught either by demonstration with an oversized papier-maché model of the teeth and a large toothbrush or by showing a motion picture of the technique. Both can be used with fairly large groups, although individual personalized instruction is better. The demonstrations, whenever possible, should be followed by child participation. Much more can be learned, and more quickly, by doing than by observing.

Dietary Factors.   The role played by carbohydrates in producing dental caries must be stressed, and means of limiting their usage, especially between meals, should be discussed. The fact that a well balanced diet containing all of the essential foods is necessary for oral health as well as for general body health should be made clear in any dental health education program.

Fluoride Prophylaxis.   The need for preventive programs such as topical fluoride applications are presented to the public not merely as an educational endeavor but with the thought of establishing a topical fluoride clinical program in the community.

A concerted communal effort to initiate a program of water fluoridation for a community which has a fluoride-deficient communal water supply requires a well planned and executed campaign. The opposition to fluoridation may be impassioned and bitter, and may employ unlimited exaggeration and distortion of facts to mislead the public and to confuse the uninformed. Even after several decades of demonstration of the efficacy and safety of water fluoridation, the opposition is relentless in its efforts to stifle this health measure. Workers in a campaign for fluoridation should be forewarned of the nature of some of the opposition and must be armed with all of the effective arguments. Stress the fact that communal water fluoridation will benefit the indigent child as well as the non-indigent child, and that no other caries preventive measure has proved as effective on a mass scale. All evidence as to its complete safety is conveyed to the public.

Prevention of Malocclusion.   In any preventive program, malocclusion must be taken into account. Studies have shown that from 35 to 50 per cent of all children suffer from some form of malocclusion. The public must be educated to the deleterious effect on occlusion of the early loss of the primary teeth unless remedial measures are taken.

Sources of Educational Materials

A preventive program requires not only speakers but educational material as well. A great deal of material is available for this purpose.

Many agencies, local, state and national, can offer aid of varying types, from helpful suggestions to assistance in securing the necessary personnel and supplies.

They may also contribute actual monetary support. Monies from Federal sources are now available to establish indigent programs for both correction and prevention. In a number of states Medicaid programs are in operation. In establishing a preventive program, it is advisable to set up a steering committee of persons interested in child welfare. Among them may be members from the medical, dental and hospital personnel of the community, school principals and staff, health departments, health councils, Parent-Teacher Associations, welfare agencies, Red Feather organizations, service organizations, women's clubs, and interested civic-minded individuals from the community.

There are many ways of approaching the public in an educational program. Some are: (1) talks before school groups, Parent-Teacher Associations, service organizations, women's clubs, union meetings, hospital staff meetings, church groups, etc.; (2) school projects such as health clubs and instructional programs in oral hygiene; (3) poster, essay, "Perfect Smile," and other types of contests; (4) free x-rays or dental examinations at state or county fairs or other large public gatherings; (5) posters on trucks (milk delivery, express company, department store, etc.); (6) newspaper articles, radio and television programs, and spot announcements; (7) moving pictures and puppet shows. Each will have an additive effect and together they will result in a campaign having considerable impact on the population.

The success of this type of program can be judged by the overall motivation it produces in the community.

CORRECTIVE PROGRAMS

Corrective programs generally imply treatment of dental caries. Although preventive measures now available will reduce the prevalence of dental caries, they will not completely eliminate the need for dental care programs. However, as more preventive measures come into being and the amount of necessary work to be done on each patient decreases, more children can be treated with the present limited number of available dentists. It will be possible for the private practitioner to treat a larger number of children in his office. In this way, greater numbers of non-indigent children will receive necessary care. Programs providing care for the indigent and underprivileged are receiving greater recognition. If this can be provided, the entire child population possibly could be handled.

An educational program can go a long way in motivating those who can afford dental care to seek it from the private dentist. A large segment of the population, however, earn only enough money to give their children the barest of necessities. These are the dentally indigent. There is also a large group that is completely indigent. Dental public health programs should be organized to provide care for these underprivileged children. The children's dentist can help by activating the community to think along these lines.

There are many types of care programs dependent upon the availability of dental personnel and space and equipment, and the amount of financial aid obtained. Dental personnel is limited. Public dental care programs may be conducted in the private dental office or in a clinic established for the purpose. Although some endowed clinics have their own buildings, modest clinics may be set up in a public health building, school, hospital, church, or any place with adequate space and utilities.

A correction program consisting only of dental examinations does very little in the way of preserving teeth and is to be avoided in favor of a program that includes fewer patients but does actual restorative work. With a limited program, not all teeth can be treated. In this situation, attention should be placed on saving the first permanent molars, since they are the most vulnerable permanent teeth.

If a more extensive program is contemplated, all of the necessary dental work can be done for the 6 year olds. The second year, the entire 6 year age group is completed plus the yearly increment necessary for the 7 year olds who received complete treatment the previous year. The plan can be expanded until all ages of grade school children are included. This type of program is flexible and may also include preschool children. An early grade school program is more effective and less costly than one starting with teen-age children because there is not as great a backlog of untreated teeth.

A dental corrective care program that is frequently neglected is that for the handicapped child, yet these children are especially in need of dental attention because of their handicaps. The cleft palate or epileptic child can be handled in the dental office, as can the moderately spastic child. The markedly cerebral palsied child may be handled better under general anesthesia.

Whatever type of program is contemplated by the community, whether it be preventive or corrective, the children's dentist should make his experience and training available in whatever capacity his altruism directs him.

REFERENCES

1. Berdon, J. K., and Griffin, J. A.: A survey of toothbrushing habits of dental school students. W. Va. Dent. J., *42*:6, 1968.
2. Blayney, J. R., and Hill, I. N.: Fluorine and dental caries. Special issue. J.A.D.A., *74*, 1967.
3. Brock, D. W., Hodges, F. T., Castaldi, C. R., Waterman, G. E., and Ingle, J. I.: Sixth national dental health conference symposium. J.A.D.A., *52*:663, 1956.
4. Gutman, R. E.: Why dental health education? Clinical pediatrics, *10*:669, 1971.
5. Hammons, P. E., and Jamison, H. C.: New duties for dental auxiliaries—the Alabama experience. Am. J. Public Health, *58*:882, 1968.
6. Henning, F. R., and Fanning, E. A.: Instruction in oral hygiene. Australian Dent. J., *13*:40, 1968.
7. Law, F. E.: Appraisal—A national authority assesses Philadelphia. Public Health Views, Philadelphia Department of Public Health, p. 14.
8. Mack, E. S.: Practical pedodontic practice. J. Dent. Child., *23*:13, 1956.
9. Pelton, W. J.: The problem of making dental care available to all areas. Ala. Jour. Med. Sci., *5*:167, 1968.
10. Robinson, G. E., Wuehrmann, A. H., Sinnett, G. M., et al.: Four handed dentistry: The whys and wherefores. J.A.D.A., *77*:573, 1968.
11. Roder, D. M.: A study of dental knowledge and behavior in 1000 Australian school children. Australian Dent. J., *14*:327, 1969.
12. Shiller, W. R., and Dittmer, J. W.: An evaluation of some current oral hygiene motivation methods. J. Periodont., *39*:83, 1968.
13. Teuscher, G.: The role of the clinician. J. Dent. Child., *20*:37, 1953.
14. Williford, J. W., Muhler, J. C., and Stookey, G. K.: Study demonstrating improved oral health through education. J.A.D.A., *75*:896, 1967.
15. Young, W. O.: The organization of effective community dental health programs. J. Dent. Child., *26*:220, 1959.

2

PARENT COUNSELING AND CHILD BEHAVIOR

by SIDNEY B. FINN

Children begin by loving their parents; as they grow older,
they judge them; sometimes they forgive them.

OSCAR WILDE.

The intent of this chapter is to discuss the emotional problems of children, particularly in relation to dental treatment, and to offer the dentist an insight into parental influences which may produce unnecessary anxieties in children. With this basic information, it is hoped the reader will be encouraged to pursue the subject further and will eventually be in a position to advise and guide parents intelligently.

A child's behavior pattern in any situation is governed by his inherited physical and mental endowment, and as he develops, by the conditioning he receives through contact with his environment. The former, except within certain narrow limits, cannot be altered. The latter can be controlled and developed so that the child will grow to have a well adjusted personality suited to the society in which he finds himself. One of the adjustments all children must make is developing a pattern of behavior which will be socially acceptable and which will satisfy their physical and emotional needs. One of their physical needs may be dental attention. Whether children accept dental treatment gracefully or refuse it entirely will depend on how they have been conditioned. The emotional conditioning of children toward dentistry, as toward other experiences which make up childhood, is formed primarily in the home and under parental guidance.

If the dentist is to perform satisfactory dental work for his child patients he must have their full cooperation. He can secure this cooperation only if he understands the emotional make-up of children and of their parents. Without this understanding he may find managing children difficult. The dentist must acknowledge that he is emotionally involved with his patients and to handle them successfully he must be aware of those psychological and sociological factors that have formed their attitudes and behavior patterns toward dentistry. A study of the sciences which help understand the development of fears, anxieties and anger as it applies to the child in the dental situation can be designated as Behavioral Pedodontics. The proper handling of children in the dental office is the dentist's responsibility, and it is one that he should assume without hesitation if he is to fulfill his obligation to his patients and to his profession. It is equally clear that the conditioning of children toward the dentist and dental services is entirely the parents' responsibility. They should accept this obligation as a parental duty. If children enter the office for the first time with undue fear and an unwillingness to cooperate, one can assume that parental conditioning has been faulty. Although it is the parents' responsibility to inculcate in their children proper attitudes toward dentistry, the dentist can help by making sure the parents are fully informed of and educated in the necessary fundamentals of child psychology. The practitioner should accept this obligation as a routine part of his practice. *If we are to have good child patients we must first educate parents. A dentist who fails to do this is not using every means available to him in the management of the child.*

Before a dentist is in a position to advise parents regarding the proper psychological preparation of their children, he must understand the problems involved. He must understand the nature of fear and have an awareness of how parental attitudes may modify behavior patterns. He should be familiar with personality formation and how anxieties develop. He should also have the diplomacy and tact to transmit this information to parents in an acceptable and professional manner. If the dentist can counsel parents in an enlightened manner the advice, in most instances, will be willingly and even eagerly accepted. If the dentist is to be a respected member of the health profession he should certainly be competent to discuss problems related to his field. Parents are eager to give their children all the advantages of life even though they themselves may not have been so rewarded in childhood. Intelligent emotional training of the child provides one of these essential advantages, for it may govern whether he is to be successful or not. The dentist should be as competent to offer advice on child behavior as the physician. Certainly management problems are of greater importance to the dentist, who may see children under considerable emotional stress—yet dentists hesitate to give advice to parents on child behavior. It is time for the dentist of today to realize his full responsibilities as a professional man.

The parents will in turn apply this knowledge to their children, who will look with favor on dentistry rather than with unwarranted fear. This knowledge will help the child as well as the dentist. The information in this chapter applies not only to child patients but to adult patients as well, for if we understand the emotional problems of children we can understand those of adults. The anxieties we find in adulthood are formed primarily in childhood. In adults, the fears and anxieties are of longer duration and are usually latent and well hidden. Yet marked phobias related to dental treatment do exist among adults, and they account for the avoidance of dental treatment by a segment of our population.

THE NATURE OF FEAR

The parents' responsibility in psychologically preparing the child for dental treatment is primarily in the emotional problem of *fear*. Fear presents the greatest management problem to the dentist and is one of the reasons why people neglect dental treatment. For this reason it is well to discuss this emotion and the way parental as well as other environmental influences act in creating good child patients or difficult ones.

Fear is one of the primary emotions acquired soon after birth, although the startle response is present at birth, and the reflex response to stimuli is also demonstrable before birth. The infant, however, is unaware of the nature of the stimulus producing fear. As the child grows and his mental capacity increases. he becomes aware of the stimuli producing fear and can identify each individually. The child tries to adjust to these isolated experiences by resorting to flight if he cannot solve the problem otherwise. If the child feels inadequate to cope with the situation and flight is a physical impossibility, fear is intensified.

Fear and rage are primitive responses developed to protect the individual from harm and self-destruction. The emotional stimulation is discharged by way of the autonomic nervous system through the hypothalamus and needs very little cortical integration. This is well illustrated by the uninhibited behavior of a decorticated animal. However, in man, discharges from the hypothalamus may be modified by cortical interference so that man with his highly developed cortex can control his emotions, to a degree, through rationalization and determination. In young children, too young for much rationalization, behavior is produced which is difficult to control. The infant in many respects behaves in a primitive manner in an effort to either fight or flee the situation. When this cannot be done, fear increases so that communicating with the child by the dentist may be extremely difficult. Even in older children this situation may exist in which fear is so marked that the child cannot rationalize clearly. Generally, as the child's mental age increases these responses can be controlled more and more by the cortex through higher psychic functions. (See Chapter 7.)

THE VALUE OF FEAR

Contrary to popular belief, fears are of great value when given proper direction and control. Since fear-producing stimuli can cause actual harm to the child, fear is a protective mechanism for self-preservation. The very nature of this emotion can be utilized to keep the child away from dangerous situations of either a social or a physical nature. If the child does not fear punishment or parental disfavor his behavior may make him a threat to society and ultimately lead to incarceration. If the child is not taught to fear fire his chances of being burned are greatly increased. Therefore, the proper training of the child by the parent should be not in the direction of eradicating fear, but rather in that of channeling it toward dangers that really exist, and away from situations where no danger lies. In this way it will serve as a protective mechanism against real danger and as a deterrent against antisocial behavior.

The child should be taught that the dental office is not a place to fear. Dentistry should never be employed by the parents as a threat. Taking the child to the dentist should never be used to imply punishment. Using it in this manner unquestionably creates fear of the dentist. On the other hand, if the child has become attached to the dentist, fear of the loss of his approval may have some value in motivating the child to accept office discipline.

TYPES OF FEAR

The majority of fears evident in children may have been acquired either objectively or subjectively.

OBJECTIVE FEARS

Objective fears are those produced by direct physical stimulation of the sense organs and are generally not of parental origin. Objective fears are responses to stimuli that are felt, seen, heard, smelled or tasted, and are of a disagreeable or unpleasant nature. A child who has had previous contact with a dentist and has been managed so poorly that undue and unnecessary pain has been inflicted, necessarily develops a fear of future dental treatment. It is difficult to get a child so hurt to return to the dentist of his own volition. When he is induced to return, the dentist must realize his emotional state and proceed slowly to re-establish the child's confidence in the dentist and in dental treatment.

Objective fears may be associative in nature. Dental fears may be associated with unrelated experiences. A child who has been improperly handled or subjected to intense pain in a hospital by persons in white uniforms may develop an intense fear of similar uniforms on dentists or dental hygienists. Even the characteristic smell of certain drugs or chemicals previously associated with unpleasantness may arouse unwarranted fear. An aching tooth can associate pain with dentistry and cause apprehension in connection with the dental appointment. Fear also lowers the threshold of pain so that any pain produced during dental treatment becomes magnified and leads to even greater apprehension.

SUBJECTIVE FEARS

Subjective fears are those based on feelings and attitudes that have been suggested to the child by others about him without the child's having had the experience personally. A young child is prone to suggestion. The young inexperienced child, hearing of some unpleasant or pain-producing situation undergone by a parent or others, soon develops a fear of that experience. The mental picture producing the fear is retained in the child's mind and, with the vivid imagination of childhood, becomes magnified and formidable. A child hearing from parents or playmates of the supposed terror of the dental office soon accepts it as real and to be avoided if at all possible. Shoban and Borland[15] reported that fear of dentistry in adults was based more on what they heard about dentistry from their parents than on anything else. In children, as in adults, the greatest producer of fear is hearing of unpleasant experiences in the dental office from parents or friends.

Children have an intense fear of the unknown. Any experience that is new and unknown to the child will produce fear until the child has proof that there is no threat to his well-being from that direction. His fear is an attempt to adjust to a situation which he feels may be painful to him. Until he can be convinced that there is no reason to be frightened, fear will persist. The influence of parents is most important in the child's attitude toward dentistry. It is imperative that parents inform their children of what to expect in the dental office. The child should be familiarized *in a general way* with the procedures that will be encountered and the appearance and description of the office equipment before the first dental appointment. With present day dentistry, it is not necessary to inflict undue pain. No parent therefore should tell his child that there will be intense pain experienced. Nor should any parent minimize or tell an untruth about the discomfort of dentistry. Honesty without emotional exaggeration should be employed.

Suggestive fears may be acquired by imitation. A child observing fear in others may soon acquire a fear for the same object or event as real and genuine as that observed by the child in others. This is especially true if the fear is observed in parents. Children frequently identify themselves with parents. If the parent is sad the child feels sad. If the parent displays fear the child is fearful. Child anxiety and overt negative behavior are closely correlated with parental anxiety.

Imitative fears may be transmitted subtly and may be displayed by the parent and acquired by the child without either being aware of it. They are generally recurrent fears and therefore are more deep-seated and difficult to eradicate. Displayed emotion, such as anxiety observed in the parent's face, may create more of an impression than verbal suggestion. A mother who fears going to the dentist and goes only under great emotional stress transmits this fear unconsciously to her child who is observing her. It is easy to realize how even a tight clenching of the child's hand in the dental office in an unconscious gesture of encouragement for what is to transpire may be enough to create suspicion and untoward fear in the child. Generally, the longer subjective fears exist in the mind, the more they are magnified. As a consequence, these fears may be much more intense and out of all proportion to the objective fear which would have been produced by the actual experience. Hence long-standing fears, generally subjective, may be the most difficult to overcome and eradicate. Fear of objective stimuli, such as the pain of an injection, is not too difficult for the child to overcome by using logic and understanding if the pain has been endured before. The child knows that the amount and length of the pain can and has been endured previously without undue injury. Suggestive fear of the pain of dentistry, on the other hand, is not circumscribed by any real personal experience, so there is no limit to the intensity of fear that can be produced. For most children, fear of dentistry is subjective and is not the result of previous dental care.

Although parents have the most profound influence on their children in matters of suggestion, suggested fears may be acquired from friends or playmates or from materials such as books, periodicals, cartoons, radio, television, and the theatre. How effective these influences will be will depend upon the potency and repetition of the stimuli and the suggestibility of the child. Generally, a fearful child is fearful of everyone and everything.

Suggestive fears may become so magnified that they may approach irrationality. Jersild[10, 11, 12] has studied the experiences feared most by children and found no correlation between them and the worst experiences encountered in their own lives. Their greatest fears were imaginary events or objects.

As the imaginative capacities of the child develop, imaginary fears become more intense. Imaginary fears therefore become greater with age and mental development, up to a certain age, when reason shows them to be ill founded.

Fears may be irrational in the sense that the child may not know why he is frightened. Memories of past experiences may fade entirely from his consciousness, but the emotion associated with the forgotten experience determines, to a large measure, his reaction to a similar event in the future.

The intensity of children's fears varies. These differences in manifestation may be explained as simply as the child's need or desire for sleep. The sleepy child tends to show more fear and irritation than does the wide-awake child, because he has a reduced ability to rationalize and control his fears and has a lower tolerance to discomfort.

The pattern of fear may be unpredictable, for not all fears expressed by children are genuine. Frequently they will use fear for ulterior purposes. Perhaps, by using fear of the dentist as a protective mechanism, the child will not be required to keep his dental appointment or have dental work done. It is for the parent and the dentist to judge what is genuine fear and what is faking.

It is well to remember that, regardless of conditioning, normal children with similar previous experiences will show a great variation in their acquisition of and response to fear. Each child is an individual and responds in an individual manner. Much of the response must depend on the innate physical and mental capacities of the individual. The physically healthy child with normal endocrine function will respond more actively than the child with glandular hypofunction. The mentally alert child will respond more intelligently and rapidly than the mentally retarded individual. It is not uncommon to find that two children subjected to the same stimulus or experience and with the same mental capacity react in opposite directions; for example, one will show courage and attempt to battle the causative agent while the other will respond with trepidation and flight. These human variations should be understood by parents in training individual children to accept a standardized procedure such as dentistry, and to accept it as a normal health experience.

FEAR AND GROWTH

Parents can be taught that age is an important delineator of fear and modifies the effectiveness of conditioning. A child's fears and the way he handles them change with age. Emotional behavior, like any other behavior, undergoes a process of maturation which is dependent on the total growth of the individual.

A study by Hess[8] points up the early age at which emotional events and experiences can influence individuals. He has admirably demonstrated that one can imprint an experience or object on 16 hour old fowl so that they will later respond to the object imprinted. For example, a jungle fowl cock, imprinted at a very young age and kept away from his own species for the first month, even after five years spent mostly with his own species, courts human beings with typical behavior but not females of his own species.

Imprinting is a rigid form of learning, occurs even before the onset of fear, and is of lasting duration. Painful experiences increase its effectiveness. The usual association learning, according to Hess, generally develops later in life, after the time of imprintability.

The role of mothers in overcoming early fears is well documented. Arsenian[1] has demonstrated the role of the mother as the source of safety and security for the child even at one year of age.

Harlow and Zimmerman[7] demonstrated with very young orphaned monkeys that a satisfactory mother surrogate could overcome induced fear in a very short time, while an unsatisfactory mother surrogate produced marked emotional disturbances which persisted for an indefinite time when exposed to a fear-promoting object.

The possible relation between imprinting cuddling and mother attention before one year of age on the child's personality and reaction to fear later in life may be greater than previously believed.

A child who senses a threat to the security of his routine pattern of life by being thrust into a new situation will respond with fear if he is too young to understand the reason for the change. As a child grows older and his ability to reason develops, these acquired fears are discarded, one by one, as experience and intellect teach him that there is little to be feared. What frightens a child at 2 years of age may not frighten him at 6 years of age. Therefore age is a potent delineator of what produces fear in a child. The parent and the dentist must be aware of these variations with age and interpret all responses to stimuli in the light of the child's emotional, mental, and chronological ages.

Since between 2 and 3 years of age is the appropriate time to introduce the child to dentistry, it is well to consider the stimuli with dental importance that produce fear from this age to adolescence. Obviously one cannot expect from a child responses and understanding which at any given age he is not mentally equipped to comprehend.

The child's earliest fears associated with dentistry are those of the unknown and the unexpected. Any intense or sudden stimulation of the sense organs is fear-promoting to the child, for it is unexpected. The noise and vibration of the dental drill and the pressure exerted in the use of hand instruments in cavity preparation are conducive to fear in the very young child. Unless the pain is severe he generally fears the noise of dental procedures more than he does any attendant pain.

Since the young child also fears falling or sudden and unexpected movements, suddenly being lowered or being tilted back in the dental chair without warning may arouse fear. Quick and jerky movements of the hands are frightening. Bright lights, especially the intense light of the operating unit if allowed to shine in the child's eyes, are fear producing.

Preschool children may have a fear of separation from a parent. If the child is thrust into a new situation where he must be separated from his parent, whom he has learned to depend upon for security, he has a feeling of being abandoned, of being left alone. Along with the fear of being abandoned is the fear of not having satisfied the parent. He feels that this may be the reason for his abandonment. He may feel that dentistry is his punishment.

Since some children fear being separated from their parents, it might be preferable to have the parent accompany the child to the operating room if the child is very young. Certainly the parent should be in the operatory during the first visit. The sight of the unfamiliar dental chair or the dental unit with its strange projections may be fear-inciting to the very young.

Several years ago Frankl[5] demonstrated in a carefully controlled study that children under 50 months of age benefited considerably by the presence of the mother in the operatory during dental treatment, even when such involved treatment as cavity preparation was undertaken. Children over 50 months of age showed no difference in behavior whether the mother was present or absent from the operatory. It is interesting that in neither of these age groups was the mother's presence in the operating room harmful to the child's behavior and certainly under four years of age it was desirable. If the mother can be with the child without projecting her feelings to the child, there is no reason for the parent's not being admitted to the operatory. This assumes that the children are well adjusted.

Frequently infants are brought to the office by parents immediately after they have had accidents involving injury to the anterior teeth. Because her presence gives comfort and reduces fear, the mother should be requested to hold the child in her arms in the chair while emergency treatment by the dentist is performed. Although the child may still cry, the dentist should keep on doing the necessary work with dispatch and a minimum of pain.

Unfamiliar persons wearing white gowns will arouse fear, especially if the environment is suggestive of painful experiences in the past. To the very young child accustomed to the activity and noise of a family, the extreme quietness of the waiting room may be strange and disturbing. Overenthusiasm arouses suspicion and fear. As the child becomes more familiar with the dental office this fear of the unfamiliar should disappear.

At 4 years of age, the peak of definite fears is reached and from 4 to 6 there is a gradual decline in the earliest fears such as fear of falling, of noise, and of strangers. As the child acquires the ability to evaluate fear-producing situations, both from his own experience and from his ability to ascertain the severity of the danger, many of the earlier fears are lost and forgotten. Fear of strangers, which is most intense between 2 and 3 years of age, is lost through broad association with others. For this reason children attending nursery school become more sociable and willing to make up with strangers, while children raised on a farm without many social contacts may be shy and diffident until they identify with the dentist. Jersild and Holmes[11] state that the average number of fears at 3 years of age is 5.5 while at 6 years of age it has decreased to only 3.2. The decrease in fears may have been due to (*a*) realization that there is nothing to fear, (*b*) social pressure to conceal fear, (*c*) social imitation, and (*d*) adult guidance.

Intelligent children have been observed to display more fear than others, perhaps because of their greater awareness of danger and more defined reluctance to accept verbal assurance without proof. At these ages boys tend to be aggressive and adventuresome and to have a friendly attitude. Girls, on the other hand, are likely to be much more reserved.

One fear that may become rather general is that of bodily injury. Sometimes a child will go completely to pieces from a minor injury. Even the prick of a hypodermic needle or the sight of blood following his own tooth extraction may produce a response out of all proportion to the degree of pain. The fear of injury is often associated with dentistry because he has learned that the dentist can hurt. Often the fear of pain is associated in the child's mind with being bad, for at some time when he was bad he was hurt in some way as a punishment. Since the dentist can hurt, the child may interpret his visit to the dentist as punishment for being bad.

At this age, the child is developing a fear of his own conscience which is formed through corrective discipline by the parents. The "yes's" and "no's" become a part of him and may lead to anxieties if discipline has been faulty, or they may be conducive to good behavior when discipline is moderate and just.

From ages 4 to 6 the child enters a period of marked conflicts and emotional instability. The child is in constant turmoil between his developing ego and his desire to conform. As the ego develops it becomes of sufficient strength to tolerate many unpleasant inner tensions and suppress them until satisfaction is possible. It is during this period that fantasy, perhaps as a protective mechanism, plays an important role. It serves as a buffer for emotional problems. Children will combat on an imaginative level things they fear in reality. By so doing the child not only gains comfort but also develops the necessary courage and poise to meet the real situation. Children will do with pleasure in fantasy what they dislike doing in reality, if it can be brought into the realm of play. Since fears can be overcome by subjecting the individual to the fear-promoting situation, doing this by imaginative play and through fantasy might help overcome undue fear. In the home where the child has an intense subjective fear of dentistry, the make-believe play of going to the dentist and having his teeth worked on might go a long way in dispelling undue fear and instilling courage for the dental appointment. At this age the safety valve of fantasy is important and can be used by the dentist as a tool in managing the young child. Even at these ages the child is uncertain of his ability to cope with a potential danger and is given to some shyness, although children in this age bracket obey commands more quickly than do 3 year olds.

By the time a child reaches school age most of the fears of dentistry established by suggestion, imitation or actual previous unpleasant dental experience have become easily manageable. Only a few children retain marked phobias. The youngster of this age is becoming less demanding and more conforming. He is developing a marked curiosity about his environment. At school age the child's ego is at its zenith.

At 7 years of age the child has improved his ability to resolve his fears although he may react in a manner that appears alternately cowardly and brave. He is at the worrisome age but he is resolving the real fears. Family support is all-important in understanding and overcoming his fears. The child of this age can generally resolve his fears of dental operative procedures because the dentist can reason with him and explain what is being done. If pain is inflicted the child of 7 can be encouraged to convey dissatisfaction to the dentist either by raising his hand or by some other gesture. As children become older their fears become more variable and individual.

At ages 8 to 14 the child has learned to tolerate unpleasant situations and has marked desires to be obedient. He carries his frustrations well, is carefree and easily adjusts to the situations in which he finds himself. He develops considerable emotional control. However, he objects to people making light of his suffering. He dislikes bullying, injustice or cajoling, whether it be from a friend or from the dentist in his office.

Children of teen age, especially girls, become concerned about their appearance. They would all like to be as attractive as possible. This interest in cosmetic effects can be used by the dentist as motivation for seeking dental attention. To satisfy their ego they are willing to cooperate. Management problems occur only in those considerably maladjusted.

INTERPERSONAL RELATIONSHIPS

The nature of fear has been considered at some length. Although it is one of the major emotions of concern to the dentist, it does not fully explain the overt behavior of the child in the dental chair. There are a vast number of interpersonal influences which alter the behavior pattern of every child who comes to the dentist. Each child will respond to fear in a different manner based on these environmental influences and his inheritance since there are hereditary factors in basic personality formation as documented by Wenger.[16] Primary among the child's interpersonal relationships are those with parents. Since parent-to-child relationships are the most intimate and hence the most potent in determining the emotional behavior of the child, these will be given some emphasis. When one considers the number and variety of emotional factors manifest in parental attitudes such as affection, indifference, hostility, rivalry, dependency, domination, submission, one becomes impressed with the wide variety of factors which can modify the individual child's personality. If parental attitudes are faulty, the child's behavior may be so altered as to make him an unsatisfactory dental patient. On the other hand, if parents have healthy attitudes toward their children, the children will be properly reared, well behaved, and generally good dental patients. Parental attitudes, therefore, can determine whether a child will be amenable or hostile, cooperative or rebellious. In most cases, the child's behavior in the dental office is an excellent indicator of his parents' attitudes toward him.

One cannot overemphasize the need for children to live with emotionally mature adults. Since children acquire emotional maturity from their parents, one cannot expect mature emotional behavior from a child who has been raised by emotionally immature parents. One cannot expect a child to develop an acceptable personality of his own if the parents are trying to resolve their own psychological conflicts through him. The growing and developing child learns by example, and if these necessary patterns are not furnished him by the parents, he may acquire less desirable ones elsewhere. But if the parents are emotionally mature and live a well adjusted and happy life, the child will generally grow up emotionally mature.

Frequently parents adopt one attitude toward themselves and another toward their children. Parents often attempt to be different from what they really are in order to impress their children. This pretense is ineffective. Children have keen powers of observation and cannot be fooled for long. No parent has to be perfect in order to be a good parent. If both parents are perfect beyond reproach, the child has no opportunity to observe mistakes and their rectification. If both parents are perfect, the child will have no experience in combating the vicissitudes in life and will be unable to deal satisfactorily with members of the not-too-perfect genus *Homo sapiens.*

Every child has fundamental emotional needs such as for love, protection, acceptance, self-esteem, independence, authority, discipline, limitations, consolation and comfort. Every child should have these needs fulfilled in order to reach maturity as a well adjusted individual. Love is necessary to give the child a sense of being wanted. It instills confidence in himself and in his ability to cope with his environment. Discipline, on the other hand, indicates to the child how far he can go. It places a limit to the boundaries of his freedom, but within these he should have complete freedom. The undisciplined child does not possess this freedom of action because he does not know at what point his actions may cause untoward difficulties.

When behavior is unrestrained, feelings of guilt often arise which in turn may lead to sullenness, fear and anxiety. Parents are the child's first contact with authority. How he is handled will determine his behavior toward authority elsewhere. Authority must be asserted in a loving and protective manner, never in an overbearing way. Authority properly exercised will give confidence. Loving and consistent authority is desirable over that which is rigid, punitive or inconsistent.

When the emotional needs are fulfilled to extremes by parents the child is apt to grow up with emotional conflicts and present problems both to his parents and to those with whom he has contact. When a child comes to the dental office with parents who are bedraggled and bewildered and complain that their child will not cooperate although they have been ideal parents, a great deal of the difficulty can be traced to the emotional atmosphere of the home. It is in every child's bill of rights to have a home atmosphere conducive to normal emotional development, for human behavior is determined more on an emotional basis than on an intellectual one. For a child to grow in behavior, he must have a reasonably normal emotional environment.

There are definite reasons for the extreme attitudes some parents take toward their children. Some attitudes are displayed with full realization that they are not producing a healthy environment for the child, yet the parents are not too greatly concerned with the consequences. Other parents may display these faulty attitudes, totally unaware of their feelings toward their offspring and oblivious to the fact that they may be harming the child emotionally. Suffice it to say that erroneous parental attitudes do exist and may so alter the child's behavior as to make management in the dental office a difficult procedure.

EXTREMES OF PARENTAL BEHAVIOR

Among the extremes of parental behavior toward the child may be mentioned the following:

Overprotection

Every child has a need for love and affection. However, because of a number of emotional factors related to past experiences or present difficulties, the parents' protective drive may become excessive and interfere with the normal rearing of the child. Generally the overprotected child is not permitted to use his own initiative or make decisions for himself. Assistance is forced on the child in every minute task attempted. The mother assists in dressing and feeding the child and takes an active part in his social activities. The child's play is restricted as well as his work for fear of injury, disease, or the acquisition of undesirable habits from his playmates.

This maternal overprotectiveness may be manifested either in extreme dominance or in extreme indulgence. According to Bakwin and Bakwin,[2] there seems to be no happy medium. Whether the parent becomes overindulgent or overdominant depends on the innate disposition of the child and how he reacts to his mother's early behavior toward him. There appears to be an inverse behavior response to parental attitudes.

Dominating parents generally present children who are very shy, delicate, submissive and fearful. These children are not aggressive and lack conceit and social drive. They are humble with feelings of inferiority and many fears and deep-seated anxieties. As can be imagined, these children may make ideal dental patients, if not overtaxed, because are obedient, polite, and respond well to discipline. Frequently, however, because of the child's shyness, the dentist must break through the "shyness barrier" by building the child's confidence in his ability to be a good dental patient.

Overindulging or luxury-heaping parents present children who have a difficult time conforming to their social environment. These children are not forced to face moral realities, so they become demanding in attention, affection, and service. Because they are made to feel superior to others, they become inconsiderate, selfish, stubborn, and tyrannical. If their demands are not met they become impatient, release outbursts of temper and even attempt to battle those who do not accede to their wishes. With a strange dentist they can use charm and coaxing, even bullying, to get their way and avoid dental treatment, and if this fails they display extreme anger and may resist even forcibly the dentist's attempts at management. They are indeed spoiled children and, although not incorrigible, are very difficult to manage in the dental office. Some display of discipline should be used as a means of getting their cooperation in a large percentage of the cases. Once they have learned the meaning of compliance they turn out to be excellent patients. The method of handling these patients will be described in the next chapter.

It is not unusual for the overindulgent parent to bring the child to the dentist in a hostile manner, insisting upon being allowed to accompany the child to the operating room. No amount of reason will dissuade her from doing so. Once in the operating room any attempt on the part of the dentist at discipline will be interpreted by her as brutality. Generally it is these children who are most in need of office discipline. It would be well for the dentist to bear in mind in counseling parents of overindulged children that they rate their children significantly more well behaved than general observers do, so that extreme tact must be used.

Overindulgence is a common fault of grandparents, who, having already reared a family, wish to re-experience the joy of being loved again by young children without the responsibility of having to discipline them. The behavior of a child reared in a home where grandparents reside is generally that of an overindulged child. This is especially true if both parents work and are away from home all day.

Rejection

There are many gradations of rejection, from mild indifference because of work or other interests, to complete rejection because of emotional problems. The mildly indifferent parent has children who feel inferior and neglected. They are unsure of themselves and their place in society. They develop resentment, become uncooperative, and completely withdraw into a shell, loving no one and taking an interest in no one.

Unwanted or rejected children not only suffer from a lack of love and affection but they may be treated with obvious scorn and even violent brutality. These children may be constantly criticized, nagged, and continually tormented with overt displays of displeasure. They may be severely punished and pitifully neglected. It is little wonder that these children develop a lack of self-esteem and a feeling of helplessness leading to deep anxieties. Since the child has no home security, he becomes suspicious, aggressive, revengeful, pugnacious, disobedient, unpopular, restless and overactive. Because of his attitude he is found undesirable by other members of his age group and must seek the companionship of others like himself. Many of today's delinquent children come from this category.

In the dental office this child may be difficult to control. Certainly any manifest disobedience on the child's part should be met not with rejection but with an effort at friendliness and understanding. These children are generally demanding and their demands should be respected as much as possible, for these children are in need of attention and kindness. In many instances the rejected child misbehaves to call attention to himself. The child should receive this attention when he decides to behave but not when he misbehaves. The child should be taught that when he is behaving well dental treatment is much more pleasant.

Overanxiety

This attitude is characterized by undue concern for the child as a result of some previous family tragedy following upon accident or illness. It is usually associated with overaffection, overprotection, and overindulgence. The child is, therefore, not permitted to work or play alone. Minor illnesses are greatly exaggerated and frequently the child is bedridden unnecessarily. These children are usually shy, timid and fearful. They become increasingly concerned about their health and lack the ability to make decisions for themselves. They are generally good dental patients when admonished to be so. The dentist, however, may have some difficulty overcoming their fears. With encouragement and assurance the child usually responds in a satisfactory manner.

Domination

Parents exemplifying this attitude demand of their children excessive responsibility which is incompatible with their chronological age. They cannot accept the child as he is, but put the child on a competitive basis with other children older or farther advanced. They force the child in an effort to train him, generally by being unduly critical, strict, and often even rejecting. This constant nagging and criticizing develops in the child resentment and evasion, submission and restlessness. Negativism may be common. Fearful of resisting openly, they will obey commands slowly and with as much delay as possible. With kindness and consideration they generally develop into good dental patients. Their response is like that produced by demanding parents.

Identification

In certain instances parents try to relive their own lives in those of their children. In so doing they attempt to give the child every advantage denied them. If the child does not respond favorably the parent displays overt disappointment. The observant child senses this parental disappointment and has feelings of guilt which are mirrored in shyness, retirement and unsureness. He cries easily and lacks confidence, attempting very little for fear of failure. These children respond in the dental office in the same manner as children of dominating parents and should be handled in the same manner.

Considering parental attitudes in general it appears that, within just limits, a certain amount of dominance by parents and submissiveness in children is necessary for a successful adjustment to the culture pattern of this age. The children with some suppression at home appear to accept outside experiences with more zest and interest. If parental dominance is just and properly administered, the child will tend to be a good dental patient as well as fit into a world in which adjustments are always necessary. Certainly the group lacking parental pressure will grow up deficient in acquiring the ability to adjust themselves to the situations of life, of which dental treatment is but one. If parental dominance is more evident in one parent than in the other, the one showing the least indulgence should be the one to bring the child to the dental office. Because of fear no young child should come to the dental office for the first visit unattended. The dental office is a new experience for the child. He, therefore, needs the confidence and reassurance that only a parent can give.

The attitudes children have toward others are formed primarily by the parents. These attitudes may vary depending on the number of children and their position in the family. The last born child has the most difficulty with parental attitudes. The oldest child, on the other hand, is born in a position of command, for, although the parents may lack the knowledge learned from previous experience, they have the enthusiasm and youthful endurance sometimes necessary for administering proper and just discipline. The oldest child often is conservative and moderate in his behavior. He is well behaved if his parents are intelligent and understanding of their own attitudes. The youngest child, if born some years after the others, has a tendency to be spoiled by the parents or older siblings.

The only child or the adopted child may be overindulged by his parents, and tends to be antagonistic, disobedient, selfish and given to temper tantrums. This need not be. If parental attitudes toward the child are moderate in application, the child may be fairly well adjusted.

Sibling relationships, although not as important as those with parents, do influence the child's behavior. Dominance by an older sibling and the child's dictatorial dominance of a younger sibling enter into forming the child's personality. Rivalry and jealousy between siblings for the affection of parents and other members of the family may influence the behavior pattern of the child.

There are many factors, aside from parental and sibling relationships, that form the personality of the child. Among these may be mentioned innate individual personalities, family rapport, leisure, relaxation, morale, etc. All of these have a bearing on the final personality pattern. They can make the difference between a happy child and a sullen and confused one.

Broken homes may be deleterious to a good personality. They may lead to feelings of insecurity, inferiority, apathy and depression. Yet broken homes may not be any more destructive to character formation than homes with chronic conflicts and complete maladjustment. Harmonious homes are homes where children are wanted. A high-rating home in building character and personality is a warm and friendly place where happiness is continuously pursued and where sociability is emphasized.

As the child grows older and enrolls in school, the teachers play an important role in molding personalities, as do playmates. The influence of playmates on dental matters is considerable. Children love to dramatize situations, especially if it makes them heroic in the eyes of other children. They will exaggerate the pain of an extraction or of a dental operation, producing deleterious effects on the child listening who has yet to go to the dentist for his first appointment. But the home is by far the most important factor in sculpturing the overall personality of the child. It is the home that governs the child's destiny in his social milieu.

PARENTAL BEHAVIOR IN THE DENTAL OFFICE

One cannot conclude a chapter on parental responsibility in child management without saying a word about the parents' behavior in the dental office. Parents can be led to understand that once the child is in the office the dentist knows best how to prepare the child emotionally for the necessary treatment. The parent must have complete confidence in the dentist and entrust her child to his care. When the child is taken to the treatment room the parent should make no gesture toward following or leading the child into the room unless invited to do so by the dentist. Some school children behave better away from their parents, especially if parental training has been faulty. However, there are times when the mere presence of a parent instills confidence in a child, especially in one under 4 years of age. If the parent of an older child is invited into the treatment room he must assume the role of a passive guest and either sit or stand away from the chair. He should not speak to the dentist or child unless asked to do so by the dentist, nor should he hold the child's hand or look sympathetically at the child, while at the same time displaying dread in his expression. Nothing is more disturbing to the successful management of a child than to have the parent either giving false information to the child or extending sympathy to the child. Not only will this divided obedience lead to distrust of the dentist, but it will create fear of dental procedures. The American Dental Association has pleasant posters that can be framed and placed on the reception room wall notifying the parent that she should not accompany the child into the operatory if the dentist prefers to work with the parent out of the room.

INSTRUCTIONS TO THE PARENT

It is indeed unusual to find a parent bringing a child to the dental office without some misgiving and apprehension concerning his reaction to dental treatment. The dentist can do a great deal in parent education that will assure the parent that his child will not enter the dental office with hesitation or fear. It will be a great comfort to the parent to know that extreme disciplinary measures will not be necessary and the child will participate willingly in his new experience. The parent will become enthusiastic about the dental well-being of his child and is less apt to wait until his teeth ache before bringing him for dental treatment. A more satisfactory rapport will thus exist between the entire family and the dentist. By counseling the parent in a few simple rules to follow before bringing the child to the dentist for the first time, a great service can be rendered to the parent and the child. Counseling parents about dental treatment should begin preferably before children are old enough to be impressed adversely by outside influences. Counseling can be done on a mass scale through various media, or individually.

1. Tell the parents not to voice their own personal fears in front of the child. The primary cause of fear in children is hearing their parents complain about their own dental experiences. Aside from not mentioning their own unpleasant experiences, they can prevent fear by explaining in a matter-of-fact and pleasant manner what dentistry is and how nice the dentist will be. For those parents who still have fear of dental treatment it should be pointed out that with modern anesthesia, our better understanding of child management and improved operative techniques

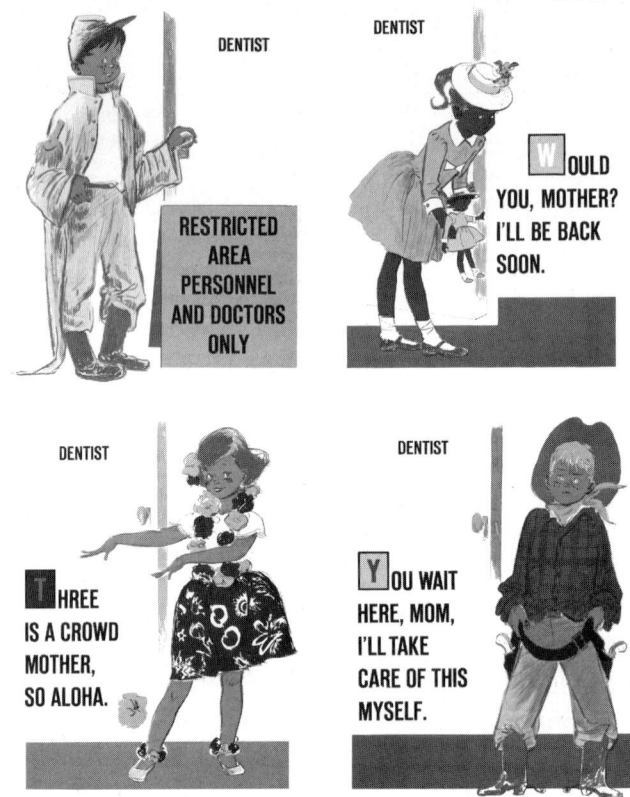

Figure 2–1   A montage of four posters available from the American Dental Association.

there is no need for any child to fear dental treatment. Great strides have been made in alleviating most of the pain of dentistry. The parent who educates his child to be receptive to dental treatment will find that it pays dividends in the child's enjoyment of dentistry. It is usually when great fear has been inculcated in the child by parents and others that difficulty is encountered. The parent must also conceal feelings of anxiety, especially in facial expression, when taking the child to the dentist.

2. Tell the parent never to use dentistry as a threat of punishment. Punishment in the child's mind is associated with unpleasantness and pain.

3. Tell the parents to familiarize their child with dentistry by taking the child to the dentist to become accustomed to the dental office and to become acquainted with the dentist. The dentist should cooperate fully by greeting the child cordially and conducting him on a tour of the office, explaining and demonstrating the equipment. Some small gift at the end of the tour would make the child feel he had made a friend.

4. Explain to the parent that an occasional display of courage on his part in dental matters will build courage in the child. There is a correlation between child and parent fears.

5. Counsel the parent about the home environment and the importance of

moderate parental attitudes in building well adjusted children. A well adjusted child is generally a good dental patient.

6. Stress to the parent the value of regular dental care, not only in preserving the teeth but also in the formation of good dental patients. The poorest time psychologically to bring a child to the dentist is when he is suffering with a toothache.

7. Discourage parents from bribing their child to go to the dentist. This method will signify to the child that there must be danger ahead.

8. The parent should be instructed never to shame, scold, or ridicule to overcome the fear of dental treatment. At best it only builds resentment toward the dentist and makes the dentist's efforts more difficult.

9. The parent should be informed of the need for combating all deleterious impressions of dentistry from outside the home.

10. The parent should not promise the child what the dentist is or is not going to do. The dentist should not be placed in a compromising situation where he is limited in what he can do for the child. Nor should the parent promise the child that the dentist will not hurt. Lying only leads to disappointment and mistrust.

11. Several days before the appointment the parent should be instructed to convey to the child in a casual manner that they have been invited to visit the dentist. The parent should never force the issue, be oversympathetic to the child, or display any fear or misgivings in his voice or manner.

12. The parent should commit the child to the dentist's care once the office is reached and should not enter the treatment room unless requested to do so by the dentist. Once in the treatment room he should act as an invited spectator only.

REFERENCES

1. Arsenian, J. M.: Young children in an insecure situation. J. Abnorm. & Social Psychol., *38*:225, 1943.
2. Bakwin, H., and Bakwin, R. M.: Clinical Management of Behavior Disorders in Children, 3rd ed. Philadelphia, W. B. Saunders Co., 1966.
3. Breckenridge, M. E., and Murphy, M. N.: Growth and Development of the Young Child, 8th ed. Philadelphia, W. B. Saunders, 1969.
4. Davies, G. N.: The management of children. New Zealand D. J., *53*:71–77, April, 1957.
5. Frankl, S. N.: The Effects of Separation and Nonseparation of the Mother and the Pre-School Child in the Dental Office. Thesis, Tufts University, January, 1961.
6. Gesell, A., and Ilg, F. L.: The Child from 5 to 10. New York, Harper & Bros., 1946.
7. Harlow, J. F., and Zimmerman, R. R.: Affectional responses in the infant monkey. Science, *130*:421, 1959.
8. Hess, E. H.: Imprinting. Science, *130*:133, 1959.
9. Hurlock, E. B.: Developmental Psychology. New York, McGraw-Hill Book Co., 1953.
10. Jersild, A. T.: Child Psychology. New York, Prentice-Hall, Inc., 6th ed., 1968.
11. Jersild, A. T., and Holmes, F. B.: Children's Fears. Child Development Monog. No. 20. New York, Teachers College Columbia University, 1935.
12. Jersild, A. T., Markey, F. V., and Jersild, C. L.: Children's Fears, Dreams, Wishes, Day Dreams, Likes, Dislikes, Pleasant and Unpleasant Memories. Child Development Monog. No. 12. New York, Teachers College Columbia University, 1933.
13. Lampshire, E. L.: Understanding the two-to-five-year-old child dental patient. Texas Dent. J., *83*:6, February, 1965.
14. Shirley, H. F.: The Child, His Parents, and the Physician. Springfield, Illinois, Charles C Thomas, 1954.
15. Shoban, E. J., and Borland, L.: An empirical study of the etiology of dental fears. J. Clin. Psychol., *10*:171, 1954.
16. Wenger, M. A.: Preliminary study of the significance of measures of autonomic balance. Psychosom. Med., *9*:301, 1947.

3

CHILD MANAGEMENT IN THE DENTAL OFFICE

by SIDNEY B. FINN

> No one can be successful in the management of little children who has not acquired the art of hiding from them their power to disturb.
>
> HECTOR C. CAMERON, LANCET, 1928.

In the previous chapter the emotional development of the child was discussed in conjunction with the promotion of fear of dentistry. Also considered were means of educating parents to eradicate or minimize these fears in their own children. This chapter will be concerned with the management of the child patient once he enters the dental office.

It is gratifying to observe that the vast majority of children coming to the dental office for corrective care can be classified as good patients. It is equally true that most children enter the office with some apprehension and fear but that, as clinical experience shows, they can control this fear by rationalization. A relatively few children in all age brackets, because of fears instilled at home or because of faulty parental attitudes, will not or cannot conform to the discipline and discomfort attendant upon dental routine. Illingsworth[9] succinctly stated that "problem children are children with problems." One will have more enduring success in handling the patient if he attempts to recognize these problems and adjust his psychological approach with reference to this knowledge.

It is interesting that child behavior may fluctuate over rather narrow ranges of time. At 2 years of age he may be cooperative and well behaved, while at 2½ years of age he may become contrary and difficult. At 3 years of age he is amiable and has good control of himself, while at 4 or 4½ he may regress in behavior so as to be dogmatic and difficult to control.

32

A child's uncooperative behavior in the dental office is motivated generally by a desire to avoid unpleasantness and pain and what might be interpreted by him as a threat to his well-being. Since children act on impulse, fear of pain may manifest itself in untoward behavior regardless of rationalization and knowledge that there is little reason to be frightened. In spite of the child's desire to please, he finds complacency untenable in the presence of the unbearable fear of pain. This attitude is sometimes difficult for the dentist to understand, and indeed it is sometimes difficult for the child himself to account for his behavior. Since fear comes from a lower brain level than reason, it is quite understandable that fear is manifested more on an emotional basis than on an intellectual one and therefore cannot be interpreted on the basis of reason alone. Although the child's behavior may not be well understood and may seem unreasonable, it is completely purposive and is based on experiences acquired both subjectively and objectively during the child's entire lifetime. His logic is based entirely on his feelings. It is the total conditioning of the child which will govern his emotional behavior in the dental office.

One can carry this reasoning a step further and state that the child will behave in the dental office in a manner which in the past has given him the greatest freedom from unpleasantness. If unpleasantness can be avoided at home by negativism and temper tantrums, he will attempt to act the same way in the dental office. If by forcibly resisting his parents he has had his desires gratified, then he will attempt to avoid dental work by the same means. However, a child's behavior is modifiable. If these emotional outbursts are made unprofitable to him his behavior will change. Once the child learns that in your office undesirable behavior is unrewarding the motivation for its continuance will be lost. One cannot bargain with a young child about behavior problems. It is better in these situations to be a benevolent authority than to give him his own choice of action.

The importance of bringing the child to the dentist early so that he can become familiar with the dentist and dental surroundings has already been discussed. Once the child appears for dental correction his behavior will depend not only on his previous conditioning but on the dentist's ability to manage him. With proper handling it is indeed rare that cooperation cannot be obtained. A great deal depends on how the dentist impresses the child and how he gains his complete confidence. Once rapport has been established, corrective work should proceed without undue delay.

This might be a good time to remind the reader that children think in terms of extremes. A child's feelings cannot be ambivalent. When he is frightened, he is frightened. He cannot be frightened of someone and yet feel kindly toward him. He cannot be angry with someone and still like him. Therefore, if one is dealing with a frightened and fearful child one must first eliminate fear and then substitute delight and a liking for the dentist. Even if you eradicate fear only to a point at which he has some skepticism and reservations, he can like you sufficiently to trust you. When this point is reached the greater portion of the battle is won in the management of the child.

If it is at all possible, the dentist should establish a good relation with the patient before separating the child from the parent, for otherwise the child may feel that you are forcing him to abandon his parent. The fear of abandonment is critical in a young child.

There is a proper approach to the psychological management of children in the dental office. Procrastination is not a part of it, for it does little to eradicate fear.

To cite a hypothetical case, the child is brought into the office at a young age with necessary dental work to be done. He begins to cry—sometimes with considerable volume—when seated in the dental chair. The dentist, somewhat bewildered and not knowing how to cope with the situation, dismisses the child with an apologetic suggestion to the mother to bring the child back when he is a little older. In six months the child returns and there is a repetition of the first visit with the same behavior pattern. Since in young children subjective fears do not diminish of their own accord, the child's fears and resultant behavior have not improved. As a matter of fact, his fear of dentistry may have intensified as a vivid imagination exaggerates the basic need for flight. Postponement of a situation such as this might go on indefinitely with dire consequences to his teeth. With the development of aching teeth the pain may lead to the establishment of a true phobia for dentistry. If the dentist had used a more positive approach during the first appointment, this unnecessary delay and neglect of teeth would not have occurred. In this instance the patient's fear increases with the dentist's fear of handling him, for the cautious child reasons that if the dentist is afraid to do the work, there must be a reason for the delay. Any unexplained reason promotes fear in children. Do not wait for a child to outgrow an undesirable response; it may take years. Although procrastination is not desirable, a visit to the dental office previous to dental treatment is desirable.

Since children have a great fear of the unfamiliar and are unprepared and apprehensive about encountering new situations, a visit to the dentist before treatment is started might render the unfamiliar more familiar and mitigate any future need for fear and flight. This method works well with preschool children and to a lesser degree with older children. Although a preliminary trip to the dentist has value, continued repetition may not increase the effectiveness of the procedure unless some actual dental work is undertaken.

The use of a derisive and scornful attitude toward the child in order to shame him into good office behavior is contraindicated. Although many practicing dentists employ ridicule in an attempt to improve office behavior, it is a waste of time and has little value. The method is not only inadequate but fraught with danger when applied to children. A child who seats himself in the dental chair is desirous of winning the approval of the dentist. However, if the fear mechanism is so strong that cooperation is impossible, his better judgment is overruled and his behavior becomes undesirable. Ridicule may produce frustration and resentment in the child, so that an increased dislike for the dentist and dental treatment may result. The end product of ridicule is not diminished fear but increased resentment.

Children do not like being different and desire to conform to a social pattern. Children like to do things other children or persons do. They enjoy participation on a competitive basis. If the child is allowed to watch dental work being done on others it will serve as a challenge to him. Observing an older sibling or parent in the chair instills more confidence than does watching a stranger but may have little effect, as stated by Ghose and associates,[8] on children under 3 years of age. If the child sees the work being done without evident pain, he will frequently be willing and even anxious to have the same dental procedures repeated on himself. Quite often he will jump into the dental chair without being asked to do so. *In this enthusiasm lies a danger.* If he observes no expression of discomfort on the person preceding him but discovers, to his surprise, that he is being hurt when he sits in the chair, his enthusiasm may turn to disillusionment and he may completely lose confidence in the dentist. It is difficult to rewin the confidence of a child hurt in this manner. If the operative procedure is to be the least bit painful it is better to forewarn the child and maintain his confidence than to let him think that he has been deceived.

To attempt to talk a child out of his fears without giving him any concrete evidence of why he should not be frightened is not very effective. Since fears develop on an emotional level, verbal appeal on an intellectual level is generally ineffective. Once the child is in actual contact with the fear-provoking situation, verbal appeal is useless. To tell a child he has no right to feel as he does indicates a lack of knowledge of emotional problems, for the child cannot help feeling as he does. In a fearful situation the desire for flight takes precedence over reason, and verbal assurances usually fall on deaf ears. Don't expend energy telling the patient he should not be afraid without first giving him reason to believe so.

TECHNIQUES IN RECONDITIONING

By reconditioning through guidance from the dentist, the child learns to accept and to enjoy dental procedures. He loses his fear of dentistry because he learns that the unfamiliar holds no danger to his security. Through empathy and tact good rapport is established and operative procedures become pleasant interludes anticipated with pleasure by both the child and the dentist. Because this method has been so successful, the remainder of this chapter will be devoted to a discussion of the techniques employed in reconditioning the child's attitude toward dentistry.

The first step in reconditioning is to determine if the child has undue fear of dentistry and if so, the reasons for it. This can be discovered by questioning the parents about their own feelings toward dentistry, their parental attitudes and by closely observing the child. Once the cause of fear is known, controlling it becomes a much easier procedure.

The next step is to familiarize the child with the dental treatment room and all its equipment without producing undue alarm. By this means the child's confidence is gained, and fear is changed to curiosity and cooperation. Most children can be approached by arousing their curiosity. All children are gadgeteers. Any new equipment or mechanism interests and even delights them. What better place is there to find gadgets to stimulate a child's interest than the equipment in the treatment room? Fear can be allayed by permitting and encouraging the child, perhaps subtly, to try out each piece of equipment. The dentist should explain how each piece functions, so the child will become familiar with the sounds and actions of each accessory. The engine is run on his fingernail, so he can feel for himself the harmlessness of a rubber polishing cup. The air syringe is demonstrated, and then casually placed on the child's lap for him to try out. The foot control for the engine is explained, so the child will know the drill is not uncontrolled but, when necessary, *can be stopped at any time.*

After familiarizing the patient with the equipment, the next objective should be to gain his complete confidence. By carefully choosing words and ideas for conversation, an understanding can be reached without much loss of time. When establishing confidence the dentist must convey to the child the idea that he is sympathetic and familiar with his problems. In establishing rapport the conversation should be directed away from emotional problems and toward objects familiar to the child. Talk about pets or playmates or school subjects. Relate how badly you feel that your dog cannot come to the office every day with you. If the child likes dogs a sympathetic understanding will soon flourish between you. If the child has had difficulty with a school subject, remark how difficult you found that subject too. Say that you can understand his problems because you had the same ones when you attended school. In this way mutual understanding and trust will be built. A dentist must humanize his relationships with children. He cannot leave himself out of the picture and still be their friend.

It is now time to broach the subject of dental treatment. The dentist can remark that as a child he had to go to the dentist, because "fixing" teeth is necessary. And that he found as a child that the best way of doing this generally turned out to be the easiest, but he could not know the easiest way without the dentist's telling him. At this stage the child will generally be receptive to his first indoctrination to dental treatment.

During this first appointment only minor and painless procedures should be done. A history is obtained. Toothbrush instruction is given. The patient is informed that his teeth are going to be brushed with the little rubber cup he played with earlier. The teeth are cleaned and a fluoride solution is painted on them. Roentgenograms can then be taken. If the child is first permitted to touch and feel the machine and if its function is explained, there should be very little difficulty. The x-ray unit can be described as a large camera and the small film as the place where the picture will appear. When the child sees the developed x-rays, it will give him pride in his achievement.

It is good practice to work from the simpler operation to the more complex unless emergency treatment is necessary. The dentist can work with the parent in the operating room, or the parent can be barred from the room, depending upon the dentist's wishes. The parent is generally invited into the operatory at the first visit to obtain an understanding of the parental role in seeing that the child acquires good oral hygiene habits and adequate dietary control knowledge for the prevention of dental disease. Staining the teeth with erythrosine or other plaque disclosing agents before and after thorough brushing can be demonstrated at this time. If there is set aside for this purpose a health education room with visual aids and reading material, a more extensive period of indoctrination into dental health can be given to parent and child. (See Chapter 1.)

Unfortunately, children frequently come to the dental office for their first visit suffering from a toothache and in need of more extensive treatment. In these situations, as in all others, truthfulness in the dentist is essential. Frankness and honesty will pay dividends in child behavior. The child should be told in a matter-of-fact manner that sometimes there is slight pain connected with what has to be done. The child can be told that if he will say when it hurts too much, the dentist will stop, or fix it so it won't hurt so much, or try to be a lot gentler. This sincerity should prevail through all future dental appointments and the child should be so reminded before each dental operation.

In handling children too young to understand difficult explanations, rapport should be attempted through conversation about objects or events in the child's own experience. Speak in a pleasant and natural voice. The demeanor should also be a natural and understanding one. It may be necessary, however, to work with the child crying.

Occasionally preschool children scream loudly and for some time when seated in the dental chair. With continual screaming it is difficult to make yourself understood. The threat of sending a parent out of the room may be sufficient to quiet the child. At other times giving the child sufficient time to cry it out may prove adequate. However, there are a few cases in every dentist's experience, when parental attitudes have been faulty or when undue fear has been induced, in which these methods will not work and the child gradually works himself into hysteria. It is then that physical means must be resorted to in order to calm the patient sufficiently to listen to what you have to say.

The simplest method of doing this is by gently placing your hand over the child's mouth, indicating that this is not punishment but is used only so he can hear what you have to say. No attempt should be made to block oral breathing. While the child is crying talk into his ear in a casual and gentle voice, telling him you will remove your hand when he stops screaming. There must be no trace of malice in your voice. The verbalization may stick even though you think the patient does not hear you. Once he has stopped crying, remove your hand from his mouth and talk to the child about some other experience entirely apart from dentistry. It is surprising how effective this can be and what ideal patients these children become. They hold no resentment and realize that what was done, was done for their own good. Generally they turn out to be most cooperative, and even become your buddies. Placing one's hand over the patient's mouth is an extreme measure and should be employed only as a last resort and only on the hysterical patient, when all other means have failed. It may also be necessary to employ this technique on overindulged and spoiled children. As stated by Craig,[4] this technique requires considerable skill.

Disciplinary procedures like this may be time consuming. Dentists frequently remark that they do not have the time to spend in training children. If an hour given to training a child to be a good dental patient will insure that the child will be your patient for his entire lifetime, that hour will be most profitable in your practice. Patience and consideration are excellent practice builders.

The method of reconditioning has been discussed briefly. It embodies many of the features of the technique used by Addelston[1] of "tell . . . show . . . do." The author feels that no psychological trauma will be produced by using this method and that the child, as time goes on, will look forward to his dental appointment with delightful anticipation. It is not claimed that this is the only technique or the best one. It merely presents a procedure that will work satisfactorily and serve as a guide for each dentist to use in formulating his own procedures, since every child responds differently.

In expanding the technique of reconditioning, a few suggestions might help to clarify many points of procedure.

THE APPEARANCE OF THE DENTAL OFFICE

Since the child may enter the dental office with some fear, the first objective of the dentist should be to put the child at his ease and make him realize that his experience is not unusual. If the practice is not limited to children an effective method of inducing this feeling is by making the waiting room similar in many respects to his own home environment. Make the reception room comfortable and warm with the feeling that children frequent the place routinely and therefore the room is not foreign to them. By so doing, a great deal of the suspicion every child possesses will be overcome. One of the simplest ways of doing this is to have one corner of the waiting room set aside for their own use. Have children's chairs and table available where they can sit and read. Have on hand a small library with books for children of all ages. There are some fine children's magazines; one of the dentist's yearly subscriptions should be for a child's periodical. Provide a small lamp on the table with an interesting shade. A few simple but sturdy toys might be kept in the room to amuse the very young. A handy record player with well chosen records or a tape recorder and amplification system will provide comfort to frightened children. Appointment cards and appointment announcements should be made attractive to children so the child will feel that these are addressed to him. A sketch of some character of fantasy on the card will help in doing this. Suggest to the parent of a patient with a 2 year old sibling that an appointment be made now for the near future — that it is time for an oral inspection, instruction in oral hygiene, a prophylaxis and topical application of fluoride solution to the teeth. In all dealings with parents impress upon them the necessity of early contact with the dentist and the value of dental guidance in order to preserve the child's teeth.

The operating room may be made more appealing to the child if a few pictures on the wall are suggestive of children at play. A portrait of a carefree and laughing child is always good. Have the assistant skilled in making animals or other objects out of cotton rolls. These prove very amusing to children.

Try to avoid having child patients see adults in pain or the sight of blood on others. Persons with eyes reddened from crying, or emotionally upset patients, will unnerve children. Prevent children from seeing these patients by having them leave through another door if possible or by scheduling children's appointments all at one time of day.

THE PERSONALITY OF THE DENTIST AND HIS ANCILLARY HELP

It is very important that confidence be instilled in the child by everyone he meets in the office. This applies to the office assistant, the receptionist and the dental hygienist as well as the dentist himself. Since children are extremely sensitive to hidden emotions, any lack of enthusiasm for child patients will soon be recognized and only add to the child's wariness. If a dentist is going to accept child patients, he should make sure that he has sufficient knowledge of child psychology to manage children without producing psychological trauma. The dentist should also make sure that his ancillary personnel feel and act kindly toward children and know how to handle them. If the auxiliary help mishandle a child, the dentist's chances of being successful are greatly diminished. It is good psychology for the dentist to greet the child in the reception room at the time of the first visit.

When first approaching a new child patient always call him by his first name. If this is not known, ask him what his name is. Never call him "young fellow" or some other unfamiliar name. Whenever possible all conversation should be directed toward the child. In taking a history occasionally ask a question for the child to answer. If the child is forced to sit silently through a conversation that is uninteresting to him, his thoughts may naturally turn to what might befall him in the dental chair. To a child with no previous dental experience, what might befall him may seem ominous. Approaching the child should be done in an easy everyday manner. Don't be overenthusiastic or overbearing. Don't forcefully shake the child's hand, greeting him with a loud voice. Approach the child with confidence in your voice and actions, but in a matter-of-fact manner and with a warm and friendly greeting. Remember that many children are frightened by unfamiliar faces, especially if they appear to jump at them from nowhere. A casual and friendly manner and voice are most assuring because they display a warmth which is not suggestive of any impending unpleasantness.

Frequently a young child will refuse to go with the dentist to the treatment room and will cling to his mother's arm. If verbal appeal is ineffectual, the dentist should approach the child in a friendly manner and put his arms around him in a hugging motion. The child is then firmly held and can be picked up and carried to the treatment room without danger of the child's hands or feet hurting anyone. Make the child feel that you are strong enough to hold him and protect him but not strong enough to hurt him. Once in the treatment room the child can be managed as has been described earlier.

If the dentist has confidence in himself, a little of this feeling is sure to spill over on the patient. If the dentist lacks confidence, it will be reflected in the child's behavior. There is no mysterious formula or secret approach to child management. Successful handling of children is based on knowledge, common sense, and experience.

THE TIME AND LENGTH OF APPOINTMENT

In dealing with children, both the hour of the day and length of each appointment are important. Both may affect the child's behavior. Whenever possible children should not be kept in the chair for periods longer than half an hour. With longer appointments, children may be less cooperative toward the end of the period. Completely cooperative patients, if overtaxed by lengthy appointments, can reach a saturation point at which they will break down and cry. Once a child loses his self-composure, however phlegmatic and willing to cooperate he is, his cooperation is very difficult to regain.

The time of day for a child's appointment is also correlated with his behavior. A recent study has indicated that the time of day and length of appointment are not critical factors influencing child behavior. However, preschool children should not be given appointments during their regular nap time. Children brought to the dentist at this hour are usually sleepy, irritable, and difficult to manage. They cry easily and have a reduced ability to cooperate and tolerate discomfort. An uncooperative child brought to the dentist during a nap period may turn out to be completely cooperative when brought at some other time. It is suggested that when the parent calls for an appointment the child's nap time be determined and no appointment given at this time of day.

Children should not be brought to the dentist soon after a serious emotional experience, such as the birth of a brother or sister or the death of someone close. The child at these times is experiencing emotional trauma and the dental appointment will only add to his anxieties and bewilderment. At these times cooperation may be difficult to secure and emotional difficulties are likely to be encountered.

THE DENTIST'S CONVERSATION

In talking to a child the dentist must get down to the patient's own level in position and in conversation, in both words and ideas. It is of little value to use words too difficult for the child to comprehend. Verbosity will confuse the child and, like any subject not understood, be a cause for distrust and some apprehension. Use simple everyday words generally used by children at the patient's age level. In selecting subjects for conversation, choose objects and situations familiar to him. In speaking of football to a young boy, do not discuss complicated rules of college football; rather, talk about the child's own experiences in scoring a touchdown at the playground. Let the child lead the conversation. In very young children it is advisable to add a little fantasy for zest. One must also beware of talking down to children. It is a greater offense to talk down to children than above them. Do not use baby talk to a 4 or 5 year old. It flatters children if adults judge them older than they really are. Talk to them at their own or slightly older age level. Never underestimate the intelligence of a child. Almost all enjoy hearing the dentist talk about some subject that is interesting. It gets their mind off dental procedures by keeping them preoccupied with what is being said. When working on a child do not ask questions that require an answer when both hands and a few dental instruments are in the mouth. Children are apt to use your question as an excuse for interrupting dental treatment for a few moments. Some adults prefer silence when being worked upon. Most children, however, enjoy hearing the dentist talk. They do not feel as completely ignored and neglected as they would otherwise. Sometimes a monotonous tone and constant repetition will induce a fearful child to submit to an injection if there is no change in inflection or timbre of the voice while changing from a monologue about something interesting to the child to the procedure of injection. The technique will succeed, particularly if the monotone is continued as the injection is given. If children ask questions, try to answer them to the fullest extent. However, do not let children use questions as a delaying tactic.

KNOWLEDGE ABOUT THE PATIENT

It is a wise policy to know the child patient before he is seated in the chair. When the parent first phones to make the appointment, pertinent information can be obtained about the child. Ask the parent what the child knows about the dentist and dental procedures. Does the child fear going to the dentist? Is the child nervous? Does he get along well with adults? Has he spent any time in a hospital? Is he afraid of the physician? These questions can provide an insight into the child's possible behavior. A great deal can be learned about the child's emotional behavior by observing him in the reception room. If he is sitting on his mother's lap or cuddled close to her, one can anticipate management difficulties at the first visit. However, if the child sits by himself reading a book or playing with toys away from the parent, one can assume that the child is well adjusted for dental treatment and emotionally mature. During the first visit complete information can be secured from the history. Get to know the family as well as the child at this time. With this patient knowledge one can anticipate the reaction to dental treatment. It is much simpler from a management aspect if one can foretell even remotely how the patient is going to respond when he is approached. Knowing the patient is half the victory. How he acts will govern how he will be handled. It is valuable to be able to predict his behavior.

ATTENTION TO THE PATIENT

Every child should have the dentist's undivided attention. Always treat the child as though he were the only patient seen that day. Never leave a very young child alone in the chair, for his fears, not yet completely dissipated, will become magnified. If it is necessary to leave the operating room even for a minute or two, always make sure that your assistant is present. However, when the child is markedly fearful it is far better for the dentist not to leave the room at all. It is also a poor policy to transfer the same child from one treatment room to another for a different type of procedure, such as surgery. This will present a new situation to the child and be the cause for anxiety. If possible do all the work necessary on the child in the same room.

THE DENTIST'S SKILL AND SPEED

The dentist should perform his duties with dexterity, dispatch and a minimum of pain. In working with children an assistant is a valuable asset. She can be invaluable in helping to control the child and in making operative procedures easier for the dentist. In doing operative work the simplest and easiest way is generally the correct way. This does not imply sloppy technique or work of inferior quality. However, operative techniques can be made to run smoothly. By so arranging the instruments, fumbling and searching for equipment once the operation has begun will not be necessary. Chapter 1 describes the successful utilization of an assistant. A child can tell very quickly, after only a few visits to the office, when inefficiency exists. Children are more observant than adults, perhaps because they are more inquisitive and interested in their surroundings. An inefficient operator will soon be spotted and will lose the confidence of his patient. Work smoothly and carefully and do not waste time or motions. A child can endure discomfort if he knows that it is soon going to end. In industry, time and motion studies are made to increase efficiency. Each dental office can profit by a similar study. One would be surprised at the countless unnecessary motions that are made during the course of a day's work.

THE USE OF FEAR-PROMOTING WORDS

The dentist should avoid using words that might arouse fear in the child. Many suggestive fears are not of the procedure itself, but rather of the fear-producing connotation of a word. Some children may cringe in fear when the word "needle" or "drill" is mentioned, yet object very little to the actual experience if another name is attached to the procedure. Deception should be avoided in working with children, yet descriptive words without the connotation of pain should be used when possible, words familiar to them and used in their everyday conversation. The exact substitution of words should be governed by the age of the patient. Each dentist can make his own preferred selection. Instead of words like "injection," "needle," "stick," etc., one might say, "We are going to put something on your gums that will feel like a mosquito bite." All children have had mosquito bites. They know that mosquito bites produce a little discomfort, but the pain is not great enough or of long enough duration to produce marked anxiety. Instead of the word "drill," which means to a child going down into the tooth, indicate to him that you are going to brush the bad bugs out of the tooth. At the same time run a large inverted cone bur over his fingernail, mentioning that the bur is flat so it cannot dig into the tooth. Addelston[1] demonstrates the use of a spoon excavator. He then takes a large round bur and shows that the blades are many spoons and therefore can do the job more easily and quickly. By this means the dentist has informed the child what is about to be done without the production of fear. If the dentist feels that considerable pain will be inflicted, this might be explained to the child as indicated earlier in the chapter. In dealing with children it is always a good policy to inform the child of what is to be done, but avoid frightening him by using poorly selected words that suggest pain to him.

THE USE OF ADMIRATION, SUBTLE FLATTERY, PRAISE, AND REWARD

In the learning process punishment and reward are basic. Even the laboratory animal learns to travel through a complicated maze to find a reward of food at the other end. There are many types of reward for the well behaved patient. One of the most important rewards sought by the child is the approval of the dentist. It is, therefore, conducive to good behavior for the dentist to acknowledge exemplary conduct in a child. Let the child know when he is a good patient, and it will set a goal for his future behavior. He will try his best to live up to the standard he has established for himself. In praising a child, praise the behavior rather than the individual. For example, rather than say to the child that he is a good boy, state that he behaved very well in the chair today.

Gifts make fine rewards. It is good child management to give the child some gift after good behavior. There are many varieties of gifts. Some dentists give a small trinket or toy. Many give cards entitling the bearer to one ice cream cone at the corner drug store. Giving children gold stars to be pasted on a bulletin board mounted on the waiting room wall is very effective. The gamut of rewards extends from pony rides to plaster models. It is the recognition more than the gift that favorably impresses the child.

BRIBERY AND THE PATIENT

One can state categorically: never bribe a child. Bribery will rarely accomplish any good. The result will be simply that the child will keep on behaving badly in order to get more bribes and concessions. Bribery is an admission that the dentist does not know how to handle the situation. An alert child will soon take advantage of his predicament. It is well to understand the distinction between bribery and reward. Indeed the dividing line is a tenuous one. A reward after one appointment may serve as the bribe that will bring the child back for the next appointment. Generally speaking, however, a bribe is promised or given to induce good behavior. A reward is recognition of good behavior after completion of the operation, without any previously implied promise. Bribery has no place in dentistry.

COMMANDS VERSUS SUGGESTIONS

In the course of dental treatment it is necessary to secure patient cooperation. To produce the desired responses one never asks the child to comply with a request. By asking him if he will do something the dentist is actually giving him his choice of either complying or refusing. If you give the child a choice, the refusal to comply cannot be considered wrong behavior. By telling him to obey a command, no choice is implied except to do it. If he refuses, his behavior automatically becomes unacceptable. When ordering a child to comply with your wishes, state your wishes in a pleasant yet determined way. Do not hesitate to smile and enjoy your patient, yet be firm if the situation demands.

REASONABLENESS OF THE DENTIST

In dealing with children be realistic and reasonable. Do not condemn a child because he is frightened. Try to put yourself in the child's place and understand why he behaves as he does. Respect his emotions, but if they are not in conformity with the desired pattern for dental work, try to alter them. The child's ego will permit him to adjust to stress. Give the child an opportunity to participate in the procedures. If he can hold a cotton roll or assist in some other small way, he will feel that he is a part of the service rendered and will be more interested and cooperative. Treat him as an individual with feelings and emotions and not as an inanimate object in the chair.

THE DENTIST'S SELF-CONTROL

A dentist should never lose his temper and become angry. Like fear, anger is a primitive and immature emotional response. It is a mark of defeat and an indication to the child that he has succeeded in undermining your dignity. The patient has you at a marked disadvantage because anger lessens your ability to rationalize clearly and make the proper responses. If the dentist loses his self-control and raises his voice it will only frighten the child more and make conformity increasingly difficult. If you cannot help becoming angry, it is better to dismiss the child and let some other dentist test his ability. Maybe he can succeed where your temperament leads to failure. If the dentist has tried to the best of his ability and cannot reach the child, it is better to admit defeat than ruin the child for all future dental work.

GRACEFULNESS OF THE DENTIST

In carrying out dental procedures it is well to remember that young children become frightened at the unexpected. All your motions, both in handling the patients and in operative procedures, should be smooth and graceful. Quick and jerky movements tend to create fear in the very young. When lowering a child in the chair or lowering the back of the chair, do it slowly. Don't drop the child suddenly or tip him back in the chair so rapidly that he has the sensation of falling. In giving an injection, as an example, do not bring the syringe to the mouth so rapidly that the act in itself frightens the child. The syringe should be raised in a casual but deliberate manner. Be natural and graceful in all your actions and a great deal of unnecessary fright can be avoided. Dentistry is a graceful profession. Use this grace to your advantage. If one were to define the requisites of a good children's dentist, they would be grace, skill, knowledge, and intelligence.

* * * * *

In subjecting children to dentistry one must always weigh the possibility of psychological trauma against the necessity of treatment. Since dentistry is needed by almost every child, it is imperative that the psychological trauma produced be minimal. Of all the problems associated with dentistry for children, that of management is by far the most important, for without proper patient cooperation dental procedures become difficult if not impossible. There are many methods of increasing patient cooperation and decreasing discomfort such as sedatives, analgesics, hypnosis, tranquilizers and general anesthesia. The use of some of these aids will be discussed later in the book.

REFERENCES

1. Addelston, H. K.: Your child's first visit to his dentist. Child Study, *31*:33, 1954.
2. Adelson, R., and Goldfried, M. R.: Modeling the fearful child patient. J. Dent. Child., *37*:34, Nov.-Dec. 1970.
3. Carpenter, C. H.: What technics may be used to secure relaxation in a child patient? J. Dent. Child., *8*:233, 1941.
4. Craig, W.: Hand Over Mouth Technique. J. Dent. Child., *38*:23, Nov.-Dec. 1971.
5. Eduss, H., Bane, R. S., and Land, L. L.: Pedodontic psychology and premedication. J. Dent. Child., *28*:73–83, 1st quart. 1961.
6. Fadden, L. A.: What the child thinks of dental practice. New York D. J., *19*:124, 1953.
7. Finn, S. B.: The management of the normal child. Bul. Alabama D. A., *38*:20, 1954.
8. Ghose, L. J., Giddon, D. B., Shiere, F. R., and Fogels, H. R.: Evaluation of Sibling Support. J. Dent. Child., *36*:35, Jan., 1969.
9. Illingsworth, R. S., The Normal Child, 4th ed. Boston, Little, Brown & Co., 1968.
10. Johnson, R., and Baldwin, D. W., Jr.: Maternal anxiety and child behavior. J. Dent. Child., *36*:87, March-April, 1969.
11. Klein, A. I.: Control of the dentist in the management of the child patient. J. Indiana D. A., *35*:9, 1956.
12. Lenchner, V.: The effect of appointment length on behavior of the pedodontic patient and his attitude toward dentistry. J. Dent. Child., *33*:61, March, 1966.
13. McSwain, E. T.: The dentist and his young patient. J. D. Educ. *12*:216, 1947.
14. Olsen, N. H.: The first appointment—a mutual evaluation session. J. Dent. Child., *32*:208, 4th quart., 1965.
15. Watson, E. H., and Lowrey, G. H.: Growth and Development of Children. 5th ed. Chicago, Year Book Medical Publishing Company, Inc., 1967.

4

MORPHOLOGY OF THE PRIMARY TEETH

by SIDNEY B. FINN

One of the factors that distinguish children's dentistry from adult dentistry is that the dentist, when treating children, is dealing with two dentitions, a primary set and a permanent set. The primary teeth are 20 in number and consist of a central incisor, a lateral incisor, a cuspid, a first molar, and a second molar in each quadrant of the mouth from the midline posteriorly. The permanent teeth are 32 in number and consist of the succedaneous central incisors, lateral incisors, and cuspids, which replace similar primary teeth; the first bicuspids and second bicuspids, which replace the primary molars; and the first, second, and third molars, which displace no primary teeth but erupt posterior to them.

FUNCTION OF THE PRIMARY TEETH

Since the primary teeth are used for the mechanical preparation of the child's food for *digestion* and *assimilation* during one of his most active periods of growth and development, they serve a very important and indeed critical function. Another outstanding role played by these teeth is in the *maintenance of space* in the dental arches for the permanent teeth. This function will be discussed in detail in a later chapter. The primary teeth also perform a function of *stimulation of growth of the jaws* through mastication, especially in the development of the height of the dental arches. One is also prone to overlook the important function of the primary teeth in the *development of speech*. Ability to use the teeth for pronunciation is acquired entirely with the aid of the primary dentition. Early and accidental loss of the primary anterior teeth may lead to difficulty in pronouncing the sounds "f," "v," "s," "z" and "th." Even after the permanent teeth erupt, difficulty in pronouncing "s," "z" and "th" may persist to the point of requiring speech correction. In most instances, however, with complete eruption of the permanent incisors the difficulty is self-correcting (See Chapter 26.) Primary teeth also serve a *cosmetic function* by improving the appearance of the child. Indirectly a child's speech may be affected if self-consciousness about his disfiguring teeth inhibits him from opening his mouth sufficiently when talking.

LIFE CYCLE OF THE TEETH

Each tooth, whether primary or permanent, in achieving morphologic and functional maturity evolves through a well defined and characteristic life cycle composed of many stages. These progressive stages, however, should not be construed as plateaus of development but rather as observation points of a continually evolving physiologic process in which histologic and biochemical changes are progressively and simultaneously taking place. These stages of development are: (1) growth, (2) calcification, (3) eruption, (4) attrition, and (5) resorption and exfoliation (primary teeth). The growth stage may be further divided into (*a*) initiation, (*b*) proliferation, (*c*) histodifferentiation, (*d*) morphodifferentiation, and (*e*) apposition.

A brief description of the growth and calcification processes may stimulate the reader to pursue further this phase of histology in one of the excellent texts available.

The teeth are derived from and consist of highly specialized cells of ectodermal and mesodermal origin. The ectodermal cells perform special functions such as enamel formation, odontoblastic stimulation, and determination of the shape of the crown and root. Under normal conditions, after performing their functions these cells disappear. The mesodermal or mesenchymal cells, on the other hand, persist throughout the life of the tooth and form the dentin, pulpal tissue, cementum, periodontal membrane and alveolar bone.

The first stage of growth is evident during the sixth week of embryonic life. The tooth bud begins with a proliferation of cells in the basal layer of the oral epithelium from what is to become the dental arch. These cells continue to proliferate and through differential growth extend downward into the mesenchyma, assuming an invaginated appearance with the folds directed away from the oral epithelium.

By the tenth week of embryonic life rapid proliferation has continued to deepen the enamel organ into a somewhat cap-shaped appearance. Ten buds in all arise from the dental lamina of each arch to become the future primary teeth. At this stage the invaginated enamel organ consists of two layers—an outer enamel epithelium corresponding to the covering, and an inner enamel epithelium corresponding to the lining of a cap. A separation begins between these two layers with an increase in intercellular fluid in which there are star-shaped or stellate cells bearing processes which anastomose with similar cells, forming a mesh or reticulum (the stellate reticulum), which will serve later as a cushion for the developing enamel-forming cells.

During this stage within the confines of the invagination in the enamel organ the mesenchymal cells are proliferating and condensing into a visible concentration of cells—the dental papilla, which will form the future dental pulp and dentin.

A change in cellular concentration also occurs in the mesenchymal tissue enveloping the enamel organ and papilla, resulting in a denser and more fibrous tissue—the dental sac which will eventuate in cementum, periodontal membrane and alveolar bone. This beginning and growth constitute the stages of initiation and proliferation.

As the cells of the enamel organ increase in number and the organ grows progressively larger with increasing invagination, several layers of low squamous cells differentiate between the stellate reticulum and the inner enamel epithelium to form the stratum intermedium, whose presence is necessary for enamel formation (histodifferentiation).

During this stage a budding takes place from the dental lamina lingual to the developing primary tooth to form the permanent tooth bud. Distal to the second primary molar the anlages for the permanent molars develop.

During the next stage (morphodifferentiation) the cells of the developing tooth became independent of the dental lamina by the invasion of mesenchymal cells into the central portion of this tissue. The cells of the inner enamel epithelium assume a tall columnar appearance with their bases oriented opposite the developing odontoblasts. They now function as ameloblasts and are capable of forming enamel. The peripheral cells of the dental papilla near the basement membrane, which separates the ameloblasts from the odontoblasts, differentiate into high columnar cells, the odontoblasts, which, together with Korff's fibers, are capable of forming dentin.

The contour of the root is designed by the extension of the united enamel epithelium, termed Hertwig's sheath, into the mesenchymal tissue surrounding the dental papilla.

During the stage of apposition the ameloblasts move peripherally from their base and lay down in their travel enamel matrix which is only from 25 to 30 per cent calcified. This material is laid down in the same shape as the ameloblasts and designated enamel prisms. The enamel matrix is deposited in incremental layers paralleling the dentino-enamel junction. However, enamel matrix deposition cannot occur without dentin formation. The odontoblasts move inward away from the dentino-enamel junction, leaving protoplasmic extensions, Tomes' fibers. The odontoblasts together with Korff's fibers form a collagenous uncalcified material called predentin. This material is laid down in incremental layers also.

In the predentin, calcification takes place by coalescence of globules of inorganic material created by the deposition of apatite crystals in the collagenous matrix. A layer of predentin always precedes calcification in the developing tooth.

Maturation of the enamel begins with the deposition of apatite crystals within the existing enamel matrix. Although there is some difference of opinion about the way maturation progresses, studies utilizing radioactive isotopes indicate that it begins from the dentino-enamel junction peripherally, progressing from the cusps cervically. The teeth erupt into the oral cavity and are subject to the forces of attrition.

Many defects and aberrations of the teeth occur during the various developmental stages in their life cycle. The manifest nature of the defect is governed by the germ layer affected and the stage of development at which it occurs. Reference will be made later in the book to the various abnormalities which occur in children.

Table 4–1 presents the chronology of the development of the teeth.

Kraus gives the following order of beginning calcification of the primary teeth:
1. Central incisors (upper before lower)
2. First molars (upper before lower)
3. Lateral incisors (upper before lower)
4. Cuspids (lower may be slightly earlier)
5. Second molars (simultaneously)

Among the 95 human fetuses studied there was considerable variation in the time of beginning calcification. It is of interest that Kraus observed the primary central incisors developed from a single lobe and not from three centers as formerly believed. Nolla has studied the serial roentgenograms of 50 children. Her results as to the ages at which crown and root formation are completed differ somewhat from those presented in Table 4–1.

Correlated with the physiologic development of the primary teeth is their subsequent root resorption and exfoliation. Root resorption generally begins about a year after eruption. In Table 4–2 is presented the age of shedding the specific primary teeth.

There is a direct time relationship between loss of a primary tooth and the eruption of its permanent successor. This time interval may be disturbed by early extraction, resulting in premature eruption.

The order of eruption of specific teeth is presented in Table 4–3. A difference in eruption time exists between the sexes.

There is a great variation in the length of the period from the time a tooth first pierces the gingiva to the time it reaches occlusion. The period also varies markedly in length among the several types of teeth. The cuspids appear to reach occlusion more slowly than the others, while the first molars reach occlusion in the least time. The time necessary to reach occlusion is shown in Table 4–4.

If one learns the sequence of eruption it will be easy to estimate the other stages of formation. It should be easy to remember that the primary teeth begin to calcify between the fourth and sixth months in utero and erupt between 6 and 24 months of age. The roots complete their formation approximately one year after the teeth erupt. The teeth are shed between 6 and 11 years of age. The eruption age of the succedaneous teeth is on the average about 6 months later than the exfoliation age of the primary teeth.

Calcification of the permanent teeth begins between birth and 3 years of age (third molars omitted), although much later calcification has been observed for the mandibular second bicuspids. One must bear in mind that tables present only averages with wide variations occurring occasionally. Eruption takes place between ages 6 and 12, and the enamel is completely formed about 3 years previous to eruption. The roots are completely formed about 3 years after eruption. Although these figures may oversimplify the chronology of the development of the teeth, they will aid somewhat in remembering more exact figures.

MORPHOLOGIC DIFFERENCES BETWEEN PRIMARY AND PERMANENT DENTITIONS

Morphologic differences exist between the primary and the permanent dentitions, both in size of the teeth and in their general external and internal design. A cross section of a primary and a permanent molar will clearly illustrate these differences (Fig. 4–1).

These differences may be listed as follows:

1. The primary teeth are smaller in all dimensions than the corresponding permanent teeth. The measurements can be found in Figures 4–2, 4–3, 4–4, 4–5.

2. The crowns of the primary teeth are wider in their mesiodistal diameter in relation to their cervico-occlusal height, giving the anterior teeth a cup-shaped appearance and the molars a squat appearance.

TABLE 4-1   CHRONOLOGY OF THE HUMAN DENTITION

Tooth	Hard Tissue Formation Begins	Amount of Enamel Formed at Birth	Enamel Completed	Eruption	Root Completed
Primary Dentition					
Maxillary					
Central incisor	4 mos. in utero	Five sixths	1½ mos.	7½ mos.	1½ yrs.
Lateral incisor	4½ mos. in utero	Two thirds	2½ mos.	9 mos.	2 yrs.
Cuspid	5 mos. in utero	One third	9 mos.	18 mos.	3¼ yrs.
First molar	5 mos. in utero	Cusps united	6 mos.	14 mos.	2½ yrs.
Second molar	6 mos. in utero	Cusp tips still isolated	11 mos.	24 mos.	3 yrs.
Mandibular					
Central incisor	4½ mos. in utero	Three fifths	2½ mos.	6 mos.	1½ yrs.
Lateral incisor	4½ mos. in utero	Three fifths	3 mos.	7 mos.	1½ yrs.
Cuspid	5 mos. in utero	One third	9 mos.	16 mos.	3¼ yrs.
First molar	5 mos. in utero	Cusps united	5½ mos.	12 mos.	2¼ yrs.
Second molar	6 mos. in utero	Cusp tips still isolated	10 mos.	20 mos.	3 yrs.
Permanent Dentition					
Maxillary					
Central incisor	3 – 4 mos.	......	4 –5 yrs.	7– 8 yrs.	10 yrs.
Lateral incisor	10 –12 mos.	......	4 –5 yrs.	8– 9 yrs.	11 yrs.
Cuspid	4 – 5 mos.	......	6 –7 yrs.	11–12 yrs.	13–15 yrs.
First bicuspid	1½– 1¾ yrs.	......	5 –6 yrs.	10–11 yrs.	12–13 yrs.
Second bicuspid	2 – 2¼ yrs.	......	6 –7 yrs.	10–12 yrs.	12–14 yrs.
First molar	at birth	Sometimes a trace	2½–3 yrs.	6– 7 yrs.	9–10 yrs.
Second molar	2½– 3 yrs.	......	7 –8 yrs.	12–13 yrs.	14–16 yrs.
Mandibular					
Central incisor	3 – 4 mos.	......	4 –5 yrs.	6– 7 yrs.	9 yrs.
Lateral incisor	3 – 4 mos.	......	4 –5 yrs.	7– 8 yrs.	10 yrs.
Cuspid	4 – 5 mos.	......	6 –7 yrs.	9–10 yrs.	12–14 yrs.
First bicuspid	1¾– 2 yrs.	......	5 –6 yrs.	10–12 yrs.	12–13 yrs.
Second bicuspid	2¼– 2½ yrs.	......	6 –7 yrs.	11–12 yrs.	13–14 yrs.
First molar	at birth	Sometimes a trace	2½–3 yrs.	6– 7 yrs.	9–10 yrs.
Second molar	2½– 3 yrs.	......	7 –8 yrs.	11–13 yrs.	14–15 yrs.

After Logan and Kronfeld: J.A.D.A., 20, 1933 (slightly modified by McCall and Schour).

TABLE 4–2   AGES AT WHICH FIFTY PER CENT OF SPECIFIED
PRIMARY TEETH ARE LOST*

Age (Years)	Maxillary	Mandibular
6		Central incisors
7	Central incisors	Lateral incisors
8	Lateral incisors	
9	First molars	First molars
10		Cuspids
		Second molars
11	Cuspids	
	Second molars	

*Parfitt: D. Record, *74*, 1954.

TABLE 4–3   AGES AT WHICH FIFTY PER CENT OF
SPECIFIED PERMANENT TEETH ERUPT*

Age (Years)	Female		Male	
	Maxillary	*Mandibular*	*Maxillary*	*Mandibular*
6	First molars	Central incisors	First molars	Central incisors
		First molars		First molars
7	Central incisors	Lateral incisors	Central incisors	
8	Lateral incisors		Lateral incisors	Lateral incisors
9				
10	First premolars	Cuspids	First premolars	
		First premolars		
11	Cuspids	Second premolars	Second premolars	Cuspids
	Second premolars			First premolars
12	Second molars	Second molars	Cuspids	Second premolars
			Second molars	Second molars

*Parfitt: D. Record, *74*, 1954.

TABLE 4–4   TIME TAKEN FOR ERUPTION OF THE PERMANENT TEETH FROM
PIERCING THE GUM TO OCCLUSION (BOYS AND GIRLS)*

Teeth	No. of Cases	Percentage of Teeth in Months		
		0–6	*7–12*	*12 and Over*
$\frac{1}{1}$	72	15	67	18
	56	29	57	14
$\frac{2}{2}$	83	27	54	19
	78	9	59	32
$\frac{3}{3}$	43	2	40	58
	58	12	52	36
$\frac{4}{4}$	65	31	45	24
	61	26	46	28
$\frac{5}{5}$	56	63	37	0
	60	64	33	3
$\frac{6}{6}$	66	44	47	9
	67	52	40	8
$\frac{7}{7}$	75	57	37	6
	72	21	47	32

*Parfitt: D. Record, *74*, 1954.

TABLE 4–5 DENTIN DIMENSIONS OF PRIMARY MOLAR TEETH*

	Max. 1st Range in mm.			Max. 2nd Range in mm.			Mand. 1st Range in mm.			Mand. 2nd Range in mm.		
	Mean	Min.	Max.	Mean	Min.	Max.	Mean	Min.	Max.	Mean	Min.	Max.
Mesiodistal diameter at cervix	4.72	4.0	5.6	5.63	4.8	7.6	5.89	4.8	7.0	7.36	6.30	8.90
Buccolingual diameter at cervix	6.59	5.5	8.0	8.29	7.0	10.1	4.66	3.8	6.6	6.91	5.25	8.50
Height of dentinal crown from cervix	5.05	4.1	5.9	5.73	4.2	6.8	5.44	4.9	6.6	...	...	...
Mesiobuccal pulp horn to cusp tip	1.83	0.8	2.5	2.90	1.8	3.8	2.14	1.4	3.1	2.92	1.80	3.70
Mesiobuccal pulp horn to buccal	1.57	1.0	2.2	2.29	1.1	2.7	1.42	0.8	2.7	2.47	1.50	3.80
Mesiobuccal pulp horn to mesial	1.54	0.9	2.6	1.76	1.3	2.5	1.62	0.7	2.2	1.75	1.30	2.50
Mesiolingual pulp horn to cusp tip	...	...	...	2.90	2.2	4.2	2.44	1.4	4.2	3.17	2.20	4.20
Mesiolingual pulp horn to mesial	...	...	...	2.18	1.5	3.9	1.54	0.9	2.8	1.88	1.40	2.50
Mesiolingual pulp horn to lingual	...	...	...	2.44	1.0	3.8	1.29	0.9	1.8	1.89	1.20	2.50
Distobuccal pulp horn to cusp tip	2.11	1.3	3.1	2.89	2.1	3.9	2.38	1.2	5.6	3.06	2.00	3.80
Distobuccal pulp horn to buccal	1.34	0.8	1.8	2.01	1.3	2.7	1.32	1.0	2.0	2.68	1.60	3.50
Distobuccal pulp horn to distal	1.31	1.1	1.5	1.88	1.4	2.5	1.35	1.0	2.1	1.80	1.40	2.20
Distolingual pulp horn to cusp tip	...	...	...	2.83	2.2	3.9	2.33	1.2	4.7	3.30	1.70	4.10
Distolingual pulp horn to distal	...	...	...	1.77	1.2	2.7	1.49	1.1	2.6	2.30	1.60	3.10
Distolingual pulp horn to lingual	...	...	...	2.05	1.2	2.8	1.09	0.9	1.7	1.97	1.30	2.70
Lingual pulp horn to cusp tip	2.05	1.2	3.8	...	...	...	...	...	...	...	...	...
Lingual pulp horn to mesial	1.49	1.0	2.8	...	...	...	...	...	...	...	...	...
Lingual pulp horn to distal	2.12	1.2	2.8	...	...	...	...	...	...	...	...	...
Lingual pulp horn to lingual	1.57	1.1	2.1	...	...	...	...	...	...	...	...	...
Centrobuccal pulp horn to cusp tip	...	...	...	...	...	...	...	...	...	3.11	1.60	3.80
Centrobuccal pulp horn to buccal	...	...	...	...	...	...	...	...	...	2.34	1.50	3.50
Pulp to mesial at cervix	0.99	0.5	1.4	1.45	1.0	2.3	1.01	0.7	1.5	1.86	1.30	2.60
Pulp to distal at cervix	1.16	0.9	1.5	1.51	1.0	2.5	1.15	0.7	1.6	1.84	1.30	2.60
Pulp to buccal at cervix	1.22	0.9	1.9	1.67	1.1	2.5	1.20	0.7	1.9	2.00	1.30	2.80
Pulp to lingual at cervix	1.39	1.0	2.0	1.72	1.3	2.4	1.12	0.7	1.9	1.89	1.30	2.30

*Table condensed from Arnim and Doyle: J. Dent. Child., 26, 3rd quart., 1959.

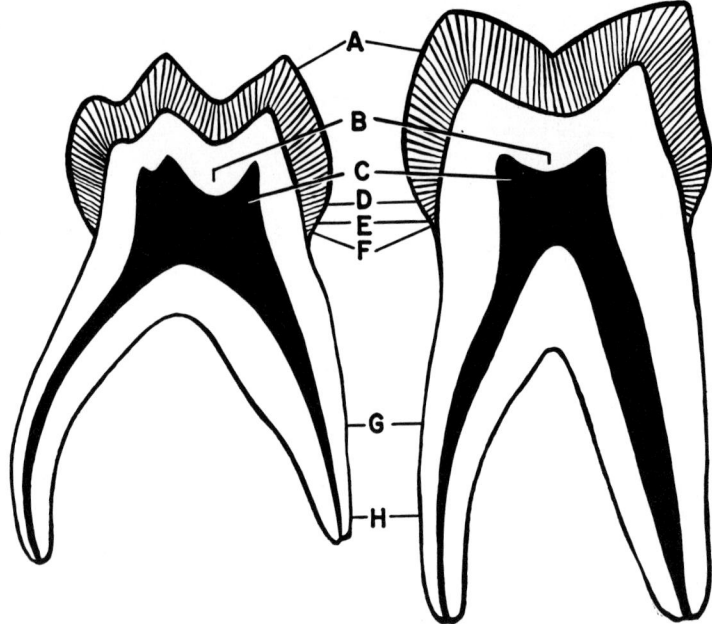

Figure 4–1 Comparison of maxillary second primary and permanent molars, linguobuccal cross section. (See text for references to labels.)

3. The cervical ridges are more pronounced, especially on the buccal aspect of the first primary molars (Fig. 4–1D).

4. The buccal and lingual surfaces of the primary molars are flatter about the cervical bulge than those of the permanent molars.

5. The buccal and lingual surfaces of the molars, especially the first molars, converge toward the occlusal surfaces so that the buccolingual diameter of the occlusal surface is much less than the cervical diameter.

6. The primary teeth have a markedly constricted neck compared to the permanent molars (Fig. 4–1F).

7. The enamel cap ends in a marked ridge in primary molars rather than tapering off to a feather edge as in the permanent molars.

8. The enamel cap is thinner and has a more consistent depth, being about 1 mm. thick throughout the entire crown (Fig. 4–1A).

9. The enamel rods at the cervix slope occlusally instead of being oriented gingivally as in the permanent teeth (Fig. 4–1E).

10. There is comparatively less tooth structure protecting the pulp in primary teeth. The thicknesses of the dentin from the pulp chambers to the dentino-enamel junction are presented in Table 4–5. In cavity preparation a knowledge of the relative thickness of the dentin is important, although there appears to be considerable variation among individual teeth possessing the same morphology.

11. The pulpal horns are higher in primary molars, especially the mesial horns, and the pulp chambers are proportionately larger (Fig. 4–1C).

12. There is a comparatively greater thickness of dentin over the pulpal wall at the occlusal fossa of primary molars. (Fig. 4–1B).

13. The roots of the primary anterior teeth are narrower mesiodistally than the permanent anteriors. This, together with the markedly constricted cervix and

(Text continued on page 57.)

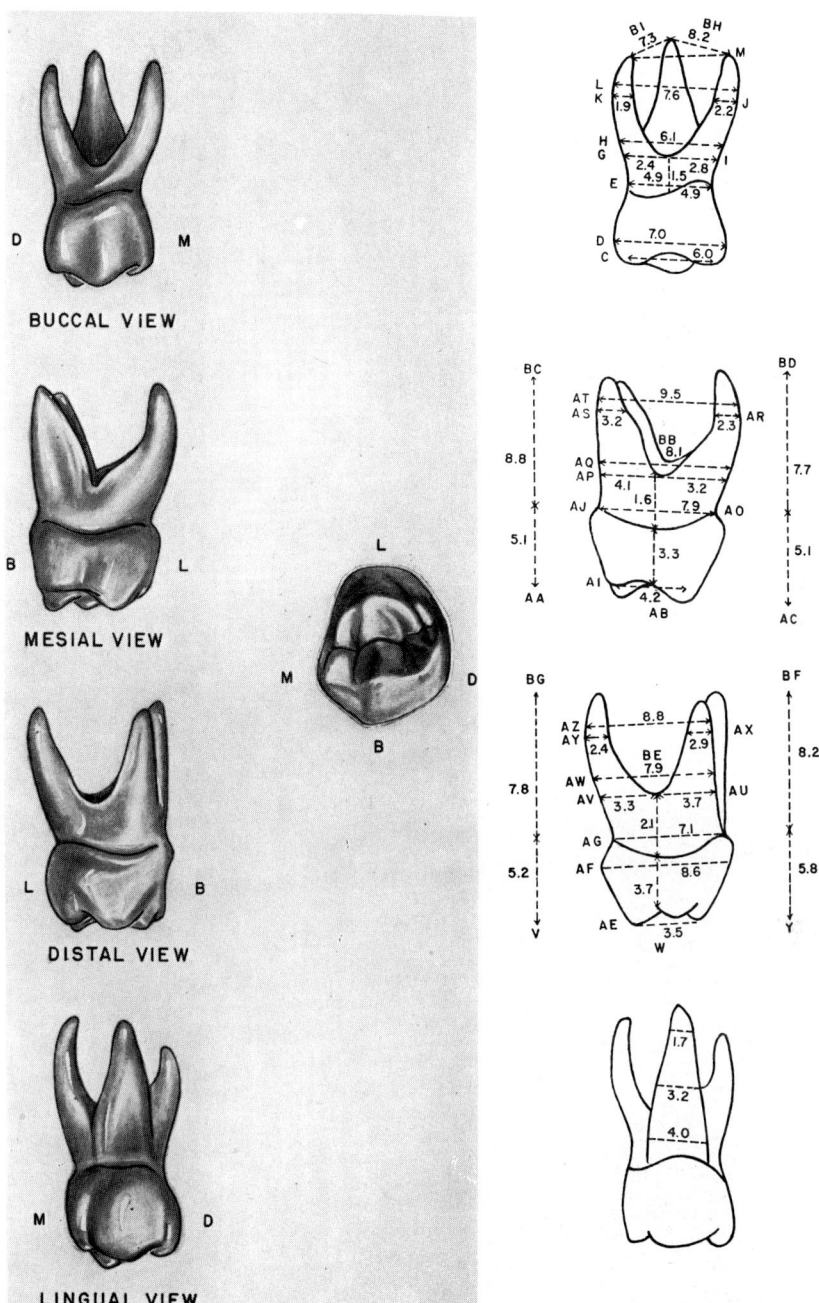

Figure 4–2 Maxillary right first primary molar. (Modified from Zeisz and Nuckolls: Dental Anatomy, C. V. Mosby Co. Measurements from Kramer and Ireland: J. Dent. Child., 26:1959.) (*See pages 57 and 58 for legend.*)

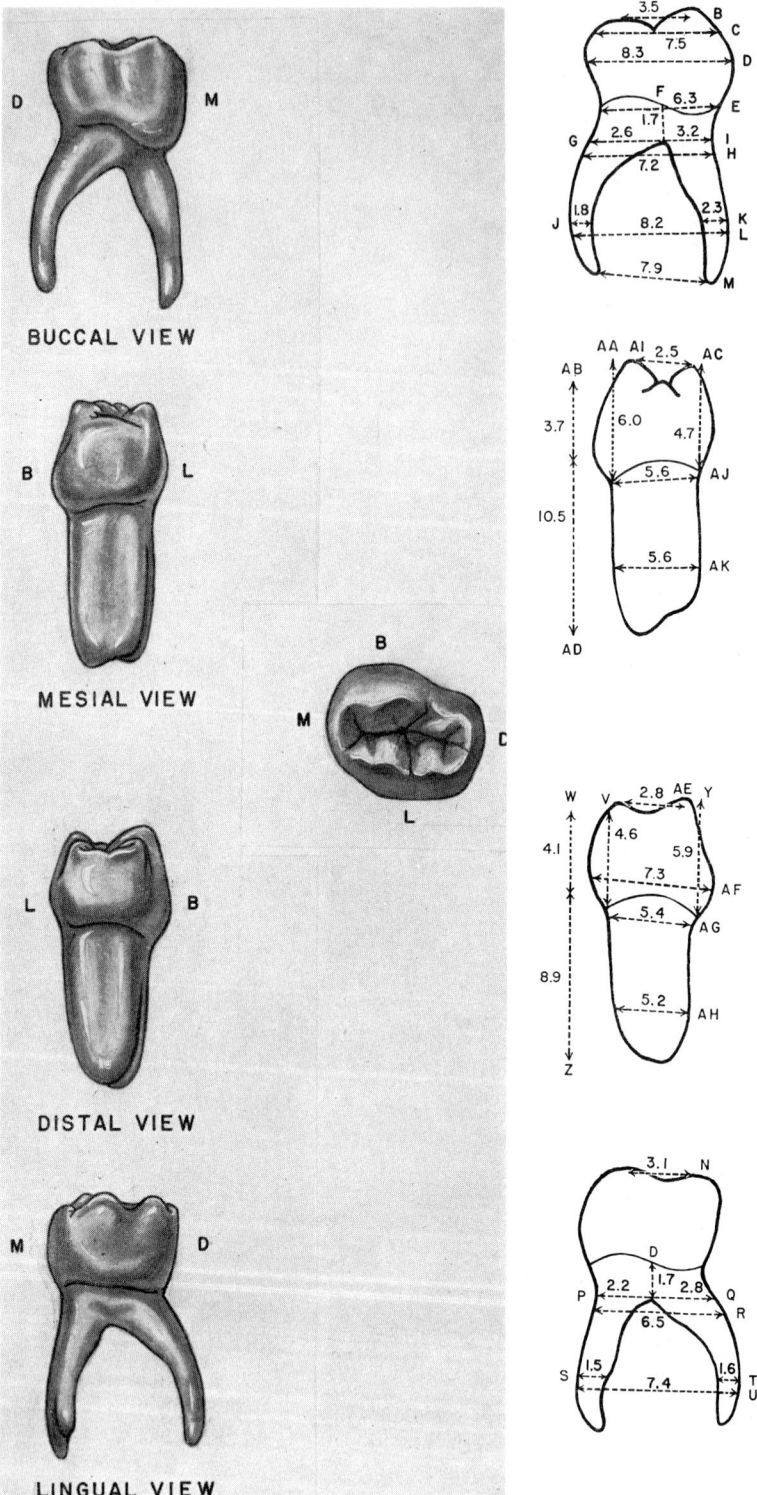

BUCCAL VIEW

MESIAL VIEW

DISTAL VIEW

LINGUAL VIEW

Figure 4–3 Mandibular right first primary molar. (Modified from Zeisz and Nuckolls: Dental Anatomy, C. V. Mosby Co. Measurements from Kramer and Ireland: J. Dent. Child., *26*:1959.) (*See pages 57 and 58 for legend.*)

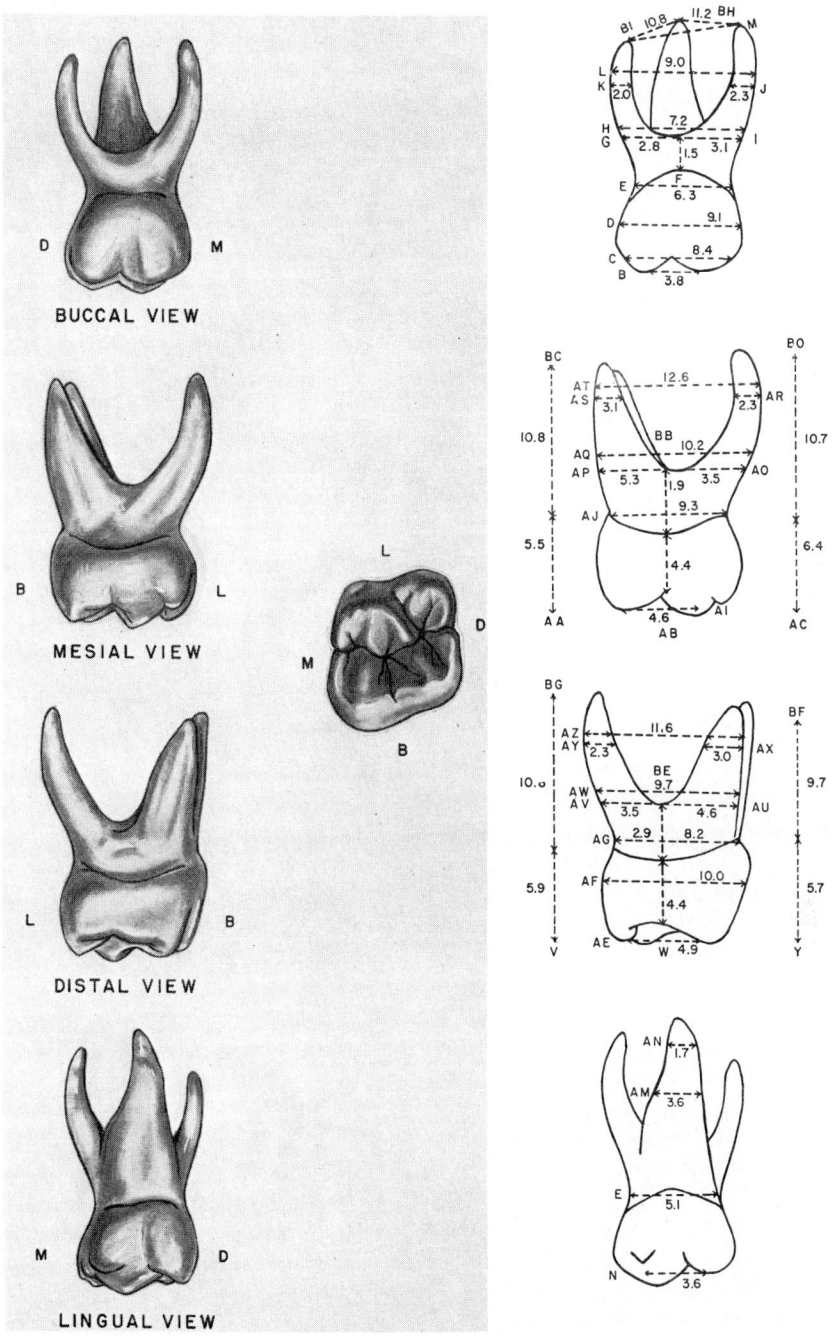

Figure 4–4   Maxillary right second primary molar. (Modified from Zeisz and Nuckolls: Dental Anatomy, C. V. Mosby Co. Measurements from Kramer and Ireland: J. Dent. Child., *26*, 1959.) (*See pages 57 and 58 for legend.*)

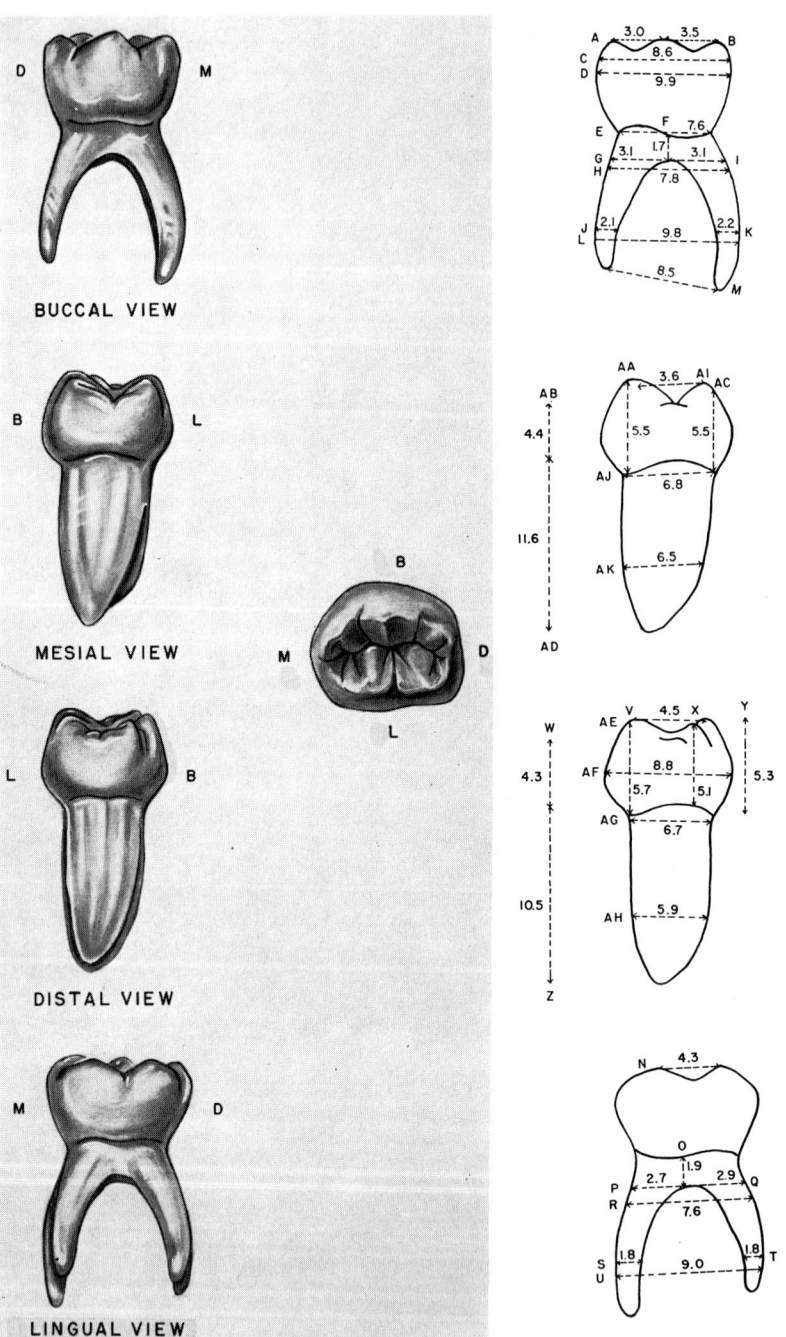

Figure 4–5   Mandibular right second primary molar. (Modified from Zeisz and Nuckolls: Dental Anatomy, C. V. Mosby Co. Measurements from Kramer and Ireland: J. Dent. Child., 26, 1959.) (*See pages 57 and 58 for legend.*)

the prominent enamel ridges, gives the characteristic picture of the crown fitting over the root as the cap of an acorn.

14. The roots of the primary teeth are longer and more slender in comparison with crown size than those of the permanent teeth (Fig. 4–1G).

15. The roots of the primary molars flare out nearer the cervix than do those of the permanent teeth (Fig. 4–1H).

16. The roots of the primary molars flare more as they approach the apices than do permanent molars. This affords the necessary room for the development of the permanent tooth buds within the confines of these roots.

17. The primary teeth are usually lighter in color.

MORPHOLOGY OF INDIVIDUAL PRIMARY TEETH

In pedodontics one deals with the primary teeth for the first time. It is well, therefore, to describe the morphology of these teeth individually, as well as their external dimensions. The description of the measurements of four primary molars is listed in Table 4–5.

MAXILLARY FIRST PRIMARY MOLAR

This tooth (Fig. 4–2) more nearly resembles the tooth that will replace it than any other primary molar, not only in diameter but in shape as well. The upper primary molar presents four well defined surfaces: buccal, lingual, mesial, and distal. The root is formed of three well defined diverging prongs.

LEGEND TO MEASUREMENTS OF THE FOUR PRIMARY MOLARS, *Figures 4–2, 4–3, 4–4, 4–5*

A	Apex of distal cusp to apex of distal buccal cusp
B	Apex of distal buccal cusp to apex of mesial buccal cusp
C	Mesial distal width of crown at marginal ridges
D	Greatest mesiodistal width of crown
E	Mesiodistal width of crown at cervix
F	Buccal surface from cervical line to bifurcation of mesial root and distal root
G	Mesiodistal width of distal root at level of bifurcation
H	From distal of distal root to mesial of mesial root at level of bifurcation
I	Mesiodistal width of mesial root at level of bifurcation
J	Mesiodistal width of distal root at level of greatest spread
K	Mesiodistal width of mesial root at level of greatest spread
L	From distal of distal root to mesial of mesial root at level of greatest spread of roots
M	Apex of mesial root to apex of distal root
N	Apex of mesiolingual cusp to apex of distolingual cusp
O	Lingual surface from cervical line to bifurcation of mesial root and distal root
P	Mesiodistal width of mesial root at level of bifurcation
Q	Mesiodistal width of distal root at level of bifurcation
R	From mesial of mesial root to distal of distal root at level of bifurcation
S	Mesiodistal width of mesial root at level of greatest spread
T	Mesiodistal width of distal root at level of greatest spread
U	From mesial of mesial root to distal of distal root at level of greatest spread
V	Cervical line to apex of distolingual cusp
W	Cervical line to distal marginal ridge

X	Cervical line to apex of distal cusp
Y	Cervical line to apex of distobuccal cusp
Z	Cervical line to apex of distal root
AA	Cervical line to apex of mesiobuccal cusp
AB	Cervical line to mesial marginal ridge
AC	Cervical line to apex of mesiolingual cusp
AD	Cervical line to apex of mesial root
AE	Apex of distolingual cusp to apex of distobuccal cusp
AF	Greatest buccolingual width of crown
AG	Buccolingual width of crown at cervix
AH	Buccolingual width of distal root in middle portion
AI	Apex of mesiobuccal cusp to apex of mesiolingual cusp
AJ	Buccolingual width of crown at cervix
AK	Buccolingual width of mesial root in middle portion
AL	Greatest mesiodistal width of lingual root
AM	Mesiodistal width of lingual root at middle portion
AN	Mesiodistal width of lingual root at apical portion
AO	Buccolingual width of lingual root at level of bifurcation of lingual root and mesiobuccal root
AP	Buccolingual width of mesiobuccal root at level of bifurcation of lingual and mesiobuccal roots
AQ	From lingual surface of lingual root to buccal surface of mesiobuccal root at level of bifurcation
AR	Buccolingual width of lingual root at level of greatest spread
AS	Buccolingual width of mesiobuccal root at level of greatest spread
AT	From lingual surface of lingual root to buccal surface of mesiobuccal root at level of greatest spread
AU	Buccolingual width of distobuccal root at level of bifurcation of distobuccal and lingual roots
AV	Buccolingual width of lingual root at level of bifurcation at distobuccal root and lingual root
AW	From buccal of distobuccal root to lingual root at level of bifurcation
AX	Buccolingual width of distobuccal root at level of greatest spread
AY	Buccolingual width of distobuccal root at level of greatest spread
AZ	From buccal of distobuccal root to lingual of lingual root at level of greatest spread
BA	Cervical line to apex of mesiobuccal cusp
BB	Cervical line to bifurcation of mesiobuccal root and lingual root
BC	Cervical line to apex of mesiobuccal root
BD	Cervical line to apex of lingual root
BE	Cervical line to bifurcation of distobuccal root and lingual root
BF	Cervical line to apex of distobuccal root
BG	Cervical line to apex of distolingual root
BH	Apex of mesiobuccal root to apex of lingual root
BI	Apex of distobuccal root to apex of lingual root

The Crown

The buccal surface is convex in all directions with the greatest convexity occlusogingivally at the cervical ridge, which is very prominently developed. From the cervical ridge the tooth slopes abruptly to the neck of the tooth and less abruptly toward the occlusal surface. The buccal surface is divided by the buccal groove, which is poorly defined and is situated distal to the center of the tooth, making the mesiobuccal cusp larger than the distobuccal one. The mesiobuccal cusp extends further cervically and hence has a longer and more prominent cervico-occlusal diameter. There is a well developed buccal ridge on this cusp which extends from the tip of the cusp to the cervical margin, and a less developed ridge on the distobuccal cusp.

The lingual surface is slightly convex occlusocervically, but is markedly convex mesiodistally. The entire lingual surface generally is made up of one definite mesiolingual cusp which is more rounded and less acute in its junction with the mesial and distal surfaces than are the buccal cusps. The shorter diameter of the lingual cusp, as compared to the diameter of the two combined buccal cusps, leads to a narrower lingual diameter. When there is a distolingual cusp the lingual surface may be crossed by a not-too-well-defined distolingual groove.

The mesial surface is greater in diameter at the cervical border than at the occlusal and slopes distally from the mesiobuccal line angle toward the mesiolingual cusp, the mesiobuccal angle being more acute while the mesiolingual line angle is obtuse. Contact with the primary cuspid is in the form of a small circular area on the occlusobuccal third of the tooth.

The distal surface is slightly convex in both directions, joining the buccal and lingual cusps at almost right angles. It is narrower than the mesial surface and narrower occlusally than cervically. The marginal ridge is fairly well developed and is crossed by a prominent distal groove. Contact with the primary second molar is broad and in the shape of an inverted crescent in the occlusolingual half of the distal surface.

The occlusal surface presents a longer buccal margin than a lingual one. The mesial margin joins the buccal margin at an acute angle and the lingual margin at an obtuse angle. Both buccal and lingual margins of the distal surface are joined at almost right angles. The occlusal surface is made up of three cusps: the mesiobuccal, the distobuccal, and the mesiolingual. The buccal aspect comprises the mesiobuccal and the distobuccal cusps; the mesiobuccal cusp, being the larger and more prominent, occupies the major portion of the bucco-occlusal surface. In some teeth the distobuccal cusp may be poorly developed or may be absent entirely. The lingual portion of the occlusal surface is formed by the mesiolingual cusp, which has many modifications. Some lingual cusps are crescent shaped, others are bisected by a lingual groove which may set off a small distolingual cusp. The junction of the lingual ridge of the distobuccal cusp with the buccal ridge of the mesiolingual cusp presents a not-too-prominent transverse ridge which in a three-cusped tooth forms the distal marginal ridge of the occlusal surface.

The occlusal surface has three pits, central, mesial, and distal. The central pit is found in the central portion of the occlusal surface and forms the hub of the three primary grooves: the buccal groove, which extends buccally onto the buccal surface, dividing the buccal cusps; a mesial groove, which extends mesially to the mesial pit; and a distal groove, which traverses to the distal pit. The mesial pit is the deepest and best defined, the distal pit the shallowest and most poorly defined. In preparing occlusal portions of class II cavities it is not necessary to include the distal pit in the outline form of the mesial preparations.

The Roots

The roots are three in number: a mesiobuccal, a distobuccal and a lingual branch. The lingual root is the longest and diverges in a lingual direction. The distobuccal root is the shortest.

The Pulp Cavity

The pulp cavity consists of a chamber and three pulpal canals corresponding to the three roots, although according to Hibbard and Ireland variations from this basic canal design are not uncommon in all the root canals of the primary molars. There may be many anastomoses and branchings. The *pulp chamber* consists of three or four pulpal horns, which are more sharply pointed than the outer contour of the cusps would indicate, although in general they follow the surface contour of the tooth (Fig. 4–6). The largest of the pulpal horns is the mesiobuccal which occupies a prominent portion of the pulp chamber. The apex of the horn lies

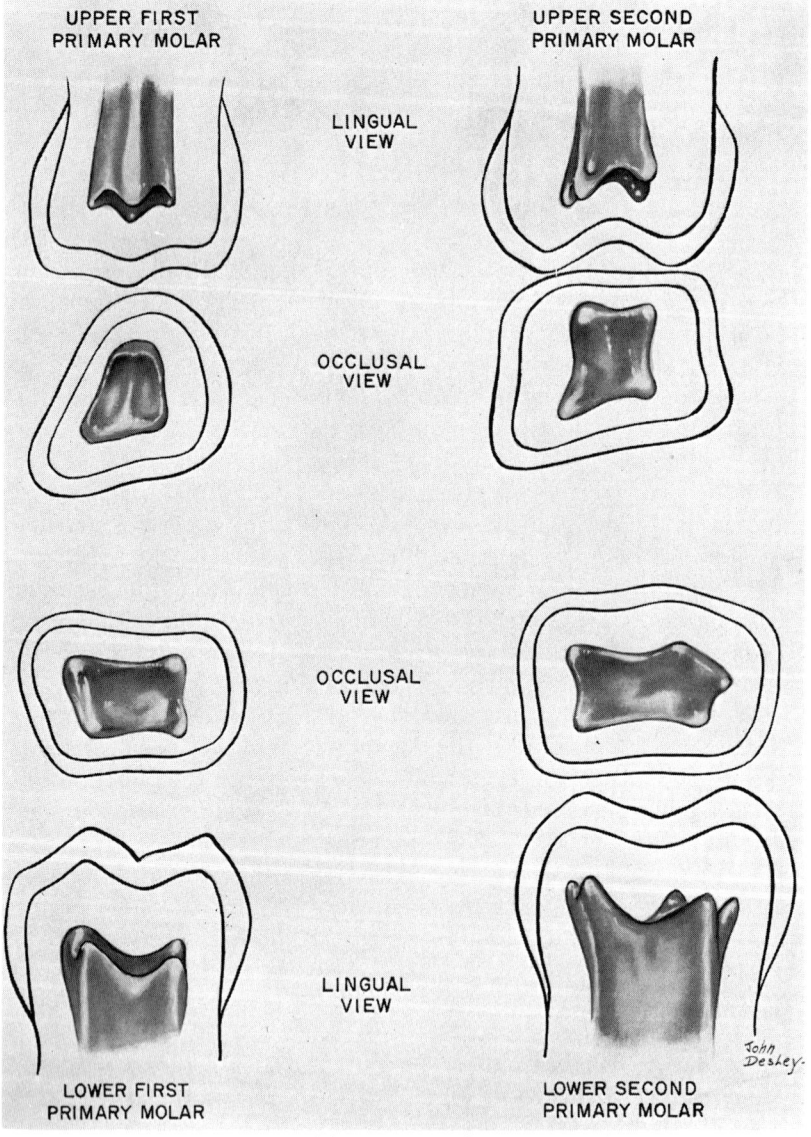

UPPER FIRST PRIMARY MOLAR

UPPER SECOND PRIMARY MOLAR

LINGUAL VIEW

OCCLUSAL VIEW

OCCLUSAL VIEW

LINGUAL VIEW

LOWER FIRST PRIMARY MOLAR

LOWER SECOND PRIMARY MOLAR

Figure 4–6 Pulp chamber outlines of the primary molars. Distances from pulp chamber to proximal walls are given in Table 4–5.

slightly mesial to the body of the pulp chamber. The mesiolingual pulpal horn is second in size and is quite angular and sharp, although not as high as the mesiobuccal horn. The distobuccal horn is the smallest. It is sharp and occupies the extreme distobuccal angle. The occlusal view of the pulp chamber follows the general surface contour of the tooth and resembles somewhat a triangle with rounded corners, the mesiolingual angle being obtuse and the distobuccal and mesiobuccal angles being acute. The pulp canals extend from the floor of the chamber near the distobuccal and mesiobuccal angles, and at the lingual-most area of the chamber.

MANDIBULAR FIRST PRIMARY MOLAR

This tooth is morphologically unique among the primary molars (Fig. 4–3). Its outline form differs considerably from that of the other primary teeth and from that of any of the permanent molars. Its chief differing characteristic is its overdeveloped mesial marginal ridge. This ridge somewhat resembles a fifth cusp; it is not found in other molars, and its presence, together with the large mesiobuccal pulpal horn, makes preparation of a classic mesio-occlusal cavity difficult. The outline of the tooth is in the shape of a rhomboid.

The Crown

The buccal surface presents a prominent and well developed cervical ridge which extends across the entire buccal surface just above the neck of the tooth but is more pronounced on the mesiobuccal. This pronounced ridge joins the mesial surface at an acute angle and the distal surface at an obtuse angle. The buccal surface is convex in a mesiodistal direction but slopes abruptly toward the occlusal surface, especially on the mesial aspect, where it is carried lingually to a marked degree. Buccolingually, the gingival diameter of the tooth is much greater than the occlusal diameter, giving a constricted appearance. Above the cervical bulge the buccal surface flattens out. The buccal surface is composed of two cusps, the larger and longer mesiobuccal cusp and the much smaller distobuccal cusp. These cusps are divided by a buccal depression, an extension of the buccal groove.

The lingual surface is convex in both aspects and slopes from the prominent cervical margin toward the midline of the tooth as it approaches the occlusal surface. The cervico-occlusal contour is parallel to the long axis of the tooth. The lingual surface is traversed by a lingual groove which arises in the central pit and ends as a depression on the lingual surface near the cervical border. The groove divides the lingual surface into a mesiolingual and a distolingual cusp, the mesiolingual cusp being the larger.

The mesial surface is quite flat in both aspects. A convexity is created in the mesial marginal ridge, which is very prominent at the junction of the mesiobuccal cusp and slopes more gingivally as it approaches the mesiolingual cusp.

The distal surface is convex in all aspects and the distal marginal ridge is crossed by a distal groove which ends abruptly on the distal surface.

The occlusal surface may be defined as a rhomboid divided by the prominent mesiobuccal and mesiolingual cusps to resemble a figure 8 laid on its side, the smaller loop representing the mesial aspect and the larger loop the larger distal aspect. The occlusal surface is longer mesiodistally than it is buccolingually, and it contains the mesiobuccal, distobuccal, mesiolingual, and distolingual cusps. The mesio-lingual and mesiobuccal cusps are the largest; the distal cusps are much smaller.

There are three pits located on the occlusal surface: a medium-sized mesial pit located mesial to the mesiobuccal and mesiolingual cusps and rather isolated by them, a central pit which lies in the center of the crown and is the deepest of the three, and a distal pit which is very shallow and lies distal to the distobuccal and dis-tolingual cusps. These pits are connected by the central developmental groove. The mesial marginal groove extends from the mesial pit lingually to separate the large mesial marginal ridge (mesial cusp) from the mesiolingual cusp. There is also a mesiobuccal triangular groove which separates the mesial marginal ridge from the mesiobuccal cusp. The other grooves are not as prominent.

The Roots

The root of the mandibular first primary molar is divided into two prongs, a mesial and a distal root. Although the roots resemble those of the mandibular first permanent molar, they are thinner and flare as they approach the apex to allow for the developing permanent tooth bud.

The Pulp Cavity

The pulp cavity contains a pulp chamber which, viewed from the occlusal, is rhomboidal in shape and closely follows the contour of the surface of the crown. The pulp chamber has four pulpal horns. The mesiobuccal horn, the largest of the pulpal horns, occupies a considerable part of the pulp chamber. It is rounded and connects with the mesiolingual pulpal horn in a high ridge, making the mesial area especially vulnerable to mechanical exposure. The distobuccal pulpal horn is sec-ond in area but lacks the height of the mesial horns. The mesiolingual pulpal horn, because of the contour of the pulp chamber, lies slightly mesial to the corre-sponding cusp. Although this pulpal horn is third in size it is second in height; it is long and pointed. The distolingual pulpal horn is the smallest. It is more pointed than the buccal horns and relatively small as compared to the other three pulpal horns.

There are three pulp canals. A mesiobuccal and a mesiolingual canal are confluent and leave the chamber widened buccolingually in the form of a ribbon. The two canals soon separate to form a buccal and a lingual canal which gradually taper to the apical foramen. The distal pulp canal projects in ribbon fashion from the floor of the chamber in the distal aspect. This canal is wide buccolingually and may be constricted in its center, reflecting the outside contour of the root.

THE MAXILLARY SECOND PRIMARY MOLAR

The maxillary second primary molar is essentially a four-cusped tooth, al-though a fifth cusp is frequently present on the mesiolingual aspect (Fig. 4–4).

The Crown

The external appearance of the crown is similar in many respects to the corre-sponding first permanent molar, having the same pit, groove, and cuspal arrangement. The crown differs, however, in being smaller and more angular, and in converging more toward the occlusal. It also has a more pronounced cervical ridge on the buccal surface. This molar is intermediate in size between the smaller first primary molar and the larger first permanent molar. The crown of the second primary molar is trapezoidal in outline.

The buccal surface presents a well defined cervical ridge which extends the full diameter of the buccal surface. It is, however, somewhat less prominent than those found on the primary first molars. The cervical ridge attains its greatest magnitude where it joins the mesiobuccal cusp. The buccal surface is divided by the buccal groove into a mesiobuccal and a distobuccal cusp, the mesiobuccal being the larger.

The lingual surface is convex, inclining slightly as it approaches the occlusal border. The inclination is greater on the mesial aspect than on the distal. The lingual surface is divided by the lingual groove, which is deep on the occlusal aspect but gradually is obliterated as it joins the cervical third of the tooth. This groove divides the surface into a mesiolingual and a distolingual cusp. The mesiolingual cusp is higher and more extensive than the distolingual cusp. A fifth cusp, when present, occupies the mesiolingual area at the middle third of the crown. It is frequently referred to as Carabelli's cusp.

The mesial surface presents a fairly high marginal ridge which is indented by the mesial groove, extending from the occlusal surface. The mesiobuccal angle of the tooth is rather acute and the mesiolingual angle is more or less obtuse. The surface is convex occlusocervically and less so buccolingually, being somewhat flattened and forming a broad contact with the first primary molar in the form of an inverted crescent.

The distal surface is convex occlusocervically but less so buccolingually, and flattened in its central portion. Contact with the upper first permanent molar is in the form of an inverted crescent with the convexity toward the occlusal.

The occlusal surface of this molar closely resembles the corresponding surface on the first permanent molar. There are four well defined cusps and a smaller, sometimes absent, fifth cusp. The mesiobuccal cusp is the second largest in size but is not as prominent as the distobuccal cusp. The mesiobuccal cusp has a steeper inclination to its lingual ridge in approaching the central developmental groove. The distobuccal cusp is third in size, but has a very prominent lingual ridge with a slight mesial inclination. The prominent lingual ridge makes contact with the large mesiolingual cusp to form an elevated oblique ridge. The mesiolingual cusp is the largest and occupies the greater portion of the occlusolingual area, extending farther buccally than the distolingual cusp. It joints in the formation of the oblique ridge, which is an outstanding characteristic of this tooth. The distolingual cusp is the smallest of the four and is separated from the mesiolingual cusp by the markedly accentuated distolingual groove.

The occlusal surface presents three pits. The central pit is large and deep and is the junction point of the buccal groove, the mesial groove, which joins the shallow mesial pit, and the distal groove, which traverses the oblique ridge to join the distal pit. The distal pit is deep and flanked with well defined triangular grooves. The distolingual groove is deep, with a mesial inclination, and it produces a definite indentation as it joins the lingual surface. Because of the pronounced oblique ridge, cavity preparation is usually confined to the area on either side of the ridge and does not traverse the ridge unless it is undermined or carious or additional area is needed for retention.

The Roots

The root of the maxillary second molar is divided into three prongs: a mesio-buccal, a distobuccal and a lingual root. Although the roots resemble somewhat those of the maxillary permanent molar, they are thinner and flare more as they approach the apex. The distobuccal root is the shortest and narrowest of the three.

The Pulp Cavity

The pulp cavity consists of a pulp chamber and three pulp canals. The pulp chamber conforms to the general outline of the tooth and has four pulpal horns. A fifth horn projecting from the lingual aspect of the mesiolingual horn may be present, and when present is small. The mesiobuccal pulpal horn is the largest. It extends occlusally above the other cusps and is pointed. The mesiolingual pulpal horn is second in size, but only slightly longer than the distobuccal pulpal horn. When combined with the fifth pulpal horn, it presents quite a bulky appearance. The distobuccal pulpal horn is third in size. Its general contour is such that it joins the mesiolingual pulpal horn as a slight elevation and separates a central pit and a distal pit corresponding to the occlusal outline of the tooth in this area.

The distolingual pulpal horn is the smallest and shortest and extends only slightly above the occlusal level. There are three pulp canals, corresponding to the three roots. These leave the floor of the chamber at the mesiobuccal and distobuc-cal corners and from the lingual area. The pulp canals follow the general contour of the roots.

THE MANDIBULAR SECOND PRIMARY MOLAR

The mandibular second primary molar is a five-cusped tooth corresponding to the first permanent molar (Fig. 4–5). The primary molar, although having the same general contour and surface pattern, presents a more rounded axial contour, is narrower buccolingually in comparison to its mesiodistal diameter, and has a more pronounced cervical ridge on the buccal surface. The tooth is larger than the first primary molar and smaller than the first permanent molar, which stand in juxtaposition.

The Crown

The buccal surface presents three well defined cusps: a mesiobuccal cusp, second in size; a distobuccal cusp, the largest; and a distal cusp, the smallest of the three, al-though the difference in size of the cusps is slight. These three cusps coalesce into a well developed cervical ridge which extends the entire width of the buccal surface just above the neck of the tooth. The distal cusp extends lingually at the occlusal border more than the other buccal cusps to give a smaller occlusal area at the disto-occlusal surface. The mesiobuccal and distobuccal cusps are divided by the mesio-buccal groove, which traverses the crest of the ridge to join the mesial groove. The distobuccal and distal cusps are separated by the distobuccal groove, which tra-verses the crest and joins the distal groove on the occlusal surface.

The lingual surface is convex in all directions and is crossed on the occlusal border by the lingual groove, which separates the mesiolingual and distolingual cusps. These cusps are of about equal height. The convexity of this surface is greatest as it approaches the neck of the tooth.

The mesial surface is generally convex, but flattens considerably cervically. It is crossed near its center by the mesial groove, which traverses the occlusal border to extend about one third of the distance down the mesial surface. The surface is constricted at the occlusal border. Contact with the first primary molar is broad and in the shape of an inverted crescent just below the notch of the mesial groove.

The distal surface is generally convex, but flattens somewhat buccolingually as it approaches the cervical border. It is smaller than the mesial surface. Contact with the first permanent molar is not as broad as contact on the mesial surface, being in the form of a round contact just buccal and cervical to the distal groove.

The occlusal surface has a wider diameter on its buccal than on its lingual border because of the convergence of the mesial and distal walls as they approach the lingual. The buccal aspect is made up of three cusps: a mesiobuccal cusp, which is second in size; a distobuccal cusp, which is the largest cusp and is separated from the mesiobuccal cusp by the mesiobuccal groove; and a distal cusp, the smallest of the three, which lies slightly lingual to the other two and is separated from the distobuccal cusp by the distobuccal groove. The lingual aspect is made up of two cusps of about equal size, the mesiolingual and distolingual cusps, which are divided by the distolingual groove and are larger than the buccal cusps. There are three pits on this surface, of which the central pit is the deepest and best defined, followed by the mesial pit, and the least well defined distal pit. Connecting these pits are grooves which pursue an angular course weaving between the inclined planes of the buccal and lingual cusps, forming the pattern of an elongated W when viewed from the occlusobuccal aspect.

The Roots

The root of the second primary molar is larger than that of the first primary molar although, in general, it has the same contour. The root is composed of a mesial branch and a distal branch. Both branches diverge as they approach the apices so that the mesiodistal space occupied is greater than the mesiodistal diameter of the crown, to allow for the developing succedaneous tooth.

The Pulp Cavity

The pulp cavity is made up of a chamber and usually three pulp canals (Fig. 4–6). The pulp chamber has five pulpal horns corresponding to the five cusps. In fact, the chamber itself conforms to the outside contour of the tooth, the roof of the chamber being extremely concave toward the apices. The mesiobuccal and mesiolingual pulpal horns are the largest, the mesiolingual pulpal horn being slightly less pointed but of the same height. These horns are connected by a higher ridge of pulpal tissue than is found connecting the distal horns of the pulp. The distobuccal pulpal horn is not as large as the mesiobuccal pulpal horn, but somewhat larger than either the distolingual or distal horns. The distal pulpal horn is the shortest and smallest and occupies a position distal to the distobuccal horn, and its distal inclination carries the apex distal to the distolingual horn.

The two mesial pulpal canals are confluent as they leave the floor of the pulp chamber through a common orifice that is wide buccolingually but narrow mesio-distally. The common canal soon divides into a larger mesiobuccal canal and a smaller mesiolingual canal. The distal canal is somewhat constricted in the center. All three canals taper as they approach the apical foramen, and conform in general to the shape of the roots.

THE MAXILLARY PRIMARY INCISORS

The maxillary primary incisors are quite similar in morphology (Fig. 4–7). They will, therefore, be considered collectively, and at the same time the differences between the central incisors and the lateral incisors will be pointed out.

The Crown

The primary central incisors are proportionately shorter incisocervically than mesiodistally. *The incisal edge* is, therefore, proportionately long, joining the mesial surface at an acute angle and the distal surface at a more rounded, obtuse angle. The incisal edge is formed from one developmental lobe.

As in all anterior teeth, the proximal surfaces are markedly convex labiolingually. They have a pronounced cervical ridge which is concave toward the root. *The labial surface* is convex mesiodistally and slightly less so incisocervically. *The lingual surface* presents a well defined cingulum and marginal ridges which are elevated above the surrounding tooth surface. The depression between the marginal ridges and the cingulum forms the lingual fossa. The cingulum is convex and occupies the cervical one half to one third of the surface.

The Root

The root is single and conical in shape. It is fairly regular in form, ending in a well rounded apex.

The Pulp Cavity

The pulp cavity conforms to the general outside surface of the tooth. The pulp chamber has three slight projections on its incisal border. The chamber tapers cervically in its mesiodistal diameter, but it is widest at the cervical ridge labiolingually. The single pulp canal continues from the chamber with no distinct demarcation between the two. Both pulp chamber and canal are relatively large when compared with their permanent successors. The pulp canal tapers evenly until it ends at the apical foramen.

The maxillary lateral incisors are quite similar in contour to the maxillary central incisors except that they are not as wide mesiodistally. Their cervicoincisal length about equals that of the central incisors. Their labial surfaces are a little more flattened. The cingulum on the lingual surface is not as pronounced and blends with the lingual marginal ridges. The root of the lateral incisor is thin and tapering. The pulp chamber follows the contour of the tooth, as does the canal. In the lateral incisor there is a light demarcation between the pulp chamber and the canal, especially on the labial and lingual aspects.

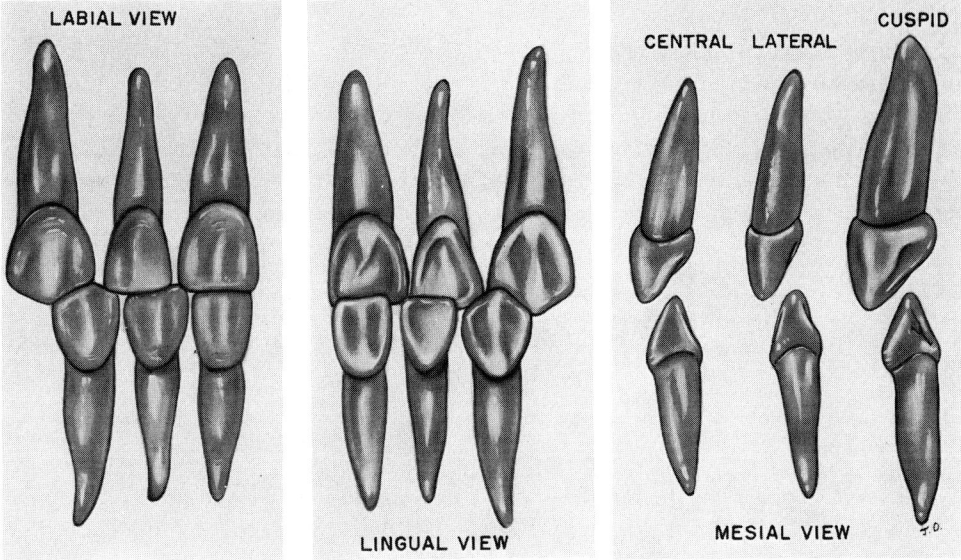

Figure 4–7 Primary anterior teeth in normal occlusion.

THE MANDIBULAR PRIMARY INCISORS

The mandibular primary incisors are narrow and are the smallest incisors in the mouth, although the lateral incisor is both slightly broader and longer than the central incisor and has a longer root.

The Crown

The labial surface of the mandibular incisors is convex in all directions, with the greatest convexity at the cervical border and a tendency to flatten somewhat as it approaches the incisal edge.

The incisal edge joins the proximal surfaces at almost right angles in the central incisor. The lateral incisor is less angular than the central incisor, with the incisal edge joining the mesial surface at an acute angle and the distal surface at an obtuse angle. The incisal edge slopes cervically slightly as it approaches the distal border to make contact with the mesial surface of the mandibular canine.

The mesial and distal surfaces are convex labiolingually and less so incisocervically. These surfaces are convex labiolingually at their cervical third, with the convexity toward the incisal edge. Contact with adjacent teeth is on the incisal third of the proximal surfaces.

The lingual surfaces are narrower in diameter than the labial, the proximal walls sloping lingually as the cervical area is approached. The mesial and distal marginal ridges are not especially well developed, and they join the convex cingulum with no definite demarcation. The cingulum occupies the cervical third of the lingual surface.

The Root

The root of the central incisor is only slightly flattened on its mesial and distal aspects and tapers toward the apex. The root of the lateral incisor is longer and also tapers toward the apex.

The Pulp Cavity

The pulp cavity conforms to the general surface contour of the tooth. The pulp chamber is widest mesiodistally at the roof of the chamber. Labiolingually the chamber is widest at the cingulum or cervical line. The pulp canal is oval in appearance and tapers as it approaches the apex. There is a definite demarcation between the pulp chamber and canal in the central incisor, which is not present in the lateral incisor.

THE MAXILLARY PRIMARY CUSPID

Like the permanent cuspids, the primary cuspids are larger than the central or lateral incisors.

The Crown

The labial surface of the cuspid is convex, bending lingually from a central developmental lobe. This developmental lobe extends occlusally to form the cusp. The cusp extends incisally from the center of the labial aspect of the tooth, yet the mesio-incisal edge is longer than the disto-incisal edge for intercuspation with the disto-incisal edge of the lower cuspid.

The mesial and distal surfaces are convex, sloping lingually and extending more lingually than the incisors. The mesial surface is not as high cervico-incisally as the distal surface because of the increased length of the mesio-incisal edge. Both surfaces converge as they approach the cervical area. The tooth is broader labiolingually than any of the incisors. Because of the heavy cervical, labial, and lingual ridges, a slight concavity is formed on the mesial surface between these ridges.

The lingual surface is convex in all directions. There is a lingual ridge which extends from the center of the tip of the cusp lingually, traversing the lingual surface and separating the mesiolingual and distolingual developmental grooves or depressions. The ridge is more prominent in the incisal area and decreases in prominence to a point at the cingulum. The cingulum is not as large or broad as on the upper incisors, but it is sharper in outline, projecting incisally to a point. The mesial marginal ridge is prominent but shorter than the distal marginal ridge, which is also prominent.

The Root

The root of the maxillary primary cuspid is long, thick in diameter, and slightly flattened on its mesial and distal surfaces. The root is tapering, however; there is a slight increase in diameter as it progresses from the cervical margin. The apex of the tooth is rounded.

The Pulp Cavity

The pulp cavity conforms to the general surface contour of the tooth. The pulp chamber closely follows the external contour of the tooth, the central pulpal horn projecting incisally considerably farther than the remainder of the pulp chamber. Because of the greater length of the distal surface this horn is larger than the mesial projection. The chamber walls correspond to the outside contour of these surfaces. There is very little demarcation between the pulp chamber and the canal. The canal tapers as it approaches the apex.

THE MANDIBULAR PRIMARY CUSPID

The mandibular primary cuspid has the same general contour form as the maxillary cuspid, but is not as bulbous labiolingually or as broad mesiodistally.

The Crown

The labial surface is convex in all directions. Like the maxillary cuspid it has a prominent central lobe which terminates incisally in the labial portion of the cusp and extends cervically to the cervical ridge, where it attains its greatest curvature.

The incisal edge is highest at the apex of the cusp and proceeds cervically both distally and mesially. The distal incisal edge is the longer and intercuspates with the mesio-incisal edge of the upper cuspid.

The mesial and distal surfaces are convex in the cervical third, but the mesial surface may become concave as it approaches the cervical ridge, because of the thickness of the marginal ridges. The mandibular canines are not as wide labiolingually as the maxillary canine, resulting in smaller proximal surfaces. Contact with adjacent teeth is on the incisal third of the tooth.

The lingual surface is made up of three ridges. The lingual ridge aids in the formation of the apex of the cusp and extends the length of the lingual surface, fusing with the cingulum at the cervical third. The marginal ridges are less prominent than on the maxillary cuspids, but are evident as extending from the incisal edge to the cervical border where they blend with the cingulum. The distal marginal ridge is slightly longer than the mesial. The cingulum is narrow because of the convergence of the proximal surfaces as they approach the lingual surface. The cingulum is convex in all directions. Between the marginal ridge and the lingual ridge one finds concavities which are the mesiolingual and distolingual developmental grooves.

The Root

The root is single, with a broader labial than lingual diameter. The mesial and distal surfaces are slightly flattened. The root tapers to a rather pointed apex.

The Pulp Cavity

The pulp cavity conforms to the general surface contour of the tooth. The pulp chamber follows the external contour of the tooth, being approximately as wide mesiodistally as labiolingually. There is no differentiation between chamber and canal. The canal follows the surface form of the root in general and ends in a marked constriction at the apical end.

* * * * *

A description of the primary teeth gives ample evidence that their morphology is designed to perform specific functions in mastication. The incisors are designed to produce a shearing action upon closing the jaws, and are used for biting and cutting. The cuspids are designed for tearing or holding food. The molars serve for grinding and macerating and for the mulling of food in incorporating oral fluids into the mass of food. When there is normal occlusion these functions are performed to a maximum. When there is malocclusion with improper overbite and overjet and improper contact and intercuspation the functioning of the teeth is greatly impaired and faulty preparation of the food for digestion may result.

REFERENCES

1. Arnim, S. S., and Doyle, M. P.: Dentin dimensions of primary teeth. J. Dent. Child., *26*:191, 3rd quart, 1959.
2. Cohen, H. J., and Diner, H.: The significance of developmented dental enamel defects in neurological diagnosis. Pediatrics, *46*:737, Nov. 1970.
3. Jorgensen, K. D.: The deciduous dentition. Acta. Odont. Scandinavica, *14*:Supp. 20, 1956.
4. Kessler, H. E.: The relationship of dentistry to speech. J.A.D.A., *48*:44, 1954.
5. Kramer, W. S., and Ireland, R. L.: Measurements of the primary teeth. J. Dent. Child., *26*:252, 3rd quart., 1959.
6. Kraus, B.: Calcification of the human deciduous teeth. J.A.D.A., *59*:1128, 1959.
7. Kraus, B. S., and Jordan, R. E.: The Human Dentition Before Birth. Philadelphia, Lea & Febiger, 1965.
8. Logan, W. H. G., and Kronfeld, R.: Development of the human jaws and surrounding structures from birth to age fifteen years. J.A.D.A., *20*:379, 1933.
9. McGehee, H. O., True, H. A., and Inskipp, E. F.: A Textbook of Operative Dentistry. 4th ed. New York, McGraw-Hill Book Co., 1956.
10. Nolla, C. M.: The development of the permanent teeth. J. Dent. Child., *27*:254, 4th quart., 1960.
11. Orban, D. J.: Orban's Oral Histology and Embryology, 6th ed. Ed. by Harry Sicher. St. Louis, C. V. Mosby Co., 1966.
12. Parfitt, G. J.: The distribution of caries on different sites of the teeth in English children from the age of 2–15 years. Brit. D. J., *95*:423, 1955.
13. Parfitt, G. J.: Variation in the age of shedding of deciduous and eruption of permanent teeth. D. Record, *74*:279, 1954.
14. Schour, I.: Noyes' Oral Histology and Embryology. 7th ed. Philadelphia, Lea & Febiger, 1953.
15. Wheeler, R. C.: A Textbook of Dental Anatomy and Physiology. 4th ed. Philadelphia, W. B. Saunders Co., 1965.
16. Zeisz, R. C., and Nuckolls, J.: Dental Anatomy. St. Louis, C. V. Mosby Co., 1949.

5

DIAGNOSIS AND TREATMENT PLANNING FOR THE CHILD PATIENT

*by STANLEY E. KELLER
and LINCOLN R. MANSON-HING*

Successful dental care for children is best achieved after a thorough examination, thoughtful diagnosis, and the formulation of a proper treatment plan. The manner in which these can be accomplished during the child's first visits to the dental office colors the whole relationship for the dentist, the child, and the parent. A warm, friendly approach by the dentist quickly makes a friend of the apprehensive child, and an interested listener of the parent. The whole examination routine should be accomplished with slow, easy movements, utilizing a minimum of instruments to avoid alarming the child. The dentist's questions and statements should take the form of easy conversation. In this way time is saved and both the child and parent are properly prepared for any dental care which may follow. Once friendly, easy cooperation is assured, the dentist proceeds with the steps in the examination.

DIAGNOSTIC ARMAMENTARIUM

The child should be seated comfortably in either a dental chair designed for children or an adult chair properly adjusted for him. Besides the dental light and air syringe, only a front surface mirror and a sharp right angled explorer need be in evidence at the start of the examination. The name of each instrument should be told the child if he is curious.

For a complete examination the following list of instruments should be available but *out of sight* of the child. A capable assistant will have them ready as needed.

Alcohol	Fixing solution
Alginate impression material	Gutta percha
Articulator	Impression trays
Articulating paper	Mixing bowl and spatula
Bunsen burner	Periodontal probe
Clean glass microscopic slides	Rubber dam, 5″ × 5″
Cotton pellets	Sponges, 2″ × 2″
Cotton pliers	Stainless steel spatula
Cotton rolls	Tongue blades
Dental floss	28 gauge wax
Ethyl chloride or ice	Vitalometer

EXAMINATION OF THE CHILD

The initial contact with the parent is usually by telephone. The dental receptionist can ascertain, at this time, the nature of the future appointment. Three types of examination appointments are common: emergency, recall, and complete.

The *emergency examination* is usually limited to the site of injury and is basically designed to arrive at an immediate diagnosis leading to early therapy and elimination of the chief complaint. The *recall or periodic examination* is a thorough follow-up after an initial complete examination. Its objective is to measure the changes that have occurred since the completion of treatment. The periodic examination is done, in most cases, every four to six months. The following outline is an example of the thoroughness with which a *complete examination* should be done:

1. Case history
   a. Patient's chief complaint
   b. Prenatal, natal, postnatal, and infancy history
2. Clinical examination
   a. General appraisal of the patient
   b. Detailed oral examination
   c. Supplementary examinations and special tests
3. Diagnosis
   a. Summary of all abnormalities, their nature, etiology, and significance

THE CASE HISTORY

The recorded history of a pedodontic patient can be divided into vital statistics, parental history, prenatal and natal history, and postnatal and infancy history.

Vital statistics are essential for office records. From this information, the dentist obtains some insight into the social stratum of the family. The child's physician should be noted in case of future emergency or if additional medical information is needed. The chief complaint is recorded in the mother's or child's own words. This may be an acute problem or merely a desire for routine care.

The *parental history* provides some indication of the hereditary development of the patient. It is designed also to tell the dentist what value the parents place on their own teeth, since the attitude of the parents toward dentistry may be reflected in the apprehensiveness of the child and the desires of the parents as regards his dental care.

The *prenatal* and *natal histories* often provide clues to the origin of abnormal color, shape, and structure of deciduous and permanent teeth. The pedodontist sees the effects of drugs and metabolic disturbances which occurred during the formative stages of the teeth.

The *postnatal* and *infancy history* review the vital systems of the patient. It also records such information as previous preventive treatments for dental caries, developmental disturbances of dental significance, allergies, nervous habits, and the child's behavior and attitude toward his environment.

The length and direction of the history depend upon the circumstances surrounding each case. In emergency situations, the history is usually limited to essentials regarding the offending lesion or condition and the presence or absence of systemic disease of importance to immediate therapy. In most other cases, a self-administered history questionnaire can be of great value. Ideally, the parent can complete such a form in the waiting room at the initial visit. A parental questionnaire, such as the one in Figure 5-1, can save time for busy office personnel and at the same time instruct the parents of the dentist's concern for the children he treats.

The pedodontist needs only to glance over the completed questionnaire to spot significant findings. Affirmative answers can be elaborated upon by further questioning of the parent and patient. Special notations are made of this additional information in the patient's records.

THE CLINICAL EXAMINATION

The clinical examination of the child is done with a logical and orderly sequence of observations and examination procedures and in a smiling, kindly manner. A systematic approach, more often than not, produces far more information about unsuspected disease processes than a more haphazard method of examination.

In emergency cases, the examination will focus on the site of the complaint and enlist those diagnostic aids (e.g., radiographs) necessary to arrive at an immediate diagnosis. In such an examination, there is no routine or set pattern of procedures; existing circumstances and the cooperation of the child determine the course of action. However, a complete examination should be done after the emergency condition is alleviated.

Clinical procedures for the health maintenance examination include routine bite-wing and necessary additional single radiographs. All data are compared with the initial or preceding examination, and if necessary, a treatment plan is formulated.

The complete examination should be a thorough evaluation; the following outline demonstrates the scope of this examination:

(Text continued on page 79.)

CHILD'S HISTORY

Vital Statistics

Date_____

Name of child_____

Birth date of child_____

Race_____Sex_____

Name of person supplying the information of this history

_____

Relationship: Mother_____Father_____Other_____

Occupation of father_____

Occupation of mother_____

Home address of child_____

With whom does the child live?_____

Child's present physician_____

Who referred child?_____

Chief complaint_____

What prompted you to bring your child to the dentist?_____

_____

Parental History　　　　　　　　　　　　　　　　　　　　Yes　　No

Are you wearing dentures?　　　　　　　　　　　　　　____　____

Is your spouse wearing dentures?　　　　　　　　　　　____　____

If above yes, at what age were your teeth removed?_____

Your spouse's?_____

Why were your teeth removed?_____

_____

Figure 5–1　Questionnaire for parents.

	Yes	No

Your spouse's?_____

_____

Do you have what is called soft teeth? ____ ____

Your spouse? ____ ____

Were your or your spouse's teeth gray, yellow, or brownish in color? ____ ____

If yes, explain_____

_____

Did your teeth wear down excessively? ____ ____

Your spouse's? ____ ____

Are you or your spouse frightened of a dental appointment? ____ ____

Prenatal History

Did you have any illness during this pregnancy? ____ ____

If yes, what sort and when?_____

_____

Were you on drug therapy at this time? ____ ____

Were you taking antibiotics during this time? ____ ____

If yes, what?_____

How long and how often did you take this?_____

_____

Were you on a high vitamin or calcium diet during pregnancy? ____ ____

Is there blood incompatibility between you and your spouse? ____ ____

Have you been told that you are Rh negative by a physician? ____ ____

Did you have fluoride tablets, or was there fluoride in the drinking water supply where you lived during pregnancy? ____ ____

Figure 5–1 (Continued)

Natal History	Yes	No
Was the child a premature baby?	——	——
Was he jaundiced at birth?	——	——
Was he given blood transfusions?	——	——
Was he a "blue" baby?	——	——

Postnatal and Infancy History

	Yes	No
Did he have any convulsions during infancy?	——	——
Was he breast fed?	——	——

For how long?_____

	Yes	No
Was he bottle fed?	——	——

For how long?_____

	Yes	No
Was he given supplements of fluoride, fluorides in the drinking water, vitamins, calcium, iron, or other minerals?	——	——

If yes, explain_____

_____

Was the vitamin in the form of syrup or drops?_____

For how long a period of time was it given?_____

_____How often?_____

	Yes	No
Did he suck a sugar teat?	——	——
Did your child have any childhood diseases during infancy?	——	——

If yes, name them_____

_____

	Yes	No
Did he have rheumatic fever?	——	——
Did he have pain in the joints (growing pains)?	——	——
Has he had diabetes?	——	——
Has he had kidney trouble?	——	——

Figure 5–1 (Continued)

	Yes	No
Has he had heart trouble?	___	___
Were you ever told by a physician that your child was anemic?	___	___
Did your child ever receive antibiotics?	___	___

If yes, at what age?_____

If yes, how long?_____

What antibiotic was given?_____

	Yes	No
Did your child have any difficulty in learning to walk?	___	___
Did he have any operations in infancy?	___	___

If yes, for what reason?_____

	Yes	No
Has he broken any bones?	___	___

If yes, how often?_____

If yes, how did it happen?_____

_____

	Yes	No
Does he frequently have minor accidents or injuries?	___	___
Is there anything unusual about your child?	___	___

If yes, explain_____

_____

	Yes	No
Would you call your child a sickly child?	___	___

Why?_____

	Yes	No
Does he fail to perspire in hot weather?	___	___
Does he have any mental or physical disability or disease?	___	___

If yes, explain_____

_____

	Yes	No
Does your child eat between-meal snacks?	___	___

Figure 5–1 (Continued)

	Yes	No
If yes, what kind of food?_____		
_____		
Does he suffer from frequent toothaches?	___	___
Do his gums bleed easily?	___	___
Has he ever injured his front teeth?	___	___
Does he frequently break out in a rash?	___	___
Is he allergic to any foods, local anesthetics, penicillin, or other drugs?	___	___
Does he have asthma?	___	___
Is there difficulty stopping bleeding when he cuts himself?	___	___
Does he bruise easily?	___	___
Have you been told by a physician that your child is a hemophiliac?	___	___
Is he a thumb or finger sucker?	___	___
If yes, when does he do this?_____		
_____		
Does he have difficulty making friends?	___	___
Does he fail to get along with other children?	___	___
Would he rather play indoors than outdoors?	___	___
Does he have brothers or sisters?	___	___
If yes, what are their ages?_____		
_____		
Does he have difficulty keeping up with his schoolwork?	___	___
Does he fear the dentist?	___	___
If yes, do you know why?_____		
_____		
Has he ever been to the dentist before?	___	___

Figure 5–1 *(Continued)*

Outline of Pedodontic Clinical Examination

1. General survey of the patient (including stature, gait, speech, hands, temperature)
2. Examination of the head and neck
   Size and shape of head
   Hair and skin
   Facial swelling and asymmetry
   Temporomandibular joint
   Ears
   Eyes
   Nose
   Neck
3. Examination of the oral cavity
   Breath
   Lips, labial and buccal mucosa
   Saliva
   Gingiva and sublingual space
   Palate
   Pharynx and tonsils
   Teeth
4. Speech, swallowing, and perioral musculature
   Tongue positions during speech
   Anterior or lateral lisping
   Tongue carriage at rest
   Mentalis action on swallowing
   Lip positioning at rest

The General Survey

Stature

The general survey is done quickly as the child enters the reception room or operatory. Probably the first observation is whether the patient is overly tall or short for his age. A child's height may be compared to that of others by reference to a percentile growth table or chart. For practical purposes, the child can be classified in one of three categories, normal height for his age, too short, or too tall. Suspected deviations can be measured by a long-term record of the child's growth to determine whether the present stature is the result of a constant growth pattern or whether it is a growth change occurring at some definite point in the child's development. An understanding of stature requires a working knowledge of linear growths. This includes the characteristics of growth at various age periods and the effects of heredity, environment, nutrition, disease, developmental anomalies, and endocrine secretions.

Gait

As the child walks into the dental office, the examiner can quickly ascertain whether the gait is normal or affected. Probably the most common abnormal gait is that of a sick child walking with the unsteady gait of weakness. Other types include: waddling, equinus, scissors, hemiplegic, steppage, shuffling, wobbly, staggering, and ataxic gaits. When observed, such gaits require that a careful evaluation be made. The mother should be questioned about any recent change in gait she may have noticed.

Speech

Speech development is dependent upon the ability to reproduce sounds that one has heard; for example, infants with severe hearing problems may have abnormally slow language development. Between the ages of 21 and 24 months, children begin to use phrases. Between 2 and 3 years, children usually begin to speak in sentences. It should be remembered that there is a great normal variation in the time at which these stages occur. The child's conversation with the assistant or dentist permits an informal appraisal of his speech.

Four types of speech disorders should be considered: (1) aphasia, (2) delayed speech, (3) stuttering, and (4) articulatory speech disorders.

Motor aphasia is rare and usually denotes loss of speech secondary to central nervous system damage. Speech retardation can be considered if the child does not talk by the age of 3. Some common causes of delayed speech are as follows: hearing loss, intellectual retardation, general developmental retardation, severe prolonged illness, sensory defects, lack of motivation, and poor environmental stimulation. The overdependent and the neurologically injured child also may be slow in talking.

A speech pathologist can help determine the etiology and therapy necessary in cases of suspected speech disorders. Early referral can many times mean the subsequent difference between normal and persistently abnormal speech patterns.

Stuttering or repetitive speech occurs in almost all children at some time during the preschool period. Overconcern and apprehension about speaking may block the normal flow of speech. Stuttering is more common in boys than in girls. Psychologic stresses play an important part in the development and persistence of this problem. "Cluttering" is an unusual type of speech characterized by repetition of words or phrases, false starts, changes in context in the middle of the sentence, and general verbal confusion.

Articulatory speech disorders of importance are substitution, omission, insertion, and distortion. Substitution of the "th" sound for the "s" sound produces lisping. Some articulatory defects occur within the limits of normal development; however, children with cerebral palsy, central neurological damage, cleft palate, or malocclusion often have articulatory difficulty. Paralysis of the laryngeal and pharyngeal muscles, for example, cerebral palsy, may alter the quality of speech and produce a voice with a nasal twang. Hoarseness may be due to excessive shouting or singing, chronic or acute sinusitis, laryngitis, laryngeal foreign body, papilloma of the larynx, paralysis, measles, or in boys, precocious sexual development.

Hands

By taking the child's hand in his, the dentist not only establishes a warm communication but also is afforded an opportunity to further appraise the general health. In most cases, the hands will feel normal, but occasionally there will be a feeling of increased temperature, moisture, or dryness. The hands are one of the few areas of the child's body normally exposed to the dentist. All primary and secondary skin lesions such as macules, papules, vesicles, ulcerations, crusts, and scales can be observed here. Many causative factors such as exanthematous diseases, vitamin deficiencies, hormonal and developmental disturbances may produce these changes.

The number, shape, and size of the child's fingers should be noted. The nails may be bitten short as evidence of his anxiety or tension; they may be spoon shaped, pitted, brittle, scaly, thickened, covered with skin, discolored, or even be absent as sometimes seen in ectodermal dysplasia.

When the dentist is examining a child whom he suspects to be too large or too small for his age, a 5 inch by 7 inch radiograph of the left hand can be taken with the dental x-ray machine. The roentgenogram may then be compared with standard carpal indices to determine the bone age of the patient. Since the dentist may be the only member of the health team to see a child in a period of several years, his appraisal of the growth and development of the child may indicate a need for further medical evaluation. By *growth* is meant the physical maturation of the child, while development means functional maturation.

Temperature

Fever, or an elevation in temperature at rest, is one of the most common symptoms experienced by children. There may be a temporary rise in temperature after eating, exercise, or when the environment is not conducive to body cooling. No single temperature reading can be given as normal for all children at all times. Most mothers regard a temperature of 98.6° F. as a sacrosanct point, a rise above which must be regarded as illness. However, the interested practitioner can help them to understand that there is, instead, a range of normality. In those unusual cases in which there is a partial or complete lack of sweat glands, as in the anhidrotic type of ectodermal dysplasia, the child may be uncomfortably warm during hot weather. Dental abscesses or acute gingival diseases, as well as numerous other oral and respiratory infections, result in a febrile condition in children.

Specific diseases cannot be diagnosed by fever alone. However, the degree of fever, its pattern, and the child's response are often factors indicative of certain pathoses.

Examination of the Head and Neck

After the general survey of the child's stature, gait, speech, hands, and body temperature, attention is automatically focused on the child's head and particularly the oral cavity. In order that no sign is overlooked, a systematic survey of the region is essential.

Size and Shape of the Head

The size of the child's head can be either normal, too large, or too small. Macrocephaly, or enlarged head, is frequently due to a developmental or early traumatic disturbance. Microcephaly, or small head, may be due to a growth disturbance, a disease, or trauma affecting the central nervous system. Abnormal head shapes may be caused by premature closure of the sutures, an interference in the growth of cranial bones, or abnormal pressures within the skull. Care must be exercised, however, to avoid a hasty judgment in head size. The heads of both parents and other siblings should be seen first before the thought is voiced. It may save the dentist an embarrassment.

Hair and Skin

Alopecia, or loss of hair, may occasionally be seen in young patients. A common baldness is a small, discrete, round area edged by a raised, indurated, inflamed line, a description almost diagnostic of ringworm. In the rare child who has congenital ectodermal dysplasia, the hair may be absent or scanty, fine and light in color. This is more often seen in boys than in girls. Certain other hormonal imbalances may cause hair losses, while the addition of hormonal medications may cause hirsutism, or excessive growth of hair.

The skin of the face, like that of the hands, should be observed for signs of disease. A number of primary and secondary skin lesions may be found on the face. While the child's face tends to reflect the general health, the observed changes may not necessarily be directly related to a dental problem. The careful dentist may wish to postpone a dental visit for the child who has a large, painful herpes lesion or other type of sore on the lip or face.

Facial Swelling and Asymmetry

Asymmetry of the face can be physiological or pathological. The two sides of the normal face are never exactly alike. Infant sleeping habits, particularly in children born at less than full term, have been shown to affect the shape of the face permanently. Pathologic facial asymmetry may be produced by abnormal intra-uterine pressures, cranial nerve paralysis, fibrous dysplasia, and familial developmental disturbances. Infections, bacterial or viral, and trauma are by far the principal causes of facial swelling in the child. The history and oral examination are important in making a diagnosis of the etiology of any swelling of the face. Any unilateral, painless facial enlargement which is slow growing with no apparent causative agent warrants special attention by the dentist, by referral to a pediatrician, since neoplasia presents such a pattern.

Temporomandibular Joint

Two valuable diagnostic methods of discerning limitation of movement, subluxation, dislocation, or mandibular deviations are the following: (1) While standing as nearly in front of the child as the dental chair will permit, the dentist may place his hands lightly on the child's cheeks in the area of the temporomandibular joint. Have the child open and close his mouth slowly, then from closed centric, have him move into the lateral excursions by asking him to "chew slowly on his back teeth." (2) With a 15 inch to 18 inch piece of dental floss, press against his face in the midline connecting forehead, point of nose, and chin point. Have him open and close his mouth slowly, showing his teeth as he does so.

These two simple aids will show discrepancies of the temporomandibular joint as well as muscular imbalances and anatomic deviations from the midline. Swelling or redness over the joint region should be gently palpated to determine the degree of firmness and extension.

Trismus, or spasm of the masticatory muscles, can be seen when there is infection following a mandibular permanent molar extraction. It is less commonly seen during the eruption of a lower permanent molar, but may develop following pericoronitis. Tetanus, a rare disease in modern life, may produce trismus, as many neoplasms and other rarer disturbances.

Ears

The dentist should certainly be aware of any deficiency of hearing in the child patient. Observation of the external auditory meatus may reveal a discharge. Usually, however, the chief complaint will be pain in the oral cavity radiating to the ear; this necessitates a thorough examination of the teeth. The dentist must be able to determine if referred pain from the dentition is the possible cause of earache. If, by clinical and radiological examination, no dental problem is found, the child should be referred to a physician for a thorough examination of the ear. Palpation of the external ear and of the mastoid process may reveal some tenderness which would indicate to the dentist that inflammation does exist within the ear itself.

Eyes

The dentist should observe whether or not the child has difficulty in seeing and whether or not he wears glasses. Observation of the child's eyes should include the action of the lids, the presence or absence of inflammation, swelling or puffiness around the eye, the presence or absence of any crusting or lesions on the eyelids, the presence or absence of conjunctivitis, any defect in the iris, and any abnormal lacrimation. Inflammation associated with maxillary teeth may extend to the orbital region, causing swelling of the eyelids and conjunctivitis. Some systemic diseases may produce changes in both the ocular and the oral tissues. Developmental defects of the oral cavity may have their counterpart in the eye. Frequently, children with upper respiratory infection, chronic sinusitis, and allergy have puffiness of the eyelids and periorbital tissues.

In general, the dentist should observe and recognize any abnormalities of the structures of the eye and the surrounding tissues. He should rule out any oral conditions as etiologic factors and refer the patient to a reputable oculist for a complete examination.

Nose

Due to its prominent location, any abnormalities in the size, shape, or color of the nose automatically call attention to this organ. In children the dentist frequently encounters nasal drainage indicative of upper respiratory infection. Scars may be evident on the nose, indicating surgical repair of a developmental anomaly or trauma. Certain infectious diseases may leave their mark on the nose, as for example, the saddle nose in congenital syphilis. Because of the close proximity of the nose to the oral cavity, extension of inflammation via the maxilla may alter the size, shape, and color of the nose. The extension of cysts or tumors from within the oral cavity, particularly the maxilla, may encroach upon the nasal passages.

Neck

The examination of the neck is done both by observation and palpation. As the dentist observes the facial asymmetry of the child, he likewise notes any abnormal configurations of the neck. The skin of the neck is subject to all primary and secondary skin lesions as well as scars of surgical repair. In the course of the examination, the dentist should stand in back of the child patient and casually pass the flat of his fingers over the parotid region, down under the body of the mandible to the submaxillary and sublingual regions, and thence palpate the triangles of the neck.Frequently, submaxillary lymph node enlargement is evident in the child patient which may be associated with enlarged infected tonsils and chronic respiratory infection. Palpable nodes may also be due to drainage from oral infection or neoplasms. Since exanthematous diseases are prevalent in children and the salivary glands are likely to be involved, the pedodontist should be acutely aware of any tenderness or enlargement of these organs.

Examination of the Oral Cavity

The oral cavity is the goal of the diagnostic survey. The general appraisal and systematic survey of the head and neck serve as an introduction to the oral cavity of the child. The dentist must guard against any tendency to focus his attention directly on the teeth, neglecting to observe other areas. By concentrating his efforts on examining the soft tissues of the mouth and oral pharynx *first*, the dentist protects his reputation as a careful diagnostician. A rule to remember might be, "A good diagnostician counts the cavities *last*, not first."

Breath

The breath of the healthy child is usually pleasant and even sweet. "Bad breath," or halitosis, may be attributable to either local or systemic causes. Local factors would include poor oral hygiene, the presence of blood in the mouth, or strong smelling volatile food. Systemic factors might include dehydration, sinusitis, hypertrophy and infection of the adenoid tissue, malignancies of the upper alimentary tract, typhoid fever, and other enteric infections and gastrointestinal disturbances. Acidosis usually produces an odor of acetone on the breath. Frequently, children with an elevation in temperature have a characteristic fetid breath.

Lips, Labial and Buccal Mucosa

The lips are the gateway to the oral cavity and should not be overlooked by the dentist in his haste to examine the teeth. After observation of size, shape, color, and surface texture, they should be palpated using thumb and forefinger. Ulcerations, vesicles, fissures, crusts, and abrasions are frequently seen on the lips. The lips protect the teeth from trauma and are, therefore, the frequent site of contusions in children. Nutritional and allergic reactions may cause dramatic changes in the lips. Scars may be evidence of surgical repair of developmental anomalies or past trauma. Any swelling or mass in the lips should be palpated between the thumb and first finger to note size and consistency. As the lips are drawn back, the dentist should note the labial mucosa. Any lesions or changes in color or consistency of the mucous membrane should be carefully evaluated. Continuing into the mouth, the buccal mucosa can be observed, noting the normal anatomic landmarks which are in the area. The most conspicuous of these is the papilla at the orifice of Stensen's duct from the parotid gland. This papilla may be inflamed or enlarged and during the onset of measles may be surrounded by small, red-rimmed, bluish white spots. Swellings in the cheek also may be palpated with thumb and forefinger. The most common lesions seen in the labial and buccal mucosa of children are those associated with herpes simplex virus. These may be relatively mild with small painful ulcerations or may be more general extending to the gingiva and palate and producing severely tender, painful gingivae with multiple shallow ulcers. With this condition, there is frequently a history of some systemic disturbance.

Normally, the buccal and labial mucosa are pink. However, melanin may cause a normal physiologic brownish pigmentation frequently seen in the Negroid race. On the other hand, Addison's disease and intestinal polyposis may cause a pathologic brownish or bluish-black pigmentation of this tissue.

Saliva

Examination procedures within the oral cavity usually stimulate profuse salivation in children. The quality of the saliva may be very thin, normal, or extremely viscous. Epidemic parotitis or mumps is characterized by a tender, somewhat painful, unilateral or bilateral swelling of the salivary glands. An excess secretion or purulent discharge from Stensen's duct may be indicative of other disturbances of the parotid gland. The submaxillary and sublingual salivary glands may also become tender, swollen, and have altered secretions in systemic infections.

Gingiva

After examining the labial and buccal mucosa, the dentist should observe the gingiva and muscle attachments. The labial frenula located in the midline of both the upper and lower jaw may be responsible for abnormal spacing between the central incisors. The gingival color, size, form, consistency, and capillary fragility should be noted. Redness and swelling may be due to inflammation from poor oral hygiene. However, the dentist should constantly be aware that the gingiva is sensitively responsive to metabolic and nutritional changes, certain drugs, and developmental disturbances. As a tooth erupts, the overlying gingiva may be swollen, painful, and inflamed. These areas are frequently traumatized by the opposing teeth. Draining fistulae on the attached gingivae accompanied by tenderness, pain, and some tooth mobility are usually diagnostic of abscessed teeth. Although true Vincent's stomatitis with eroded gingival papillae is not usually seen in children, a similar but milder condition may exist. The combination of poor oral hygiene, malnutrition, and general malaise may contribute to the severity of this disease.

Tongue and Sublingual Space

The child should be asked to extend the tongue so that the examiner may note its size, shape, color, and movement. Pathologic enlargement of the tongue may be due to cretinism or mongolism, or may be associated with a cyst or neoplasm. A desquamation of the surface papillae associated with change in color and tenderness may be due to certain avitaminoses, anemias, or stress disorders. An abnormally short lingual frenum may prevent the tip of the tongue from coming forward. Such frenula can be responsible for certain speech defects. To examine the dorsum of the tongue in detail, the tip should be grasped with a cotton gauze square between the thumb and first finger and gently drawn out of the mouth. Any masses or ulcerations can then be examined bidigitally for size, shape, and consistency. The surface of the tongue is fairly smooth and slick in the small child. Although the filiform papillae are present at birth, they are relatively short and do not become elongated until the late preschool period.

Dryness of the tongue may be due to dehydration or may occur in children who are mouth breathers. The tongue may be coated white, grayish, or brownish-white in the febrile state or in early stages of exanthematous diseases. The coating consists of desquamated cells, food debris, and bacteria. Tongue habits should be observed for possible association with malocclusion. The underside of the tongue is often overlooked by the dentist. This protected area should be examined for any cystlike swelling or ulceration. Swellings in the floor of the mouth may cause the tongue to be elevated and affect the speech and tongue movement of the child. The openings of the sublingual and submaxillary salivary glands and minor salivary glands may become clogged, causing a mucous retention cyst or ranula.

Palate

The child's head should be tipped back slightly for direct observation of the shape, color, and presence of any lesions on the hard and soft palate. The consistency of deformities or swellings should be investigated carefully by palpation. Scars on the palate may be evidence of past trauma or surgical repair of developmental anomalies. Color changes may be caused by neoplasms, infectious or systemic diseases, trauma, or chemical agents.

Pharynx and Tonsils

To observe the pharynx and tonsil area, the examiner must depress the tongue with either a mouth mirror or a tongue blade to note any color changes, ulcerations, or swelling. Proliferation of the laryngeal tonsil tissue may be so extensive that very little space exists in the throat for the passage of food and air. It is often advisable for the pedodontist to suggest that the child be examined by his physician if it is felt that the tonsils are badly infected and might be contributing to ill health.

Teeth

Certain basic observations of the overall dentition can be made quickly before individual teeth are diagnosed. These include the number of teeth and their size, color, occlusion, and malformations.

Number of Teeth. Rarely does the pedodontist see a child with complete absence of teeth (anodontia). However, with some developmental disturbances, partial anodontia or oligodontia is a diagnostic factor. Missing single teeth are far more important in the permanent dentition than in the primary. Exclusive of the third molars, the mandibular second premolar and the maxillary lateral incisors are the teeth most often missing. Often called congenital, this condition is more often hereditary, as the interested dentist may prove for himself by careful questioning of the parents. Extra teeth (supernumerary) are observed most often in the midline of the maxilla but may occur anywhere in either arch. A dentist may be alerted to the possible presence of a mesiodens by an extremely wide diastema between the upper permanent central incisors.

A disturbance in the eruption of the dentition may cause too few or too many teeth to be present, depending on whether a retarded or precocious eruption pattern exists. Certain developmental and hormonal disturbances may cause a disruption of the normal eruption pattern of the dentition. Retarded or precocious dentitions may result, with the number of teeth present varying widely.

Size of Teeth. True macrodontia (large teeth) or microdontia (small teeth) is rare. However, single teeth may be judged small, i.e., peg laterals. Also, single teeth may appear large as in gemination and fusion. Heredity probably plays the greatest role in predetermination of the size of teeth. Hormonal and developmental anomalies would be further factors to consider.

Color of Teeth. Abnormal staining of children's teeth may be divided into two types, extrinsic and intrinsic. Extrinsic stains can be caused by chromogenic bacteria which may invade deposits of materia alba and calculus, causing an array of colors on children's teeth. Generalized discoloration of the enamel and dentin is more likely to be due to intrinsic factors such as blood dyscrasias, amelogenesis imperfecta, dentinogenesis imperfecta, internal resorption, and drugs such as the tetracycline series.

Occlusion of Teeth. At this stage of the examination, the occlusion of the child may be checked by asking the child, "Will you bite down on your back teeth, please?" As the child closes down, the dentist guides the mandible gently but firmly into the most retruded comfortable position of the condyles. Molar and cuspid interdigitation should be carefully checked bilaterally. Early recognition of malocclusions alerts the parent to possible orthodontic referral later. One should be familiar with the classification of malocclusions shown on pp. 333 to 341.

Malformations of Teeth. Physical injuries and enamel hypoplasia are the most common causes of malformed teeth. In addition, teeth may be dilacerated, dwarfed, geminated, fused, notched, and peg shaped from various hereditary, systemic, or developmental disturbances. Special terms have been given to many of these anomalies such as dens in dente, Hutchinsonian incisor, bifid crown, Turner's hypoplasia, and mulberry molar.

The ravages of caries are responsible for more destruction of dental tissues than any other condition. It behooves the pedodontist to detect this disease process in its earliest stages by both clinical and radiographic means. Instrumentation and technique for detection of caries is given in Chapter 8, pp. 146 to 147.

Laboratory tests useful in oral diagnosis are mentioned in Chapter 18, pp. 428, 429, and Chapter 23, pp. 530 to 534. The biopsy technique as a diagnostic procedure is given in Chapter 18, pp. 419 to 424. Special dental diagnostic tests would include the use of the electric pulp tester, dental radiographs (Chapter 6) and the articulation of study casts.

THE DIAGNOSTIC METHOD

COLLECTING THE FACTS

Certain pathognomonic signs may lead to an early diagnostic decision. For example, an obvious swelling and drainage may be associated with a single, badly carious, tender primary molar; however, all historical facts about the child should be systematically collected and correlated. It is often necessary for the dentist to make a diagnosis before all the facts have been collected to prevent the disease process from progressing. For example, acute necrotizing gingivitis needs immediate drug and clinical therapy; a newly fractured central incisor needs instant care. In some cases, a period of observation may be necessary before the final diagnosis and institution of correct therapy. Pulpitis in restored teeth is often difficult to diagnose. If all tests fail to distinguish the offending tooth, the dentist may elect to wait for several days before making the diagnosis and instituting therapy.

EVALUATION OF THE FACTS

There must be a critical evaluation of the collected facts in relation to the overall picture and the chief complaint. Not infrequently parents are poor historians, and clinical signs and symptoms elicited by the dentist outweigh the reported facts. Interrogation of the parent concerning dental pain is not always satisfactory. The dentist must often excavate large carious lesions to arrive at a diagnosis and determine the course of treatment.

MAKING THE DIAGNOSIS

The history, clinical examination, and laboratory diagnostic aids will provide the essential facts necessary to make a diagnosis. From the facts collected, several disease processes might be suggested. There is always the possibility that more than one disease may be present at the same time. However, usually the examiner is able to sift the facts to identify a disease entity which can be properly treated. In unusual cases, consultation with specialists or other general practitioners is sometimes necessary before a final diagnosis can be made and treatment prescribed.

A febrile child with unilateral facial swelling and severely carious teeth may be suffering from either an acute alveolar abscess or mumps or both. The history, a radiographic survey, and a thorough clinical examination will aid the dentist in making a diagnosis. If the carious teeth can be ruled out as the offending factor, the child should be referred to his family physician for systemic therapy.

TREATMENT PLANNING

Successful dental treatment is based on an accurate diagnosis and careful treatment planning. Three considerations, urgency, sequence, and probable results, must be evaluated before any treatment is performed. A well organized sequence of treatment avoids many false starts, repetition of treatment, and a waste of time, energy, and money. A pattern of sequence serves as a reminder of the phases of treatment which must be considered in caring for the total needs of the child. The following general outline is suggested for pedodontic treatment planning.

OUTLINE FOR PEDODONTIC TREATMENT PLANNING

1. Medical treatment
   a. Referral to a physician
2. Systemic treatment
   a. Premedication
   b. Therapy for oral infection
3. Preparatory treatment
   a. Oral prophylaxis
   b. Caries control
   c. Orthodontic consultation
   d. Oral surgery
   e. Endodontic therapy
4. Corrective treatment
   a. Operative dentistry
   b. Prosthetic dentistry
   c. Orthodontic therapy
5. Periodic recall examination and maintenance treatment

THE IDEAL TREATMENT PLAN

Medical Treatment

A great many families today have pediatricians or family physicians who are familiar with the medical history of the child. Occasionally the child has been under the care of other medical specialists (psychiatrist, ophthalmologist, plastic surgeon, otolaryngologist, cardiologist, etc.). When the history and examination suggest a medical problem, the dentist should consult the child's physician to insure the health and safety of the child during treatment. If a parent is uncertain about a past disease (e.g., rheumatic fever), but has answered questions affirmatively that suggest such a disease, the child should be referred to a physician for evaluation. The need for such information is evidenced by the fact that antibiotics would be prescribed even before oral prophylaxis if a history of rheumatic fever were confirmed.

The dentist has an excellent opportunity to x-ray the child's hand with his dental x-ray machine. Comparing the hand films of under- or over-statured children with published standards, the dentist may suspect a developmental or nutritional anomaly. Such information should be discussed with the child's physician, who may suggest further laboratory studies.

Blood dyscrasias are often reflected in the oral cavity by changes in color, size, shape, and consistency of oral soft tissues. The dentist frequently has the opportunity of examining the child's mucosa more frequently than the physician. Therefore, it behooves the dentist to evaluate tissue changes and relay any pertinent information to the child's physician.

Patients should be referred to medical specialists through or by consultation with the family physician or pediatrician. Rarely is the dentist qualified to order and evaluate complex medical diagnostic tests. This responsibility is handled better by medical specialists who can advise the dentist about handling the dental needs of the child safely.

Systemic Treatment

Premedication of apprehensive children, spastic patients, or those with cardiac problems is frequently necessary. Such premedication should be done only after consultation with the child's physician. The exact dosages of all drugs to be used should be entered on the treatment plan. When assistants arrange the child's appointment schedule for premedication, the auxiliary personnel must be made aware of the premedication regime to be followed for each appointment. Valuable chair time can be lost if the dentist must wait for drugs to act.

Systemic drug therapy may cause oral tissue changes which make restorative work difficult or even impossible. The physician is oftentimes unaware that a child taking Dilantin sodium has developed severely hypertrophic gingivae. Such a problem should be discussed with the physician in the hope that drug substitution may alleviate the problem and dental treatment can proceed.

Preparatory Treatment

After the medical status and premedication regime of the child are established, his teeth should be thoroughly cleaned. This affords the dentist a splendid opportunity to teach him toothbrushing and other elements of home care. Also, much can be learned about the patient's temperament, apprehensiveness, and oral health status during the oral prophylaxis and the home care instruction. Treatment of acute inflammatory conditions, such as alveolar abscesses, traumatic ulcerations, herpetic gingivostomatitis, and the occasional case of necrotizing gingivitis, can usually be deferred, pending favorable results from drugs or surgical therapy.

Closely following the initial prophylaxis, an evaluation should be made of the caries susceptibility of the child. If active caries is evident, the child's mother should be questioned closely about his diet. With the proper approach the concerned dentist can offer the parent an interesting and challenging opportunity to facilitate the reduction of caries in the child (and other siblings). Several means are available, among which are topical and systemic fluorides, diet substitutions, and more regular meals without in-between snacks. These measures can be instituted concurrent with caries removal and placement of temporary or permanent restorations.

It is sometimes necessary to consult with dental specialists; for example, when crowding or malalignment is evident, an orthodontist should be consulted immediately. Frequently, preventive orthodontic measures can be performed concurrently with restorative procedures. The advice of an orthodontist may be sought before performing operative care on questionable teeth in cases of unsatisfactory occlusion.

Badly carious essential teeth should be excavated during the first appointments. Whether a tooth is to be extracted or is to be retained for endodontic therapy is a decision both parent and dentist must weigh carefully. All possibilities of alternate future treatment, such as replacement problems with removable or fixed prostheses, must be considered from a practical and a dental health standpoint. If economics is a factor with the parent, the dentist must be very careful to explain the possible sequelae of choices of treatment which might be less than ideal.

Corrective Treatment

Only after the medical and preparatory phases have been initiated can final corrective treatment be started. Even in this phase of the treatment plan, sequence is important. For example, all caries should be eliminated from the teeth and the restorations polished before orthodontic care is initiated.

While corrective treatment is being rendered to the child, the dentist has an opportunity to observe the results of oral hygiene instruction which was given during the initial appointments. Upon completion of treatment, the wise dentist gives an explicit appointment for the next recall visit. The interval may vary from three months (in unusually active caries cases) to six months (for the average child).

ALTERNATE TREATMENT PLANS

There is an ideal treatment plan for every child. This should be presented to the parent using models, x-rays, and other aids the dentist may have prepared. At this point there is a tremendous opportunity for patient education which is a continuing challenge for every conscientious dentist. The fees for carrying out the suggested treatment plan should be outlined to avoid any misunderstanding at a later date. Unlike adult treatment, dental care for children must not be delayed or even spaced over a long period of time. Also, there are few opportunities for alternate treatment plans in pedodontics.

When an alternate plan is suggested, the dentist must be sure that the results will be as beneficial as possible and not in any way detrimental to the future dental health of the child.

REVISIONS OF A TREATMENT PLAN

Once a treatment plan is approved, any revisions or alterations that arise should be explained to the parent and noted on the child's records. The parent will accept better a change in treatment if the dentist takes the time to explain the cause of action. In some instances, the treatment plan may have to be revised during corrective treatment; for example, an unsuspected pathologic pulp exposure of a tooth might necessitate extraction and the placement of a space maintainer. Treatment plan revisions must be anticipated in mixed dentition cases and when the child's growth pattern is likely to be unusual or in such cases as children with a severe handicap or skeletal disharmony.

REFERENCES

1. Blakely, R. W.: Speech as a landmark in development. Pub. Health Rep., *80*(10):880–884, October, 1965.
2. Gellis, M. D., and Kagan, B. M.: Current Pediatric Therapy. Philadelphia, W. B. Saunders Co., 1970.
3. Graber, T. M.: Orthodontics, Principles and Practice. 2nd ed. Philadelphia, W. B. Saunders Co., 1966.
4. Green, M., and Richmond, J. B.: Pediatric Diagnosis. 2nd ed. Philadelphia, W. B. Saunders Co., 1962.
5. Greulich, W. W., and Pyle, S. I.: Radiographic Atlas of Skeletal Development of the Hand and Wrist. 2nd ed. Stanford, California, Stanford University Press, 1959.
6. Judge, R. D., and Zuidema, G. D.: Physical Diagnosis. 1st ed. Boston, Little, Brown and Co., 1963.
7. Kerr, D. A., Ash, M. M., and Millard, H. D.: Oral Diagnosis. 3rd ed. St. Louis, C. V. Mosby Co., 1970.
8. Mitchell, D. F., Standish, S. M., and Fast, T. B.: Oral Diagnosis/Oral Medicine. 2nd ed. Philadelphia, Lea & Febiger, 1971.
9. Shirkey, H. C.: Pediatric Therapy. 3rd ed. St. Louis, C. V. Mosby Co., 1968.
10. Witkop, C. J.: Genetics and Dental Health. New York, McGraw-Hill Book Company, Inc., 1962.

6

ROENTGENOGRAPHY

by LINCOLN R. MANSON-HING
and SIDNEY B. FINN

Although it is often neglected, roentgenography is the most important adjunct to the successful practice of dentistry for children. During the first visit to the dental office it provides a pleasant and painless means of introducing the child to dental treatment. Any subjective fears of roentgenography on the patient's part can easily be dissipated by demonstrating the taking of roentgenograms. The confidence gained by the patient at this time is very valuable in future visits. As an aid to the dentist, roentgenography is one of the most important diagnostic tools available for the detection of disease and the interception of malocclusion.

So few children escape the ravages of dental disease that most persons have their first contact with dentistry during childhood. Since first impressions are lasting ones, it is exceedingly important that any service rendered the child be of high quality. The state of a patient's dentition upon reaching adulthood depends in large measure on the amount and quality of dental care he received during childhood. By judiciously employing roentgenography to enhance the value of dental service, many teeth can be saved which might otherwise be lost, and many malocclusions can be prevented. Dedicated dental care for young children calls for the most extensive use of this diagnostic aid so that dentistry may fulfill the ideal of a truly preventive science.

DIAGNOSTIC VALUE OF ROENTGENOGRAMS

Roentgenography has extremely wide application in pedodontic practice. Children have perhaps a greater need for roentgenography than do adults, for in children one is greatly concerned in every instance with the problems of growth and development and the factors that alter them. It is upon the foundation of roentgenography that success in pedodontic practice is achieved.

The role of the roentgenogram is too often only thought to be that of an adjunct to diagnosis. Its role during treatment, such as in endodontics where it is invaluable, in patient follow-up, as in fracture cases, and in record keeping, should not be overlooked. Basically the roentgenogram of any area provides information on the shape, size, position, relative density, and number of objects present in the area. In gathering this information the diagnostician must be aware of the limitations of the roentgenogram. The major shortcomings of the usual dental roentgenogram are that the roentgenogram shows a two-dimensional picture of a three-dimensional object and that changes in the soft tissues are not shown. The first shortcoming makes the evaluation of an area or object difficult when it is superimposed upon another area or object on the roentgenogram. The second shortcoming emphasizes the fact that the information provided by roentgenograms pertains mostly to the calcified structures. Regardless of these shortcomings, the information gained about the underlying structures is extremely valuable, since this information cannot for the most part be obtained by any other means available to the dentist.

The roentgenogram should be employed to supply the following eight categories of information.

INCIPIENT CARIOUS LESIONS

A great number of incipient interproximal lesions cannot be detected by the usual mirror and explorer examination and must be located by roentgenography. Because of broad contacts, especially between the primary molars, the tine of a fine explorer frequently cannot penetrate the narrow area below the contact point to detect a roughened area or the presence of a definite catch. If one relies entirely on the explorer to find cavities, by the time they are detectable they may frequently have grown so large and so deep as to jeopardize the integrity of the tooth. Because of the large pulp chambers and rapid progress of caries in children, early detection is imperative (Fig. 6–1). It is axiomatic in dentistry that the most satisfactory resto-

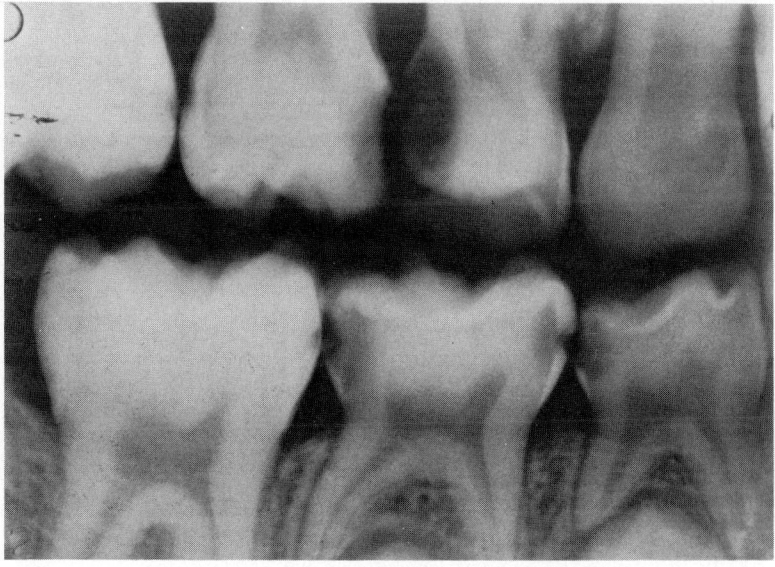

Figure 6–1 Interproximal carious lesions.

ration of a tooth is one that preserves, both in depth and in area, as much of the natural tooth structure as possible, consistent with good cavity preparation. All things being equal, the smaller the lesion, the smaller and potentially more enduring can be the final restoration. Early detection, therefore, is most desirable. In an assessment by Blayney and Greco of the value of roentgenograms in revealing cavities, between 40 and 50 per cent of all lesions detectable would have been overlooked using only an explorer. It is evident that no examination for carious lesions can be considered complete without the use of roentgenography.

ANOMALIES

There are anomalies of the teeth that are asymptomatic and also not visible in the mouth. Many of these anomalies are hazards to the development of a normally functioning occlusion. Such anomalies can be detected only by roentgenography; thereafter they may possibly be corrected. In the majority of instances early detection and interception are advisable.

Among these anomalies that may alter the development of a normal occlusion may be mentioned supernumerary teeth (mesiodens, Figs. 6–2 and 6–3), macro- and microdontia, fused, ankylosed and geminated teeth (Fig. 6–4), malpositioned and impacted teeth, and missing teeth. Other anomalies of importance include dens in dente (Fig. 6–5), odontomas (Fig. 6–6), hypoplasias (Fig. 6–7), and pulp stones (Fig. 6–8).

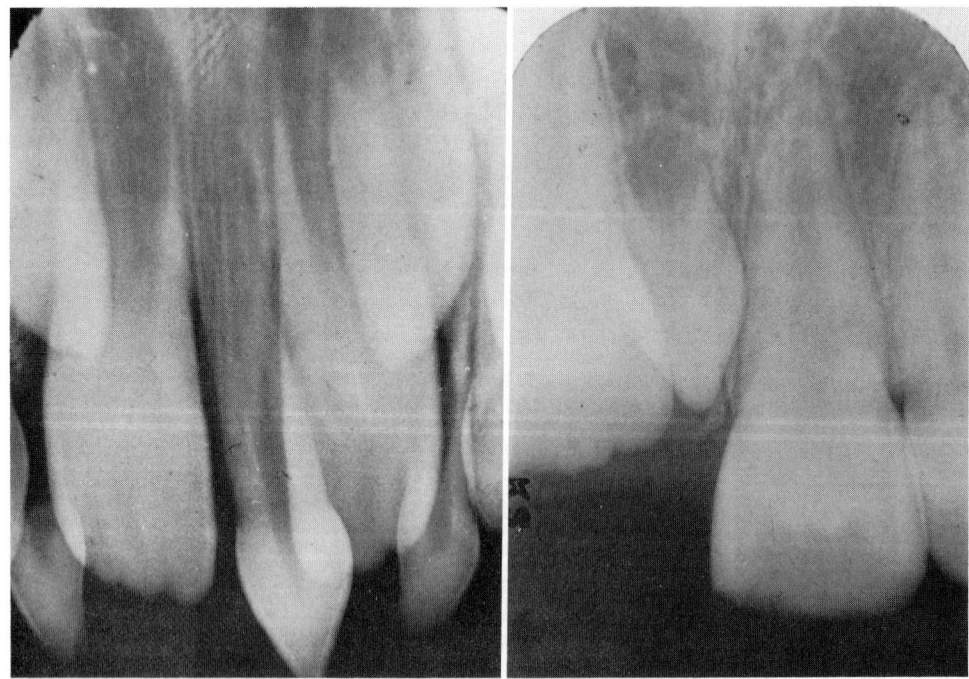

Figure 6–2.   **Figure 6–3.**

Figure 6–2 Mesiodens with normally erupting permanent central incisors.
Figure 6–3 Mesiodens with interference of one erupting permanent central incisor.

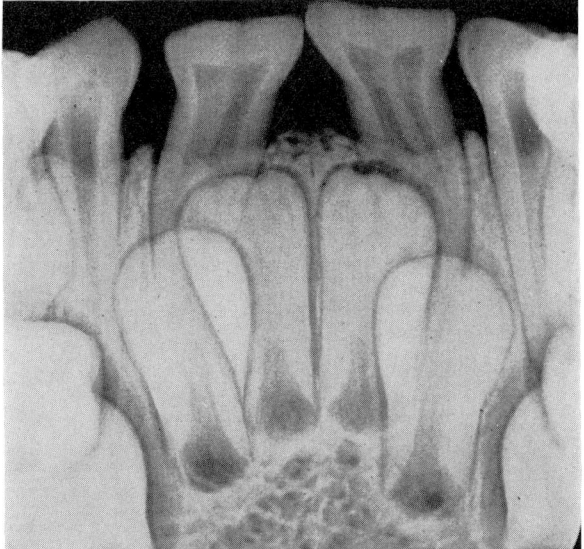

Figure 6–4 Gemination of the primary mandibular incisors.

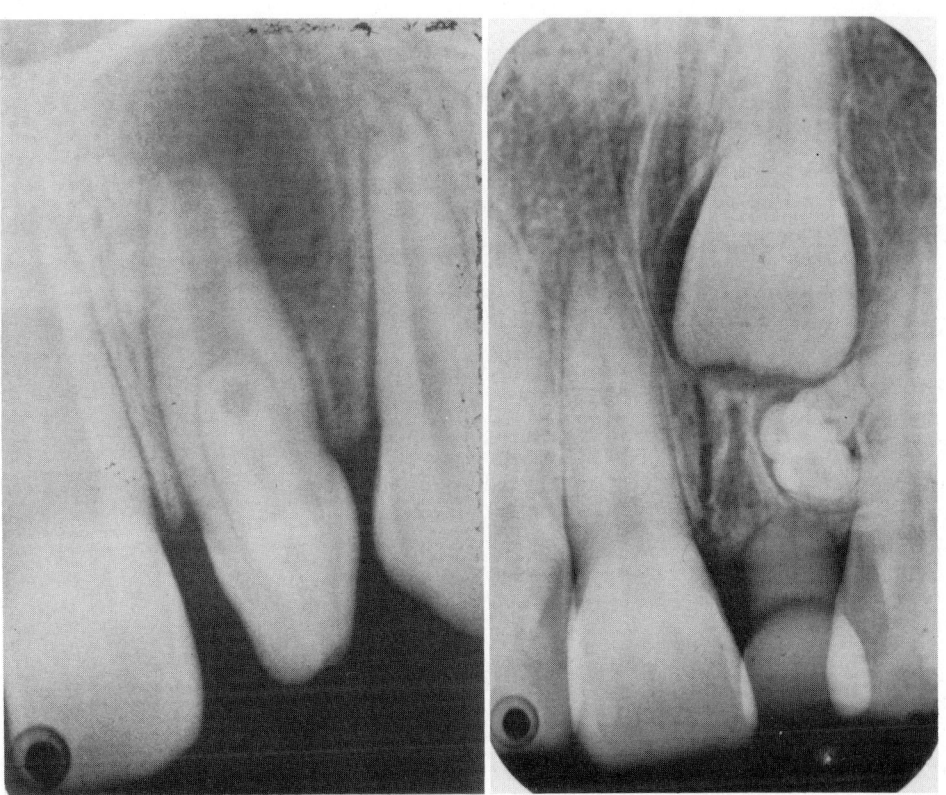

Figure 6–5.   **Figure 6–6.**

Figure 6–5   Dens in dente of a lateral incisor with associated periapical pathology.
Figure 6–6   Odontoma with retention of deciduous central incisor and impaction of permanent successor.

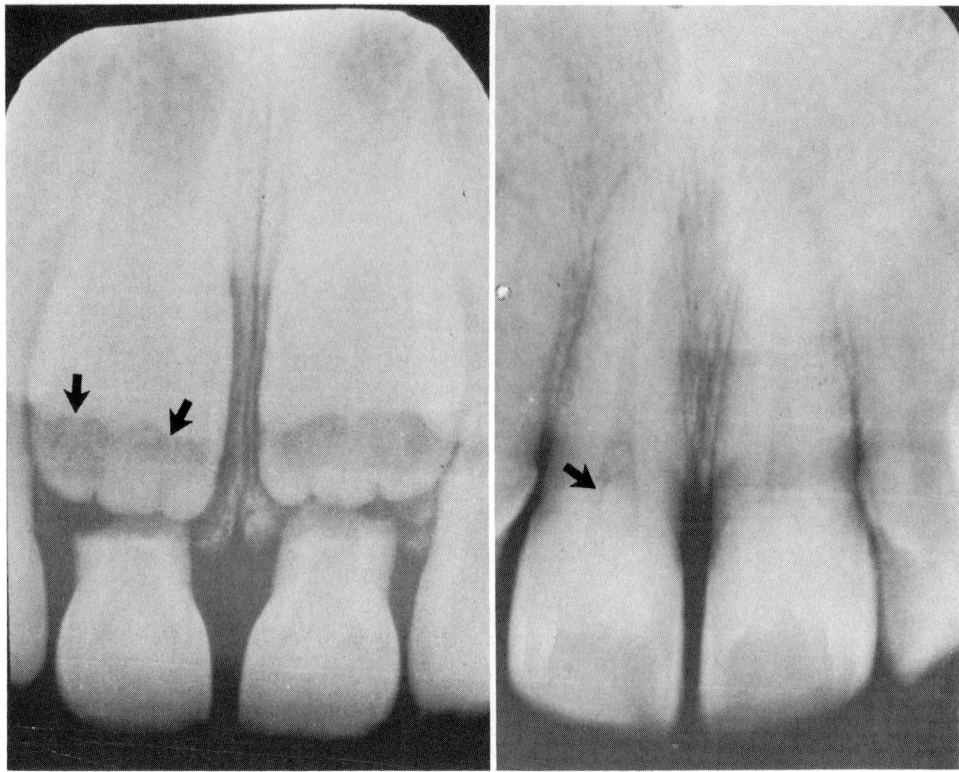

Figure 6–7.   **Figure 6–8.**

Figure 6–7 Hypoplasia of unerupted permanent central incisors.
Figure 6–8 Pulp stones present in incisor tooth.

ALTERATIONS IN CALCIFICATION OF THE TEETH

Early detection of alterations in calcification of the teeth is important.
Roentgenograms aid in the recognition and diagnosis of systemic disease with dental manifestations. They also lead to the identification of disease peculiar to the teeth alone. Among the systemic diseases which may be manifested in the teeth are osteogenesis imperfecta, congenital syphilis, chronic fluorosis, rickets and ectodermal dysplasia. Among the diseases peculiar to the teeth producing alterations in calcification are amelogenesis imperfecta, dentinogenesis imperfecta, dentinal dysplasia and pulp stones.

ALTERATIONS IN GROWTH AND DEVELOPMENT

Although there may be a wide variation in the eruption age of teeth among physically normal children, a deviation of more than three years from the average eruption time should be looked upon with suspicion. Roentgenography may furnish an early clue to a delay in development, and it may also indicate the extent of the delay or the precocity of eruption. The most common cause of aberrant eruption is abnormal glandular function. Delayed eruption may indicate impaired glandular activity as observed in hypothyroidism and hypopituitarism. Metabolic diseases such as cleidocranial dysostosis may also lead to delayed eruption. Precocious eruption is a common observance in hyperpituitarism. Occasionally a tooth erupted into occlusion becomes submerged (Fig. 6–9).

Roentgenography of the bones of the hand and forearm is another method of determining the physical or bone age of the child. The age at ossification of the eight carpal bones is utilized by pediatricians and should be used by dentists as an accurate index of a child's physical development. It is certainly more reliable than the actual chronologic age. A marked delay in eruption time may be correlated with a delayed appearance and growth of the carpal bones.

Cephalometric roentgenograms provide an accurate method of evaluating growth and development of the skull and, more important, the tooth-bearing areas of the skull.

ALTERATIONS IN THE INTEGRITY OF THE PERIODONTAL MEMBRANE

Roentgenograms can be very helpful in diagnosing apical pathosis. One of the cardinal characteristics of periapical infection is a thickening of the adjacent periodontal membrane. Local and systemic factors may damage or destroy this tissue. Among the factors that may be local in nature are irritation, traumatic occlusion, lack of functional stimulation, and caries. Among the systemic factors may be listed bacterial or viral infections, avitaminoses and blood dyscrasias. Roentgenograms can help not only in diagnosing these conditions, but also in establishing a prognosis as well as assessing the success of any treatment. The diagnostician must remember that the initial acute periapical abscess often presents no roentgenographic change because a significant amount of bone must first be resorbed before a change can be demonstrated on the roentgenogram.

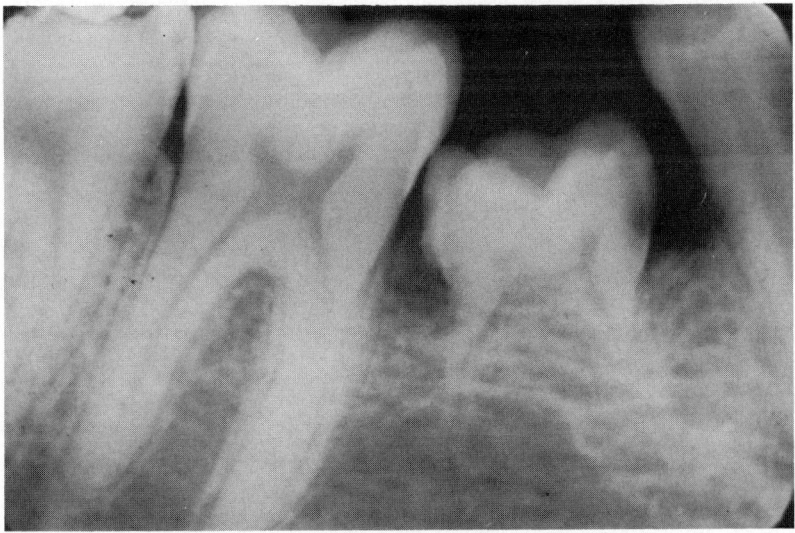

Figure 6–9 A submerged second primary molar.

ALTERATIONS IN THE SUPPORTING BONE

Many changes in the bony structure of the maxilla and mandible observed roentgenographically are indicative of either local or systemic disease. Local bone destruction may indicate abscesses, cysts, tumors, osteomyelitis or periodontal disease. Among the systemic diseases producing bone destruction are rickets, scurvy, hyperparathyroidism, cleidocranial dysostosis, blood dyscrasias such as agranulocytosis, Paget's disease, diabetes, eosinophilic granuloma and related metabolic diseases, and chronic poisoning. Localized roentgenopacities can occur in periostitis ossificans, fibrous dysplasias, Paget's disease, enostoses, and exostoses. A generalized roentgenopacity occurs in Albers-Schönberg's disease (marble bone). In many instances, the first indication that a child has a chronic disease is the discovery of bone changes in a roentgenogram by the dentist.

CHANGES IN THE INTEGRITY OF THE TEETH

Concussion of a tooth frequently produces the gradual death of the pulp with abscess formation. Routine roentgenograms frequently reveal the first evidence that makes the dentist suspect that the pulp has died, e. g., incomplete root formation. Roentgenograms are useful in detecting fractured and resorbed roots, encroachment of primary teeth on permanent tooth buds, dilacerations, displacements, ankylosis, bone fractures, and foreign bodies. The use of roentgenography in locating foreign bodies is classic.

PULPAL EVALUATION

Roentgenography plays a major role in pulpal evaluation and therapy. In assessing the need for pulpal therapy, it aids in determining, within certain limits, the relative depth of a carious lesion and its proximity to the pulp. It assists in evaluating the condition of the periapical tissues. It shows the shape of the pulp and forms the most reliable guide available in filling root canals and in evaluating the final fillings. The success of pulp capping, or pulpotomy, may be observed in many teeth by the formation of a dentin bridge subjacent to the area of treatment. Failures can be observed in the destruction of the lamina dura, as periapical abscesses and occasionally in the internal resorption of the root.

TYPES OF EXAMINATION

Roentgenography for children can be divided arbitrarily into three general categories: (1) the general survey of the mouth; (2) the examination of specific areas; and (3) special surveys.

THE GENERAL SURVEY

Children should have a complete survey of the mouth taken as part of their first regular visit to the dentist and periodically thereafter.

The frequency of these surveys should be governed by the caries susceptibility and growth pattern of the individual. As a supplement to the general survey, bite-wing roentgenograms should be made every six months and possibly every three months in the caries-susceptible child. At these visits, if the child has large and deep cavities or restorations, where the possibility of periapical involvement exists, the survey should consist of periapical as well as bite-wing films.

Although the child's age and behavior may determine the type of survey made, they should not govern the need for a survey. Infants or very young children are sometimes uncooperative; in these instances lateral jaw films can generally be obtained with the aid of a parent or assistant. Although extra-oral films are less effective in locating incipient interproximal lesions, they are useful in locating the larger cavities, and are highly effective, among other things, in finding periapical pathosis, dental anomalies, aberrant growth patterns, changes due to systemic diseases, and injuries.

THE EXAMINATION OF SPECIFIC AREAS

Local pathosis or injury can be examined with intra- as well as extraoral films. The examination may consist of a single periapical film such as is used to confirm the presence of periapical pathosis, or a group of films such as is used in the examination of the sinuses. In the main, specific area examinations consist of examinations for the localization of bone lesions and objects within the soft tissues, evaluation for multiple roots and pulp canals, and examinations of the sinuses and temporomandibular joints.

SPECIAL SURVEYS

Special surveys are generally made for one of two reasons: (1) to provide some specific bit of information, or (2) to show structures not shown on the usual dental roentgenograms.

In pedodontics two roentgenograms made to secure specific information are of special importance: the cephalometric roentgenogram used to follow the growth and development of the child's skull, and the hand and wrist roentgenogram used in the determination of the patient's bone age. Cephalometric roentgenograms are usually lateral projections of the skull. These pictures are made with the child's head positioned in a stabilizing device or cephalostat so that future pictures can be made under reproducible conditions. Tracings made of these roentgenograms depict mathematically the development of the child's skull; such roentgenograms are made by most orthodontists. The hand and wrist or carpal index roentgenogram is made on any screen or nonscreen film large enough to show the entire area in question. The palm of the hand is placed flat on the film away from the child's body, and the x-ray beam directed perpendicular to the film. With a 30 inch tube to film distance, 10 MA, and 65 KVP, the average exposure time for nonscreen film is 1 second and for screen film in par-speed cassettes $\frac{1}{5}$ second. The number of carpal bones present and their corresponding size indicate the stage of development of the child (see Table 6–1 and Chapter 30). The roentgenograms can be compared with a standard atlas of bone development such as that by Greulich and Pyle. If a

TABLE 6–1   AGE AT ONSET OF OSSIFICATION

| | BOYS | | | GIRLS | | |
| | MEAN | | S.D.* | MEAN | | S.D.* |
BONES	YRS.	MOS.	MOS.	YRS.	MOS.	MOS.
Capitate	0	2	2	0	2	2
Hamate	0	3	2	0	2	2
Distal epiphysis, radius	1	1	5	0	10	4
Triquetral	2	6	16	1	9	14
Lunate	3	6	19	2	10	13
Greater multangular	5	7	19	3	11	14
Lesser multangular	5	9	15	4	1	12
Navicular	5	6	15	4	3	12
Distal epiphysis, ulna	6	10	14	5	9	13
Pisiform	..	..	..	..	..	..

* Standard deviation, adjusted to nearest month. The range included between minus 1 and plus 1 standard deviation for any ossification center will usually include 68 per cent of a population of healthy children.

Adapted from Nelson, W. E.: Textbook of Pediatrics.

marked variation exists between the carpal index of the child and that of a standard bone atlas, the child's pediatrician should be notified and provision made for a complete physical examination.

Roentgenograms made to show structures not seen in the usual dental projections include roentgenograms made of soft tissue lesions and roentgenograms made of areas other than the facial areas. Soft tissue roentgenograms are made with less exposure time and/or kilovoltage to show such things as sialoliths or calcified lymph nodes. Roentgenopaque media can also be used to show soft tissue cavities such as the salivary gland ducts in sialography, cysts, the oropharynx, and the sinuses. The visualization of areas other than the facial area is called for when the diagnostician feels that he is not seeing the complete pathologic picture, or enough of it. More often than not this survey consists of skull pictures, and examples of conditions wherein these roentgenograms are helpful include eosinophilic granuloma, hyperpituitarism, sickle cell anemia, thalassemia, and fractures.

TYPES OF FILM

Intra-oral and extra-oral pedodontic roentgenography requires a number of films of various sizes and speeds. Such films are commercially available and may be purchased under a variety of trade names.

INTRA-ORAL FILMS

The smallest intra-oral film, No. 1.0,* measures 0.81 by 1.25 inches. Although it has been designed specifically as a child's film, it is used generally for children with small oral cavities. It may be used as a periapical film or in combination with a

---

*The American Standard Size Designations and Dimensions for Intraoral Dental Radiographic Film, Diagnostic Grade, PH 6.2–1962.

bite-wing tab as a bite-wing film. The pre-school child of three to five will generally tolerate these small films if given proper indoctrination.

The anterior periapical film, No. 1.1, measures 0.94 by 1.56 inches. This film may be used for periapical pictures of permanent anterior teeth or as a periapical or bite-wing film in younger children.

The most generally used film is the No. 1.2. It is the adult size periapical film measuring 1.22 by 1.61 inches. This packet is also used as an occlusal film in preschool children. In school children it can serve as a periapical film, and used with a bite-wing tab it makes an ideal bite-wing film.

Bite-wing films are available with tabs attached as part of the film packets. They have no added advantage over the use of periapical film with bite-wing tabs and usually only add to the storage and inventory problem.

The occlusal film measures $2\frac{1}{4}$ by 3 inches. It can be used to take occlusal pictures of both arches in older children and can also be used in some instances as a lateral jaw film in infants.

There are many films with various emulsion speeds on the market. A film's speed is classified by the American Standards Association as being A, B, C, D, E, or F; A is the slowest film available and F is the fastest.

EXTRA-ORAL FILMS

There are two types of extra-oral films: the nonscreen and the screen film. These films come in various sizes, but the most common sizes used are the 5 by 7 and 8 by 10 inches. The 5 by 7 inch nonscreen film is the extra-oral film most widely used in children's dentistry. This film in its cardboard film holder is preferred by the authors for taking lateral jaw pictures on children because it is lightweight, is easy to handle, and has a greater range or scale of contrast than screen films. Screen films, used with screen cassettes, have greater speed and are used mainly where the x-ray beam has to penetrate a great amount of tissue; for example, skull pictures and pictures of the temporomandibular joint.

ROENTGENOGRAPHIC FACTORS

Aside from the alignment of the x-ray beam, patient, and film, five variable roentgenographic factors must be controlled in the making of a roentgenogram. These factors are (1) film exposure time, (2) film speed, (3) kilovoltage (peak), (4) milliamperage, and (5) tube to film distance. In this discussion it is assumed that film processing is done under optimum conditions and that the operator has taken the size of the patient into consideration.

FILM EXPOSURE TIME

Most dentists find it convenient to keep all other factors constant while varying the film exposure time to provide the proper density in a roentgenogram. In working with children it is better to take all roentgenograms as fast as possible in order to minimize the effects of any motion of the patient. When film speed, kilovoltage, and milliamperage are increased, the exposure time can be considerably reduced, but special timers are needed. There are timers available that give exposure times as short as $1/20$ second. Short exposure times are very helpful in making roentgenograms on spastics, children with cerebral palsy and other crippling conditions.

When a change is made in any factor affecting exposure time, it is often necessary to conduct a test to determine the new exposure time. For periapical roentgenograms it is unnecessary to test for each area of the mouth. Three roentgenograms of the same area made with different exposure times will usually establish the correct exposure time for that particular area. From this correct exposure time the exposure times for other areas can be calculated. The relationship between the different areas in the mouth are: upper anterior teeth 1, upper bicuspids $1\frac{1}{4}$, upper molars $1\frac{1}{2}$, lower anterior teeth $3/4$, lower bicuspids 1, and lower molars $1\frac{1}{4}$.

FILM SPEED

The faster the film speed, the shorter can be the exposure time. Manufacturers are constantly increasing film speeds since this is the greatest single method of reducing the radiation dose or exposure of the patient. It is important that the operator follow the manufacturer's directions for exposure time in order to avoid over- or underexposure. If it is not possible to obtain very short exposure times on the x-ray machine, the fast films can still be used if less milliamperage or a greater tube to film distance is utilized.

KILOVOLTAGE PEAK

The higher the KVP, the more penetrating are the x-rays produced, and less exposure time is needed. The usual dental machine is operated at 65 KVP, but machines are available with KVP's varying from 60 to 100. An increase of about 12 KVP requires a 50 per cent reduction in exposure time and vice versa. The effect of increased KVP upon the quality of roentgenograms is an increase in the scale of contrast. *When high contrast is needed, for example, to detect small carious lesions, the lower kilovoltages are used.*

MILLIAMPERAGE

Milliamperage has almost a direct correlation with exposure time, and the two are often multiplied together to form a single factor (MAS). The greater the MA is, the less exposure time needed. Changes in milliamperage also affect the effective KVP, and many machines have two separate KVP scales for different milliamperage settings.

TUBE TO FILM DISTANCE

When the tube of film distance is increased and all other factors remain constant, the exposure time must also be increased. If all the other variable factors are kept constant, the exposure times for any two tube to film distances is directly proportional to the squares of these distances. For instance, when the tube to film distance is increased from 8 inches to 16 inches, the exposure time must be multiplied by four.

ROENTGENOGRAPHIC TECHNIQUES

INTRA-ORAL TECHNIQUES

There are two techniques for intra-oral roentgenography: the paralleling technique and the bisecting angle technique. Both have merit in children's dentistry. A comparison of the two shows that the paralleling technique provides better diagnostic roentgenograms but is not always practical for children. The paralleling technique can be used only with a 16 to 20 inch tube to film distance (long cone), while the bisecting angle technique can be used with both the extended distance or the 8 inch distance (short cone). When the long cone is used with very fast films, the exposure time with 65 KVP and 10 MA is between $1/2$ and $1\frac{1}{2}$ seconds. This gives the operator enough exposure time latitude to expose properly the various areas of the mouth. When the fast films are used with a short cone with 65 KVP and 10 MA, the exposure time is approximately $1/5$ second, and little exposure time latitude is available. The authors favor the long-cone paralleling technique in older children, the long-cone bisecting angle technique in younger children, and the short-cone bisecting angle technique when very short film exposure times are needed.

The paralleling technique requires placing the film parallel to the long axis of the teeth in the vertical plane and parallel to the buccal surfaces of the teeth in the horizontal plane. The beam of radiation is directed perpendicular to the film and teeth in the vertical plane, and between the teeth in the horizontal plane. This technique produces roentgenographic images that have a minimum of magnification and distortion, and shows the proper relationship of deciduous teeth to permanent tooth buds (Fig. 6–10). To assist in properly positioning the film, a variety of film holders are available. These include bite blocks made of wood or rubber, hemostats with rubber blocks, plastic holders with extensions to direct the beam of radiation, and throat sticks to which the films can be attached with cellophane tape.

The bisecting angle technique is based on the principle of isometric triangulation. When the film and the teeth form an angle, and the central ray is directed perpendicular to the bisector of this angle, the image of the tooth on the film will have the same length as the tooth being examined (see Fig. 6–10). The film is commonly held in place by the patient; thumbs are used for the upper teeth and forefingers for the lower. When fingers are used to retain the film in the mouth, the film is curved, and the result is a distorted image. It is advisable to use some form of film holder to insure a flat film surface when the film is in the mouth.

Both paralleling and bisecting angle techniques are sometimes unsuccessful with a very apprehensive child. In these instances it is often possible to get a film in the child's mouth if neither a film holder nor the child's hand is used; the film can be held by the teeth themselves. The anterior teeth can be examined using the intra-oral film like an occlusal film. In the posterior areas $1/3$ inch of an adult periapical film can be bent at right angles to the film and placed in the mouth like a bite-wing film.

Bite-wing pictures are taken to examine the crowns of the teeth and alveolar ridges in both arches. The x-ray beam is directed between the teeth in the horizon-

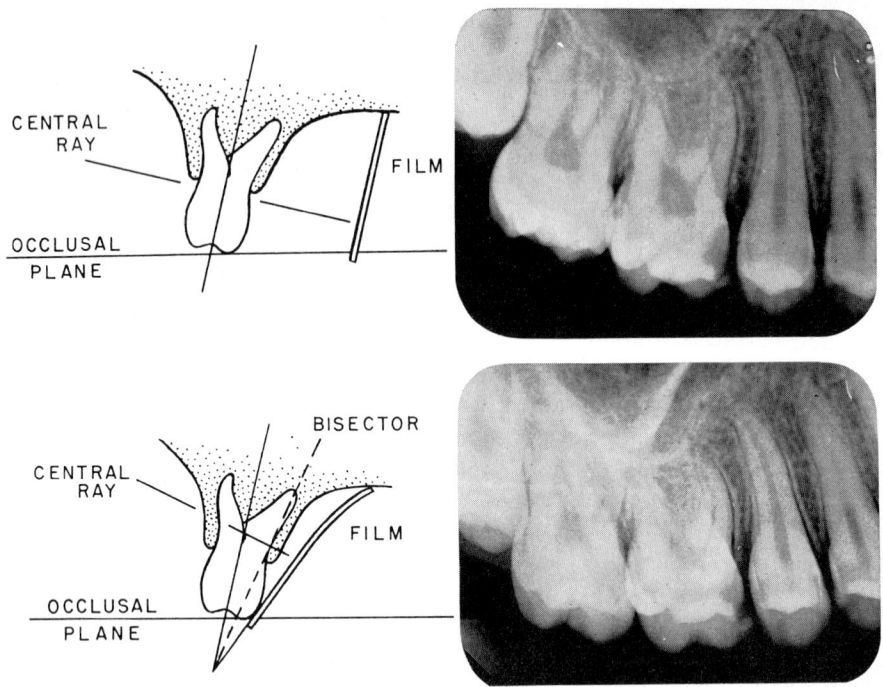

Figure 6–10   Above: Relationship of x-rays, film, and tooth in the paralleling technique, and a typical roentgenogram of the upper posterior teeth. Below: Relationship of x-rays, film and tooth in the bisecting angle technique, and a typical roentgenogram of the upper posterior teeth.

tal plane. On the vertical plane the x-ray beam is directed slightly downward to form an 8 to 10 degree angle with the occlusal plane.

COMPLETE MOUTH SURVEYS

The complete or full-mouth x-ray survey should examine the teeth and their supporting structures. The survey is basically dependent upon the size of the oral cavity and cooperation of the child being examined. It is reasonable to assume that the greater the number of pictures taken, the more information will be revealed, but radiation dose, time, and cost must be considered, and a compromise in the number of films to be used must be achieved. Whenever the films indicate that the complete pathologic picture is not being seen, the making of extra films and possibly extra-oral films becomes mandatory. Because of differences in patient cooperation, size of the mouth, and the number of teeth present, further discussion will be based on the arbitrary division of pedodontic patients into four age groups: infancy, primary dentition age, changing dentition age, and adolescence.

AGES 1 TO 3

In this age bracket the patient is often unable to cooperate. With the exception of early interproximal caries, lateral jaw films will provide the information most pertinent to this age group; this includes development and calcification of the teeth, anomalies, and any gross pathosis. An example of a child's lateral jaw roentgenogram is shown in Figure 6–12 Right. Also of assistance in this age group is the intra-oral film used like an occlusal in the anterior area. It is possible for these films plus two bite wings to constitute a complete mouth survey. Figure 6–12 Left shows a modified occlusal film technique. These films demonstrate a practical x-ray survey for difficult cases.

AGES 3 TO 6

The child at this age level can learn to tolerate intra-oral films. The No. 1.0 and No. 1.1 films may be used. A full survey can be accomplished with 12 films consisting of six anterior, four posterior and two bite-wing films. It is important that this survey show the deciduous dentition and the tooth buds of the developing permanent teeth.

AGES 6 TO 12

Children in this age bracket are usually very cooperative and tolerate intra-oral films satisfactorily. A 14 film survey is recommended for this age group, and an example of such a survey is shown in Figure 6–11. No. 1.1 film is used for anterior teeth and No. 1.2 for the posteriors and bite-wings.

AGES OVER 12

The complete mouth survey in this age group should consist of at least 20 pictures. In addition to the films shown in Figure 6–11, four periapical and two bite-wing pictures of the permanent molar teeth are needed.

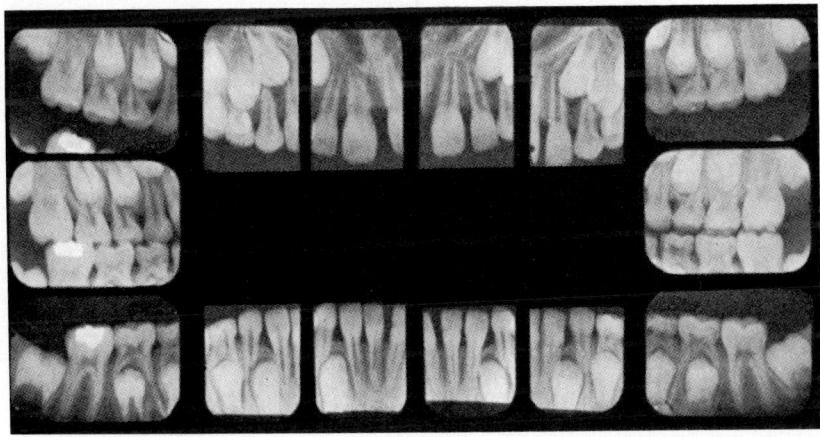

Figure 6–11 A 12 film periapical survey plus two bite-wing films.

OCCLUSAL ROENTGENOGRAPHY

The occlusal or sandwich film is used mainly on older children, but an adult periapical film can be used on infants and young children, using the same technique. These films are used to examine areas of the dentition greater than those normally seen on regular periapical films. An eight-inch tube to film distance is generally used, but greater distances can be utilized. The film is held in the occlusal plane between the teeth like a sandwich, and the x-ray beam is directed perpendicular to the bisector of the angle formed by the film and the teeth in the area being examined. Such topographic projections can be made of the upper arch and the lower anterior areas. Cross section projections can be made of the lower jaw with this film, and these roentgenograms are very useful in localizing objects in and around the lower jaw.

When topographical views of both upper and lower anterior teeth are needed in young or uncooperative patients a modified technique is suggested. The occlusal film is bent upon itself completely and positioned in the mouth so that half of the exposure side faces upward and half downward. The film is exposed twice, once for the upper teeth and once for the lower. The double thickness of lead foil in the back of the film packet makes this technique practical and reduces patient management time. Figure 6–12 (Left) shows this roentgenogram.

LATERAL JAW TECHNIQUES

The film usually used for this projection is the 5 by 7 inch nonscreen film in a cardboard film holder. On very small children an occlusal film may be substituted. All films should be marked with lead letters indicating right and left.

The child is seated with the sagittal plane perpendicular to the floor and the occlusal plane parallel to the floor. The chin is thrust forward to increase the distance between the jaws and the vertebral column. A short cone is used, and the central ray of the beam of radiation directed to enter at a point just superior and medial to the angle of the mandible opposite the side being examined. The central ray is positioned so that it exits just anterior to the area being examined and at or a little above the occlusal plane. The film is held between the heel of the patient's hand and the malar or cheekbone with the fingers curved over the top of the film and touching the cranium for stability. The nose in the anterior areas and the zygomatic arch in the posterior areas can assist in stabilizing the film. The film is positioned so that it is perpendicular as far as possible to the central ray in both horizontal and vertical planes (Fig. 6–13*A*). With 65 KVP and 10 MA the average exposure time is 1 second.

In very young or uncooperative patients the film can be placed on the headrest of the chair, and the patient simply rests his head upon it. The central ray is directed from behind the ramus of the opposite mandible if possible, and if not, it is directed beneath the body of the opposite mandible (Fig. 6–13*B*). These alternative projections provide usable roentgenograms but suffer more from distortion of the images. Figure 6–12 (Right) shows a lateral jaw roentgenogram.

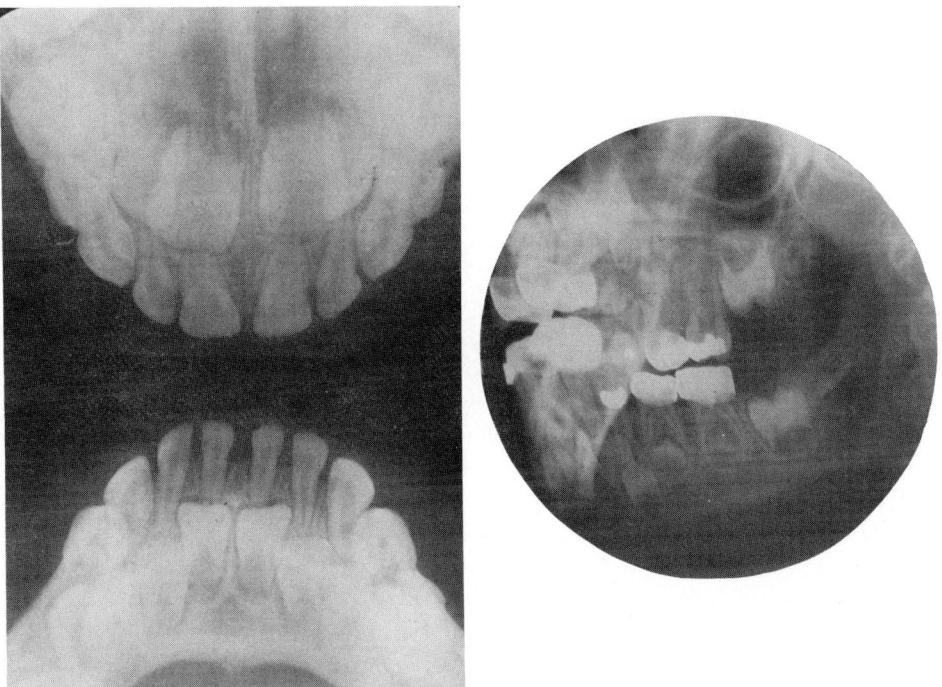

Figure 6–12   Left: Topographical projections of a child's upper and lower anterior teeth made on a single occlusal film. Right: Lateral jaw roentgenogram of a child showing the developing teeth.

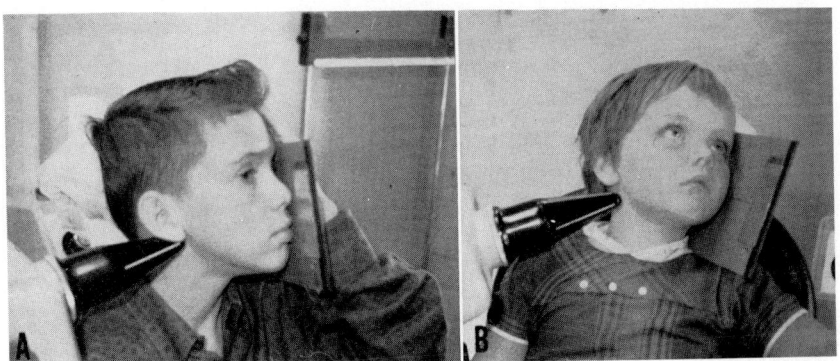

Figure 6–13   *A:* Lateral jaw technique. *B:* Lateral jaw technique for a young child.

PANORAMIC RADIOGRAPHY

In the last two decades, x-ray machines capable of taking large areas or panoramic views of the jaws have been developed. To examine both jaws, a series of still pictures are made with the Panoramix and Status-X machines that place the x-ray tube in the patient's mouth and have the film extraorally positioned. Machines using a laminagraphic or tomographic principle have also been developed, for example, the Rotagraph, the Panorex, the Orthopantomograph and the General Electric 3000. These machines examine both jaws on one film. At present, the Panorex and Orthopantomograph are the machines most widely used with the GE-3000 recently being made available to the profession.

The first commercially available panoramic-tomographic machine, the Panorex, appeared in 1957. The machine used a slitlike opening in the collimator which produced a thin beam of x-rays. The x-ray tube head and film cassette carrier rotated around the patient's head about a fixed axis. The axis was located at a point just medial to the third molar area. The patient was seated in a chair that shifted laterally, after one side of the jaws was examined, so that the rotational axis of the tube head cassette carrier assembly was repositioned at a similar point on the opposite side during the film exposure of the other side of the jaws. Synchronization of the movement of the cassette, behind an opening in the cassette carrier, with the speed of rotation of the tube head cassette carrier assembly produced the panoramic radiograph of the jaws. The radiograph showed a view from condyle to condyle with a break in the middle which was created during the chair shift.

The Orthopantomograph, like the Panorex, places the patient in a stationary

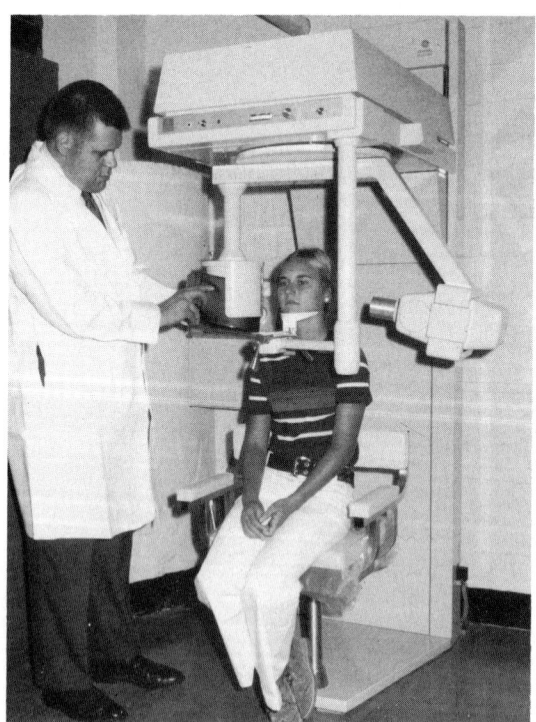

Figure 6–14 The GE-3000 panoramic x-ray machine. The film in a flexible cassette is placed on the rotating drum of the tube head cassette assembly. The chin-rest rotates on a vertical post attached to the canopy like over-head section that is counterbalanced and controlled with electric locks.

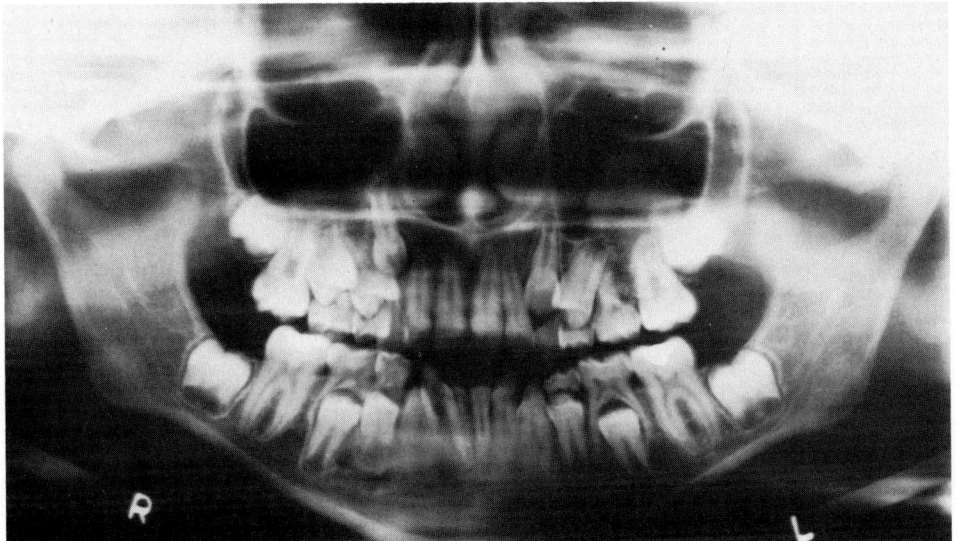

Figure 6–15 Panoramic radiograph of a pedodontic patient made with the GE-3000.

position and rotates the tube head and cassette holder. Unlike the Panorex, this machine uses a curved film cassette, does not use a built-in chair, and does not have a lateral patient shift to change the rotational axis of the tube head cassette holder assembly. The Orthopantomograph uses three rotational axes (two posterior and one anterior) instead of two, as in the Panorex, and shifts from one axis to the other when the x-ray beam is aligned with two axis points. The resultant radiograph shows a continuous image from condyle to condyle without a break in the midline anterior area.

The GE-3000, like the Panorex and the Orthopantomograph, places the patient in a stationary position and rotates the tube head cassette holder assembly. The fundamental difference is in the movement of the rotational axis of this assembly, which is continuously moving and follows the arc of the mandible and maxilla; the arc is not of fixed size but can be adjusted for different-sized jaws. The GE-3000 panoramic machine is shown in Figure 6–14, and an example of the panoramic radiograph is shown in Figure 6–15.

Panoramic radiographs examine not only the teeth and the supporting bone in the area but the entire maxilla and mandible. However, the sharpness of structures is not as well defined as with intraoral radiographs. The usefulness of these radiographs must therefore be restricted to surveys for relatively large lesions of teeth and bone. In addition, it must be remembered that these machines examine a layer of tissue and deliberately blur out other areas; the dentist must thus be aware that he is not viewing a superimposition of all structures as is seen in periapical radiographs. The midline palatal area may be portraited twice, Figure 6–16, and unusual artifacts may occur, Figure 6–17. The great advantages of panoramic radiography include the facts that the entire jaw areas are examined, the radiography is done quickly, and the film is positioned outside the patient's mouth. Panoramic radiographs are thus very useful for examining patients with bad gag reflexes or trismus, children who are uncooperative in opening the mouth for one

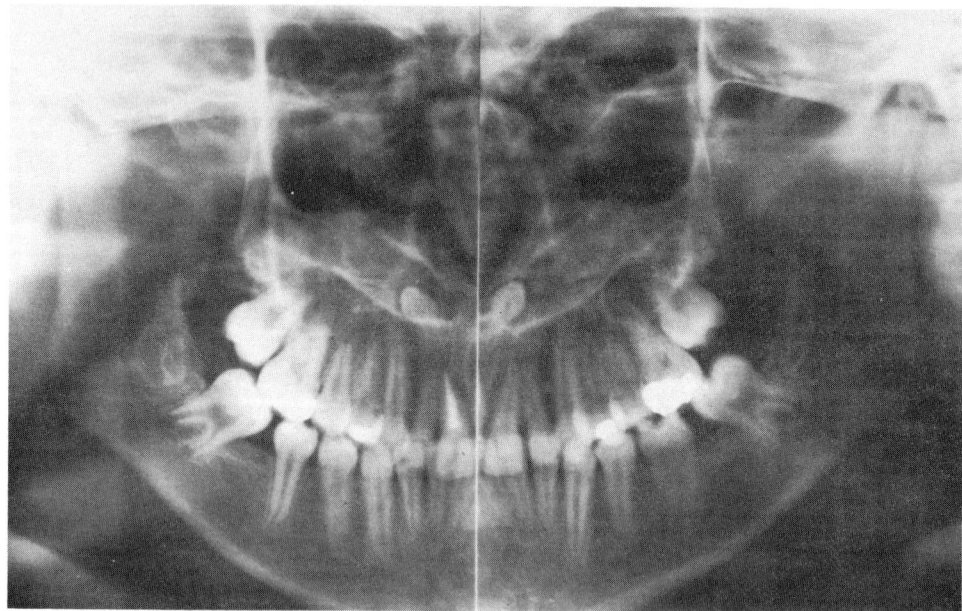

Figure 6–16 Panoramic radiograph made with the Panorex showing duplication of the midline palatal area which contains a single impacted tooth. An occlusal radiograph of this area is helpful in identifying individual teeth.

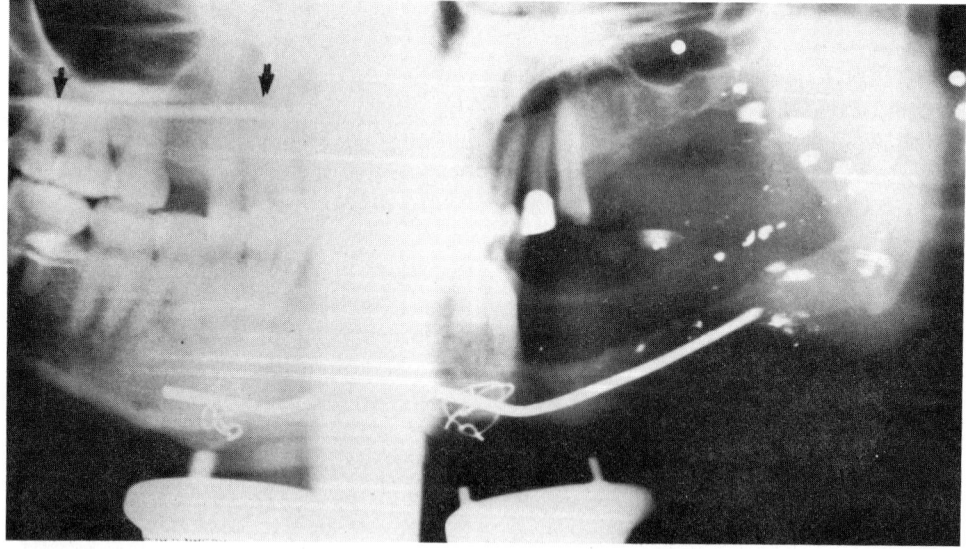

Figure 6–17 Panoramic radiograph showing a linear radiopaque artifact on one side (arrows). The artifact was produced by a lead pellet situated in the center of rotation located on the opposite side during examination of the side containing the artifact.

reason or another, and for mass children surveys. Depending on the type of machine used, special projections of preselected layers such as the TMJ or an area of the sinus are possible through repositioning the patient's head or changing the rotational axis path of the machine.

DARKROOM PROCEDURES

The darkroom should be light-tight, clean, free of dust, and well ventilated. Equipment must include a safelight, processing tanks, film racks, and a work bench. Processing solutions should be kept at full strength by frequent replenishing and changing. It is recommended that film processing be done by the time-temperature method, as only by this method can optimum and consistent film quality be obtained. Cleanliness is essential, as chemicals such as the fluorides can cause artifacts on roentgenograms when they come in contact with the film before processing. All too often good film-exposure technique is ruined by poor darkroom procedures.

All finished roentgenograms should be mounted for ready reference; mounts can be obtained to fit any number and type of survey.

The importance of saving roentgenograms cannot be stressed too highly. Not only will these films have future diagnostic value for later comparisons, but they are also important for legal reasons.

X-RAY HAZARDS AND PROTECTION

X-ray hazards are due to the fact that the x-ray is an ionizing radiation. These radiations are known to have deleterious biologic effects when absorbed in large doses. However, the doses used in diagnostic dental roentgenography are so small that the benefit obtained through the use of roentgenograms far outweighs any possible risk. There is no recorded case where the proper use of dental x-rays has caused any clinically observable change in a patient. The continued use of radiation for diagnosis is essential in modern dentistry, and the dentist should not hesitate to make roentgenograms on children whenever they are needed. However, since these rays have undesirable effects, the indiscriminate and improper use of x-rays is inexcusable. Dentists have a professional responsibility, for no matter how small the amount of radiation used, it adds to the total radiation exposure of human beings.

Although properly used dental x-rays produce no clinical changes it is possible that they assist in producing some of the more subtle effects of ionizing radiations. These effects include genetic changes, leukemia, and life shortening. At the dose levels used, dental x-rays contribute very little to these changes. However, since the rapidly developing tissues of children may be more sensitive to x-rays, and since the distance between the gonads and the teeth is less in children, extreme caution is desirable. It is recommended that the gonads of children be shielded during dental x-ray examinations.

Most states in the United States require x-ray machines to be registered. X-rays can be controlled. Dental x-ray machines must meet certain requirements in design and construction to eliminate unnecessary exposure of the patient and operator.

Radiation exposure during oral diagnostic roentgenography can be reduced by practical methods. The operator should rigidly observe certain rules. He should never hold the film for the patient or have any part of his body in the primary beam of radiation. He should never hold the head of the x-ray machine while it is being operated. He should stand at least six feet from the patient and x-ray machine; if this is not possible, some protective barrier should be provided.

Much can be done to reduce the patient's exposure to x-rays. In the main, any reduction in patient dose is accompanied by a reduction in exposure to the operator. Patient-protection measures are as follows: (1) Use fast films. Fast film is the greatest single factor in patient-dose reduction. (2) Filter the x-ray beam. The use of 2 to 2½ mm. of aluminum (equivalent) total filtration removes the soft x-rays that irradiate the patient but do not reach the film. (3) Collimate the x-ray beam. This is done with lead washers or diaphragms. A beam 2¾ inches in diameter at the patient's skin provides ample coverage for intra-oral films without unnecessarily irradiating tissue outside of the field of interest. (4) Increase the tube to patient distance. An increase in this distance, while maintaining the 2¾ inch beam size at the patient's face with proper diaphragms, will reduce the patient's skin dose and also reduce the amount of tissue in the primary beam of radiation. (5) Use a properly constructed x-ray machine. (6) Use good chairside and darkroom techniques. When retakes are required, the child is unnecessarily exposed to x-rays. (7) Use open end cones and if possible a recessed filter. X-ray scatter from the cone and filter should be avoided. Lastly, (8) use a shield for the gonads. Leaded shields are commercially available, and when used give extra protection to the child and calm any apprehension in the parents about radiation damage.

X-ray rooms should be monitored or have a radiation survey at least once. Film badge monitoring services are available in the United States, and some states have public health radiation survey teams. Also available are personnel ion chambers for measuring radiation dose to the operator.

REFERENCES

1. The Biological Effects of Atomic Radiation. National Academy of Sciences, National Research Council, Washington, D.C., 1960.
2. Alvares, L. C.: Periapical examination for preschool children. Oral Surg., Oral Med. & Oral Path., 21:47, 1966.
3. Blackman, S.: Rotational tomography of the face. Brit. Radiol., 33:408–418, 1960.
4. Blackman, S.: Radiology in child and adolescent stomatology. Dent. Pract. and Dent. Rec., 12:77, 1961.
5. Blayney, J. R., and Greco, J. F.: Recognition of early proximal caries: X-ray versus clinical procedures. D. Radiog. & Photog., 26:33, 1953.
6. Budowsky, J.: The x-ray and diagnosis in pedodontics. New York J. Den., 22:330, 1952.
7. Feasby, W. F.: The number and types of films necessary for a satisfactory radiological survey for children. J. Dent. Child., 27:91, 2nd Quart., 1960.
8. Graber, T. M.: Problems and limitations of cephalometric analysis in orthodontics. J.A.D.A., 53:439, 1956.
9. Graber, T. M.: Panoramic radiography. Angle Orthodont., 36:293–311, 1966.
10. Greulich, W. W., and Pyle, S. I. (after Todd, T. W.): Radiographic Atlas of Skeletal Development of the Hand and Wrist. Stanford, Calif., Stanford University Press, 1950.
11. Hatton, M. E., and Grainger, R. M.: Reliability of measurements from cephalograms at the Burlington Orthodontic Research Center. J. D. Res., 37:853, 1958.

12. Hayden, J., and Richards, A. G.: Procedures for adequate radiographs of preschool children. J. Dent. Child., *22*:70, 2nd Quart., 1955.
13. Hudson, D. C., Kumpula, J. W., and Dickson, G. A.: Panoramic x-ray dental machine. U. S. Armed Forces M. J., *8*:46–55, 1957.
14. Kumpula, J. W.: Present status of panoramic roentgenography. J.A.D.A., *63*:194–200, 1961.
15. McCall, J. A., and Wald, S. S.: Clinical Dental Roentgenology, 4th ed. Philadelphia, W. B. Saunders Co., 1957.
16. Manson-Hing, L. R.: Advances in dental pantomography: The GE-3000. Oral Surg., Oral Med., and Oral Path., *31*:430, 1971.
17. Manson-Hing, L. R.: Basic x-ray protection in dental radiology. J. Ala. Dent. Assn., *55*:15, 1971.
18. Mortell, J. F.: Morphologic considerations of primary teeth in diagnosing radiographs. J. Dent. Child., *21*:89, 2nd Quart., 1954.
19. The Nature of Radioactive Fallout and Its Effects on Man. Parts 1 and 2. Joint Committee on Atomic Energy, Congress of the United States. Washington, D.C., U.S. Government Printing Office, 1957.
20. Paatero, Y. V.: Use of mobile source of light in radiography. Acta Radiol., *29*:221–227, 1948.
21. Paatero, Y. V.: New tomographical method for radiographing curved outer surfaces. Acta Radiol., *32*:177–184, 1949.
22. Paatero, Y. V.: Pantomography in theory and use. Acta Radiol., *41*:321–335, 1954.
23. Paatero, Y. V.: Pantomography and orthopantomography. Oral Surg., *14*:947–953, 1961.
24. Richards, A. G., and Alling, C. C.: Extra-oral radiography—mandible and temporomandibular articulation. D. Radiog. & Photog., *28*:1, 1955.
25. Rockman, M. N.: Suggestions for radiographing the young child. J. Ontario D. A., *28*:349, 1951.
26. Spear, L. B., and Ruhamah, H.: Practical and improved periapical technique. D. Radiog. & Photog., *26*:21, 1953.
27. Sweet, A. P.: Personal communication.
28. Sweet, C. A.: Radiography in dentistry for children. D. Radiog. & Photog., *22*:1, 1949.
29. Symposium on Oral Roentgenology (S. H. Yale, Ed.) Dent. Clin. N. Amer., July, 1961, pp. 353–478.
30. Updegrave, W. J.: Radiodontic technique for the child patient. J. New Jersey D. Soc., *22*:11, 1951.
31. Updegrave, W. J.: Panoramic dental radiography. D. Radiog. & Photog., *36*:75–83, 1963.
32. Waggener, D. T., and Ireland, R. L.: Intra-oral roentgenography for children. J.A.D.A., *47*:133, 1953.
33. Watson & Sons, Ltd.: Rotagraph for Rotary Tomography of the Skull. Publication 580, Wembley, England.
34. Wuehrmann, A. H., and Manson-Hing, L. R.: Dental Radiology. St. Louis, C. V. Mosby Co., 1965.

7

THE PROBLEM OF PAIN AND SEDATION

by ROLAND R. HAWES

Fear and pain are two of the most powerful influences affecting attitudes about the use of dental services. Experiences with toothaches and fear of unskilled, painful treatment in years gone by have left impressions in the minds of many grandparents and some parents about the kind of dentistry from which they want to protect their children of today. This concern for their chidren's welfare motivates some parents to seek early, preventive care for them. It moves others in the opposite direction toward deferral of care and ultimate disaster. If it is to provide for the needs of both groups, the dental profession needs all of the knowledge and skills which can be mustered to allay fear and to prevent and control the pain of oral disease as well as the pain of treatment.

The skillful management of pain is essential to the mission of the profession for the benefit of the public and for the success of the individual practitioner. However, it remains to be proved that non-users of dental services become users because their fears of pain are reduced by learning of the painless and otherwise satisfactory dental experiences of others. There is some empirical evidence that this is so from the numbers of parents who first evaluate how a new dentist deals with thier children before they will allow him to treat themselves. Such comments as "gentle," "kind," or "didn't hurt a bit" spoken of dentists by their grateful patients have a potent effect upon the growth of dental practices.

Dentists are frustrated in their efforts to prevent and control pain in the dental treatment of children when they fail to identify and deal effectively with two facts. The first of these is that the perception of pain and patients' reactions to it are not constant from one patient to the next and they are not constant from time to time for a single patient. Perceptions of painful sensations and reactions to them are molded in large part by anxiety and fear, particularly in children in threatening circumstances. Anxiety and fear, like shadows, precede and follow painful experiences. The second fact which must be dealt with in treating children is that they have limited ability to describe their experiences and feelings clearly and objectively, especially when they are fearful or in pain.

114

Before describing the means for managing pain and fear it will be useful to attempt to understand these phenomena as best we can. Authorities do not agree about what pain is. And fear, apprehension, and anxiety are enigmatic except at the most elemental levels. In spite of these problems a useful description of the relationship of emotion to pain has been given by Hardy, Wolff and Goodell (1967), who rejected the old idea that pain is a feeling state opposite to that of pleasure and the opinion that it is a result of excessive intensity of other sensations. They proposed that feeling is the most important aspect of pain to the one who suffers, and that he perceives pain by means of a special sense with its own structural, functional, and perceptual properties. They further stated that pain is composed of pain sensations and associated sensations of emotional and affective states (such as fear). They indicated that noxious stimulation of other bodily reactions, even below the conscious level, may contribute to the pain perceived and they have given an important, even dominant, role to emotions in painful experiences. But they considered all other "contributaries" secondary to the painful sensation itself. To put it briefly, pain hurts.

Pain hurts; and to the child who suffers, that is most important. It must be high in importance to the dentist also; but from a different point of view, that of the objective therapist who will apply appropriate preventives and remedies. The dentist must be prepared to deal on both a psychological and a physiological basis with the child's apprehension of and reactions to pain. The principles of psychological management of children under ordinary circumstances not involving pain and the technical aspects of injecting local anesthetics are described in detail in other chapters of this book. Here will be considered in simplified form the integration of knowledge of these subjects with knowledge of pain and the use of several adjuncts for increasing comfort and a sense of well-being for the child patient.

THE ANATOMY AND PHYSIOLOGY OF PAIN

The Afferent Sensory Pathway

The human face, mouth, and pharynx are supplied richly with sensory nerves. These neurons are derived principally from the fifth cranial nerve but there are important contributions from the seventh, ninth, and tenth nerves. A few fibers pass also from the first and second cervical nerves to the lower face.

The sensory neurons are unipolar. Their cell nuclei are located in ganglia such as the gasserian ganglion of the fifth cranial nerve. A myelinated process extends peripherally from the cell nucleus to the receptor organ or free ending of the neuron. The central process extends from the cell nucleus to the place where it makes synapse with cells in the sensory root nucleus of the nerve.

Transmission of stimuli begins at the receptor end of the afferent neuron and proceeds past the nucleus in the ganglion to the synapse in the sensory nucleus. Special receptors have been identified for such stimuli as heat and touch; but it is not generally accepted that there are special pain receptors (Merskey and Spear, 1967; Lim, 1966). Although it has been observed that fibers of larger diameters have faster conduction times it is not at all certain how this affects pain perception even though it is likely that fiber size may be selective for the transmission of a spe-

pallor (sometimes with traces of circumoral cyanosis), and even stupor and uncon-sciousness. In very severe pain the pupils may be dilated and there may be facial grimacing and physical agitation.

Description of the Pain

Pain is often described by adults and by investigators of the problem as superfi-cial—pricking, burning, aching, or itching—and deep, more characteristic of an aching type. The words chosen to describe pain offer insight into the emo-tional content of the patient's reaction or of the parent's reaction. For instance, "I thought I would die" or "He carried on like he was crazy or something" are laden with feeling, whereas "He complained after breakfast for a minute or two" may play down too much the real concern of the parent.

Young children cannot clearly describe their experiences and feelings and so parents may defer acting on their complaints until the pain becomes incapacitating when, finally, with vivid memories of recent, severe dental pain, they are brought to the dentist. Under such circumstances if the pain is no longer present it is some-times difficult to determine its cause. The child may indicate his left side and the mother the right (mirror-imaged) side in describing the problem. Even if both reports coincide, they may be inaccurate because of referral of the pain from a remote site within the affected neuraxis or the spread of the pain within a segment. Both of these need to be distinguished from pain arising as a sequel of motor and vasomotor reflexes, which are atypical for children complaining of facial pain.

It is also unusual for children to feign dental pain. Indeed, they often deny it when they have it. They are more likely to rely on a stomach ache when they malin-ger. The diagnosis of a pain problem is greatly simplified if there are clear answers to the questions of where the pain occurs, when does or did it occur, what makes it better, what makes it worse, what type of pain is it, and how bad is it.

Examination for Causes of Pain

Clinical examination of a patient in pain, or one who fears pain, must be done very considerately. Reassurance before, during, and after each procedure is essen-tial for many apprehensive patients. The "tell, show, and do" approach produces remarkably useful results.

A fairly reliable sign of an offending tooth is a localized unilateral accumula-tion of materia alba indicating avoidance of mastication and mouth cleansing because of pain in the area. The cardinal signs of inflammation as well as tooth mo-bility and open carious lesions often are present.

On the other hand, some children have numerous large carious lesions with open embrasures due to fracture of marginal ridges and even chronic draining dento-alveolar abscesses and yet there may be no present pain and no history of pain. Parents and dentists alike are perplexed by these findings; but even though there is no way to be certain of it, there is a possibility that pain does not recur because the child has carefully (and painfully) learned to avoid the painful stimuli. He does not take very hot or very cold foods, eats only soft non-fibrous foods (or does not chew), eats only a little at a time, and avoids toothbrushing. It seems rea-sonable to call this set of symptoms a pain avoidance syndrome. Parents of such children often report remarkable improvement in their eating habits following oral rehabilitation.

Autonomic Nervous System Effects of Pain

Pain and the fear of pain have effects on the autonomic nervous system as well as upon behavior. Lewis and Law (1958), showed that heart rate, face and hand temperature, and galvanic skin response, all of which are important psychomotor responses to stress, are modified in some degree by various elements of the dental treatment situation. Ship and White (1960) clearly demonstrated that differential stresses were produced by several dental procedures as indicated by decreases in the circulating blood eosinophils as stressfulness increased. According to Shannon and Isbell (1963), adrenocortical hyperactivity can be caused by oral injections. They showed increased serum content of free 17-hydroxycorticosteroids following injection of several local anesthetics. In three papers published by Howitt and Stricker (1963, 1965a, 1965b), it was shown that intelligence of children was a factor in elevation of pain thresholds and that physiological responses to several types of oral stimulation were modified by intelligence and preexisting anxiety. In the last of these three papers (1965b), Howitt and Stricker indicated that only 16 per cent of the 88 children they evaluated between the ages of 4 and 7 years were found to be apprehensive. Half of these 88 children had made dental visits, but no information is available about the nature of their experiences.

Emotions and Reactions to Pain

Birns et al. (1969) observed that infants differ from one another in their reactions to stress as early as the age of one month. These differences persisted over a three month period of observation. This finding supports the hypothesis that some aspects of behavior develop very early in a characteristic way and remain stable for the individual. This idea is consistent with the cherished belief of some parents about the behavior of their offspring. Along these same lines, Perryman et al. (1971) have observed in adults that there is a considerable variability in the autonomic responses registered in experimental subjects when a painful stimulus just exceeds a tolerable level for each subject. They suggested that characteristic emotional factors within the individual have considerable influence in setting the limits for his tolerance of pain. They felt that emotional factors accounted for the variability of the autonomic responses.

In their report on odontophobia in adults, Molin and Seeman (1970) pointed out the large part that fear plays in modifying the behavior of some adults, to the extent of preventing them from seeking needed dental care. Borland (1962) made similar observations and recommended using appropriately reassuring psychological measures, administering sedatives and, very importantly, allowing the patient to participate in controlling the treatment procedures. Many dentists wisely allow children as well as adults to stop the cavity preparations or whatever treatment is in progress to rest briefly before continuing. Experience shows that this is reassuring to the patient and that the privilege is seldom, if ever, abused. The frequency of stops declines over the first five or ten minutes. After this initial testing of the effectiveness of the practice, the child, being satisfied that his control is real, usually declines to use it even if encouraged to do so.

Just as behavior can improve during a single dental visit as the patient learns, one also finds that it improves from visit to visit as reported by Howitt and Stricker (1970) and by Johnson and Koenigsberg (1971). These investigators found reduced autonomic responses and improved behavior in the 8 to 14 year old patients they observed. Nasif (1971) suggests that the same results are seen in patients 3 to 6 years old. Growth of behavior as a result of learning is seen generally in children as they mature and gain experience. Some dentists view the learning aspect of children's dental experiences as an important reason to avoid using medications which might dull their perceptions and intellectual responses to the learning values in the treatment setting. There is no evidence that learning occurs in a child who ought to have been given a medication but was not. While the idea has an appeal to a certain Spartan view of life, it is doubtful that a worried child learns much that is worthwhile in the dental chair. It is just as likely that the learning takes place after the dental visit when he reflects on his experiences and girds up for the next one. If the visit had a positive value, then it ought to show up in subsequent behavior.

CAUSES OF PAIN IN CHILD DENTAL PATIENTS

The stimuli which result in pain are grouped here according to their origin either as symptoms of disease and injury or as results of dental treatment.

Symptomatic Oral Pain in Children

The most severe dental pains commonly experienced by children are from pulpal and dentoalveolar abscesses. These pains, when they are severe, may occur at any time; but they seem to be more common at night. They appear to begin spontaneously and are usually accompanied by signs of inflammation and infection adjacent to carious, traumatized, and restored teeth. The pain may last for several hours and prevent sleeping, eating, or any other normal activity if it is severe enough. Many primary teeth and even some permanent ones develop abscesses without ever causing the child to complain of pain.

The most common dental pain is probably the brief, sharp pain of varying severity which children experience from time to time when eating and drinking. Sometimes these are vasomotor pains resulting from sudden chilling of teeth and other oral structures by large volumes of very cold food and drink. The same kind of pain may be due to stimulation of dentin which has been exposed to the oral cavity by fracture or by dental caries. Occasionally, this type of pain arises in young permanent teeth in which hypoplastic enamel leaves areas of dentin unprotected from the oral environment in which it soon develops hypersensitivity. These spasms of pain disappear as soon as the stimulus is dissipated unless the injury to the tooth and pulp are severe, in which case there may be prolonged pain. This is the so-called "second pain," a deep, dull ache which follows the "first" bright, superficial pain. Unfortunately, there is no reliable means for determining the condition of a dental pulp from its symptoms. But, in a very general way, the sharper initial pain is, and the longer the second dull ache lasts, the more likely it is that serious trouble exists (Mumford, 1967; Tyldesley and Mumford, 1967).

Another common cause of pain in children which is often mistaken for pulpitis is the pain which is caused by food impaction in open interdental embrasures where carious lesions have destroyed marginal ridges and normal contacts. Such pain may occur while the child eats. It may not occur until several hours later. It is important to identify the cause of this pain so as to avoid unnecessary pulpal therapy or extraction of teeth which are only carious. Careful debridement of the carious lesion and placing correctly contoured restorations will resolve any doubts about the diagnosis in the absence of obvious periodontal damage.

Trauma to hard or soft tissues results in surprisingly little pain of long duration in children. The injured teeth and tissues do not usually ache or cause spontaneous pain, although they will be very painful if manipulated or debrided, especially if astringents are used on tissue.

Other pathological conditions in children which are accompanied by orofacial pain include parotitis or other salivary gland inflammation or infection, tonsillitis, tumors, and subluxations of the temporomandibular joint. Erupting teeth, both primary and permanent, are sometimes a source of pain, especially if they are impacted or develop a pericoronitis, which sometimes happens solely from trauma due to crushing of the operculum during chewing. Occlusal trauma and bruxism sometimes cause children pain.

A burning tongue is usually a symptom of systemic upset. The tongue, gingiva, and other intraoral and labial tissues are very painful in herpetic gingivostomatitis as the vesicles rupture and leave a raw surface of the corium exposed to irritation. This pain interferes seriously with eating and drinking.

A child who reports pain in the oral and facial tissues should be examined as carefully as any adult. If a thorough examination does not reveal a cause for the pain, the dentist is justified in requesting a medical evaluation. Such conscientious follow-up has led to the timely diagnosis of more than one case of leukemia and tumors of the jaws and central nervous system (Macrae, 1959).

It is probable that more pain occurs outside the dental office than occurs in it. There is not much that the dentist can do about pains in children who are not brought to him for care. Someone else must see to them. That someone else may be another dentist, a physician, or a parent. But whoever it is to be will play an important role affecting the child's feelings about dental pain and treatment.

The very first oral pains experienced by a significant number of children appear at the time of teething. Parents and pediatricians and friends and relatives deal with these problems far more often than do dentists. Treatment is directed at producing local analgesia and central sedation and analgesia. These aims are accomplished by repeated direct applications of teething lotions, paregoric, whiskey, ice, aspirin tablets, teething rings, or toast in the area of the erupting teeth. Teething lotions and paregoric are helpful if applied properly. Lotions usually contain a topical anesthetic and a counter irritant. Aspirin should not be applied topically because it burns tissues. Some teething lotions contain mercurials and should never be used (Day, 1968).

Systemic analgesia and sedation are provided by paregoric or phenobarbitol $\frac{1}{4}$ gr. to $\frac{1}{2}$ gr. and acetylsalicylic acid $1\frac{1}{4}$ gr. by mouth every three to four hours as needed for pain. According to an excellent study of the subject by Tasanen (1968), there is no clear evidence of an association between teething and other systemic symptoms, except for greater drooling before one year and greater daytime restlessness. His findings do not support old ideas of teething convulsions, fevers or constipation.

Another kind of dental pain which children experience outside of the dental office is associated with the group of signs and symptoms which we have chosen to call a pain avoidance syndrome. The child may be in acute pain when finally he arrives at the office or there may be no pain at all. There even may be denial of a history of pain. But usually these children are more than a little apprehensive, especially when approached without explanation. Since these patients have extensive carious lesions and sometimes a considerable degree of periodontitis, they have almost certainly had pain from time to time. During those episodes and from them they have learned to avoid pain-producing stimuli. They may have used a number of toothache remedies and pills, too, before seeking professional care. Most over-the-counter toothache drops contain dilute eugenol or oil of cloves. A few contain benzocaine. These agents are harmless and reasonably effective if used according to their directions. They have saved many a late night call to a dentist and many a night's sleep for patients, but in doing so they delay the needed professional treatment, sometimes disastrously long.

When patients with a history of this sort arrive in the dental office or clinic, they perceive as a threat the loss of control of the stimuli to be applied to their teeth. They fear that air, cold water, medications, and instruments will produce the dreaded pain which finally drove them to the dentist. The child's reactions to this threat are loaded with emotion and amount to a fear-flight response characterized by crying and attempts to escape or to protect the mouth and teeth with hands and feet on occasion. In these situations the dentist must first resolve this reaction to fear and pain before he can examine or treat the child effectively. This is usually accomplished gently with reassurance. The gaining of confidence by the child should be nurtured by giving him a degree of control over the proceedings. It might be well at this point to say, while raising the child's hand, "Put up *this* hand when you want to rest and I'll stop right away for a moment." Repeating this in a loud, kind, slow way will help to get the attention needed to get started.

Treating this kind of toothache is fairly simple for a cooperative patient. It is not much more difficult for an uncooperative patient. In such cases there is almost always good localization of the pain by the patient and there is usually ample evidence of dento-alveolar abscesses or pulpal abscesses. If it is at all possible, treatment should be directed at relieving pain at once without sacrificing the tooth. Often this can be done by opening the pulp chamber as quickly and as comfortably as possible. Use of a block anesthesia after premedication with an analgesic and a sedative increases patient comfort. But the operation is very short and even a fearful child in pain will often accept the brief, sharp pain needed to get the relief which invariably follows in moments. Whenever it is available nitrous oxide-oxygen relative analgesia is almost ideal for this procedure. Block anesthesia is often only partly effective in these cases and so it should be supplemented.

The extraction of such carious teeth often leaves an unhappy patient even when general anesthesia and the help of a considerate and skilled oral surgeon is available. The significance of this experience has been the subject of papers by Sosnow (1962), Baldwin (1964, 1966), and Shapiro (1967). All of these authors emphasize the need to reassure and give psychological support to the child patient. No one knows how long lived are the undesirable sequelae of such early experiences; but some adults recount them vividly, and at length.

If it is necessary to defer treating such a tooth, the patient should receive an antibiotic, penicillin being the first choice, to control infection in addition to a potent analgesic.

Pain Associated with Dental Treatment

Pain, as Hardy, Wolff, and Goodell have suggested, is more than a sensation. It has behavioral, emotional and autonomic, conscious, and unconscious components.

Young children, whose behavior is not yet differentiated, react by crying or wiggling or shouting just as vigorously about things they do not like as they do about things that hurt. The dentist with even a little clinical experience can predict the possibilities of pain accurately. However, he cannot always predict patients' perceptions of the stimuli nor their reactions to them, so he should be prepared for the worst.

The most painful stimuli are encountered in surgery and vital pulp therapy. Instrumentation of carious lesions and cavity preparation produce pain and the noxious stimuli of the noises, pressures, and vibrations of instrumentation. Next to these in sensitivity are the anesthetic injections, particularly into palatal tissue, and deep scaling and currettage. Placing rubber dams, placing bite wing radiographic film, and sometimes placing and activating appliances are of a lesser but still significant painfulness. Occasionally, pain may be inflicted during a dental examination. This should be avoided by all means unless it is done deliberately as a diagnostic procedure as in pulp testing.

Of all these causes of pain there is controversy about only one, the amount and kind of pain associated with cavity preparation in children's teeth. First of all, teeth and patients are not all equally sensitive and equally reactive to pain at all times. Second, there are some facts to guide the dentist in predicting when teeth probably will be more or less sensitive. Young teeth, whether primary or permanent, are more sensitive than old teeth. Primary teeth are young until about five years after they erupt. They are old after that. Pulp recession makes the difference. A recent injury or a new active cavity will be more sensitive usually than old or arrested ones. Teeth are very sensitive at the dentino-enamel junction, the deep layers of dentin near the pulp, on the cementum, and most sensitive of all, of course, in the pulp. So carious lesions and cavity preparations which are shallow, or in cementum, or near the pulp will be the most sensitive to instrumentation, heat, medications, and desiccation. A history of pain is an important clue to the need for pain control.

It is important that the dentist establish rapport with any patient before beginning a procedure which likely will be painful. Children want answers to three questions concerning pain: Will it hurt? How much will it hurt? How long will it hurt that much? There's nothing quite so upsetting to them as unexplained, unpredicted pain. "Will it stop or get worse or will it last forever?" they wonder. On the other hand, when injecting an anesthetic, patients sometimes have to be reminded to stop crying when it doesn't hurt anymore.

Some dentists are inclined to the view that it is unwise to treat a child whose oral hygiene is not in an acceptable status. This is very good practice for most children for whom the necessary tooth brushing and flossing can be done painlessly. But this approach is not likely to work well for children whose teeth and tissues hurt when they are cleaned. For these children dental treatment to restore comfort should accompany or precede instruction and practice of modified oral hygiene procedures to reduce discomfort. Arranging treatment in this way makes it much more likely that oral hygiene practices will be comfortable and this will improve the chances of their being done properly.

Postoperative pain is usually not very troublesome in young children even after extensive oral surgery. Dry socket, for instance, is very rare. In older children there is a tendency for greater postoperative discomfort, approaching that seen in adults. The most common postoperative pain which children experience is not caused by dental treatment, but rather by their biting and chewing their tongues, cheeks, and lips while they are insensible following block or infiltration anesthesia. Children and the adults who accompany them to treatment must be given clear instructions to protect them from this danger. A written notice to take home is an excellent preventive of this very painful and worrisome injury. Fortunately, healing is usually uneventful and recovery is complete.

METHODS AND AGENTS FOR CONTROLLING FEAR AND PAIN IN CHILD DENTAL PATIENTS

It seems reasonable to suggest that in the human being pain and fear are supplementary. If this is so, then measures which reduce fear ought to bring about an elevation of the pain threshold and a reduction of reactions to pain. Similarly, reduction of pain perceptions ought to reduce anxiety and fearful reactions. These are the twin goals of measures employed to control fear and pain in child dental patients.

Some dentists and parents feel that children should be spared all but accidental or unpreventable pain; that their anxieties should be minimized or prevented and that crying or other objections to dental treatment ought to be managed by sedation. On the other hand, there are those, equally conscientious dentists and parents, who feel that pain is a necessary part of the human experience and that the individual is strengthened by overcoming fear, pain, and other adversities. The truth probably lies somewhere between these two points of view.

Psychological Measures

When the dentist and his auxiliaries appear to be kind, competent, self-assured and appropriately interested in the welfare of their patients, their actions create confidence and reduce patients' fears. They can be especially effective at this when they know the cultural, educational, and other sociological differences among their child patients and families. These differences will be more and more important in dental offices in the future as patients are drawn from more diversified groups in our American society. An example of these differences could be seen in the reactions of mothers to preoperative sedation which might be viewed as necessary for their children by some mothers but which might be seen as a threat to her child by a mother who is concerned about narcotics abuse.

Chambers (1970) has pointed to the dangers of simplistic interpretations of human behavior, particularly in regard to the child dental patient. He has urged caution in using drugs to sedate children and has explained that there are both good and bad aspects of anxiety. He has described several techniques for guiding the learning of children. They include modeling, or setting a good example; positive and negative reinforcement, which encourage desired behavior and discourage the undesirable; and finally, positive association, which can be used to extinguish fear-producing negative-associations.

Using these and similar techniques a thoughtful dentist can build a community of confidence with the child and proceed with treatment as far as necessary and acceptable. Continuing his instruction as he proceeds from one stage to the next

keeps his patient tuned in with him so that he can reinforce good conduct and encourage associated good feelings.

For most children and dentists these psychological approaches satisfy. They
are simple to use, once they have been learned. They have the additional benefit of
positive after-effects at subsequent appointments.

Children are usually very susceptible to instruction and suggestion from
adults. It is often possible to make use of this characteristic to help children control
their reactions to pain and fear in dental treatment. This may be done by distracting their attention or by increasing their level of suggestibility which involves the
use of techniques also used in hypnosis. Even painful procedures may be done
without discomfort for some suggestible children. Because of this some authors, according to Finn (1961), believe that suggestion is a phase of hypnosis. It is possible
that on occasion highly suggestible children may slip into a hypnotic state without
anyone intending it or realizing that it has happened; however, the deep hypnotic
trance state is not readily attained by children and is very seldom used in treating
them. Many of the reassuring phrases used in calming children during dental treatment and the idea of substituting pleasant euphemisms for unpleasant terms, such
as using "shape" for "grind" or "pinch" for "hurt" have come from experience with
hypnosis. The effective use of this special vocabulary is seen by some authors
(Bartlett, 1970) as a direct contribution to many patients from knowledge gained
from the study of hypnosis.

Partly because of their suggestibility, it is almost always possible to gain a normal child's attention and a little cooperation. From such small beginnings the
thoughtful dentist, who has mastered his own anxiety, can develop a great deal of
cooperation. But, when it is impossible to gain even a little attention and the beginnings of cooperation from a normal child, the dentist should not hesitate to use appropriate physical restraints, including holding the child firmly back in the chair
while muffling his cries with one hand over his mouth while he firmly instructs the
child as described elsewhere in this text.

Pharmacological Measures

Obviously, the majority of children who have dental treatment accept it with
little or no difficulty, but there are a few who require special help. Learning to identify them and learning to select effective means to help them are of special importance to the dentist who treats children.

During the first visit the dentist and the child patient can size up one another.
The dentist can evaluate the child's responses to his instructions as well as his emotional and intellectual functioning. These direct observations of the child and also
of the parent help the dentist decide how best to manage the patient's behavior
during examination and subsequent treatment visits. He can decide at this time
which methods of behavior and pain control will be used.

Some dentists discount the value of this observation and routinely prescribe
premedication for new patients to take before they are seen in the office. Stewart
(1961) described the advantages of premedicating 98 per cent of new patients with
10 to 20 mg. of hydroxyzine. He indicated that nitrous-oxide analgesia and hydroxyzine proved successful in all but 50 of 1500 treatment visits for children. This is
equal to a failure rate of about 3 per cent. Interestingly enough, about the same
percentage of failures occur in clinics and practices where hydroxyzine and nitrous
oxide analgesia are not used routinely. That is, about 3 per cent of otherwise nor-

mal patients need some sedation in order to get through a dental visit intact.

How do dentists develop such different approaches to behavior management? Probably they evolve out of each dentist's attitudes, formal education, and practical experience. Thus it is that a dentist who is not troubled by a child's crying because of anxiety expects others to accept crying as normal behavior, also. Such a dentist would not consider his management of the patient to have failed because the child cried. Another dentist might feel differently as suggested by Kracke (1962), who reported on the effectiveness of routine preoperative sedation using a combination of barbiturate, meperidine and promethazine. He judged the procedure to have failed if the child cried or was restless during the lengthy treatment visits.

The dentist who does not use sedation routinely will find occasionally that his patients need some aid more potent than pragmatic psychology and local anesthesia. The identification of those occasions and the determination of a course of action can be done by guesswork, but good results can be achieved more consistently by following guidelines such as these:

1. Clearly identify the treatment to be done.
2. Decide how much time will be needed in reasonable circumstances.
3. Decide how much discomfort will be caused and what effect this will probably have on the patient.
4. Decide how much disruptive behavior can be accepted without sacrificing the quality of treatment.
5. If too much disruptive behavior probably will occur or if the procedure will be unduly taxing on the patient, decide whether pain or anxiety or both require special measures.
6. Select the drugs which will provide the relief needed.
7. Select the dosages, routes of administration, and times of administration which will probably achieve the desired behavior modification.

Lampshire's (1959) classification of child patients as tensely cooperative, outwardly apprehensive, fearful, and hyperemotive is a useful guide to the degree of behavioral disturbance one might expect from a given child.

The dentist must set objectives for the kind of behavior which he requires of his patients for the treatment he must do in a given length of time. Nearly all patients and dentists can get through brief painful procedures without special help, but as the technical demands, discomfort and length of the procedure increase so does the need for help to secure the patient's cooperation or passivity.

The choice of agents, or combinations of agents, will be determined after evaluating the patient's need for special help to elevate the pain threshold with analgesics and anesthetics and to reduce anxiety and fear with sedatives and tranquilizers. The dosages of analgesics, sedatives, or tranquilizers to be used before and during dental treatment are governed by all the conditions which govern their safe and effective use generally, with one additional special consideration. Most dosage recommendations given in package inserts, pharmacopeias and the like are those which are used under normal circumstances, not dental treatment situations. Thus, the normal dosage of a barbiturate for an ill child being put to bed to go to sleep, would be too small to sedate that same child if, when well, he were brought to the dental office for treatment. He might be overexcited instead of sedated in the dental setting by that low dose. The stimulation provided in dental treatment can overcome the normal effects of the customary dosages of analgesics, sedatives and tranquilizers which have been developed for the most part for non-dental purposes. In a similar way the dosages of premedication which are used prior to general anesthesia will not be effective for the patient who is to be treated while awake. The determination of the right dose begins with knowledge of the desirable and dangerous properties of the drugs available and their effects on physiology and behavior.

The required dosages of commonly used analgesics, sedatives, and tranquilizers are increased with increases in children's body size, age, weight, activity and alertness. A full stomach reduces or delays absorption of orally administered medications. Patients who are debilitated require smaller doses. Drug tolerance may raise dosage requirements or may result in no drug effect at any dose. Synergism reduces dosage and must be considered when prescribing more than one drug or when prescribing for a patient already taking another medication.

The most satisfactory guide to selection of drug dosage for children is the body surface area. Pugh (1963) has described the use of Augsberger's rule for calculating children's dosages from their body surface area. Pugh gives Augsberger's formula as: $0.7 \times$ weight in pounds = % of adult dose, by which the dosage for a child is calculated as a percentage of the adult dosage. Use of this formula results in dosages that are about 7 per cent too low for children who weigh 45 to 85 pounds. A more realistic dosage schedule for children has been prepared by Leach and Wood (1967). Table 7–1 presents the dose proportions which they determined on the basis of body surface area, but which are related to body weight in the table for easy reference.

Dosage guides and tables do not eliminate the need to calculate dosages for individual patients. The drug effects must be evaluated and the dosage corrected as needed. Album (1961) recommends what might be called titration of a drug dosage, which is accomplished by giving the calculated dose of the drug and in one hour giving up to half that dose again if satisfactory sedation is not achieved. It is important to remember that many variables affect the response to analgesics and sedatives, and therefore over- and under-dosing are bound to occur from time to time. If the dosage is within the safe range, there is no harm in this except for the inconvenience.

TABLE 7–1 DOSE AS PROPORTION OF ADULT DOSE AND IN MG. PER KG. FOR DIFFERENT AGE-GROUPS

	Weight		(A) Dose as Proportion of Adult Dose	(B) Dose in mg. per kg. If Adult Dose is 1 mg. per kg.
Age	lb.	kg.		
Adult	145	66	1	1.0
12 yr.	82	37	3/4	1.25
7 yr.	51	23	1/2	⎫
3 yr.	33	15	1/3	⎬ 1.5
1 yr.	22	10	1/4	⎭
4 mo.	14	6.5	1/5	⎫ ⎬ 2.0
2 wk.	7	3.2	1/8	⎭

From Leach, R. H. and Wood, B. S. B. Drug dosage for children. Lancet, 2:1350–1351, 1967.

In his 1961 article, Album tested ten rules for drug administration which deserve repetition here.

Rules for Drug Administration

1. An adult must accompany the patient.
2. Strict supervision in the office.
3. Wait a reasonable time after administration.
4. Parents must supervise children closely after administration of a drug.
5. A quiet environment is essential.
6. Vital reflexes must not be impaired.
7. Never use premedication during an acute illness.
8. Parents must be told of postoperative rules.
9. The dentist must know the drug's effects and side effects.
10. Emergency medications must be available.
    An eleventh rule might be:
11. Know the patient's physical condition and drug history.

Pharmacological Agents Used for the Control of Pain

Analgesics.   Agents used to reduce pain without affecting consciousness are called analgesics. They act by elevating the pain threshold or modifying central perception, interpretation and reaction or by depressing reflex activity and reducing psychogenic aspects of pain.

NARCOTIC ANALGESICS.   The only one of the several opium alkaloids which is used to any extent in dentistry for children is codeine phosphate. It is only about $1/20$ as effective as morphine. In general, the very potent and addictive morphine is reserved for intractable pain, which occurs very seldom in children.

The most widely used of the synthetic opiates is meperidine, which frequently has been used as a premedication for operative dentistry alone and in combination with promethazine. Like morphine, it is a central nervous system depressant and dangers from overdosage are cerebral stimulation, tachycardia, disorientation, muscle twitching, and respiratory depression. It is relatively inefficient when taken by mouth. The narcotics are thought to act by elevation of the pain threshold through depression of the cerebral cortex, hypothalamus and the medullary centers.

NON-NARCOTIC ANALGESICS.   Aspirin and the popular combination of aspirin, phenacetin, and caffeine, known as APC are quite effective oral analgesics. Their analgesic action is due to peripheral blockage of the algesic effect of bradykinin; there is also a central effect at the thalamic level. Propoxyphene, which is available alone in 32 mg. and 55 mg. doses, is somewhat more effective than aspirin in a 65 mg. dose in combination with aspirin, phenacetin, and caffeine.

All of these drugs are useful pre- and postoperatively for pain control. They are potentiated by sedatives, particularly the barbiturates. They are listed in Table 7–2 in descending order of potency.

OTHER ANALGESICS OF INTEREST.   Nitrous-oxide and oxygen relative analgesia is enjoying a renewed popularity. When administered in concentrations between 40 per cent and 80 per cent, nitrous-oxide produces analgesia and euphoria. It is said to produce general anesthesia only in the presence of anoxia and so its use for that purpose is discouraged. Langa (1962) and Hogue et al. (1971) have reported very satisfactory experiences with nitrous-oxide analgesia for children. Special training is needed to learn the safe use of this procedure. Everett and Allen (1971a) have recently reported that nitrous oxide-oxygen mixtures have little or no effect on cardiorespiratory function at analgesic levels.

Everett and Allen (1970, 1971b) have reported satisfactory analgesia in adults with combinations of pentobarbital, meperidine, and scopolamine with local anesthesia. Intravenous analgesia is not much used in treating normal children.

Anesthetics. General anesthesia has its proper place in dental treatment of children. It generally is used as a last resort when all alternatives have had to be rejected as unproductive. Discussion of the properties and uses of general anesthesia lies outside the scope of this chapter. Any dentist who wishes to perform these services must have special training.

Local anesthesia is the most commonly used means for pain control in dentistry. While local dental anesthesia can be produced by pressure or cold (Fritz, 1953), and even, it is claimed, by electrical methods (Brooks et al., 1970), the most popular and effective means remains the injection of a solution of a local anesthetic along a nerve trunk to block conduction or peripherally at the nerve trunk termination by infiltration of the tissues.

There are several hazards of low order involved in the use of local anesthesia for adult patients, such as accidental intravenous injections, which Schiano et al. (1964) reported to happen in up to 15 per cent of block anesthesia injections in the area of the mental, sphenopalatine and mandibular nerves. Aspiration is recommended prior to injection to control this complication. In addition to this hazard, child patients present two special problems. First, they require more careful preparation to assure their cooperation and safety during injection. No child should be injected unless his body movements are under complete control. Second, it is erroneously believed that the innervation of the child's mouth differs from the adults when in fact it does not. While distances between landmarks are slightly shorter and landmarks themselves are slightly smaller, there is little or no difference in their relationship between adults and children. It is popular to blame a missed mandibular block on a misplaced mandibular canal. It is much more likely to be due to a misplaced needle and an injection that was made too low, too far anteriorly, or too far medially. Goldberg (1961) and Berns (1962), have showed radiographically, using radiopaque material injected with local anesthetic, that the anesthetic will spread far enough to produce anesthesia providing the solution is not separated from the nerve by a layer of muscle or a fascial plane. Thus, it is not essential to hit the mandibular nerve with the tip of the needle to produce anesthesia; it is only necessary to be reasonably close. An excellent article describing techniques of administering local anesthesia to children has been published by Mink (1966). An important part of his description concerns the use of topical anesthetics. It is very good practice to apply an effective topical anesthetic for three minutes by the clock before injecting a child's oral tissues.

Epstein (1971) and Schmidt (1970) have reported very satisfactory topical anesthesia with the use of pressure jet injection of local anesthetics in adults and children. This produced excellent topical anesthesia and made it possible to inject painlessly in the area with a needle. In some instances sufficient anesthesia was obtained for painless cavity preparation when several applications were made with the jet injector on the buccal and lingual sides of the alveolus.

TABLE 7–2   BASIC ADULT DOSAGE OF SEVERAL COMMON ANALGESICS

Drug	Route of Administration	Daily Frequency	Adult Dose
Morphine SO$_4$	I.M.	4–6	10.0 mg.
	P.O.	4–6	15.0 mg.
Meperidine HCl	I.M.	4–6	50–100 mg.
	P.O.	4–6	50–100 mg.
Codeine PO$_4$	P.O.	6–8	5–10.0 mg.
A.P.C.	P.O.	4–6	1–2 tablets
Dextropropoxyphene HCl	P.O.	4–6	32–65 mg.
Aspirin	P.O.	6–8	300–600 mg.

Children's dosage is calculated by Augsberger's Rule (0.7 × weight in pounds = % of adult dose).

Table 7–2 contains a list of the more widely used local anesthetics, indicating their potency and duration of the anesthesia they produce (Reeve, 1970).

New local anesthetics are frequently reported. Some of the more recent reports have dealt with local anesthetic properties of psychotomimetic or tranquilizing drugs (Bowles, 1971) and antihistamines (Mattern 1968).

Pharmacological Agents which Modify Anxiety and Fear

Sedatives and Hypnosis.   There are many drugs which have sedative effects. The term hypnotic is given only to those sedative drugs which promote natural

TABLE 7–3   COMMON LOCAL ANESTHETICS

Duration

Short 1/2–1 Hour	Primacaine Duocaine	Nesacaine Monocaine
Medium 1–2½ Hours	Metycaine Unacaine Pontocaine	Primacaine Duocaine Dynacaine
	Citanest	
Long 2½ Hours +	Kincaine Xylocaine	Carbocaine Ravocaine

Potency Compared to Xylocaine

Less	Procaine Monocaine	Oracaine
Equal	Metycaine Kincaine Nesacaine Citanest	Dynacaine Carbocaine Unacaine Primacaine
Much Greater	Ravocaine	Pontocaine

sleep. The barbiturates, together with chloral hydrate, paraldehyde, and related drugs as well as derivatives of glutarimide and another half dozen nondescripts constitute the bulk of the hypnotic drugs.

The barbiturates and chloral hydrate are commonly used for sedation of child dental patients. They induce a calm sleep from which children are easily aroused, sometimes quite excited. According to Jones (1969), this paradoxical reaction to barbiturates, as this excitement is called, occurs in about 3 per cent of patients given $1\frac{1}{4}$ grains of secobarbitol prior to dental treatment.

Phenobarbital (Luminal), amobarbital (Amytal), pentobarbital sodium (Nembutal sodium), secobarbital (Seconal) and thiopental sodium (Pentothal sodium) are the most commonly used. The barbiturates have many uses and few side effects which usually occur only at high dosage (Krantz and Carr, 1969). They are commonly used to prepare unruly children for pediatric examinations. Barbiturates have a wide margin of safety and so are excellent for sedating ambulatory patients since the hypnotic dose is from three to six times larger than the sedative dose. Ordinarily, the short acting barbiturates, secobarbital, pentobarbital, and amobarbital, are preferred although phenobarbital is common. These drugs have the additional advantage of being very inexpensive. They are moderately addictive.

Chloral hydrate, like the barbiturates, is a drug with a wide safety margin. It is more often used at a hypnotic dosage of a little less than 1.0 gram for preschool-age children. It has less effect in safe doses in older children in need of sedation for dental treatment. It has an unpleasant taste. It is not indicated in patients with heart disease.

Paraldehyde, which is occasionally and unaccountably lethal, is not indicated in dental procedures.

Tranquilizing Drugs. Because there is some disagreement about terminology the words "tranquilizer" and "psycholeptic" are here used in the same sense, referring to drugs which have a special antipsychotic effect. The diverse effects of these drugs cannot be explained on any simple basis. It is thought that they may act by enzyme inhibition to prevent chemical transmitter destruction in the brain, or they may bring about biochemical metabolic changes at subcellular levels. Some of them also change the electrical activity of specific regions of the brain.

One group of these drugs, known as the phenothiazines includes three of the tranquilizers which have been successfully used for child dental patients. They are chlorpromazine, prochlorperazine and promazine. Promethazine, which is often used with meperidine, is related to the phenothiazines, but usually it is classified as an antihistamine rather than as a tranquilizer. These three phenothiazines are part of a larger group of major tranquilizers. Another group of tranquilizers is called the minor group; it contains some phenothiazines as well as other drugs. Two of the minor tranquilizers also are often used by the dental profession. They are a diphenylmethane derivative, hydroxyzine, and a benzodiazepine, diazepam.

The distinction between major and minor tranquilizers lies in their ability to reduce major or minor manifestations of anxiety and tension.

The drugs which have been used most frequently for dental tranquilization are the benzodiazepine, Valium; the phenothiazines, Thorazine, Mellaril and Compazine; the propane derivative, Equanil; and the diphenylmethanes, Atarax and Vistanil.

All these drugs have been shown to have beneficial effects for dental patients in controlled studies. There is no evidence whatsoever on which to base a preferential choice of one over the other, regardless of the claims of the manufacturers. All are effective; all are minor tranquilizers except the three phenothiazines, Thorazine, Mellaril and Compazine (Brown, 1968; Kopel, 1959; Lang, 1965; Rosenbaum, 1966; and Shamer, 1958).

The tranquilizers, sedatives, analgesics, and sometimes other drugs are used in combinations intended to provide balanced medication with a drug present to affect the patient's pain perception, fear reactions, and even to reduce salivation and promote euphoria.

Buckman (1956) described successful use in children of chlorpromazine and scopolamine or elixir of pentobarbital, followed by meperidine and scopolamine. Engelman (1960) also used a combination of meperidine and scopolamine, but added promethazine for tranquilization instead of pentobarbital. Foreman (1970), who is an authority on intravenous medication, reported on the effective use of several combinations of tranquilizers, analgesics, and barbiturate sedatives in a procedure of intermittent anesthesia.

Robbins, in 1967, reported effective use of chloral hydrate and promethazine for fearful children.

There is a bewildering variety of techniques, agents, drugs, and philosophies concerned with the management of pain and sedation in children. The dentist who wishes to make good use of the information is beset by the problem of trying to decide where to start. The best approach would seem to be to start by using only one drug for forty or fifty patients. In this way the variabilities of dosage and patient response can be mastered. It is likely that more useful experience will come from this approach than from using a larger number of drugs. It would be useful to select one analgesic, one sedative, and one tranquilizer to use repeatedly alone and in combinations until the results of dosage variation in different circumstances can be predicted more and more accurately. Records must be kept if this experience is to be useful.

REFERENCES

1. Baldwin, D. C. Jr.: Value of waiting period in psychological preparation for dental extraction. J. Dent. Res., 43(Suppl.):826–827, 1964. Abst.
2. Baldwin, D. C. Jr.: An investigation of psychological and behavioral responses to dental extractions in children. J. Dent. Res., 45(Suppl.):1637–1651, 1966.
3. Bartlett, K. A. Jr.: Knowledge gained from hypnosis. J.A.D.A., 80:125–132, 1970.
4. Berns, J. M., and Sandove, M. S.: Mandibular block injection: A method of study using an injected radiopaque material. J.A.D.A., 65:735–745, 1962.
5. Birns, B., Barton, S., and Bridger, W. H.: Individual differences in temperament characteristics of infants. Trans. N. Y. Acad. Sci., 31:1071–1082, 1969.
6. Borland, L. R.: Odontophobia—Inordinate fear of dental treatment. Dent. Clin. N. Amer., pp. 683–695, 1962.
7. Bowles, W. H.: Chlorpromazine as a possible local anesthetic in dentistry. J. Dent. Res., 50:906–910, 1971.
8. Brooks, B., Reiss, R. and Umans, R.: Local electroanesthesia in dentistry. J. Dent. Res., 49:298–300, 1970.
9. Brown, P. R. H. et al.: Diazepan in dentistry: Report on 108 patients. Brit. Dent. J., 125:498–501, 1968.
10. Buckman, N.: Balanced premedication in pedodontics. J. Dent. Child., 23:140–153, 1956.
11. Chambers, D. W.: Managing the anxieties of young dental patients. J. Dent. Child., 37:19–34, 1970.
12. Day, R. L.: O-T-C oral hygiene aids. J. Amer. Pharm. Assoc., 8:72–78, 1968.
13. Engelman, M. A.: An investigation of balanced premedication for children in the general practice of dentistry. N. Y. State Dent. J., 26:371–380, 1960.

14. Epstein, S.: Pressure injection of local anesthetics: clinical evaluation of an instrument. J.A.D.A., 82:374–377, 1971.

15. Everett, G. B. and Allen, G. D.: Simultaneous evaluation of cardiorespiratory and analgesic effects of intravenous analgesia in combination with local anesthesia. J.A.D.A., 81:926–931, 1970.

16. Everett, G. B., and Allen, G. D.: Simultaneous evaluation of cardiorespiratory and analgesic effects of nitrous oxide-oxygen inhalation analgesia. J.A.D.A., 83:129–133, 1971a.

17. Everett, G. B. and Allen, G. D.: Simultaneous evaluation of cardiorespiratory and pentobarbital, meperidine and scopolamine with local anesthesia. J.A.D.A., 83:155–158, 1971b.

18. Finn, S. B.: Hypnosis in the Pedodontic Practice. Dent. Clin. N. Amer., pp. 521–531, November 1961.

19. Foreman, P. A.: Pain control and patient management in dentistry – a review of current intravenous techniques. J.A.D.A., 80:101–111, 1970.

20. Fritz, J. R.: Refrigeration anesthesia of the dentition in cavity preparation. Internat. J. Anesth., 1:46–49, 1953.

21. Goldberg, A. F., and Sandove, M. S.: Further studies in spread of local anesthetics. J. Oral Surg., 19:232–236, 1961.

22. Hardy, J. D., Wolff, H. G., and Goodell, H.: Pain Sensations and Reactions. New York, Hafner Pub. Co., 1967.

23. Hogue, D. et al.: The responses to nitrous oxide analgesia in children. J. Dent. Child., 38(2):65–69, 1971.

24. Howitt, J. W., and Stricker, G.: The influence of age, sex, intelligence and modified environment upon childrens reactions to tooth pain. N. Y. Dent. J., 29:262–264, 1963.

25. Howitt, J. W., and Stricker, G.: Physiological recording during simulated dental appointments. N. Y. Dent. J., 31:204–206, 1965a.

26. Howitt, J. W. and Stricker, G.: Child response to various dental procedures. J.A.D.A., 70:70–74, 1965b.

27. Howitt, J. W. and Stricker, G.: Sequential changes in response to dental procedures. J. Dent. Res., 49(5):1074–1077, 1970.

28. Johnson, R., and Koenigsberg, S. R.: Child behavior during sequential dental visits., I.A.D.R. Abstracts, #872, p. 270, Mar. 1971.

29. Jones, K. F.: Preoperative medications in operative dentistry for children., J. Dent. Child., 36:19–28, 1969.

30. Kopel, H. M.: The use of ataractics in dentistry for children. From a Symposium on Newer Concepts on Drug Therapy and Dosage in Dentistry for Children. J. Dent. Child., 26(1):14–24, 1959.

31. Kracke, R. R.: Premedication in children undergoing single-visit, multiple cavity repair. J. Dent. Child., 29:207–210, 1962.

32. Krantz, J. C. Jr., and Carr, C. J.: Central nervous system depressants. The barbiturates. In Pharmacologic Principles of Medical Practice. 7th ed., Baltimore, The Williams & Wilkins Co., 1969, pp. 176–191.

33. Lampshire, E. L.: Balanced medication. J. Dent. Child., 26(1):25–28, 1959.

34. Lang, L. L.: An evaluation of the efficacy of hydroxyzine (Atarax-Vistaril) in controlling the behavior of child patients. J. Dent. Child., 32(4):253–258, 1965.

35. Langa, H.: Analgesia for modern pedodontists. N. Y. State Dent. J., 28:58–64, 1962.

36. Leach, R. H., and Wood, B. S. B.: Drug dosage for children. Lancet, 2:1350–1351, 1967.

37. Lewis, T. M., and Law, D. B.: Investigations of certain autonomic responses of children to a specific dental stress. J.A.D.A., 57:769–777, 1958.

38. Lim, R. K. S.: A revised concept of the mechanism of analgesia and pain. In Pain. Knighton, R. S. and Drunke, P. R. (eds.), Boston, Little Brown and Co., 1966, pp. 117–154.

39. McRae, D.: Intercranial causes of oral and facial pain. Dent. Clin. N. Amer., pp. 529–542, July 1959.

40. Mattern, J. B., and Gander, R.: Antihistamines as local anesthetic agents for allergic patients. J. Colorado Dent. Assoc., 46:26–28, 1968.

41. Merskey, H., and Spear, F. G.: Pain; Psychological and Psychiatric Aspects. London, Bailliere, Tindall and Cassell, 1967.

42. Mink, J. R., and Spedding, R. H.: An injection procedure for the child dental patient. Dent. Clin. N. Amer., pp. 309–325, July 1966.

43. Molin, C., and Seeman, K.: Disproportionate dental anxiety and clinical considerations. Acta Odont. Scand., 28:197–212, 1970.

44. Mumford, J. M.: Pain perception threshold on stimulating human teeth and the histological condition of the pulp. Brit. Dent. J., 123:427–433, 1967.

45. Perryman, J. H., Wolff, B. B., and Yerre, C.: Experimental pain: autonomic correlates of threshold and tolerance responses. I.A.D.R. Abstracts, No. 854, pp. 266, March 1971.

46. Pugh, C. E.: Drug dosages for children by Augsbergers new rule. J. Dent. Child., 30:41–45, 1963.

47. Reeve, L. W.: Modern pharmacodynamic concepts of local anesthesia. Dent. Clin. N. Amer., pp. 783–804, October, 1970.

48. Robbins, M. B.: Chloral hydrate and promethazine as premedicants for the apprehensive child. J. Dent. Child., *34*:327–331, 1967.
49. Rosenbaum, C. H.: Mellaril—an aid to behavior control. J. Dent. Child., *33*:244–245, 1966.
50. Schiano, A. M., and Strambi, R.: Frequency of accidental intravascular injection of local anesthetics in dental practice. Oral Surg., Oral Med., Oral Path., *17*:178–184, 1964.
51. Schmidt, D. A.: Jet injection: High speed infiltration anesthesia. J. Dent. Child., *37*:17–20, 1970.
52. Shamer, D. H., Sanders, D. J., and Dobbs, E. C.: Tranquilizers in dentistry for children. J. Dent. Child., *25*(4):269–273, 1958.
53. Shannon, I. L., and Isbell, G. M.: VII. Adrenocortical responses in patients receiving intraoral injections. Oral Surg., Oral Med., Oral Path., *16*:1145–1149, 1963.
54. Shapiro, D. N.: Reactions of children to oral surgery experience. J. Dent. Child., *34*(2):97–107, 1967.
55. Ship, I. I., and White, C. L.: Physiologic response to dental stress. Oral Surg., Oral Med., Oral Path., *13*:368–376, 1960.
56. Sosnow, I.: The emotional significance of the loss of teeth. Dent. Clin. N. Amer., pp. 637–650, November 1962.
57. Stewart, J. G.: Routine preoperative medication in dentistry for children. J. Dent. Child., *28*:209–212, 1961.
58. Tasanen, A.: General and local effects of the eruption of deciduous teetn. Annales Pediat. Fenn., *14*:(Suppl.)28, 1968.
59. Tyldesley, W. R. and Mumford, J. M.: Dental pain and the histological condition of the dental pulp. Dent. Pract., *20*:333–336, 1970.

8

OPERATIVE DENTISTRY FOR CHILDREN

by JOSEPH M. SIM
and SIDNEY B. FINN

For the dentist who treats children a major goal is preserving the integrity of the deciduous teeth so that normal function is maintained and normal exfoliation occurs. In achieving this goal the dentist has the satisfaction of knowing he has exerted all his skills toward preparing the way for healthy permanent teeth to erupt and assume their rightful places in the dental arches and, by so doing, contribute to the child's total health. If any of these primary teeth should be lost prematurely, a significant and lasting damage may be done to the permanent dentition.

For the child, elements of the primary dentition must remain healthy for a period from about six months of age to approximately age 11, when the maxillary cuspids are shed, in the normal course of events. During this period of about 11 years these teeth are subject to the vicissitudes of abrasion, attrition, trauma, and dental caries just as are the adult teeth.

Although in individual teeth the anatomy differs somewhat, the primary dentition functions and superficially resembles that of the adult. However, because of the child's immaturity, the differences in dental anatomy, and the timing of exfoliation, the approach to many procedures in operative dentistry for children may clearly differ from that to similar procedures in an adult. In restoring these teeth the dentist is forced to make decisions which are important to his practice and often of lasting importance to the children he treats. Operatory equipment chosen wisely and the increased utilization of his dental assistant can make a profound impact on a dentist's young patients. (See Fig. 8–1.)

Undoubtedly some of these restorative decisions are difficult to make. It is perhaps best to remember to try to treat children's teeth in view of what is best for the child, and not what is easiest for the parent or for the dentist. Treatment planning, therefore, is not always a simple procedure, and the variables which enter into decisions made by the dentist are many.

135

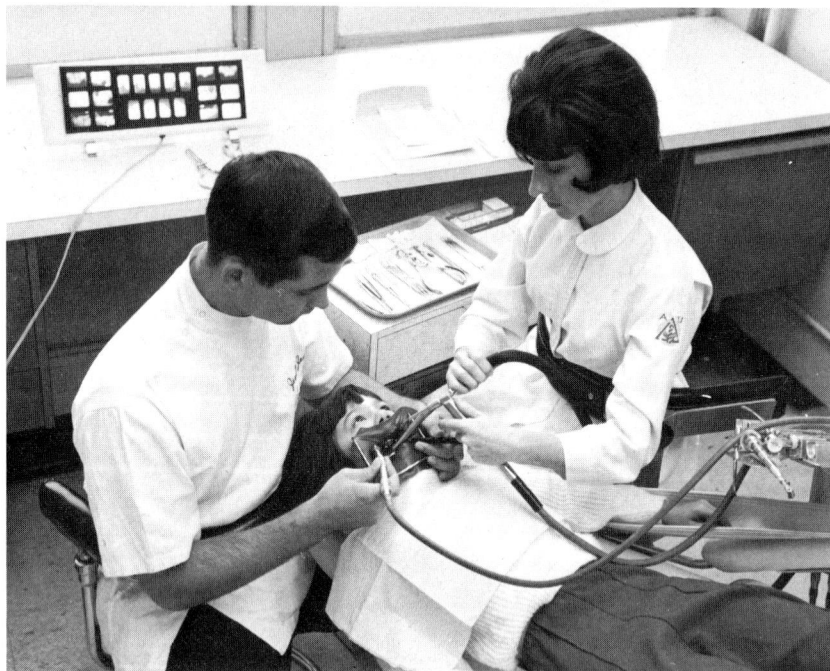

Figure 8–1   Dentist performing operative dental care fully utilizing his assistant. Restorative care can be accomplished with less fatigue for the dentist and his assistant, and with greater comfort for the child, if both the dentist and the assistant are seated and the child is in a supine position. Note the arrangement of the instruments and their accessibility to the assistant and the operator.

ADDITIONAL GOALS FOR THE DENTIST

The dentist must establish additional goals for himself if he is to be successful in the restorative care of children's teeth. He must extend himself to comprehend the *needs* of children and their parents. He must spend time and effort teaching parents and children in his practice and in his community the *value* of preserving the primary and young permanent dentition of children. He must pass on to parents the information regarding *when* children's teeth should receive restorative care.

UNDERSTANDING THE NEEDS OF PARENTS AND CHILDREN

A dentist must understand the needs of his child patients and their parents. To accomplish this it is necessary to listen to their explanations of the dental problems which they feel they have. It is all too easy to begin to present a dental diagnosis to a parent before listening but it must be remembered that the child arrived in the dental office because of some motivation or need. Listen carefully to identify these, since it will simplify the approach to caring for the child. A dentist who listens will be regarded as a warm and outstanding human being.

AGES AT WHICH RESTORATIVE CARE IS BEST ACCOMPLISHED

The maturity of the child has some bearing on the age at which good restorative care may be accomplished. Although many pedodontists suggest that children be seen for routine dental examinations as early as 18 months, it is usually at two to three years of age that restorative care will be initiated. Children who have not dispensed with the sweetened bottle feeding habit by age two years may require this care earlier.

Certainly every child should have a complete dental examination by age three years. Only by encouraging early care can a real effort toward caries prevention be realized. In families who have several children, the dentist observes that the children seen early are generally better patients and that the restorative care rendered will be more meaningful in preserving the total function of the deciduous teeth.

In his office the dentist has many means of gathering information concerning the child which will assist him in making decisions. These include a short questionnaire filled out by the parent, the health history taken by the dentist, together with direct chairside observation using mirror and explorer, palpation and percussion of the teeth, and examination of the surrounding soft tissues. To these are added the dentist's impression of the maturity of the child and his psychological as well as his physical health.

Other aids to diagnosis are good clear radiographs, transillumination, vitality tests, and hand excavating instruments to determine the extent of decay and its proximity to the pulp. All of this information should be employed in deciding whether to restore or extract a primary tooth. A dentist should not condemn a permanent or primary tooth to extraction without first exerting every effort to make a proper evaluation of the available facts acquired through the use of all the diagnostic aids at his command.

OPERATIVE PROCEDURES FOR PRIMARY TEETH

CONTROL OF PAIN AND DISCOMFORT

Most dentists with broad experience in children's dentistry agree that the proper and comfortable management of children in their offices is the key to good operative dentistry.

If use of a local anesthetic or mild premedication or both can make any procedure more comfortable and less painful, then it should be utilized. Increasingly, nitrous oxide as an analgesic measure is being administered first to lower the apprehension and discomfort associated with injections.

Careful injections following application of a paste topical anesthetic at the site of the injection can do much to allay the fears of the child and improve the quality of the operative dentistry. Infiltration of a short-acting local anesthetic buccal or labial to the maxillary teeth, and an inferior alveolar block for mandibular teeth can be used with marked success on children of all ages, even the very young. (See Fig. 8–2.)

For the handicapped or psychically unprepared children when cooperation is

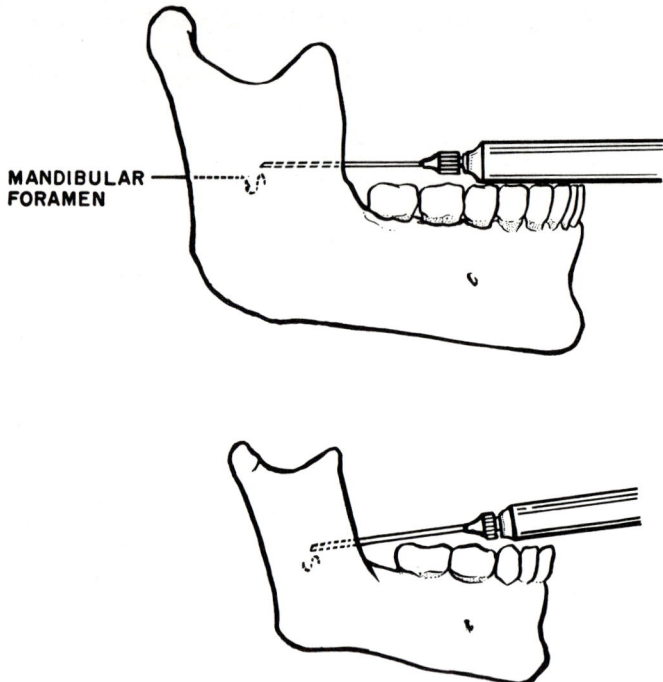

Figure 8–2   Inferior alveolar block. The mandibular foramen is *above* the plane of occlusion in the adult. It is *below* the plane of occlusion in children.

difficult to obtain, moderate or deep premedication with Elixir of Chloralhydrate, Seconal, Nembutal alone or in combination with various types of tranquilizing drugs may be used. Dosages and routes of administration are described in Chapter 7. In teen-age children who may have a high level of anxiety when undergoing dental care, controlled presedation over a period can be used to allay psychic trauma. After initial success, the dosage for each appointment may be decreased as anxiety is overcome and confidence is established. Hopefully, a time is reached when further sedation is unnecessary.

In many practices there will be some children whose work cannot be accomplished under normal office conditions. General anesthesia should be made available for the physically handicapped or psychically inadequate children. During these procedures, usually accomplished at a hospital, full mouth restorative care can be provided by the family dentist or pedodontist during one operative session.

USE OF 4-HANDED DENTISTRY TECHNIQUES

The utilization of 4-handed dentistry techniques is one of the most significant advances a dentist may incorporate into his office routine. It promotes comfort and a sense of well-being in his child patients as well as the dentist and his auxiliaries.

For many practitioners 4-handed dentistry improves the quality of dental care they may offer their patients because the positional fatigue factor is markedly lessened. It also opens many opportunities for the expansion of the roles and duties of the auxiliary personnel he employs in his office.

Children operated on in a reclining position are not only more comfortable but are more easily controlled if they try to move suddenly during a critical operative procedure. It is a rare dentist who once having operated in this way, reverts to his older method.

USE OF THE RUBBER-DAM

The use of the rubber dam is one of the most valuable approaches a dentist can develop in rendering excellent restorative care for children. Its superiority in skilled hands is unquestioned for the following reasons:

1. It gives both the inexperienced and experienced operator the key to successfully managing nearly all children.

2. It increases the quality and quantity of work produced in a unit of time, because it retracts the cheeks and tongue away from the field of operation, literally giving the operator "extra hands." It also lessens the possibility of bur injury to the tissues and the swallowing or aspiration of foreign material.

3. It provides a dry field when necessary for bases, pulp capping, or pulpotomy procedures, and for insertion and condensation of amalgam restorations.

4. It allows the use of air-water spray on high speed burs, and facilitates the use of high-volume suction tips held by the dental assistant. At the same time it obviates the necessity of using a saliva ejector because the child is operated on while reclining in a supine position.

5. It affords the operator greater total visibility and accessibility for the necessary procedures.

Many dentists have speculated why the rubber dam has such a calming effect on children after the area to be operated on has been properly anesthetized. Some children will indeed sleep through most of a dental office visit when the dam is used. Jinks and others have stated that it is because the child "seems to acquire a sense of protection from the very fact that the teeth seem to be isolated from the rest of the body."

In the authors' experience the children seem to accept the rubber dam as an *artificial cheek*, warm, slick, and non-tasting, which is gently and rather naturally pressing their tongues out of the usual resting positions. Involuntary tongue thrusting toward the isolated teeth, which appears many times when using cotton rolls, is eliminated by using the rubber dam.

With the new emphasis in recent years on horizontal patient positioning with the dentist and assistant seated, the dentist now initiates no gagging in his young patients when water sprays, air, and suction are used with the rubber dam in place.

The dentist who returns to the use of the rubber dam after relinquishing its use in the belief that it extends the operating time during any procedure longer than a simple occlusal cavity is invariably surprised, not so much at the timesaving qualities, but at the children's attitude toward his work. He will find that children are at ease and relaxed during the procedure, and that they take an active interest in the mixing of the amalgam, the condensation, and the carving. The clinician can have the patient hold an unbreakable mirror so that he can watch these fascinating procedures.

As Jinks has so ably summed up, "The rubber dam provides a security for the child that no other method can provide." The dentist directly benefits from the security in his child patient by having to spend less time on most procedures, by being at ease, and by better handpiece control during critical restorative work.

Equipment

The necessary equipment for using the rubber dam for children may be varied to suit the individual tastes of the dentist. In the following list of items, the authors' specific suggestions are in parentheses at the right: (See Fig. 8–3.)

5 × 5 inch rubber dam (dark heavy or extra heavy)
Rubber dam punch
Rubber dam forceps
Rubber dam frame (Young's)
Waxed dental floss
Scissors (Curved crown and collar)
Petroleum jelly
Clamps for partially erupted teeth (Ivory #14, #14A)
Clamps for fully erupted teeth (S.S. White #18; #206; Ivory #00)
Blue articulating paper

Most rubber dam clamps need not be altered in any fashion although Jinks and Tocchini advocate such changes as altering the wings or placing grooves in the wings of clamps to facilitate application. If the hole punched for the clamp is lubricated with petroleum jelly, the rubber slips over the wings easily with finger pressure alone. The clamps get sprung out during use, however, and one should use his fingers to squeeze them closed again, thus restoring most of the original gripping force of the clamp. Also after much use the jaws of the clamps become worn, and should be sharpened with a small tapered stone and polished so that the clamp has less tendency to slide on a tooth.

Due to the increased use of the reclined position for operative procedures with child patients, an added precaution is suggested regarding the use of clamps.

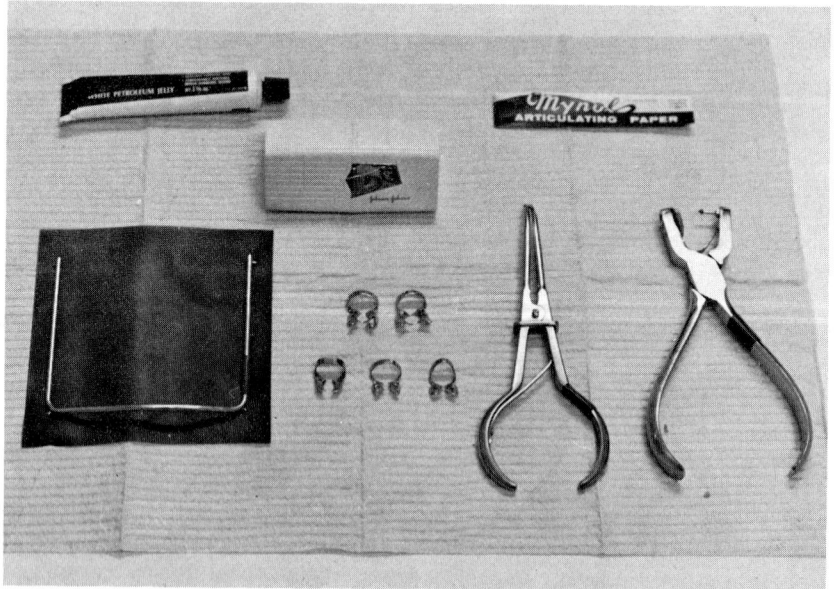

Figure 8–3 The instrument set-up for utilizing the rubber dam for children.

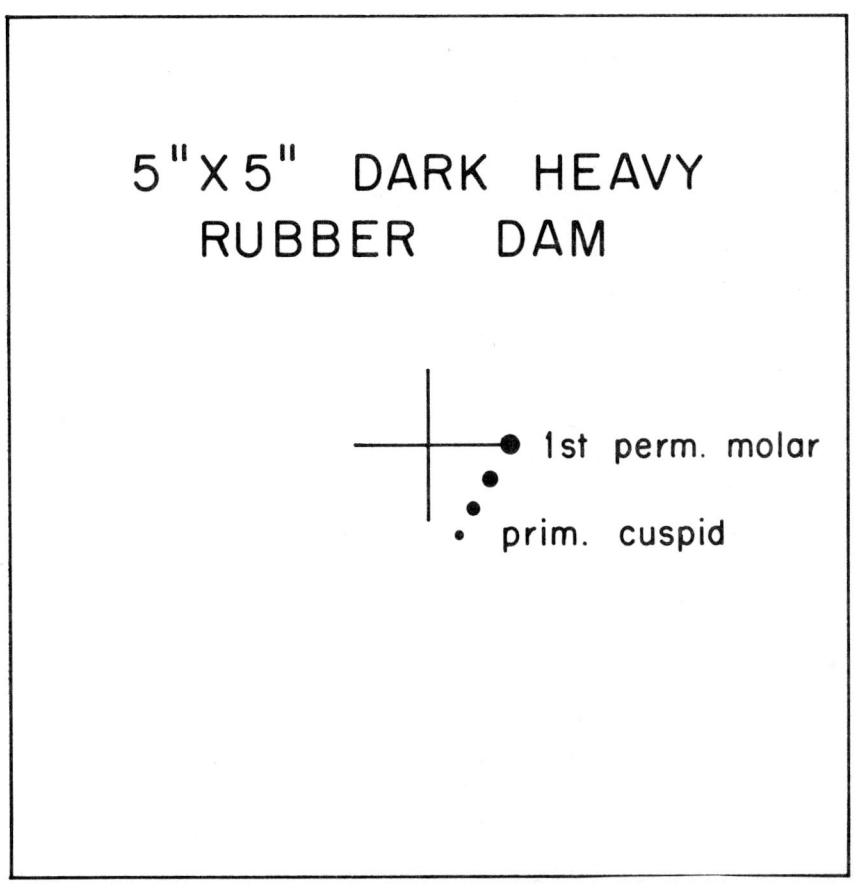

Figure 8–4 The multi-arch method for punching a rubber dam for children. This diagram can be used as a template and a rubber stamp made so the assistant may prepunch the dams correctly. Punched in this fashion, the rubber dam fits opposite arches by simply being turned over.

Each rubber dam clamp should have a 12-inch piece of doubled dental floss looped around its bow before being placed on the child's tooth. A clamp so prepared cannot be aspirated by the child.

Punching the Dam

The number of teeth one includes in the rubber dam application is optional, although it is suggested that all posterior teeth and the cuspid in one quadrant be included when possible. As previously explained, winged clamps are used because they provide a larger field of operation and will protect the dam and gingival tissues to some extent if the bur should slip from the tooth.

A simplified method of punching the dam is suggested which saves time and alleviates the multiplicity of areas on the dam to be punched. The use of this simplified system permits the beginning student or the experienced dentist an easy approach to using the rubber dam.

Basically, the system consists of four holes of graduated size, large to small, punched on an angle near the center of the dam. (See Fig. 8–4). This method has three decided advantages:

1. The dam is centered on the quadrant being worked on, not on the face of the child. This allows clear peripheral air to be breathed while the child's nostrils are protected.

2. The dam can be washed, powdered, prepunched, and stored by the assistant during times when the dentist is out of the office.

3. These prepunched dams will fit all arches, upper and lower, by simply being turned over to the other side.

However, most men will want to keep a small supply of washed and powdered* dams which have been stamped but not punched, for those patients who have missing teeth in the quadrant to be restored. In these cases, the dentist can custom punch his own dam at the chair as he sees fit. The time saved by this system is obvious and for most of those to whom this technique has been demonstrated it has been a highly significant addition to their practices.

Selection of Clamps for the Rubber Dam

The clamp selection is almost automatic. All clamps in order to be secure on primary teeth should be placed below the height of contour of the tooth. The ivory #14 can be used on all second primary molars, while the Ivory #14-A can be used on all partially erupted six-year molars. Most first primary molars can be clamped with either the S. S. White #206 or the Ivory #00. For those older children whose six-year molars have lower gingival contours, the S. S. White #18 universal molar clamp can be used. These five clamps can serve to secure the dam to the arch in all except a very few children. Indeed, the same five clamps will serve to secure the dam for most adult operative care as well.

Techniques of Applying the Rubber Dam

In general, there are three approaches to applying the rubber dam to the arch.

In the first method the most posterior tooth in the arch may be clamped, the dam slipped over this clamp, and subsequently over all other teeth to be exposed. The second method can be accomplished only when the wings of the clamp are engaged in the dam already stretched on the Young's frame, after which the whole complex is carried to the tooth to be clamped, then secured.

In the third method the bow of the clamp can be slipped through the most posterior hold of the rubber dam. Then with the forceps in one hand and the other hand holding the corners of the dam gathered above, the clamp with the dam attached is carried to the tooth and secured by the fingers pressing the lubricated material over one wing at a time to seal the tooth. The dam is stretched to receive the Young's frame; then the remaining teeth are isolated and dried to prevent dislodgment. Usually ligation with dental floss is not necessary, but if it is used, only the most anterior tooth exposed need be ligated.

Although the second method described here is recommended by experienced operators such as Jinks and Lewis, the third method is preferred because it is of the greatest assistance to the inexperienced operator for these reasons:

1. The tooth to be clamped remains at all times completely visible to the operator so he can place the jaws of the clamp. (In the second method outlined

---

*Johnson's Baby Powder.

previously the operator can see the tooth to be clamped only by looking through the hole formed by the jaws of the clamp.)

2. An extra instrument is not needed to disengage the rubber from the wings of the clamp, nor do the clamps need to be modified by special grooves, etc.

3. While a dental assistant can be helpful in all methods of rubber dam application, she is least necessary in the second and third methods described, thus permitting the dentist to apply the dam with dispatch even if his assistant is temporarily absent from the chair.

Ligation of Teeth Under the Dam

Many writers have insisted that teeth exposed through the rubber dam should be ligated by dental floss, either around each tooth exposed, or at least around the most anterior tooth exposed. Ligation is usually unnecessary if heavy or extra-heavy weight rubber dam is used. The extra "body" of the rubber, the 3 to 4 mm. separation of holes and the eversion of the dam into the sulcus around each tooth (most easily accomplished with dental floss) as the tooth is being dried with air will effectively anchor the dam in position. Only occasionally will ligation be necessary on a lower or upper primary cuspid.

Quicker than ligation is a method of wedging with a round toothpick on the mesial of the most anterior tooth exposed. This can be used to stabilize the dam, as can also several thicknesses of a small piece of rubber dam wedged into the same area.

A napkin usually need not be placed under a rubber dam if the child is semi-reclining or fully reclined. Also the saliva ejector need not be used, although occasionally the aspirator suction tip should be placed under the corner of the dam by the dental assistant and any thick ropy saliva sucked out.

To sum up the use of the rubber dam for children, it is felt that this simple addition to the dental office armamentarium will produce less trauma and more satisfaction during all restorative procedures for the children, for the parents, and for the dentist.

USE OF COTTON ROLLS

While most situations in operative dentistry are amenable to use of the rubber dam, it may be the preference of the operator to use cotton rolls. These can be held in place best by using any one of a number of cotton roll holders, some of which lock themselves in position by a sliding vertical friction lock. Cotton rolls placed so will be better tolerated by the child if sprayed with a bit of mint or otherwise flavored mouth wash. The spray can be applied after the cotton rolls are on the holder and ready to be placed in the mouth.

In placing the cotton rolls, the operator must be very gentle and make sure there is no gingival impingement inside the mouth, or excessive pressure by the portion of the holder which clasps under the child's chin. To fully block the flow of saliva from the parotid gland a cotton roll should be placed in the buccal reflection opposite the upper first permanent molar regardless of which arch is being operated on.

If saliva ejectors are to be used for children, they should be of small size, free-flowing and nonirritating to the tissues of the mouth. It is difficult for most children to tolerate an adult saliva ejector because of the very shallow depth of the floor of their mouths.

With high speed handpieces many dentists who prefer not to use the rubber dam may place a tongue guard, which closely resembles a cotton roll holder except that it has a metal cup device which holds the tongue out of the operating area. The dental assistant operates the suction tip, and a saliva ejector is not necessary.

Regardless of the preference of an operator for the method by which he protects his operating field from saliva and other contamination, that field should remain completely dry during the insertion and carving of an amalgam restoration. For it is of little use to have exquisitely accurate high speed instruments to prepare exacting cavity areas, only to place an amalgam contaminated by saliva or blood which is a potential failure before it is even carved.

EMERGENCY RESTORATIONS OF CARIOUS TEETH

Amalgam restorations accomplished in primary teeth are certainly not considered "temporary." The care with which they are done should rival that in permanent teeth. However, there will be children afflicted with rampant decay who will enter the dental office for treatment. In these cases treatment of a temporary nature can be initiated immediately to prevent continuation of the carious forces and the possibility of toothaches or abscesses which might occur during the waiting period before routine appointments can be arranged.

After radiographs are obtained, the child can be seated in the chair, and usually in less than an hour mass excavation of the carious areas can be accomplished. Generally this is done with the child under premedication (see Chapter 7, The Problem of Pain and Sedation) and anesthetized with a short-term local anesthetic. With a #2 round bur in an air rotor handpiece using water spray, the carious areas in a whole quadrant can be cleaned out in a matter of minutes. A calcium hydroxide sub-base can be placed in each area where there is deep caries. Quickly formed T-band matrices can be fitted to each tooth, and a stringy cement mix of zinc phosphate cement is mixed and flowed into each cavity area. A drop of eugenol can be added to the cement liquid for an anodyne effect. The matrices can be removed within a few minutes and the temporary restorations smoothed using a high speed diamond point under water spray.

It is important for the parent to realize that these restorations are only temporary. Properly used in those cases in which rampant caries exist, particularly in children under age four, this method will relieve the dentist of the necessity of seeing the child for a whole series of emergency appointments which can disrupt an office schedule.

CHOOSING HANDPIECES FOR OPERATIVE CARE

High Speed

With the present wide use of air driven handpieces the dentist has his choice of rotary speeds of up to 400,000 rpm. Using carbide burs at high speeds with air-water spray playing continuously on the tooth being prepared, decay may be removed and cavities can be shaped with less trauma for the patient and less time expended by the operator. The tactile sense needed to skillfully use the air driven handpieces is one which only practice can bring. The pressures exerted by the dentist against the tooth structure during cutting procedures are much lighter and more delicate than those used with the older belt-driven handpieces.

Many similarities remain, however, when low and high speed operations are compared. Carbide burs and diamond points must be sharp and clean. Above all they must not be worn to a point at which they produce more heat than the air-water spray can easily dissipate. It is poor economy to use dull burs or worn diamond instruments over and over again to reduce office expense. The time saved by using sharp instruments and the increased comfort to the patient are well worth the cost of more frequent replacement. Frequent sharpening of hand instruments also lessens the time necessary to smooth and plane cavity walls properly, and facilitates the obtaining of sharp line angles or retention areas where desired.

Low Speed

That low speed belt driven contra-angles will prepare cavities in teeth rapidly and well needs no restatement. However, many dentists now use them solely for prophylaxis and polishing procedures. In some cases the operator's unit may have no provision for a belt drive, in which case the straight handpieces driven by air will have attached to them the necessary contra-angles for prophylaxis and polishing.

As do many other dentists, the authors regret the passing of the "silent" low speed belt driven contra-angle. For some children the high pitched whine of the air rotor is extremely disturbing, and it was helpful to have the quiet low speed contra-angle available as an alternative. In spite of the increased bone conduction vibration, this handpiece was more acceptable for this small group of children. Many dentists feel that the final depths of decay in a cavity should be eradicated using only slow speed and a round bur. It is now felt by many operators that round burs used at high speeds will accomplish the same thing just as effectively and in somewhat less time, but this still remains a matter of personal preference.

DIAGNOSIS AND TREATMENT SELECTION

The decision to restore a primary tooth must be based on many other things than the fact that it may be cariously involved. What the dentist decides to do may hinge on his total knowledge of the primary dentition as well as his ability to manage the child.

Some factors he must consider before restoring a tooth are:
1. Age of the child.
2. Degree of carious involvement.
3. Condition of tooth and supporting bone in radiographs.
4. Time of normal exfoliation.
5. Effect of removal or retention on the child's health.
6. Space consideration in the arch.

The wise dentist constantly teaches the inestimable value of preserving children's primary dentition in as near its natural state as possible. In a very real sense, in a dental practice, he may be able to watch his errors of omission or commission grow and develop and return to his office as teen-age or adult dental problems directly traceable to earlier decisions he himself made concerning the primary teeth.

DETECTION OF CARIES

Certain anatomical differences in primary teeth, such as extremely large pulp chambers, prominent pulpal horns, and their proximity to the external surfaces of the tooth, make it imperative that incipient lesions be discovered early and treated promptly. There is no justification for assuming that an incipient lesion that is barely detectable need not be prepared and restored but can be allowed to wait until the following recall appointment. When one considers that in many areas of the primary teeth there is less than 2 mm. of tooth structure between the surface of the tooth and the pulp, the disastrous consequences of delaying restorative work should be obvious. Furthermore, it is apparent to all those who work with children that the larger the cavity becomes, the more difficult it is to restore satisfactorily.

The detection of incipient lesions in teeth can be approached by several methods. With the mirror and a *sharp* explorer, pit and fissure caries and cervical caries can be detected. Radiographs are essential if one is to discover the interproximal lesions, especially those between the wide contacts of primary molars. However, all lesions can be detected better if the teeth are cleaned prior to examination and if the teeth are dried during the examination. Sognnaes has assessed the value of each of these factors in a survey of 32 children averaging 9 years of age. Of a total of 879 detectable carious surfaces in these children, only 651 were detected by mirror and explorer alone. A similar mirror and explorer examination revealed 835 lesions when the teeth had been cleaned and dried prior to the examination. Only by using the foregoing procedure along with roentgenography were all 879 lesions found. Sognnaes has concluded from this study that all clinical methods available should be used to attain maximum detection, since *one-fourth of all carious surfaces found would have remained undetected without radiographs and a cleaning and drying of the teeth.* There is no valid excuse for making a cursory examination in even a very young and somewhat difficult patient. The success of any dental treatment plan depends upon how soon the lesions are discovered and treated. Any questionable pit or deep groove should be restored. Any noncarious but deep pit or fissure may be treated by prophylactic odontotomy, particularly if the child's history of caries activity shows this to be an area of potential danger to the health of the tooth.

COMMON SITES OF CARIOUS LESIONS

Seemingly, each tooth in the mouth has its own distinct caries susceptibility. If caries develops in primary teeth, those with the greatest predilection to caries are attacked first. For this reason some teeth and specific surfaces remain caries free unless the attacking force is so great (rampant caries) that all available tooth surfaces may be attacked.

In reviewing the susceptibility of the various primary teeth and comparing it with their morphology, studies have shown that second molars have the highest caries attack rate, followed by first molars, cuspids, and incisors in this order. (See Chapter 25, The Epidemiology of Dental Caries.) Regardless of attack rate, the dentist will be called upon to restore all the morphologic types of teeth with all degrees of destruction in the course of his practice.

However, on all teeth there are certain areas which become carious more rapidly and more frequently than others. These are areas where natural defects in the tooth exist, or in areas which are not self-cleansing, or areas which become non-self-cleansing through accident or disease. These general areas can be localized as the pits and fissures of the molars and anterior teeth, the cervical and proximal areas on all teeth, as well as hypoplastic or damaged areas located in otherwise resistant parts of the tooth.

It is important for parents to realize that, in an extremely susceptible child who is on a constant diet of medicinal syrups, sticky carbohydrates, or sweetened liquids in the bedtime bottle, caries can attack the primary teeth as soon as they have erupted. These children pose real problems; their treatment will be discussed later in this chapter.

CAVITY PREPARATIONS

The classification of cavity preparations in permanent teeth originated by Black[2] can be modified slightly and applied to primary teeth. These modifications can be outlined as follows:

Class I cavity preparation: Those pits and fissures of the occlusal surfaces of the molar teeth and the buccal and lingual pits of all teeth.

Class II cavity preparation: All proximal surfaces of molar teeth with access established from the occlusal surface.

Class III cavity preparation: All proximal surfaces of anterior teeth which may or may not involve a labial or a lingual extension.

Class IV cavity preparation: A restoration of the proximal of an anterior tooth which involves the restoration of an incisal angle.

Class V cavity preparation: On the cervical third of all teeth, including the proximal surface where the marginal ridge is not included in the cavity preparation (spot filling).

The same predetermined steps in cavity preparation should be followed in primary teeth as in adult. These steps are: (1) obtaining outline form, (2) obtaining resistance and retention forms, (3) obtaining convenience form, (4) removing remaining caries, (5) finishing enamel wall, and (6) performing toilet of the cavity. In carrying out these steps engineering principles and design should permit easiest access to the area, provide maximum retention and greatest resistance to the stresses placed upon the completed restoration during mastication, and provide against the possibility of secondary caries. There is a great deal of overlapping of the various steps, and many times several steps can be accomplished with one procedure. As mentioned previously, in some instances it is advantageous to excavate the carious material first with a #2 round bur or hand excavator to determine whether the tooth can be restored. Where there is the possibility that a pulpotomy may be performed, the teeth should first be isolated with a rubber dam.

The number of burs and hand instruments selected to prepare a cavity should be kept to a minimum consistent with performing the necessary operations in the minimum time. The constant changing of burs and the employment of unnecessary or unproductive hand instruments are to be eliminated as much as possible. In addition, during the cavity preparation there should be excellent visibility and constant control of all instruments used.

In preparing cavity forms for restoring primary teeth, although the basic principles of cavity preparation as just outlined apply, there are certain modifications in cavity design which make restorative care of these teeth unique. Most of these modifications have to do with the differences in anatomy of the primary molars from that of the permanent molars.

Some of these differences are the thin (1 mm.) enamel covering, the broad molar proximal contacts, the enlarged pulp chamber, the narrowed occlusal table and the enhanced cervical bulge together with the pronounced constriction at the neck of the tooth.

Although the choice of instrumentation for the preparation of a cavity depends somewhat on whether low speed or high speed is used, the following procedures can be used with either method. However, it is assumed that high speed will be used in most instances where available, and the burs and points named are carbide friction grip burs and friction grip diamond points unless otherwise noted.

Also, the constant use of an air-water spray is assumed, although, with careful attention to light pressures, air only can be used for the final finishing touches of the preparation without damage to the tooth.

Class I Cavities

In an incipient lesion, a #34 inverted cone bur is used to penetrate the enamel and 0.5 mm. or less into the dentin. After the cavity outline together with extensions for grooves or fissures is completed, a #56 or #57* fissure bur is used to smooth the walls and finish the cavity. The occlusal enamel walls will be approximately parallel to the axis of the tooth and the pulpal wall will be flat and smooth.

If the carious area is extensive, a #2 or #4 round bur can be used to enter and remove the decay. The burs should be run at a slower speed (assuming a variable speed control) and a light feather touch used to sweep out the deepest penetrations of decay. A sub-base containing calcium hydroxide is then applied to the dried cavity and allowed to set. A zinc phosphate cement or other hard setting base is applied over the sub-base. The enamel walls are then smoothed and finished with a #57 bur while at the same time the hardened base is smoothed pulpally.

The final occlusal outline form will consist of sweeping curves and be devoid of sharp angles. A bevel on the enamel should not be placed at the cavosurface angle because of the poor edge strength of amalgam. The sharp cavosurface angle also facilitates easy carving of the amalgam.

When the carious attack is so deep that an indirect calcium hydroxide pulp treatment is to be used, the foregoing procedure remains the same as outlined, except that the last remaining vestiges of decay are not removed (the removal of which would expose the pulp), but are dried thoroughly with gentle blasts of warm air. The sub-base containing calcium hydroxide is then applied in the fashion described. (See chapter on pulp treatment.)

---

*Unless specifically stated otherwise, all fissure type burs used will be the smooth, not the cross-cut type.

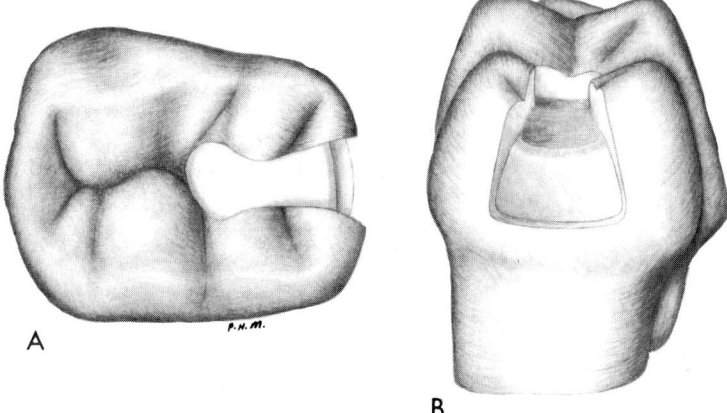

Figure 8–5 Mandibular primary first molar, a disto-occlusal cavity preparation. *A*, Occlusal view: Note the conservative isthmus and the slightly curved axial wall. *B*, Proximal view: Note the marked occlusal convergence and the slightly rounded proximal box buccogingival and linguogingival line angles.

Before amalgam is inserted into any cavity the area must be clean and dry. *It should remain dry during the entire insertion and carving procedure.*

Class II Cavities

General Modifications

Assuming that all primary molars are essentially similar in their basic anatomy, certain *general* modifications from cavity preparations in the permanent molars may be noted (Figs. 8–5 to 8–10). These include the following:

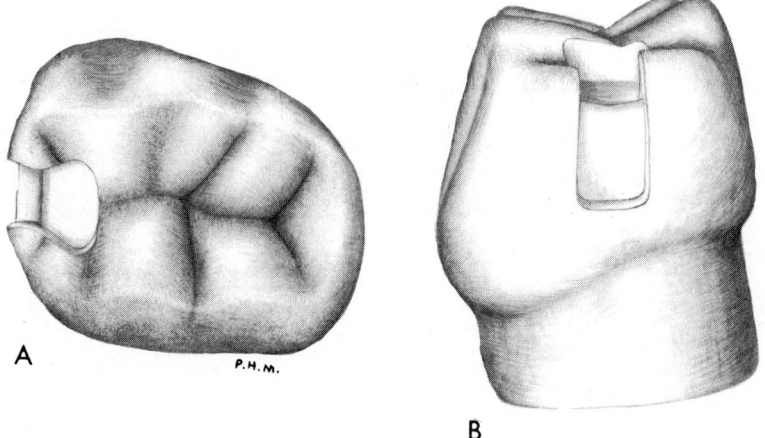

Figure 8–6 Mandibular primary first molar, a mesio-occlusal cavity preparation. *A*, Occlusal view: Note the conservation of tooth structure. *B*, Proximal view: Note parallel proximal walls.

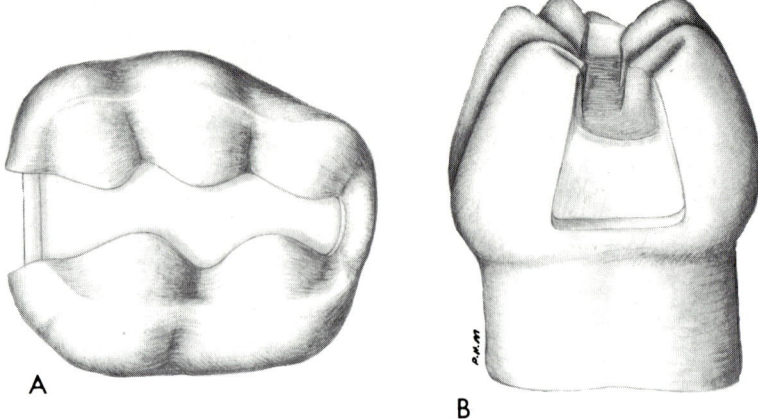

Figure 8–7   Mandibular primary second molar, a mesio-occlusal cavity preparation. *A*, Occlusal view: Note conservatism in groove extension. *B*, Proximal view: Note marked convergence of the proximal box toward the occlusal.

1. Proximal Box.   The greater constriction of the necks of primary teeth increases the danger of damaging soft tissues interproximally as the gingival wall is established preparatory to shaping the proximal box. Also, the farther the gingival wall is carried down, the deeper pulpally must be the axial wall to maintain the proper 1 mm. width. This clearly can endanger the pulp if the wall is established too far gingivally (Fig. 8–10).

2. Gingival Wall.   The width of the gingival wall should be approximately 1 mm., which is also the width of the cutting end of the #57 or #557 burs. The preparation should be cut so it relies on dentin for its support of enamel walls.

3. Axial Wall.   The axial wall may be flat on a small restoration, but should curve to parallel the outside contour of the tooth in a larger preparation. Failure to curve the axial wall may result in an exposure of the pulp.

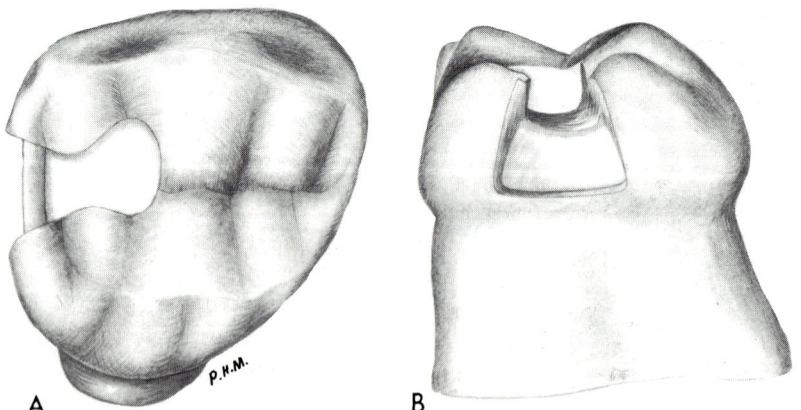

Figure 8–8   Maxillary primary first molar, a disto-occlusal cavity preparation. *A*, Occlusal view: Note the slightly curved axial wall. *B*, Proximal view: Note the slightly beveled axiopulpal line angle.

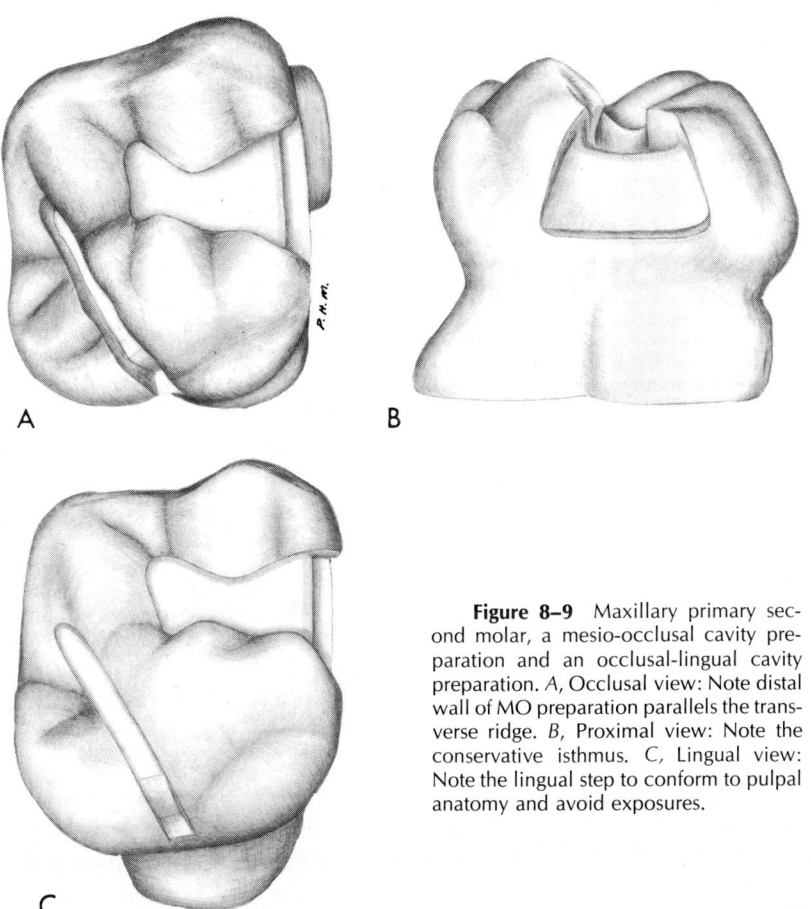

A

B

C

Figure 8–9 Maxillary primary second molar, a mesio-occlusal cavity preparation and an occlusal-lingual cavity preparation. *A*, Occlusal view: Note distal wall of MO preparation parallels the transverse ridge. *B*, Proximal view: Note the conservative isthmus. *C*, Lingual view: Note the lingual step to conform to pulpal anatomy and avoid exposures.

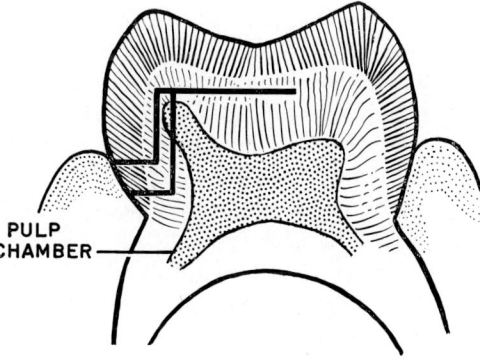

Figure 8–10 Diagram illustrating the increased danger of pulp exposure when the gingival wall is carried too deeply.

PULP CHAMBER

4. *Convergence.* The proximal box line angles and walls should converge toward the occlusal, approximately following the buccal and lingual surfaces of the tooth. This provides for increased retention, carries the preparation into self-cleansing areas, and avoids undermining the adjacent cusps. A 90 degree cavosurface angle should be maintained.

5. *Line Angles.* The buccogingival and linguogingival line angles can be very slightly rounded.

6. *Cavosurface.* The buccal and lingual cavosurface angles need not be flared too markedly to be in an entirely self-cleansing area. Divergence of the buccal and lingual walls should be reduced to the minimum consistent with bulk consideration and proper access. The buccal and lingual walls should be at right angles to the surface of the tooth and in the direction of the enamel rods. The occlusal cavosurface margins should be placed in non-stress-bearing areas.

7. *Cervical Enamel Rods.* It is not necessary to bevel any of the walls of the cavity since there is little danger of rods being unsupported. At the cervical margin the rods incline slightly toward the occlusal.

8. *Retention.* Retention grooves may be placed into the bucco-axial and lingual-axial line angles, but in a fashion which will not undermine the enamel walls.

9. *Isthmus Width.* On the occlusal surface the isthmus width should rarely exceed the width of a channel cut by a #58 or #558 straight fissure bur in a high speed handpiece (approximately one-third the dimension between buccal and lingual cusps). By making the isthmus less wide, the possibility of subsequent ditching along occlusal margins and the undermining of cusps is reduced. Adequate bulk for strength is provided by having the greatest buccolingual width of the restoration in the marginal ridge area directly above the axial wall.

While in the past it has been suggested that the isthmus be made proportionately somewhat wider than that described here, it is difficult to justify replacing sound tooth structure with potentially weaker amalgam. Recent studies have shown that isthmus fracture has not contributed to a high percentage of amalgam failures. Instead, isthmus fracture seems to occur only when there is a definite premature contact by an opposing cusp on a newly carved amalgam's marginal ridge. By checking with articulation paper *before* the restoration is begun, areas of potential danger at the marginal ridges to be restored can be ascertained, and the opposing primary tooth cusps disked slightly. Of course, articulation paper is also used after the amalgam is carved as a final check.

10. *Axiopulpal Line Angle.* This can be rounded with a bur or hand instrumented by *sharp* enamel hatchets.

11. *Pulpal Wall.* The pulpal wall may be flat or rounded slightly and should be prepared so it is about 0.5 mm. into the dentin. If it is finished by a bur such as the #57 or #557, creating a flat wall, the wall should be extended minimally in a buccolingual dimension because of the possibility of nicking pulp horns. This is especially true in the mesiobuccal pulp horn area.

12. *Occlusal Walls.* The buccal and lingual walls of the occlusal step may converge slightly as they approach the occlusal surface.

13. *Occlusal Dovetail.* This should be extended to include the susceptible or carious areas of each specific tooth. The outline form should be rounded, smooth, and graceful with a definite lock on the occlusal.

Specific Modifications

There are certain modifications which can be made in a classic class II preparation to conform to the anatomy of a particular tooth.

1. Deep Proximal Caries. If the caries extends gingivally so far below the cervical bulge that a proper gingival wall can not be established, it is permissible to round the proximal box form gingivally, as long as the wall itself is kept at approximately right angles to the axis of the tooth. This permits good resistance form and the same type of retention normally used, except that the proximal angles need not be extended buccally and lingually so far.

2. Small First Molars. Much care should be exercised to avoid the mesiobuccal pulp horn on these teeth. Many times it is advisable to step the bur sizes down, e.g., using the #33½ and #56 instead of the #34 and #57. This is particularly true when preparing mesio-occlusal cavities on the lower first primary molars (Fig. 8–6). On a small lower first molar this can pose a difficult problem, which can best be solved by keeping the extension and the gingival flare to a minimum. Since the contact is a point contact proximal to the cuspid, this can be done and still be kept in a self-cleansing area.

3. Thin Cusps. Certain teeth pose a problem with thin unsupported cusps remaining even though a very conservative cavity approach has been used. These cusps should be reduced to the level of the pulpal floor, and the cavity extended in this fashion. Research has shown that by covering these cusps an almost certain marginal failure can be avoided.

Instrumentation in Class II Cavities

Whether the cavity preparation is being done to restore an initial proximal lesion or an area of extensive proximal decay, the procedure and instrumentation remains essentially the same. This makes for a time-saving approach by the dentist and allows his assistant to prepare fewer instrument set-ups.

In this discussion it is assumed that the cavity preparations are made with a rubber dam held in place by a clamp and a Young's frame. The burs are tungsten carbide friction grip type, and the handpiece is an air rotor with an air-water spray playing on the bur as it rotates, and the dental assistant is holding a high volume vacuum suction to aspirate the water from the rubber dam. At the same time she is flowing air-water spray or water on the tooth being prepared, as the dentist directs (Fig. 8–1).

If the dentist elects to use low or medium handpiece speeds, the cavity preparation procedure and instrumentation are the same except latch-type tungsten carbide burs are used. The round burs used for removal of final decay may be of steel. Otherwise, instrument selections remain the same. Air only may be used in the low speed procedure, since there is less heat generated than with air rotor speeds.

The steps and instruments used in most class II preparations are as follows:

1. Gingival Wall Established. Using the #34 inverted cone bur the gingival wall is established first, since it governs four critical dimensions of the cavity; the gingival depth, the width of the gingival wall, and the buccal and lingual extensions into self-cleansing areas. Indeed, many dentists feel that the establishment of a well defined gingival wall is the key to a good cavity preparation. *At this stage the carious tooth structure is disregarded.* It is to be removed *last,* not first. The only exception to this rule should be when a pulpotomy is necessary. Then a #4 round bur with high speed is used to prepare the tooth for pulpal treatment.

The #34 bur is preferred for starting most cavity preparations because it has an effective cutting edge of 1 mm. and its depth and width of cutting will not damage the full length of the proximal wall if the child should move unexpectedly.

2. Proximal Box Form Roughed Out.   Using the #34 bur, the box form of the proximal is prepared by stroking the bur occlusally against the walls. This controls the extension of the box, but leaves it in rough form.

3. Occlusal Step Roughed Out.   The #34 bur then is swept across the occlusal step, still using little stroking movements, until the occlusal depth is correct and the occlusal outline is roughed out.

4. Proximal Box Smoothed.   The #57 straight fissure bur is used to smooth the proximal box form, first by gently polishing the gingival wall following the curved axial wall of the preparation, then by smoothing the buccal and lingual walls of the box.

5. Pulpal and Occlusal Walls Finished.   The #57 bur continues into the occlusal step, simultaneously smoothing and finishing the pulpal wall and the occlusal walls.

6. Proximal Box Finished.   In the upper molars, a sharp 10–8–14 D.E.* hoe can be used to do the final planing of the buccal and lingual walls of the proximal box and establish a bevel on the axiopulpal line angle. This instrument can also establish retention form if desired. In the lower molars a 15–8–14 D.E. enamel hatchet is used for these same procedures.

7. Final Decay Removed.   When the cavity preparations are complete, including retention areas, then the last vestiges of decay can be removed. To accomplish this a #4 round bur is operated at high speed with air-water spray using a very light stroking action against the remnants of decay. In this fashion all carious material is finally removed, after which the cavity is dried carefully. Always, the effectiveness of the final removal of deep caries by the round bur must be tested with a sharp spoon excavator.

8. Sub-base and Base.   If the carious area is extensive a sub-base containing calcium hydroxide should be placed over the deepest area. Then a harder base of zinc phosphate cement can be placed over the sub-base and shaped so that the cavity form in the tooth is much the same as if a preparation had been made for an initial proximal lesion.

9. Toilet of the Cavity.   The cavity preparation must be cleaned of all debris, the retention areas checked, and the cavity area dried thoroughly. There is convincing evidence in the literature that cavity sterilization is ineffective when drugs are applied for a few seconds only. Drugs so used act as surface disinfectants and do not sterilize the deeper areas. Disinfectants that do penetrate the tubules to considerable depths may cause irritation and necrosis of the pulp. Flushing out the cavity with either warm water or hydrogen peroxide and then drying thoroughly seems to be an acceptable method of insuring cleanliness.

10. Placing Cavity Sealant.   The last step before fitting the matrix is the plac-

---

*D.E. refers to a double end instrument.

ing of a cavity varnish or sealant. Abundant evidence exists to show that such a sealant reduces marginal percolation after amalgam restorations have been placed.

Use of Matrix Bands

The prominent cervical bulges and sharply converging buccal and lingual surfaces of the primary molars cause these teeth to have a squat contour which makes it difficult to adapt a matrix for class II cavities. This is especially true of the maxillary and mandibular first molars. Although there are many types of matrices which may be adapted to primary molars it is felt the following four kinds will serve most situations:

1. Spot-welded Band. This custom-made type of band provides the tightest fit and the most stability of any matrix. It is thin enough to allow quadrant dentistry for multiple restorations during one appointment, and it can be contoured easily to produce a restoration which restores the proximal contours of the original tooth.

The technique of making spot-welded bands is as follows:

A section of .002 inch by 3/16 inch stainless steel matrix material (.002 by 1/4 inch for permanent teeth) 1½ inches long is fitted around the tooth and snugged up tightly with thin flat-nosed serrated pliers. The ends may be drawn together in such a fashion on the buccal for both maxillary and mandibular molars, although occasionally it is more convenient to work from the lingual on a maxillary tooth. The band is removed, still holding it in the jaws of the pliers, then the jaws are slipped away from the band joint a bit and three spot welds placed to "sew" the band material together. The loose ends of the band material are now cut off carefully leaving a convex edge (Fig. 8–11). The edge is folded over to the distal in the operator's fingers and crimped there with the flat-nosed pliers, then fitted back over the

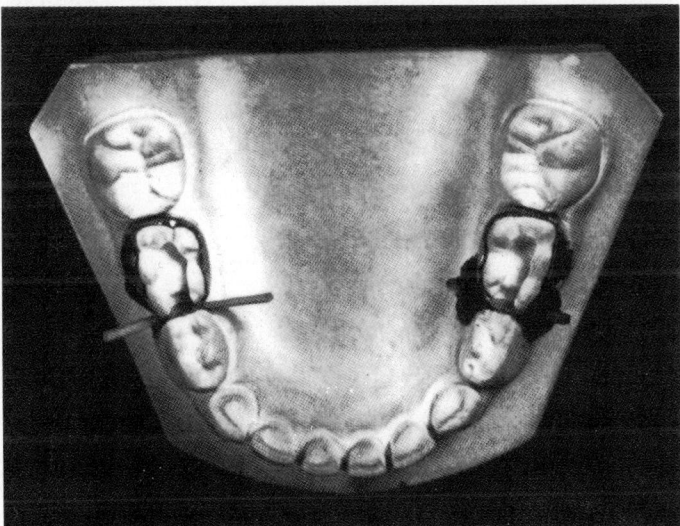

Figure 8–11 Illustration of two types of matrix bands. Left: A spot welded band adapted to the tooth; wedges have been placed both from labial and lingual to prevent gingival overhang. Right: A T-band adapted to the tooth; the band has been wedged, and the compound has been forced into the interproximal areas for additional rigidity.

molar. The band should fit snugly. The band is marked at the height of contour of the area to be restored by pressing with any sharp instrument and removed from the tooth. Then with the #112 pliers a contour is pressed quickly into the band. As it is slipped back on the tooth, a definite resistance showing extremely close adaptation is felt.

Wedging at the gingival to stabilize and adapt the matrix can be easily accomplished by pressing a round toothpick into the largest embrasure, usually the lingual. The toothpick can be wetted first in water. The flat handle of the cotton plier can serve as the pushing instrument for the wedge. In most cases the wooden wedge will provide full stability and compound is not required. The bands can be removed after condensation and carving by slitting the buccal surface with curved crown and collar scissors.

For dentists who might like to make up a supply of these stainless steel matrices ahead of time, Tocchini has suggested the projections of the lid of a Moyer copper band box be used as forms. The different sized bands can be stored in plastic boxes with compartments to accommodate three sizes of band for each tooth, which will usually be adequate.

The proper size band is fitted around each tooth to be filled. The bands should not extend above the marginal ridge of the adjacent teeth. They are wedged as previously described, forcing the teeth apart slightly so that removal of the bands on adjacent teeth will leave a satisfactory contact. The burnishing of the band should then be done with a burnisher or similarly rounded instrument, contouring the band so it contacts the approximating tooth or teeth. After condensation of the amalgam and carving of marginal ridges, the band may be cut with a curved crown and collar scissors. It is always removed by pulling the band through the contact area buccally or lingually, never occlusally.

2. T-bands. Although these bands are made in several combinations (curved or straight, large or small, brass or stainless steel) the most versatile and effective for primary molars are the small curved stainless type. For permanent teeth the large curved stainless seem to work best. The T-band matrix is formed by folding the two wings of the T so a channel results, into which is placed the band which now makes

TABLE 8–1   SPOT-WELDED BANDS

Teeth	Maxillary	Mandibular
1st primary molars	Small No. 8, medium No. 9, large No. 10, extra large No. 15	Small No. 7, medium No. 8, large No. 9, extra large No. 10
2nd primary molars	Small No. 12, medium No. 13, large No. 14	Small No. 11, medium No. 12, large No. 14, extra large No. 15
1st and 2nd bicuspids	Small No. 9, medium No. 10, large No. 11, extra large No. 12	Small No. 7, medium No. 8, large No. 9, extra large No. 11
1st molar	Small No. 17, medium No. 18, large No. 19, extra large No. 20	Small No. 17, medium No. 18, large No. 19, extra large No. 20
2nd molar	Small No. 15, medium No. 16, large No. 17, extra large No. 18	Small No. 15, medium No. 16, large No. 17, extra large No. 18

a circle. The circled band is locked in place by folding the ends tightly over the band using the cotton pliers, but the band remains adjustable until the free end of the band is bent to tighten it to fit the tooth (Fig. 8–11). The band should be wedged carefully to prevent overhangs and to withstand the force of condensation. All wedges must be placed *below* the gingival wall of the restoration to be effective. A round toothpick end (½ inch long) or commercially prepared wooden wedges are satisfactory.

3. Matrix Retainers. Matrix bands held by adjustable matrix retainers are in wide use in dental offices today. Despite this they probably form the least satisfactory matrices from the standpoint of the resulting proximal contour of the restoration. This is not to say they cannot be contoured properly, because they can with a little effort.

Just as with the spot welded stainless steel band and the T-band, the matrix retainer band should be contoured with #112 or #114 pliers to approximate the contour of the missing surfaces, then burnished after being tightened in place to contact the adjacent teeth. Retainers holding these matrices may be of the Tofflemire, Ivory, Steele, Ash, Wagner, Kerr, or other makes, but they all have one common fault. They adjust to tighten around the tooth *evenly*, so that a highly contoured tooth such as a primary molar is usually left with either a poor fit at the gingival area or a poor proximal contour or both. Even with wedging these problems remain.

To sum up, whatever type of matrix retainer or band is used, its primary purpose must be kept in mind, i.e., it must form a strong, stable, well contoured form proximal to the cavity box and in contact (unless open contacts are present) with the adjacent teeth into which the amalgam mix can be condensed. The force of condensation must not dislodge the matrix nor allow amalgam to escape gingivally to form an undetected overhang which can cause periodontal difficulties.

In widely spaced primary teeth, contact need not be established if the proximal surfaces are contoured properly and polished. The tissues will remain normal and healthy in this case.

Multiple Restorations in a Quadrant. If teeth are to remain in proper contact after being restored by quadrants, probably each tooth should be condensed separately although multiple matrices may be applied before condensation procedures. This makes the wedging and subsequent proximal contours more normal. However, as in all operative techniques this may be varied.

Gingival Trimming Instrument. A curved blunted sickle explorer may be ground flat on its superior surface to form a sharp double-edged gingival amalgam trimmer to carve any fresh amalgam overhang remaining at the gingival cavosurface after condensation. Postoperative bite-wing radiographs can dramatically show the value of this instrument which can improve the interproximal contour of nearly all restorations.

Class III Cavities

In the anterior part of the mouth esthetics is often an important consideration. One of the reasons parents may bring children to a dental office is that they show unsightly carious lesions when they smile. In these situations the dentist should consider the wishes of the parents. Esthetically acceptable and lasting interproximal restorations of amalgam can be placed in the primary anterior teeth. Or, one of the new composite restorative resins may be used. These exhibit the very qualities that have been sought so long by dentists — good color blend, comparative ease of manipulation, and ease of finishing, particularly if the newer fine diamonds are used.

When the lesion on an incisor is an incipient one, a #½ carbide bur can be used at high speed to prepare a cavity with minimal labial and lingual extension. If the caries is more extensive and the incisal angle is intact, a dovetail preparation can be made with the dovetail prepared either on the lingual (preferred) or on the labial surface of the tooth (Figs. 8–12A, 8–12B).

Since the cuspids may be retained for six years longer than the incisors, amalgam restorations are usually indicated. When these cavities are prepared in cuspids the additional retention provided by a dovetail is usually necessary. If the incisal angle has been lost, a composite resin may be used.

The technique recommended for the dovetail preparation is as follows: After gaining access with a small inverted cone bur (#33½ or 34) or a small round bur (#1) the cavity outline is established, first on the gingival, then the labial and lingual, and lastly the dovetail is cut (usually lingual, but labial if access is a problem). Care should be taken to make the lock on the dovetail at the expense of the gingival rather than the incisal, which might weaken the angle of the tooth (Fig. 8–12). With the same small bur, the point angles and slight retentive undercuts in the dovetail can be made. Usually the whole cavity can be prepared with the one bur. Loose enamel rods can be planed with a 6½–2½–9 D.E. hoe. The depth of the preparation will seldom exceed 1 mm., which will be just into the dentin on these teeth.

The matrix adaptation for the anterior primary teeth will be slightly modified

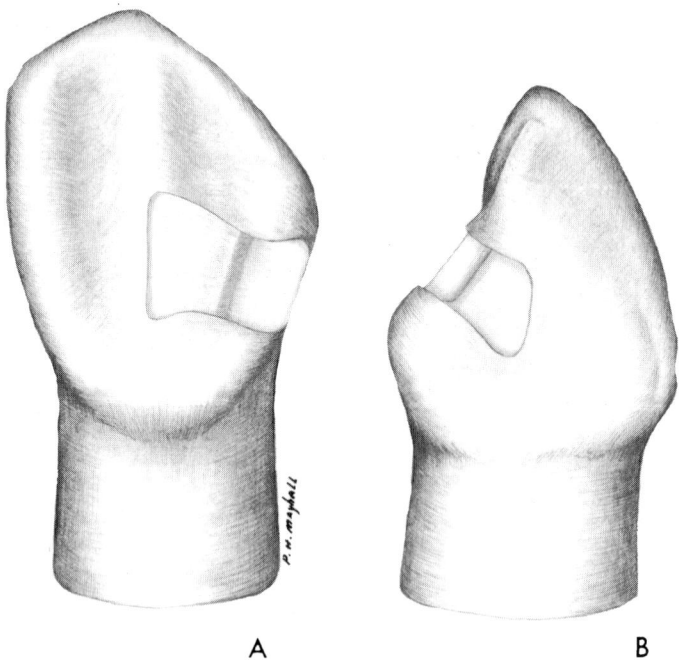

A   B

Figure 8–12 Primary cuspid, a distolingual preparation. *A,* Lingual view: Note that the dovetail is cut more at the expense of the gingival than of the incisal wall to avoid the danger of later fracture following attrition. *B,* Proximal view: Note near parallel incisal and gingival walls allowing direct access from lingual.

from that described for class II restorations. Any thin (0.002 inch) strip of metal can be wedged interproximally and wrapped around on the opposite surface from the dovetail to be held with the fingers during condensation. This permits good access through the dovetail area. As a rule, composite resins require plastic matrix strips of the mylar type.

Class IV Cavities

In the primary anterior teeth where caries is extensive and involves the incisal angles, completely esthetic restorations are possible using either composite resins or pre-formed plastic crowns. In general, four approaches to restoring badly decayed anterior teeth can be considered: composite resins, pre-formed plastic crown, stainless orthodontic bands, and stainless steel crowns.

Composite Resins

Provided a lock is accomplished in preparing the tooth, the use of composite resin materials can almost miraculously restore a deciduous incisor. None of these materials should be trusted to withstand incisor abrasion, however.

Pre-formed Plastic Crowns

Although these crowns take a bit longer to prepare, they serve as the best esthetic replacements of gross caries affecting primary anteriors. The enamel of the incisor is cut away with a tapered fissure bur such as a #169L. The pre-formed plastic crown is fitted, then cemented to place with a zinc phosphate cement. When proper contouring is utilized, these restorations can be esthetically almost perfect.

Stainless Orthodontic Bands

Remove all caries from the teeth and apply a calcium hydroxide sub-base where necessary. Fit the new commercially available stainless orthodontic bands to each tooth. Trim away the labial portion of the band so only a narrow portion (1½ to 2 mm.) of the band remains gingivally. Cement the bands in place with zinc phosphate cement, then clean out any of this cement in the proximal areas. Use the brush technique to apply restorative acrylic which is held in place by the band on the proximals much as a matrix. The result is esthetically pleasing for the parent and child and economically feasible in the dental office.

Anterior Stainless Steel Crowns

These take longer to fit properly than bands, as a rule, and the resulting esthetic effect is not nearly so good. Functionally, however, they serve as excellent restorations.

Class V Cavities

These preparations are cut much like those in permanent teeth. To make sure the gingival wall is clear of decay and decalcified tooth structure, an Ivory #00 rubber dam clamp may be used to retract the buccal or labial tissues. This facilitates condensation and carving also. In all deep preparations a protective base should be used. Since the enamel rods are directed incisally or occlusally in primary teeth, it is not necessary to bevel the gingival cavosurface.

WILLETT INLAY PREPARATIONS

Inlays for primary teeth are both practical and advisable. The limiting factor in restricting their use is a monetary one. Many families will not or cannot afford to pay the additional expense of laboratory procedures even when base metals are used. If an inlay is indicated in a particular situation, the dentist should not hesitate to recommend this restoration and explain to the patient the additional value which an inlay might offer over amalgam. Since Willett-type inlays can be prepared with so little chairtime and a number of teeth can be prepared at one sitting, the reduction of chairtime compensates for some of the cost of the laboratory work. Although a conventional inlay can be used in any situation in which amalgam can be placed, it has its greatest application for broken-down teeth where another type of restoration might not be as durable.

An inlay preparation differs from an amalgam preparation in the same respects as in permanent teeth. The walls must be parallel and all undercuts removed. The inlays may be cast out of base metal or gold. An inlay preparation that is both easy to prepare and simple in design is illustrated in Figure 8–13. Preparation of the tooth involves slicing the proximal area or areas with a safe-sided disk at low speeds, making the slice at right angles to the occlusal plane of the tooth and carrying it just below the free margin of the gingiva and laterally into self-cleansing areas, or, at high speeds, with a small diameter (0.6 mm.), tapering diamond such as Densco No. 1/2 D-L, do the same, removing the proximal surfaces from adjoining carious teeth. With a stone or a tapering diamond, a trench is cut through the enamel beginning one-third up the buccal groove, extending over the occlusal surface, and down the lingual surface for the same distance. The trench ends in a

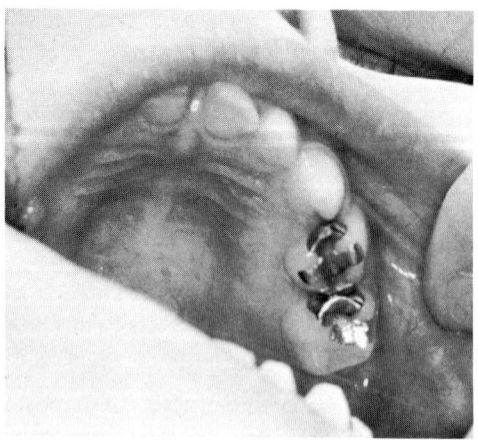

Figure 8–13   Gold cast Willett inlays on the maxillary left first and second primary molars.

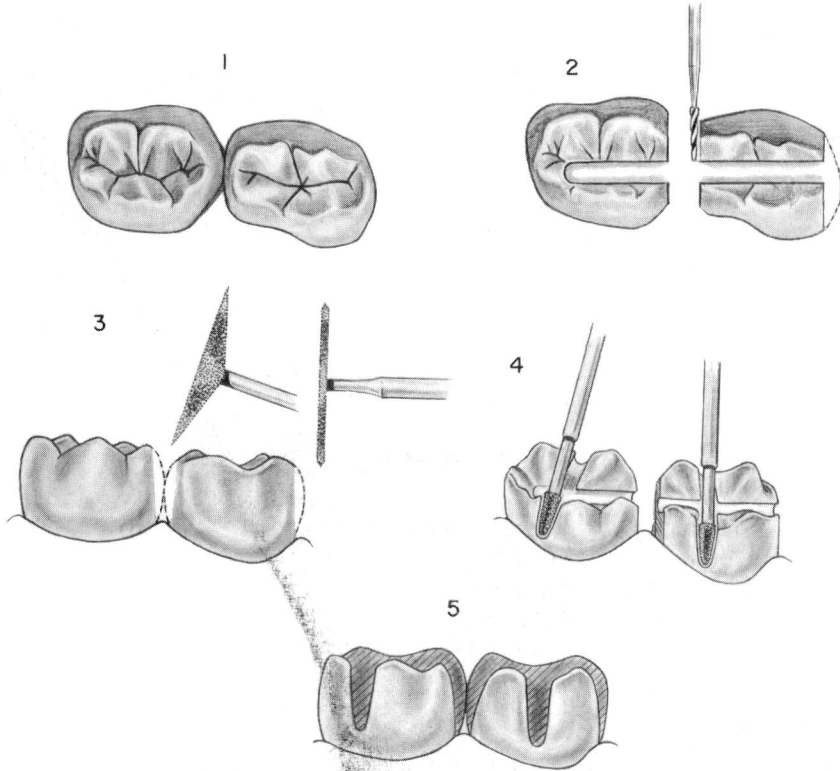

Figure 8–14 The preparation of teeth to receive the Willett inlay. *1,* Mandibular first and second primary molars. *2,* A slice preparation is made on the proximal surfaces to be restored and on the occlusal with a #70L fissure carbide bur or tapered diamond instrument. *3,* The margins of the proximal slices are accentuated with small diamond wheels. *4,* The buccal and lingual extensions are prepared with the fissure bur or tapered diamond instrument. *5,* The completed inlays as they appear in the mouth.

feather edge at the gingival third and follows the contour of the tooth. From the central trench a similar cut is made to connect with the proximal slice. The margins of the proximal slices will have a better defined finish line if the margins are disked with a diamond disk. Before the cavities are prepared, an impression is taken with compound in a small Willett tray and set aside until after the cavities are prepared. Gingival retraction cord is packed around the teeth. The teeth and gingiva are dried thoroughly and a silicone impression material mixed and placed in the tray. The tray is seated on the teeth, using the compound as a guide, and held steadily until set. Then the impression is removed and, if satisfactory, it is ready for the preparation of the models. It is imperative that all carious material be removed before cementing the inlays. (See Fig. 8–14.)

Class I and class V inlays can be prepared as in permanent teeth. All undercuts must be avoided to permit the wax pattern to separate freely and without distortion.

Inlays in the anterior teeth can be made with a dovetail and proximal box as in permanent teeth or the Willett-type inlay can be prepared, extending the grooves over the labial and lingual surfaces and connecting them with the proximal slice by removing about 1.5 mm. of the incisal edge.

BRIDGES

There are many indications for gold bridgework for the primary dentition. A bridge can serve as an excellent space maintainer, restoring occlusal function as well as esthetically benefiting the appearance of the mouth. An anterior bridge may prevent the onset of tongue thrusting and faulty speech habits. Either three-quarter or full crown coverage can be used. In preparing the teeth all undercuts are removed with disks and tapered diamond instruments. The occlusal is reduced with a small diamond wheel. Additional retention and stabilization is gained by a vertical groove placed on the labial or buccal surface with the tapered diamond instrument. The surfaces of the abutment teeth should be parallel for drawing the impression. Silicone base material is satisfactory for impressions in children as the odor is not as displeasing as a mercaptan base material. (See Fig. 8–15.)

PREFORMED STAINLESS STEEL CROWNS

Certainly in no other area of restorative materials for children's teeth has the proliferation of available products been so impressive in recent years as has that of stainless steel crowns. There are now nearly a dozen companies engaged in trying to satisfy the dentists' needs. While the multiplicity of preformed crowns is pleasing, it is also confusing, with claims and counterclaims passed indiscriminately.

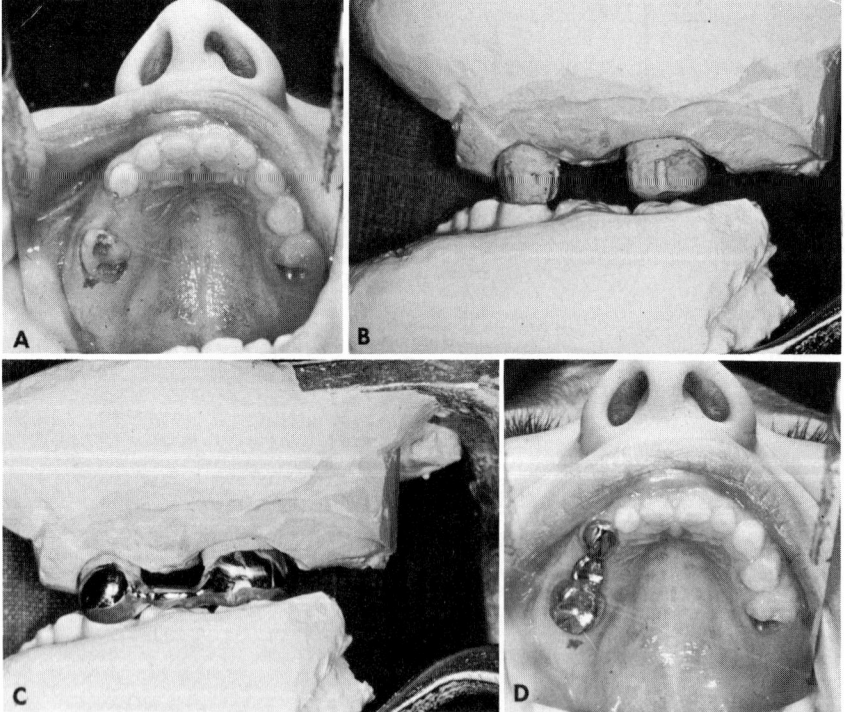

Figure 8–15   A sanitary gold bridge from cuspid to second primary molar replacing a missing first primary molar. *A,* The maxillary arch with missing right primary first molar. *B,* A model of the prepared teeth. *C,* Gold bridge cast and fitted to the model. *D,* An occlusal view of the bridge in the mouth.

It should suffice to say that while none satisfy all the criteria for a perfect custom crown, most of the new crowns can be contoured more easily and in less time than formerly. Time is saved by purchasing a crown which comes already festooned at the gingival and which by its anatomy requires less tooth reduction than formerly.

Some disadvantages remain. The interproximal contact areas are too broad and flat on some types, while others have remedied this contouring difficulty, but are made of too soft material. In general, however, the size selection, precision, and finish of these new products lend themselves to the rising tide of interest in restoring badly broken-down primary teeth and, as such, are being accepted wholeheartedly by dentists who treat children.

Preparation of a Tooth to Receive a Stainless Steel Crown

When trying to decide whether to use a crown or place an alloy restoration, the following criteria may provide useful guidelines. Crowns are indicated when:
1. A tooth has rampant caries involving three or more surfaces.
2. A primary molar has had pulp therapy.
3. A child patient has rampant caries.
4. Malformed teeth are present, such as hypoplastic enamel.
5. A handicapped child patient's oral hygiene is a factor.

A badly broken-down carious primary molar may be prepared for a stainless steel crown as follows: The decayed areas of the tooth are removed with a #2 or #4 round bur under high speed and air-water spray. A sub-base of calcium hydroxide containing material is placed, then the whole tooth is restored to nearly original contour by filling it with Zn OE cement or zinc phosphate cement. After the cement has set, a thin tapered fissure bur (#69L) or a thin tapered diamond stone is used to clear the interproximal contact areas (proximal slice). Sufficient space should be left for clearance of the crown. Then a *minimal* buccal and lingual reduction is accomplished with the same bur or stone just to the gingival margin. The occlusal reduction of 1 to 1.5 mm. is also accomplished by simply angling the same bur or stone along the occlusal planes, reducing the anatomy but retaining its general form. Lastly, all sharp angles and edges are smoothed, still using the same bur or stone, but with an extremely light and well controlled touch. The resulting preparation resembles the original tooth in outline and occlusal form but has smaller dimensions. All peripheral reduction shaping should stop approximately at the gingival contour, allowing the crown to be fitted and contoured so it "snaps" over the non-chamfered finish line and hugs the tooth subgingivally.

Contouring and Fitting the Crown

Belling and stretching of the crown, so necessary with older types of crowns, usually may be omitted with the newer types. Occasionally the #112 contouring pliers may be needed to enhance the proximal contour. The #114 (wide), the #115 (medium width), or the 007-118* (very narrow) type of plier may be used to contour the gingival edges or to tighten the fit of the crown.

---

*This number refers to the recently available ultra-thin crown contouring pliers made by Unitek Corp. All plier numbers refer to Rocky Mt. Dental Products Company except the 007-118 which is available from Unitek Corporation.

When the crown snaps into place and has the proper gingival fit (1 mm. below tissue with no excessive gingival blanching), the occlusion is tested with articulation paper. If it rocks or seems to bite high, the dried *inside* surface of the crown can be colored with a soft lead pencil and the crown reseated. When it is removed, the tooth will be marked with the black graphite where the occlusal contour is high. Slight recontouring will usually remedy the occlusal discrepancy.

Cementation

The fitted crown is removed, washed, and dried thoroughly. Festooning may have been necessary with curved crown and collar scissors. In this case burred edges may be polished with a wire brush wheel or a rubber abrasive wheel with the crown held in the fingers so the wheel rotates toward the gingival edge.

The tooth is cleansed and dried, and a fairly thick mix of crown and bridge cement is applied to the inside of the crown and to the tooth in that order. The crown is seated firmly with the fingers, then the child is asked to bite down on a tongue blade held occlusally to the crown. In this method much more force is generated with less possible harm to the child. The occlusion is checked immediately when the crown is in place, then the child again holds the tongue blade in place during the final setting of the cement. When the final set occurs, the cement particles are loosened then vacuumed out with the suction tip.

PROPHYLACTIC RESTORATIONS

Primary molar teeth contain fewer natural fissures and faults than do permanent teeth, as a rule. But when these are present, prophylactic restorations should be done if decay or the probability of decay exists. A #33½ or #34 inverted cone bur operated under high speed can be used to carefully follow the outlines of the fissure to a depth just into the dentin. The preparation may be continuous or discontinuous, but should effectively remove all dangerous faults in the occlusal anatomy. The preparations should be kept as conservative as possible to avoid weakening tooth structure and at the same time prevent any inroads of caries.

MODIFICATION OF INSTRUMENTS FOR PRIMARY TEETH

Although most dentists experienced in treating children would agree that there is now a broader choice of all instruments and materials used in pedodontic work than ever before, the careful dentist might still wish to modify a few of his instruments specifically for primary teeth.

It has been suggested that in using a one-to-one mix in amalgam a small round 0.8 mm. condenser should be used. This is a necessity in children's smaller amalgam preparations. With this as a starting point, the following suggestions are made:

a. Grind down and polish all amalgam condensers so that they fit the more convergent cavity forms in primary molars. (See Fig. 8–16.)

b. Sharpen a sickle-shaped blunted explorer as described on p. 157 in this chapter to trim overhangs before the amalgam hardens.

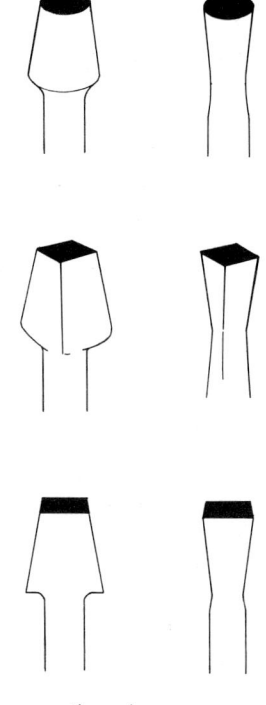

<figure>**Figure 8–16** Drawings showing amalgam hand condensing instruments. Left: Conventional type instruments showing how nibs taper improperly to condense accurately into proximal boxes of class II cavities. Right: Altered instruments (modified by the dentist) are tapered to fit the primary molar class II cavities.</figure>

Conventional   Altered

    c. Remove as much as 3 mm. of length from the noncutting end of a carbide bur to make it shorter for children's smaller mouths. This can be done with a separating disk, and the end can be polished with an abrasive rubber wheel.

    d. Constantly check to be sure of the sharpness of all instruments, especially burs, enamel hatchets, chisels and hoes, caries excavators, and all amalgam carvers. This will enable each dentist to produce the excellent results his training has prepared him to accomplish.

PIN-RETAINED AMALGAM RESTORATIONS

    It is of value to review methods of reinforcing amalgam restorations placed in young first permanent molars when the size of the restorations preclude achieving retention in the normal manner. Teeth with caries mutilated crowns, but with healthy roots, can be salvaged for many additional years of useful service by a method analogous to reinforced concrete structure which was first systematized clinically by Markley. He advocated the use of threaded, stainless steel pins cemented into holes drilled in the dentin of the tooth.

    Recently, two other methods of pin retention have been made available. The first is the self-threading pin, and the second is the friction-locked pin. In each of these techniques the drill to prepare for the holes is operated from a latch-type slow speed contra-angle handpiece. The drill size for both pins is 0.001 inch smaller than the pin which is driven into the prepared hole and held there by the friction and high elasticity of the surrounding dentin. Research has shown that the force needed to withdraw pins of the friction-locked type may be as high as 1600 psi. The pins may be placed in line with the axis of the tooth, then bent over, or they can be placed at an angle for better retention. Excess length can be removed in the mouth using high speed small round burs.

Some precautions are obviously in order when using pins secured by any of these three methods:

1. Use of the rubber dam is essential to maintain dryness whether the pin is cemented or driven to place. If any moisture is present the hydraulic pressure may split the tooth.

2. A thorough knowledge of the pulpal and dental anatomy of the young permanent molar together with good radiographs is essential.

3. Two or three pins well placed may yield an amalgam restoration that has greater strength than one in which five or more pins are placed. Research has shown that the compressive strength of the amalgam mass decreases as the number of wires increases.

4. Small diameter (0.8 mm.) round condensers are best to start the condensation of amalgam around the pins, or a poorly condensed restoration can result.

5. The matrix must be well stabilized and well contoured, otherwise much time is lost carving the anatomy of the larger amalgams.

In general, shorter pins have frequently been recommended for the friction-locked and the self-threading methods because of the forces with which they are seated. The sizes of the pins vary, and this is a consideration when a small tooth is involved. The sizes of pins, graded smallest to largest, are: friction-locked, 0.022; cemented, 0.022 and 0.025 (using a 0.027 drill); and the self-threading, 0.029 inch. Any of the methods using these pins can substantially increase the strength and versatility of large amalgam restorations.

REFERENCES

 1. Allen, W. E.: Stainless steel: Its uses in pedodontics. Dent. Clin. N. Amer., 357–363, July, 1966.
 2. Black, G. V.: A Work on Operative Dentistry. Chicago, Medico-Dental Publishing Co., 1908. 2 Vols.
 3. Brown, W. E., Jr.: A mechanical basis for the preparation of class II cavities for amalgam fillings in deciduous molars. J.A.D.A., *38*:417, 1949.
 4. Finn, S. B.: Cavity sterilization. An unnecessary step. Dent. Clin. N. Amer., p. 663, November, 1960.
 5. Going, R. E.: Pin-retained amalgam. J.A.D.A., *73*:619–624, 1966.
 6. Goldstein, P. M.: Retention pins are friction locked without use of cement. J.A.D.A., *73*:1103, 1966.
 7. Haskins, R. C., Haach, D. C., and Ireland, R. L.: A study of stress pattern variations in class II cavity restorations as a result of different cavity designs. J.D. Res., *33*:757, 1954.
 8. Ireland, R. L.: The class II cavity preparation for primary teeth and its restoration with silver amalgam. D. Practitioner and D. Record, *11*:208, 1961.
 9. Jinks, G. M.: Rubber dam technique in pedodontics. Dent. Clin. N. Amer., 327–340, July, 1966.
10. Lampshire, E. L.: An evaluation of cavity preparations in primary molars. J. Dent. Child., *22*:3, 1st quart., 1955.
11. Law, D. B., Sim, J. M., Simon, J. F., Jr.: A new look at class II restorations in primary molars. Dent. Clin. N. Amer., 341–355, July, 1966.
12. Lewis, T. M., Seattle, Wash. Personal communication.
13. Mack, E. S.: A restorative pedodontic practice without amalgam. J. Dent. Child. *47*:428–437.
14. Markley, Miles R.: Pin-retained and pin-reinforced amalgam. J.A.D.A., *73*:1295–1300, 1966.
15. Nadal, R.: Amalgam restorations: Cavity preparation, condensing and finishing. J.A.D.A., *65*:66–77, 1962.
16. Ousley, J. S., Wagner, M. J., and Taylor, P. P.: Effect of surface conditioners on amalgam marginal leakage. J. Dent. Child., *39*:62–78, 1972.

17. Redig, D. F., and Frankl, S. N.: Characteristics of anterior filling materials used in pedodontics. J. Dent. Child., *36*:369–371, 1969.
18. Schuchard, A., and Watkins, C. E.: Thermal and histologic response to high-speed and ultra-speed cutting on tooth structure. J.A.D.A., *71*:1451–1457, 1965.
19. Sognnaes, R. F.: The importance of a detailed clinical examination of carious lesions. J.D. Res., *19*:11, 1940.
20. Sweet, C. A.: Cavity preparation in deciduous teeth. J.A.D.A., *38*:423, 1949.
21. Swerdlow, H., and Stanley, H. R., Jr.: Reaction of the human dental pulp to cavity preparation. II. At 150,000 RPM with an air-water spray. J. Pros. Den., *9*:121, 1959.
22. Tocchini, J.: Preformed multiple matrix bands. J. Calif. D.A. and Nev. D. Soc., *35*:22, 1959.
23. Willett, R. C.: An improved operative technique for deciduous molars. D. Items of Interest, *53*:489, 1931.
24. Williams, Q. E., and Arnim, S. S.: Conservation of primary teeth using high speed and Willett inlays. J. Dent. Child., *26*:94, 2nd quart., 1959.

9

PROPERTIES AND USES OF RESTORATIVE MATERIALS

by SIDNEY B. FINN and LOUIS W. RIPA

This chapter includes a discussion of some dental materials which are commonly used in dentistry for children. Proper handling of these materials is essential for satisfactory clinical performance, and, when pertinent, manipulative procedures are discussed. The key to a successful dental restoration, however, also lies in the careful selection of a material which is appropriate for the intended procedure. The dentist's choice of material is predicated upon his understanding of its physical limitations and its effects upon vital dental tissue. The discussion will, therefore, include a description of those physical and biologic properties which influence the materials' desirability for use in the treatment of the young dental patient.

RESTORATIVE MATERIALS

SILVER AMALGAM

An amalgam is a special kind of alloy which contains mercury as one of its constituents. The union of mercury with an alloy of other metals is accomplished by the process of "amalgamation." Because an amalgam is weak compared to such cast materials as gold, relatively greater bulk is employed to impart strength.

Silver amalgam is the leading material used for restorations in children in both the primary and the permanent dentitions. In the primary dentition it is used in both the anterior and posterior teeth, although its frequency of use in primary incisors is decreasing. In the permanent dentition its use is generally restricted to the premolars and molars, while for the anterior teeth a more esthetic tooth-colored restoration is used.

Silver alloy is a mixture of silver and tin with small amounts of copper and zinc. Each constituent has its specific function (Table 9–1). The American Dental Association has set the standards for the composition of silver alloy, and more than four dozen commercial alloys meet these criteria. Because the composition of the approved alloy is standardized the dentist need only check that the manufacturer has complied with the recommended specifications by consulting the A.D.A.'s list of certified dental materials.

Due to the standardization of composition, the dentist generally bases his selection of silver alloy on criteria of "workability" such as setting time, ease of carving, and polishing characteristics. These factors are, in-part, influenced by the *grain size* of the alloy.

The alloy is generally prepared by filing or shaving an ingot. The filings are then available as a powder or they may be incorporated into pellets for handling convenience. Figure 9–1*A* is a microscopic enlargement of alloy filings. Note the irregular elongate outlines of the individual particles or grains. A small-grained alloy. or one which upon trituration is reduced to a small grain, is recommended because of the superior qualities imparted to the final restoration. Amalgam restorations prepared from small-grained alloys are easier to adapt to the walls of the cavity preparation, demonstrate a higher strength up to 24 hours after placement, and provide a smoother. more corrosion-resistant surface. An additional property, especially advantageous in a pedodontic practice. is the more rapid hardening of amalgam restorations which employ small-grained alloys. Because of the superior manipulative properties of the small-grained alloy, the trend in recent years has been toward their selection.

Within the past decade spherical alloy has been developed representing a departure from the conventional grain-type alloy. Spherical alloy is produced by an atomizing procedure. A molten mist of metal is sprayed into an inert atmosphere producing solidified relatively spherical droplets. In Figure 9–1*B* the spherical particles of this type of alloy are demonstrated. The size of the droplet particles in commerical spherical alloy varies from approximately 10 to 37 microns. Because of

TABLE 9–1   COMPOSITION OF SILVER ALLOY

Constituent	Approximate Proportion	Function
Silver	65%	Increases strength Increases expansion Increases resistance to tarnish Decreases flow
Tin	25%	Increases ease of amalgamation Decreases expansion Decreases strength
Copper	6%	Increases expansion Increases strength Decreases flow Compensates for variables in manufacture and handling
Zinc	2%	Provides clean alloy during manufacturing process

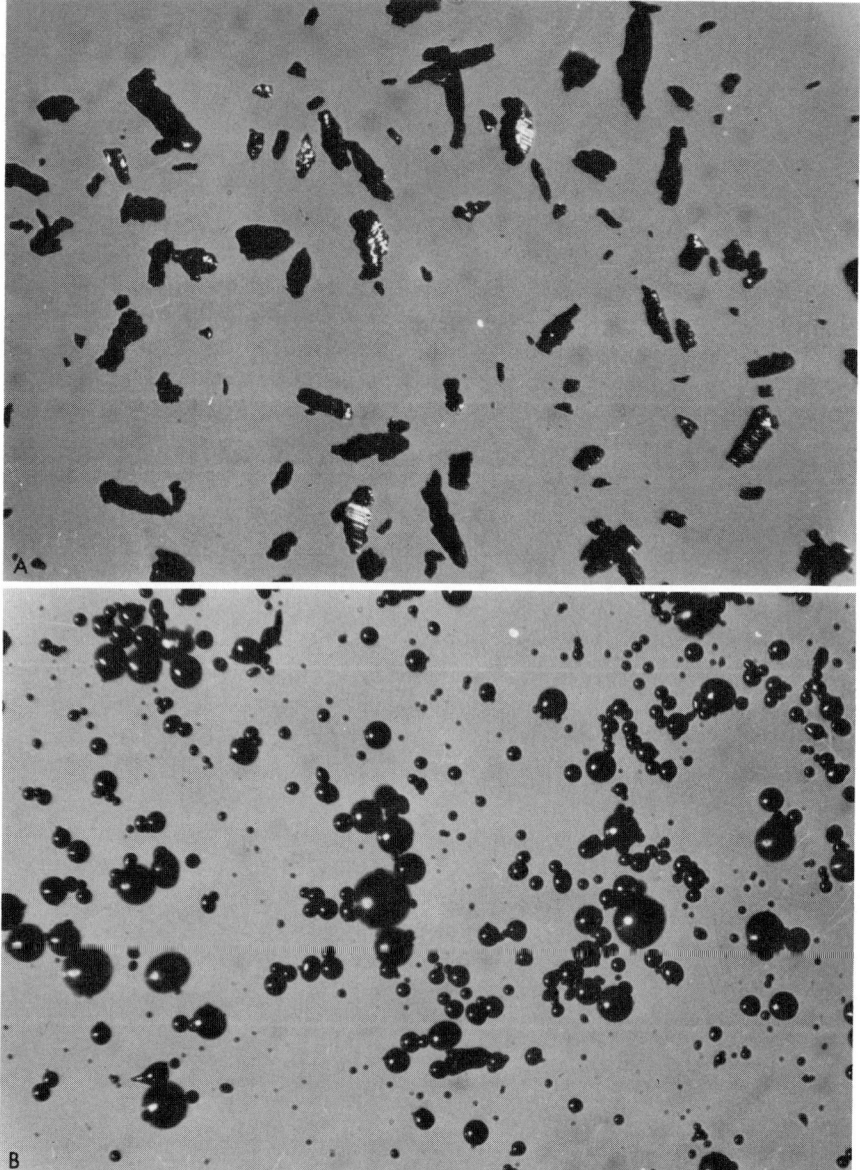

Figure 9–1   *A,* Magnified view of grain type alloy. *B,* Magnified view of spherical alloy. (Courtesy of Dr. M. Buonocore.)

the small size and spherical shape of the particles, it is recommended that manipulative techniques different from those employed with a grain-type alloy be used when restoring a tooth with a spherical alloy.

Whether a grain or spherical alloy is selected, it is the manipulation of the material by the dentist and his assistant that will ultimately determine the success or failure of the restoration in any properly prepared cavity. The steps in handling the material may be divided into (1) proportioning. (2) trituration, (3) condensation (4) carving and (5) polishing.

Proportioning

Silver alloy is amalgamated with mercury to produce a plastic material which hardens upon setting. The proportion of alloy to mercury used is an important factor in determining the clinical success of the restoration. If too little mercury is used, the compressive strength of the amalgam will be altered and proper amalgamation will be difficult to achieve. If an excess of mercury is used, the final strength of the amalgam will be reduced. Each manufacturer specifies the optimal proportions of silver alloy and mercury for his particular product. Generally, approximately five parts of the alloy to eight parts of mercury, by weight, are recommended for initial amalgamation. Excess mercury is then expressed from the mass prior to placement in the prepared cavity and by adequate condensation pressure during packing. These methods are designed to produce a finished amalgam restoration whose residual mercury content is below 55 per cent, the critical point above which there is a definite decrease in the compressive strength of the restoration. To circumvent the inexactness and subjectiveness inherent in the clinical expression of mercury, Dr. W. B. Eames has proposed a technique which initially employs an approximate 1:1 ratio of mercury and alloy, thus guaranteeing a final ratio of 50 per cent mercury or less.[21] The "Eames technique" employs mechanical trituration and a "scrubbing" method of condensation using small condenser points of 0.5 to 1.0 mm. in diameter. Excellent clinical, as well as laboratory, results have been obtained with this technique. However, when properly employed, similar compressive strengths can be obtained with either the conventional technique or the "Eames technique." It is the decision of the individual dentist, therefore, as to what technique he will employ. If a spherical alloy is used, an initial mercury content of 45 to 48 per cent is recommended. Because of the low surface area of the spherical particles even this amount of mercury is considered excessive. The final mercury content of the spherical alloy restoration is reduced to 35 to 38 per cent during the condensation procedure.

Four methods of proportioning are available:

1. Weighing   The operator may weigh the mercury and alloy in an appropriate weighing balance. Although accurate when properly done this method is inconvenient and time consuming and has generally been replaced by the other methods.

2. Mechanical Dispensers. Dispensers are available for both mercury and powder-type alloy. The accuracy of these dispensers is within acceptable limits and most are adjustable allowing the dentist to select the alloy-mercury ratio he desires.

3. Preweighed Pellets. Preweighed pellets are extremely accurate and are used with mechanical mercury dispensers. In order for the proper ratio to be secured by following the manufacturer's instructions, the pellets and mercury dispenser should be from the same manufacturer.

4. Preproportioned Capsules. Manufacturers have introduced disposable plastic capsules containing preproportioned alloy and mercury (Fig. 9–2*A*). By manipulating the cap of the capsule the contents are brought together immediately before mixing. Provided the manufacturers can secure adequate quality control these capsules should give the most consistent mercury:alloy ratios. Furthermore, the disposable nature of the capsules makes them convenient and easy to use; the major disadvantage is their greater cost.

An improper mercury:alloy ratio can adversely affect the physical properties

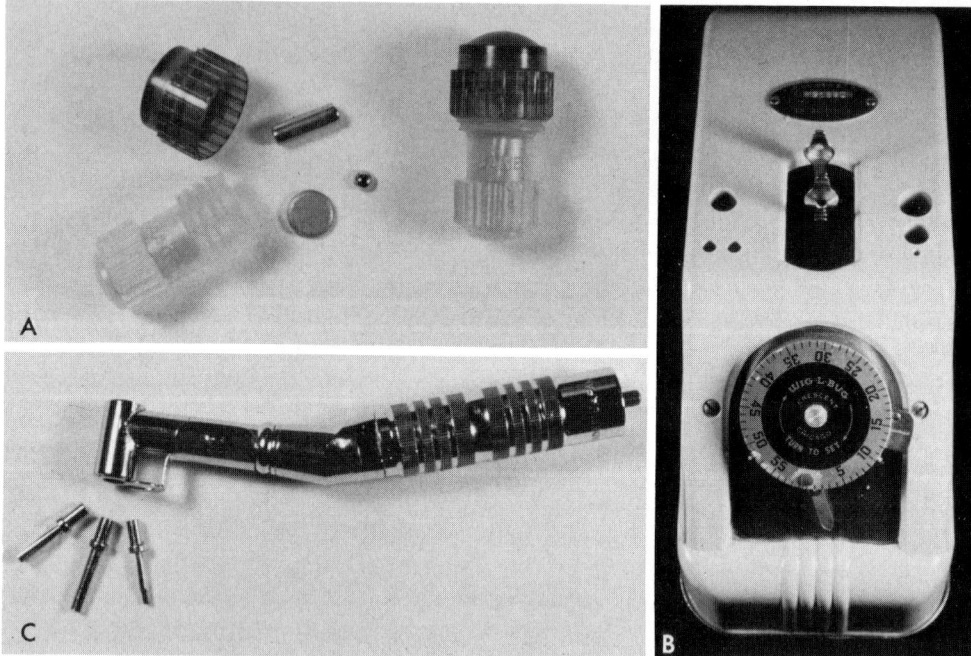

Figure 9–2 Mechanical methods of amalgam preparation. *A,* Disposable preproportioned capsules containing a pellet of alloy, appropriate amount of mercury, and pestle. Alloy and mercury come in contact by manipulating the cap immediately before trituration. *B,* Mechanical amalgamator. *C,* Mechanical condenser with selection of condenser tips.

and clinical performance of the final restoration. Present methods have reduced errors in proportioning to almost nil, thus reducing the variability in this manipulation

Trituration

The purpose of trituration is to provide complete wetting of the alloy particles with mercury While some practitioners still mix amalgam manually with mortar and pestle, most use mechanical amalgamators (Fig. 9–2*B*). The mechanically triturated amalgam has a more uniform consistency, good working and carving properties, and good dimensional stability.

Trituration has a profound effect upon the properties of the amalgam mix and the ultimate clinical course of the restoration. Undertrituration results in an amalgam that contains more residual mercury and larger incompletely alloyed particles. The restoration is weak, carves poorly, and is more susceptible to surface corrosion. Because there are a number of different mechanical amalgamators which differ in speed, amplitude, and vector a firm recommendation cannot be made regarding trituration time. Generally, conventional high speed amalgamators (e.g., Wig-L-Bug, Torit; 3000 rpm) require approximately 20 to 30 seconds while ultrahigh speed machines (Silamat; 4400 rpm) require only 3 to 5 seconds. While spherical alloys generally require less trituration time for proper wetting, they may require longer trituration when they are supplied as pellets because of the difficulty in breaking the highly compressed pellet mass. For the practicing dentist, the consistency of the mix must be the guide for determining the amount of trituration. A mix that has been properly triturated for a sufficient length of time will have a smooth, velvety surface and be plastic rather than granular. If an error in trituration is to be committed, however, it should be one of over-trituration rather than under-trituration.

Condensation

After the amalgam is triturated it should be placed in a clean squeeze cloth and excess mercury expelled by finger pressure. After it is squeezed, small increments are placed in the prepared cavity, using an amalgam carrier, and are condensed. Condensation is as important as trituration in determining the ultimate success of the amalgam restoration. Proper condensation is necessary for maximal strength, good marginal adaptation corrosion resistance, and a smooth polish.

For conventional grain-type alloys, condensation pressure should be heavy. A force of 6 pounds or more will express excess mercury from the packed mix. Amalgam should be added to the cavity in small increments. Removal of the excess mercury as condensation progresses produces an increase in the strength of the final restoration. The condenser tip should be small, since the same amount of force is translated into a higher condensing pressure within the small area of the condenser point. The condenser should not be so small, however, that it will slip through the increments of amalgam. It is recommended that condensers with points which are one-third to one-fourth of the width of the cavity be used. When spherical alloy is used, even with the initial low mercury content, the mix is plashy and less condensation pressure is required. For spherical alloy, therefore, the largest condenser tip that can effectively fit into the cavity should be used at lower packing pressures (2 to 3 lbs.). Since cavity preparations in the primary dentition are necessarily smaller—both narrower and shallower—than comparable preparations in the permanent dentition, the dentist may have to modify his condenser points to conform to the recommendations presented. Chapter 8 describes modifications that can be made in the commercially available condensers so that they can better fit the preparations in primary teeth.

Mechanical condensers are available with varying shaped plugger points (Fig. 9–2C). Mechanical condensation produces excellent adaptation of the amalgam to the surrounding cavity walls, hastens the speed of the packing process, and produces consistent results since the pressure is evenly and uniformly applied at all times and does not tend to vary with the fatigue of the operator.

The dentist should time his operation so that the mixed amalgam is used within 3 minutes after trituration. As the time between trituration and condensation increases, the ultimate strength of the restoration decreases because of the difficulty of removing excess mercury. Phillips and co-workers[56] state that use of an amalgam mix that is 5 minutes old reduces the strength of the final restoration by as much as 40 per cent. Three minutes after trituration, therefore, the old mix should be discarded and a fresh one prepared.

The effect of moisture contamination during condensation is well known. Saliva or moisture from the hand can react with zinc to produce hydrogen gas. The accumulation of hydrogen within the amalgam produces voids within the restoration, reducing the compressive strength. It also causes a delayed expansion of the amalgam so that the restoration extrudes from the cavity walls (Fig. 9–3). The malaligned cavo-surface margin serves as an area for bacteria and food debris to collect and initiate "secondary caries." The use of zinc-free alloys will eliminate this delayed expansion but may produce a surface in the final restoration which is more susceptible to tarnish. In the child patient moisture contamination from saliva can best be avoided by the routine use of a rubber dam for all operative procedures. Use of a zinc-free alloy *in a moisture contaminated tooth* is not the answer to successful restorative dentistry in children.

Carving

When carving primary molars, the intercuspal grooves should be shallow, conforming to the original anatomy of the tooth. Deep carving has a tendency to weaken the margins of the restoration by reducing the bulk of the amalgam and to make polishing difficult. Sharply carved developmental grooves produce harmful stress concentrations at the occlusal surface. Marginal ridges should be conservative in size and taken out of excessive occlusal contact. After the anatomy is carved, the presence of high areas should be located with articulating paper by having the child gently close and observing the occlusion in all excursions.

In completing the carving. the amalgam should not be burnished to attain smoothness. This can be accomplished more effectively by rubbing the surfaces with a cotton pellet dipped in an aqueous slurry of flour of pumice. Burnishing forces mercury to the surface at the margins of the restoration; when the mercury dissipates it leaves shy margins. The marginal amalgam is also weakened by the excess mercury and is prone to fracture.

The gingival margin should be carefully checked with an explorer, and any excess amalgam should be removed. After about six to eight hours, the restoration has reached 70 to 90 per cent of its maximal strength. Twenty minutes after tritura-

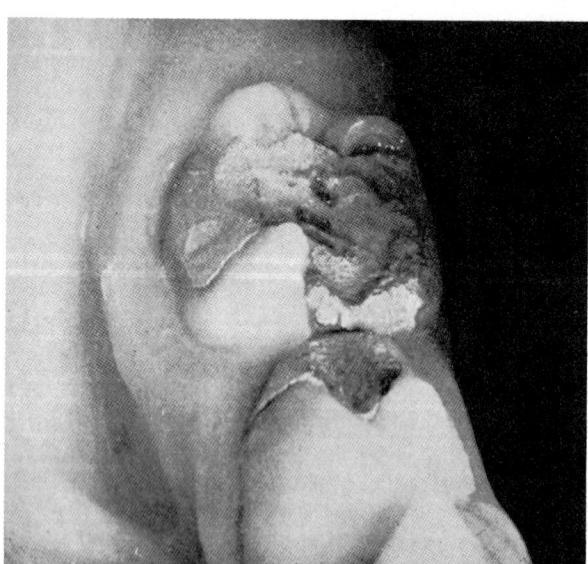

Figure 9–3 The appearance of poorly condensed and contaminated amalgam restorations. One can observe the marked expansion, faulty margins, and corrosion.

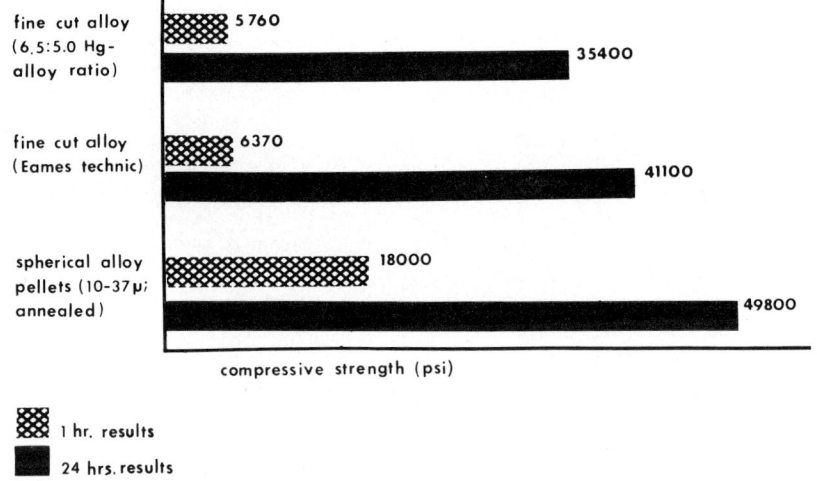

Figure 9-4 Compressive strength values of fine cut alloy and spherical alloy (adapted from Koran and Asgar, J.A.D.A., October 1967).

tion, the amalgam has achieved only about 6 per cent of its final hardness. Therefore extreme caution should be observed to prevent the child from occluding freely and fracturing the amalgam. When the restoration is completed, warn the child and parent about eating hard foods for about eight hours. Spherical alloys have the property of developing high compressive strength values early. After 1 hour the strength may be in the range of 18,000 psi[34] (Fig. 9-4). This property is advantageous when placing amalgam restorations in children since the young child is more likely to inadvertently exert biting pressure on a freshly placed restoration.

Polishing

Restorations should be carefully polished for cosmetic reasons, to limit corrosion and thus increase the life of the restoration, and to reduce deleterious occlusal stress concentrations. The final polishing should not be done for at least 48 hours after the amalgam has been inserted, to allow for attainment of the maximum degree of strength and hardness. Finishing burs, carborundum stones, rubber disks, and sandpaper strips can be used. The interproximal surfaces should be polished as well. Heat generation should be avoided in polishing because it will bring mercury to the surface and weaken the amalgam. The final luster may be imparted to the restoration with a paste of pumice and water or glycerin in a rubber cup, followed by tin oxide. or a commerically available zirconium silicate may be employed (see Fig 9-5). Zirconium silicate, made into a thick paste by the addition of a small quantity of water. imparts a high luster to the finished restoration.

Thermal and Electrical Conductivity of Amalgam Restorations

Because most metals, including amalgams, are excellent conductors of thermal changes and electrical impulses, they should never be placed in a deep-seated cavity

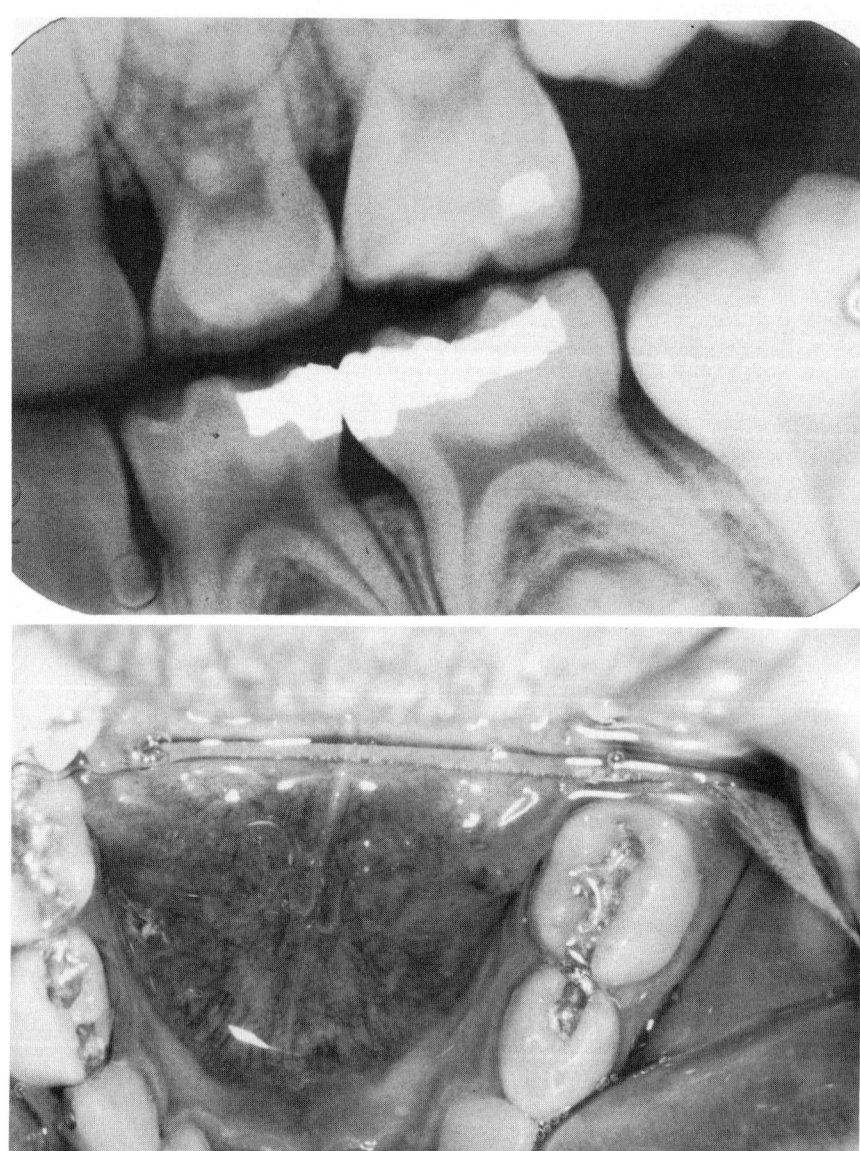

Figure 9–5 An example of well-condensed amalgam restorations prepared using the rubber dam. Notice the contour, marginal adaptation, and polish. (Courtesy of Dr. C. Brenner.)

which approaches a vital pulp without the use of an insulating layer, or base, between the restoration and the pulp chamber. Although the effect of different agents on thermal diffusion varies, it is the thickness of the base itself, rather than its conductivity, that is the significant factor in thermal insulation. It is known, for instance, that when a cement base is 0.2 mm. or less in thickness, it does not appreciably hinder thermal diffusion.

TOOTH COLORED RESTORATIONS

For reasons of esthetics, tooth colored materials are indicated for the restoration of anterior teeth. The introduction of optimal levels of fluoride to community water supplies has decreased the incidence of proximal caries in anterior teeth by as much as 90 per cent. The dentist who treats children who reside in areas with water-borne fluoride places very few anterior restorations. In patients with a high caries susceptibility however. or for those who do not receive the benefits of water-borne fluoride anterior caries is sti l a significant problem.

Three different types of tooth colored dental materials are used for most anterior restorations:

1. si icate cement
2 acry ic (polymethyl methacrylate) resin
3 composite resin

SILICATE CEMENT

The silicate cements are made from a combination of powder and liquid. The powder contains mainly silica and aluminum oxides, with some calcium and about 12 per cent fluoride The liquid is mainly phosphoric acid containing about 35 per cent water When the liquid and powder are combined in proper proportions, the resulting cement is a translucent material somewhat resembling natural tooth color. The combined mixture in the form of an irreversible gel together with unreacted particles, has reasonable strength and rigidity, a low pH, a linear coefficient of thermal expansion similar to tooth structure, and a high solubility in oral fluids and acids.

Because of the phosphoric acid component the set silicate has a low initial pH which one month after insertion sti'l remains below neutrality. The acid components of the silicate are known to penetrate the dentin[72] and can adversely affect the vitality of the pu'p. Acid penetration will be further enhanced in the young tooth with re'atively wide and unobstructed dentinal tubules. A base of calcium hydroxide or zinc oxide-eugenol will form a suitable barrier to acid penetration, while a thinner lining of cavity varnish forms only a partial barrier.[72] Preparing the tooth sufficiently to receive both a silicate restoration and the necessary protective base layer can result in a pulpal exposure if the tooth is newly erupted and the pulp chamber is large

Because of the high solubility of silicate cements in oral fluids the longevity of restorations prepared with this material is poor. The average life expectancy is usually given as 4 years. Bowen and co-workers[4] found that 42 per cent of 74 silicate restorations which they were observing required replacement in 3.5 to 6.5 years. Silicate cements have been found to be especially susceptible to erosion by citrous beverages—a common drink in the young.[81] It may be, therefore, that the life expectancy of these restorations in the child patient is even shorter than that reported for the adult. The material is definitely contraindicated in the child who mouth breathes or who exhibits markedly protruding incisors in which exposure to air with subsequent desiccation is a possibility. Silicates, upon drying out, take on a chalky appearance and undergo shrinkage and softening.

The child or adolescent who requires anterior restorations in his permanent teeth generally has a high caries attack rate. The one advantage of placing a silicate restoration in such a patient is the anticariogenic potential of the material. The clinical impression that silicate restorations, even though they leak badly and deteriorate quickly, have less new decay around their margins than other types of restorations has been substantiated by clinical and laboratory investigation. The fluoride incorporated in the silicate powder during the manufacturing process slowly leaches out of the restoration[16] and is taken up by the adjacent tooth enamel.[27] The increased fluoride level protects the tooth from acid demineralization and secondary caries.[35] The positive anticariogenic potential of the material, however, must be weighed against the pulpal irritation it can cause and its relatively short clinical life, especially in a mouth in which oral hygiene may be poor and acid conditions are present. Because of their adverse properties silicates have never been recommended for anterior restorations in primary teeth, and their usefulness in permanent teeth has been limited. With the advent of the new composite resins the use of silicate cements in the restoration of children's teeth has further declined.

ACRYLIC (POLYMETHYL METHACRYLATE) RESINS

Resin restorative materials have assumed an important place in dentistry for children They have provided the profession with a material that is cosmetically acceptable, easy to utilize, and serviceable. Their use in space maintainers, bite planes, jacket crowns, partial and full dentures, and in the restoration of fractured anterior teeth gives them a rather widespread usage throughout the many facets of dentistry for children The esthetic qualities of the resin materials are the principal indication for their use in restoring cavities in the anterior segment of the mouth.

Acrylic resin restorative materials consist of a powder and a liquid. The powder is a polymer, polymethyl methacrylate, in which is incorporated a catalyst (or initiator) such as benzoyl peroxide or p-toluene sulfinic acid. The liquid, or monomer is mainly simple chains of methyl methacrylate which are kept from forming larger chains and solidifying by an inhibitor such as hydroquinone. The liquid also contains an accelerator such as N,N-dimethyl-p-toluidine. When the powder and liquid are brought together, the dimethyl toluidine activates the catalyst in the powder and initiates polymerization. The commerical product in Figure 9–6 is an example of an acrylic (polymethyl methacrylate) resin which uses a sulfinic acid catalyst.

The principal advantages of the acrylic resin restorative materials are their excellent esthetics, their insolubility in oral fluids, their resistance to surface staining, and their low thermal conductivity. Certain inherent properties, however, limit their usefulness. These include a low hardness and compressive strength (approx. 10.000 psi), a high coefficient of thermal expansion, and contraction during polymerization The latter two properties directly affect their clinical performance. While the surface of the restoration usually does not discolor, the margins may be outlined by a dark line. This unsightly marginal discoloration is a result of leakage at the tooth-restoration interface. It is associated with two factors which affect marginal adaptation: (1) the contraction occurring during setting and (2) dimen-

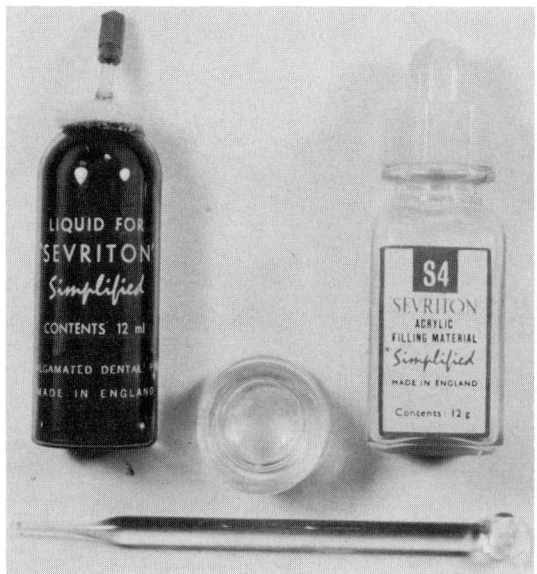

Figure 9–6 Example of an acrylic (polymethyl methacrylate) resin which uses a sulfinic acid catalyst system.

sional changes associated with intra-oral temperature variations. The Nealon or brush technique of insertion, described in the next section, is used to limit the effects of contraction during insertion.

Because of its high coefficient of thermal expansion, acrylic resin changes dimension approximately seven times as much as does tooth enamel for every one degree of change in temperature. The gross dimensional changes of the restoration associated with temperature fluctuations invariably produce an inadequate marginal seal (Fig. 9–7).

To aid in improving adaptation to cavity walls and margins, cavity "primers" (not to be confused with cavity liners or varnishes) are generally provided for use with the acrylic restorative materials. A thin coating of primer is applied to the cavity walls immediately before placement of the acrylic restoration. The primer, a low surface tension liquid, flows into the microscopic irregularities of the cavity walls. The acrylic resin will then polymerize against this thin coating or primer.

In vitro tests on extracted human and bovine teeth have demonstrated that pretreating the enamel surface with a 50 per cent phosphoric acid solution will improve adaptation at the tooth resin interface.[26, 37] The acid cleans the surface and etches the enamel to an approximate depth of 10 to 20 microns. The spaces created in the outer enamel by the acid etch are infiltrated with taglike extensions of the restorative material. The tags are believed to enhance mechanical bonding between the tooth and the resin. Acid pretreatment has been incorporated in the technique of occlusal sealing for caries prevention[9, 10] and has been reported useful in restoring fractured anterior teeth with an acrylic restoration *without* the need of pin retention.[19] To date, there are no reports in which an acid pretreatment has been used to enhance adaptation at the cavo-surface margins of Class III or Class V anterior restorations.

The acrylic liquid monomer as well as the cavity primer are potential irritants

ANTERIOR RESTORATIVE MATERIAL

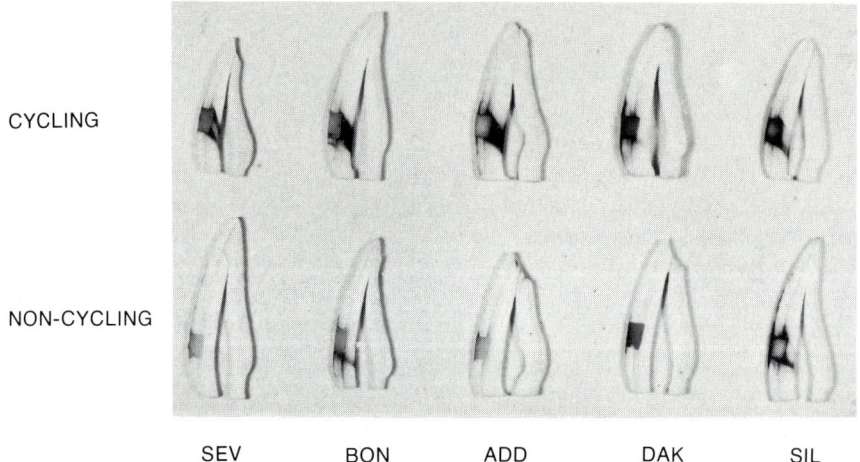

Figure 9-7   A comparison of marginal leakage associated with five anterior restorative materials. Cavities prepared in extracted bovine teeth were filled with a silicate (S.S. White New Filling Porcelain), an acrylic resin (Sevriton-simplified, Bonfil), or a composite resin (Addent-35, Dakor). Teeth were stored in water, then immersed in basic fuchsin dye and sectioned. The bottom row demonstrates leakage patterns with no temperature cycling; the top row shows the effect of 25 temperature cycles on leakage. Note that temperature cycling results in increased marginal leakage of all materials except silicate, which has a coefficient of thermal expansion similar to that of tooth structure. (Compliments of M. Buonocore and Y. Tani.)

to the pulp. A protective base must be used as a barrier to the ingress of chemical irritants. Zinc oxide-eugenol cannot be used as the base because of the reactivity between the eugenol and the acrylic. Likewise, cavity varnish or liner cannot be used because the solvent will react with, or dissolve, the resin. Calcium hydroxide is the recommended base for acrylic restorations. The base must also serve as a barrier against bacteria and fluids that enter the tooth between the cavity wall and restoration as a result of marginal leakage.

Because of the far from ideal properties of the acrylic restorative materials, there has been a tremendous effort in the past several years directed toward the improvement of these materials and the development of newer materials. The endeavors to improve the properties of the polymethyl methacrylate resins have included the addition of inert fillers of fiber glass, aluminum oxide, or silica to the polymer and the addition of cross linking agents to the monomer. Because the resin matrix does not readi y adhere to the inert fillers, the inclusion of these materials did not produce the desired effects; in addition, they served as pathways for the penetration of moisture into the restoration.

The manufacturers of certain acrylic resins (Bonfil*, Sevriton-Simplified**) have incorporated a small amount of sodium fluoride in their product in an effort to make the material anticariogenic, similar to the silicate cements. Unlike the set silicate gel, however, once the acrylic polymerizes it is quite insoluble in oral fluids.

---

*Bonfil, L. D. Caulk Co., Milford, Del.
**Sevriton—Simplified, Amalgamated Dental Trade Distributors, Ltd., London, England

Therefore, it is not known to what extent the fluoride ion is available to the tooth surface to provide the desired enamel solubility reduction.

Brush or Nealon Technique of Acrylic Application

Although there are other methods of using the acrylic resin filling materials, such as the pressure technique and the flow technique, the authors prefer the Nealon[48] or brush technique and will describe it in some detail. With this technique, the adaptation of the material to cavity walls is improved and shrinkage upon insertion is better controlled.

Two Dappen dishes are placed on the bracket table. In one is placed the liquid monomer and in the other, the polymer powder. The tooth is isolated with a rubber dam to insure dryness. After application of the recommended primer, the prepared cavity is moistened with the monomer. Then the tip of a fine camel's hair brush is dipped into the Dappen dish containing the monomer, touched to the side of the dish to remove any excess, and then dipped into the polymer. In this manner the tip of the brush picks up a pearl of the polymer, which is carried to the cavity and placed in contact with the monomer-moistened walls. This procedure is repeated until the cavity is completely filled. Sufficient time is permitted between applications to allow polymerization to begin. If too much monomer is permitted to remain in the restoration, polymerization will take longer and shrinkage will be greater. Before a fresh pearl of polymer is added to the cavity, care must be exercised to be sure that the area already filled is moist with monomer. No monomer should be permitted to drop into the Dappen dish containing the polymer or vice versa; otherwise, polymerization may occur prematurely in the Dappen dishes and thus possibly weaken the final restoration.

Previously, polishing was delayed for at least 24 hours in order to allow polymerization to be complete and the restoration to achieve its maximal strength and hardness. The newer acrylics which contain a sulfinic acid induction system have a rapid polymerization, thus permitting polishing at the insertion appointment without fear of disrupting marginal integrity. Sandpaper disks, strips, and burs may be employed in the final polishing as well as wet flour of pumice followed by tin oxide.

COMPOSITE RESINS

Composite resin restorative materials are currently packaged by the manufacturers as two separate pastes which are mixed together prior to use. One paste contains the base, the other the catalyst. The matrix of the composite resins differs from that of the polymethyl methacrylate resins. It is prepared by the reaction of bisphenol-A, an epoxy resin, with methacrylic acid and thinned with methyl methacrylate or a similar agent. Polymerization is accomplished by the benzoyl peroxide-amine system the same as described for the conventional acrylics.

The term "composite" indicates that the resin contains an inorganic filler. The filler in the composite resin, however, differs from the *inert* filler employed in some of the acrylic restorative materials discussed in the previous section in that the particles have been coated with a silane coupling agent to allow bonding between the filler and the resin matrix. The composite resins may contain as much as 75 to 80 per cent inorganic filler in the form of glass beads or rods, lithium aluminum silicate, quartz, or tricalcium phosphate.

The composite resins represent the current attempt to improve the properties and clinical performance of the tooth-colored anterior restorative materials. Their improved physical properties, compared to acrylic resins, include:[54]

1. greater compressive strength and tensile strength
2. superior hardness and abrasion resistance
3. less polymerization shrinkage
4. lower coefficient of thermal expansion.

They also have a few disadvantages:

1. possible color change
2. greater surface roughness.

The clinical implications of the physical characteristics of dental restorative materials is not always apparent. Table 9–2 attempts to correlate some of the properties of silicate cements, acrylic resins, and composite resins with their possible clinical significance. The composite resins appear to have several properties that make them more acceptable clinically.

Because the composite resins are packaged in paste form they are easier to mix than either the silicate cements or acrylic resins. They shrink less upon polymerization than do the acrylics[40, 70] and, therefore, can be inserted into the prepared cavity in bulk using a pressure technique. Because of the potential pulp irritation of the monomer a calcium hydroxide base is indicated. In spite of their lower coefficient of thermal expansion, laboratory studies have indicated that marginal leakage, with temperature cycling, is *not* less than with the conventional acrylics.[78] The clinical implications of this laboratory data are yet to be determined. However, in one clinical study which compared composite and silicate cement anterior restorations, the marginal integrity of the composite resin was superior after a three-year observation period.[43] The principal disadvantage, at this time, is the difficulty in providing a smooth polish to the surface of the composite restoration. The set mix consists of a large quantity of hard inorganic filler particles embedded in a relatively soft matrix. Finishing and polishing removes some of the particles embedded in the surface of the restoration producing depressions which maintain a rough rather than smooth finish (Fig. 9–8). The inability to obtain an ideal polish may render the composite restoration more susceptible to staining in the mouth. Dental manufacturers are currently designing special burs to finish the surface of composite restorations.

Because of the relative ease of handling and apparent superiority of composite resin, it is replacing acrylic resin and silicate cement in many dental offices. In pedodontics, it is being used more frequently not only in anterior permanent teeth but also in primary incisors. Formerly silver amalgam was widely used for restorations in primary anterior teeth. Amalgam has the disadvantage of being non-esthetic. Although acrylics are esthetic, their insertion is time consuming if the Nealon technique is used. It is always desirable to utilize a rapid, but effective, technique when treating a child patient. Composites are esthetic, may be inserted en masse, and, therefore, appear suitable for the primary anterior teeth. While the degree of clinical marginal leakage is yet to be determined, the main disadvantage appears to be the surface roughness of the restoration, even after polishing.

TABLE 9-2 TOOTH COLORED RESTORATIVE MATERIALS: ADVANTAGES AND DISADVANTAGES RELATIVE TO CLINICAL USE

Factor	A/D	Silicate	A/D	Acrylic	A/D	Composite
Method of insertion	A	Bulk	D	Incremental	A	Bulk
Color stability	D	Acquires stain	A	Color stable	U	Slightly less color stable than acrylic (in vitro)
Solubility	D	Soluble; subject to leakage and disintegration	A	Relatively insoluble	A	Relatively insoluble
Coefficient of thermal expansion	A	Similar to tooth enamel	D	Seven times greater than tooth enamel; results in marginal leakage	U	Lower than acrylic; clinical significance not known at this time
Secondary caries	A	Anticariogenic by virtue of fluoride content	D	Secondary caries may be associated with poor marginal integrity	U	Unknown at this time
Biologic status	D	Low pH; pulp irritant	D	Monomer; pulp irritant	D	Monomer; pulp irritant
Brittleness	D	Cannot be used for incisal angle repair	A	Can be used for incisal angles, but usually requires pin retention	A	Can be used for incisal angle repair but usually requires pin retention
Surface characteristics	D	Rough due to deterioration by oral fluids and acids	A	Can be polished smooth if it does not contain filler	D	Rough; cannot be polished smooth due to filler

A = advantage; D = disadvantage; U = unknown.

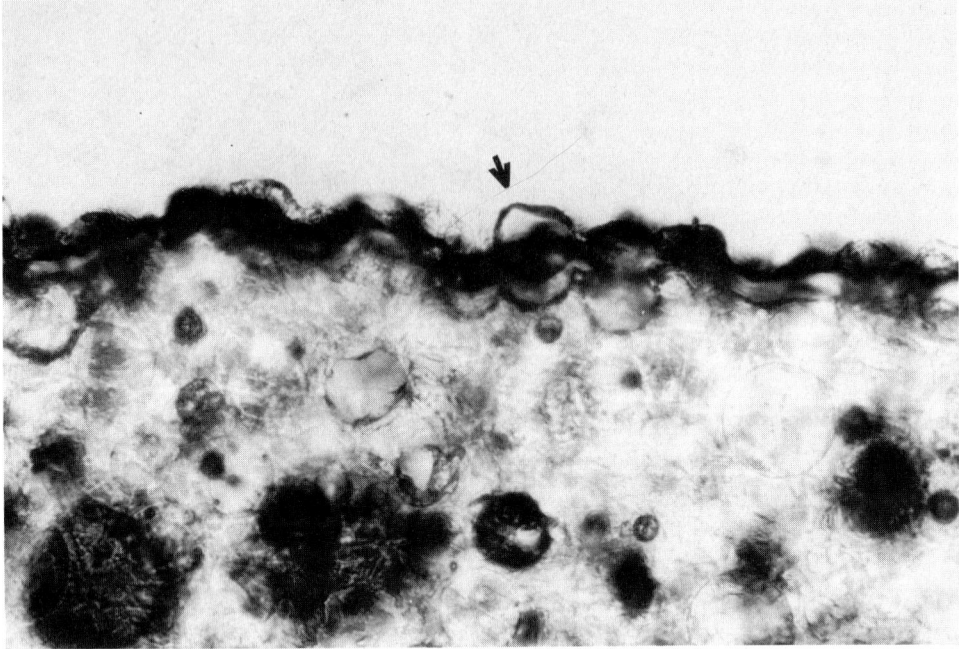

Figure 9–8 Cross section through a composite anterior restorative material which contains glass beads and fibers. Notice the roughness produced as glass particles are abraded from the surface (arrow). (Courtesy of Dr. M. Buonocore.)

LUTING AND BASE MATERIALS

Luting and base materials include zinc phosphate cement, polycarboxylate cement, zinc oxide-eugenol, and calcium hydroxide. Depending upon their physical and biologic properties these materials are used as bases in deep cavity preparations or for luting orthodontic bands, fixed pedodontic appliances, and stainless steel or other types of crowns to the teeth.

ZINC PHOSPHATE CEMENT

Zinc phosphate cement has been used both as a luting agent and as a base to provide thermal insulation in deep cavities. Its intended use determines the consistency of the mix and this, in turn, affects its physical and biologic properties.

Zinc phosphate cements are composed of a powder, mainly zinc oxide, and a liquid which is phosphoric acid with approximately 30 to 50 per cent water. Aluminum phosphate and zinc phosphate are generally added as buffers to retard the setting action when the liquid and powder are combined. Because of the extremely acid nature of the mixed cement (initial pH 1.6) it is irritating to the pulp if placed in cavities that are very deep, or which have young patent dentinal tubules. The acidity is gradually neutralized as the setting continues and the damaging qualities to the pulp are mitigated. Nevertheless, after one hour the pH is still below 7 and does not reach neutrality until approximately 48 hours.

Despite its adverse effect on the pulp, zinc phosphate cement has been used as a base because of its high compressive strength. Clinically it is possible to condense an amalgam restoration against a zinc phosphate cement base a few minutes after the base is placed in the prepared cavity. Pulp damage must be avoided by using a sub-base of calcium hydroxide or zinc oxide-eugenol over the exposed freshly cut dentinal tubules prior to the insertion of the zinc phosphate cement.

As a luting agent, zinc phosphate cement also has its deficiencies. When cementing a stainless steel crown, for instance, the problem of pulp irritation is intensified because of the relatively greater amount of free acid in the more fluid mix and the large number of exposed dentinal tubules. When used to cement bands to the teeth, the free acid has been associated with decalcification of the underlying enamel. When the bands are removed, an unsightly area of decalcification may be present as illustrated in Figure 9-9. Because zinc phosphate cement is soluble in oral fluids and provides a relatively weak mechanical interlocking between tooth and band, the band may become loose and have to be recemented at periodic intervals.

While calcium hydroxide and zinc oxide-eugenol produces milder pulpal responses, their use as a base has been limited by the low crushing strength of the commercial products available. Within the past five years, new formulations, with improved physical properties, have been marketed. The use of these biologically superior, physically improved products as bases in deep cavities is indicated rather than zinc phosphate cement. Furthermore, if they live up to expectation, the newly developed and marketed polycarboxylate cements may displace zinc phosphate cement as a luting agent. The need to use the biologically abusive zinc phosphate cement in the dental treatment of children is clearly declining.

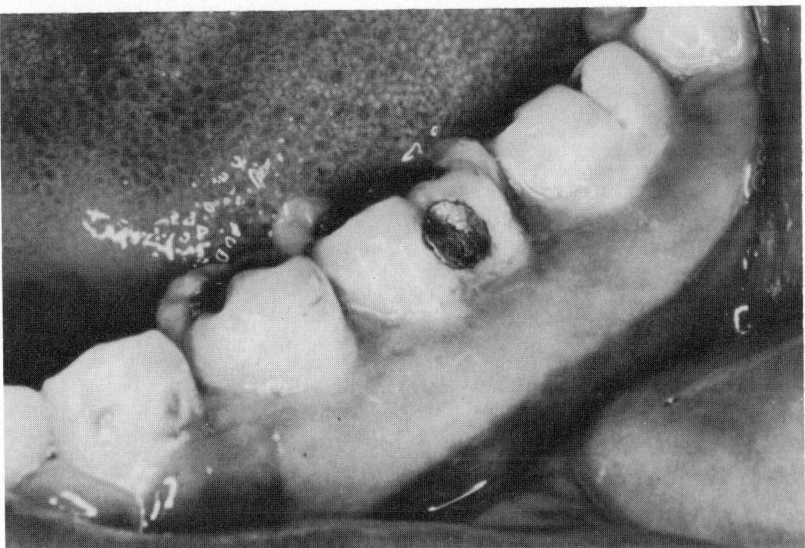

Figure 9-9 Decalcified appearance of permanent teeth after the removal of orthodontic bands which had been cemented with zinc phosphate.

POLYCARBOXYLATE CEMENT

Polycarboxylate cements represent a completely new dental material. The first published report of this material appeared in 1968.[67] Since that time several commercial dental cements with formulations based upon the polycarboxylate system have become available.

Like zinc phosphate cement the product is supplied as a powder and liquid which are mixed together prior to use. The powder is a modified zinc oxide similar to that in other dental cements. The liquid component is an aqueous solution of polyacrylic acid. Polyacrylic acid is a polymer of the three carbon acrylic acid molecule ($CH_2{=}CH{-}COOH$). It has free carboxylic acid groups on alternate carbons which are available for chelation. When the powder and liquid are mixed together, the carboxylate groups of the polyacrylic acid chelate the zinc from the powder forming a network of zinc carboxylate. According to Smith,[67] the mix wets the tooth surface and chemico-mechanical adhesion to enamel, and to a lesser extent dentin, occurs by chelation of free carboxyl groups to the calcium component of the tooth structure.

Zinc phosphate cement and polycarboxylate cement* appear to have similar properties regarding solubility in water and acetic acid, tensile strength, setting time, film thickness, and pH.[57] While zinc phosphate cement has a greater compressive strength, the polycarboxylate cement exhibits superior adhesion to both enamel and dentin. Even though both cements exhibit comparable pH values, polycarboxylate cements apparently do not produce the irritable tissue response associated with zinc phosphate cement and appear to be more biologically acceptable.[67, 79] Because of the apparent biological superiority of polycarboxylate cement, and its superior bonding potential, it is replacing zinc phosphate cement, especially as a luting agent. In children's dentistry polycarboxylate cement is used in the cementation of stainless steel crowns and orthodontic bands. Laboratory tests have been performed using this material to lute orthodontic brackets directly to teeth without an intermediate band.[44] The direct cementation is possible as long as torquing forces are not applied to the bracket. Clinical trials are currently in progress in which specially designed patch-type brackets are bonded directly to the teeth of patients undergoing orthodontic treatment with light wire techniques.[68]

The chemico-mechanical interaction between enamel and cement requires intimate contact between the two surfaces. Prior to cementation of an orthodontic band or stainless steel crown both the metal and tooth must be cleaned with an aqueous pumice slurry, the remaining film must be removed with alcohol, and the surface must be air dried. Mixing of the cement is accomplished according to the individual manufacturer's instructions, and cementation is accomplished in the usual manner. When it is necessary to remove a band, a sharp tug is required to break the bond.

Because of the short time that polycarboxylate cements have been available, their physical and biologic properties have been investigated less than for zinc phosphate cement, and there has been no long term monitoring of clinical performance. Whether decalcification of tooth structure beneath bands is eliminated

---

*Tests were conducted on Fleck's Cement (Mizzy Inc., Clifton Forge, Va.), a representative zinc phosphate cement, and Durelon (Espe, Seefield/Oberby, West Germany), a representative polycarboxylate cement.

by the use of this cement, for instance, can only be ascertained after additional reports of clinical usage become available. The practicing dentist must remain informed as additional studies of this material are reported and he must remember that future research by dental manufacturers will undoubtedly improve the properties of the products now in use.

ZINC OXIDE-EUGENOL

Zinc oxide-eugenol is a widely used material in dentistry for children. It is used (1) as a protective base beneath an amalgam restoration, (2) as a temporary filling, (3) as an anodyne dressing to aid in the recovery of an inflamed pulp, and (4) as a luting agent for stainless steel and other crowns. It also may be used as a root canal filling in primary teeth.

When zinc oxide and eugenol are mixed together elongate crystals of zinc eugenolate are formed. The zinc eugenolate matrix and the excess zinc oxide powder absorb the unreacted eugenol and form a hard mass. Non-proprietary zinc oxide-eugenol mixes have the undesirable property of having a relatively low compressive strength. The addition of o-ethoxybenzoic acid (EBA) to commercial zinc oxide-eugenol formulations considerably increases the compressive strength of the zinc oxide-eugenol mix.[8, 55] The EBA will also increase the water solubility of the mix.[8] By the incorporation of various hydrogenated rosins, this undesirable side effect is eliminated, while the high compressive strength values are retained.[7]

Zinc oxide-eugenol may be used as a protective base beneath an amalgam restoration when thermal insulation is desired. Because of its almost neutral pH zinc oxide-eugenol does not produce the pulpal irritation commonly observed with the highly acid zinc phosphate cements. Zinc oxide-eugenol also possesses an anodyne effect which is believed to be associated with its eugenol content; paradoxically, the eugenol may also be an irritant if placed in close proximity to, or in direct contact with, the pulp.[6, 46] The thicker the layer of intervening dentin, the fewer should be the irritating effects observed. Since zinc oxide-eugenol is not mixed in stoichiometric proportions, some free eugenol will always be present in the mix.[47] To avoid the chronic irritation that the free eugenol might cause, the authors prefer to use a layer of calcium hydroxide in very deep cavities where the possibility of a clinically non-detectable exposure exists. If necessary, a layer of zinc oxide-eugenol may be placed over the calcium hydroxide for the thermal insulation that the additional bulk of material will provide.

Zinc oxide-eugenol has previously not been recommended as the sole base beneath an amalgam restoration because of its low compressive strength compared to zinc phosphate cement. The addition of EBA to certain commercial formulations has considerably increased the crushing strength of the set mix. Chong and co-workers[14] compared the compressive strength of commercially available "improved" zinc oxide-eugenol cements with a representative zinc phosphate cement. As seen in Table 9–3, seven minutes after mixing, the commercial zinc oxide-eugenol products achieved relatively high crushing strengths. (Seven minutes is regarded as the time interval between initial mixing of the cement and the insertion of an amalgam restoration).[38] In the same investigation it was determined that the minimum compressive strength required of a base to resist condensation pressure was 100 to 170 psi. Using extracted teeth, one- and two-surface restorations were

TABLE 9–3 COMPRESSIVE STRENGTH VALUES OF ZINC OXIDE-EUGENOL
PREPARATIONS VERSUS ZINC PHOSPHATE CEMENT

Material	Compressive Strength (psi)		
	at 7 minutes	at 30 minutes	at 24 hours
ZnOE			
Cavitec*	400	500	750
Zinc oxide-eugenol plus			
zinc acetate	600	1200	1250
Caulk temporary cement**	900	1000	2000
Timrex***	2300	3100	3500
ZnPO$_4$			
Tenacin**	1100	12,600	16,900

*Kerr Mfg. Co., Detroit, Mich.
**L. D. Caulk Co., Milford, Del.
***Interstate Dental Co., New York, N.Y.
Adapted from Chong et al., J.A.D.A., Jan. 1967.

packed against bases made from the zinc oxide-eugenol products. The bases were approximately 0.5 or 1.0 mm. thick. The teeth were sectioned along their long axes, exposing a cross section of the restoration and base. Displacement of the base associated with packing pressure was not observed. The results indicate that zinc oxide-eugenol, especially with additives designed to improve compressive strength, may be used as the sole base directly beneath a single or multiple surface amalgam restoration without being displaced. The zinc oxide-eugenol should not, however, be used in teeth grossly destroyed by caries in which the base must provide primary support for the permanent restoration.

When EBA is added to proprietary formulations it is at the expense of the eugenol. It might be hypothesized that these cements should contain less free eugenol in the set mix, and therefore be less of a potential irritant when placed in close proximity to the pulp. Rowe,[61] in fact, found that when an EBA-zinc oxide-eugenol cement was applied to rat pulps it was less irritant than a standard zinc oxide-eugenol mix and it did not interfere with pulp repair.

Mixed to a thin consistency the "improved" zinc oxide-eugenol preparations may be used for cementation purposes. In pedodontics, they are especially useful for cementing stainless steel crowns. They should not be used for cementation of acrylic jacket crowns because the eugenol attacks the resin.

Mixing of zinc oxide-eugenol materials is not critical; however, the manufacturer's directions should be followed. Proprietary zinc oxide-eugenol formulations may be supplied in paste form, in two separate tubes, or in a powder-liquid combination. Since the reaction is not exothermic a glass slab is not necessary for mixing. If the powder-liquid combination is used, several drops are placed on a mixing pad and powder is incorporated quickly in increments until a heavy, nonsticky consistency is produced. Mixing is complete in approximately 1 minute. The base is carried to its desired location in the tooth with a smooth flat ended instrument (Fig. 9–10A,B). The instrument may be dipped in a small amount of zinc oxide powder and used to mold the base to its desired shape. If the material is to be used for luting, a more fluid mix is prepared (Fig. 9–10C). Because these cements set quickly, the crown should be seated as rapidly as possible before the viscosity of the mix increases and interferes with correct seating. The paste system is used when a thin base is required. Approximately equal lengths of paste are extruded from each tube (usually ¼ inch or less is required), mixed on a mixing pad, and flowed onto the floor of the cavity with a special ball-ended instrument provided by the manu-facturer. Because eugenol will adversely affect resin materials, zinc oxide-eugenol products should not be used as bases beneath acrylic resins, composite resins, or acrylic jacket crowns.

CALCIUM HYDROXIDE

Calcium hydroxide is a powder which, when mixed with distilled water, forms a creamy paste of high alkalinity (pH 11 to 13). A suspension of calcium hydroxide in methyl cellulose paste (Pulpdent Paste*), which is more viscous and easier to manipulate is available commercially. Other proprietary calcium hydroxide preparations which contain selected resins that cause the mix to set quickly to a relatively hard consistency (Hydrex**, Dycal***) are also available.

Because of its biologic properties, calcium hydroxide is of value in a variety of clinical situations in which the integrity of vital pulp tissue may be compromised.

Calcium hydroxide has been recommended as a base or sub-base in teeth in which there is danger of pulpal exposure due to deep caries. It is applied over sound dentin following complete excavation of carious material, or, if the indirect

---

*Pulpdent Paste: Pulpdent Corp. of America, Boston, Mass.
**Hydrex: Kerr Mfg. Co., Detroit, Mich.
***Dycal: L. D. Caulk, Milford, Del.

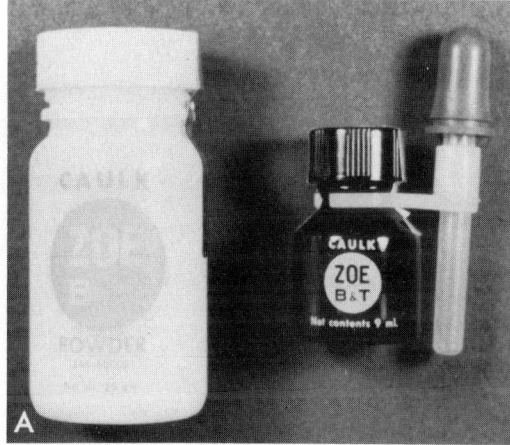
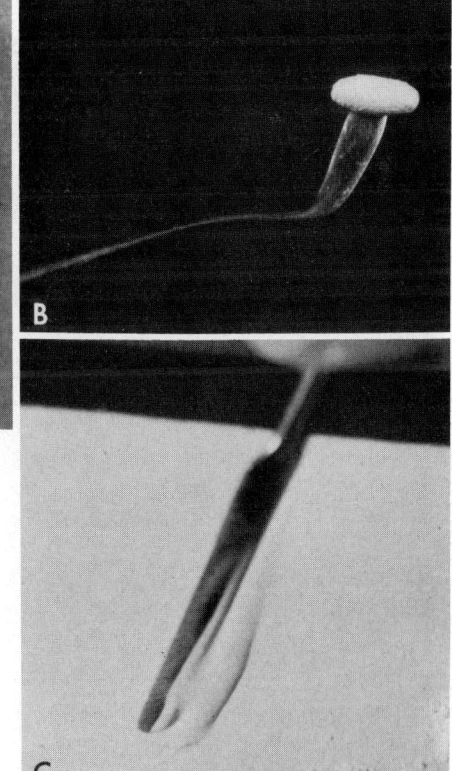

Figure 9–10 *A*, An example of an "im-proved" zinc oxide-eugenol product. *B*, Consis-tency of the material for use as a base beneath an amalgam restoration. *C*, Consistency of the mate-rial for luting a stainless steel crown.

pulp treatment technique is used, it may be applied over a residual layer of carious dentin (see Chapter 10). Convincing evidence from the work of Mjor,[45] Klein,[33] and Eidelman and co-workers[23] indicates that calcium hydroxide will increase the density and hardness of underlying dentin in primary and permanent teeth. Increased hardness of the dentin between the floor of the cavity and the pulp chamber has been observed as early as 15 days following application of calcium hydroxide. The changes are believed to be produced by intratubular deposition of calcified material as well as by intertubular calcification of secondary dentin (Fig. 9–11). These changes are considered beneficial and protective to the pulp. The greater the increase in density of the dentin between the floor of the cavity and the pulp, the better the pulp will be protected from the ingress of chemical and bacterial irritants. When calcium hydroxide is used in the indirect pulp treatment technique it appears to arrest the lesion,[66] sterilize the residual deep layer of caries,[32] remineralize the carious dentin,[31, 36] and produce secondary dentin deposition.[63]

In primary or permanent teeth in which direct pulp capping is indicated, and in cases in which the pulp of a permanent tooth has been exposed due to trauma

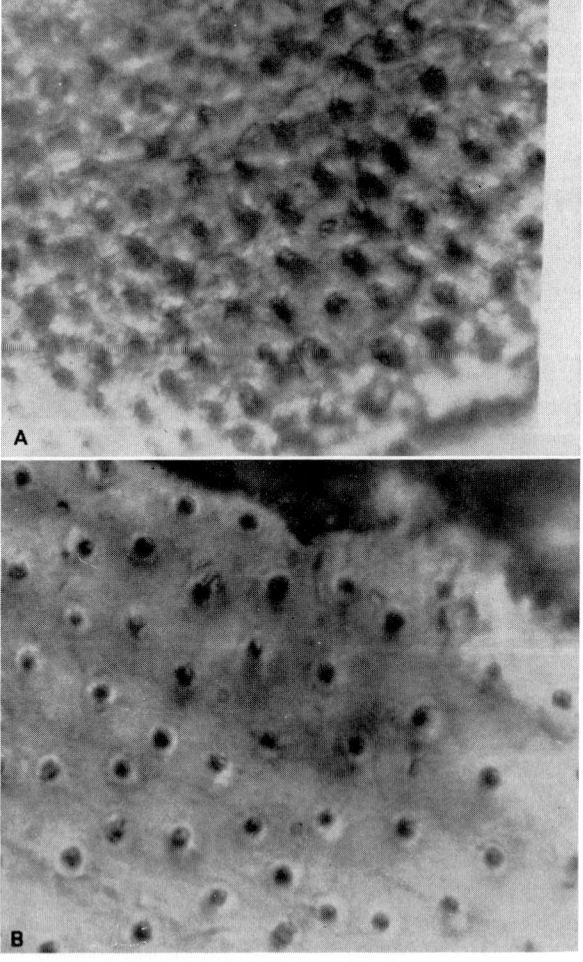

Figure 9–11 *A,* Cross section of normal dentin shows dark-appearing dentinal tubules and a diffuse intertubular matrix. *B,* Cross section of dentin beneath calcium hydroxide shows homogeneous and greater calcified intertubular matrix, and the highly calcified areas on the peripheral walls of the tubules which are reminiscent of sclerosed dentin.

TABLE 9–4 COMPRESSIVE STRENGTH VALUES OF CALCIUM HYDROXIDE
PREPARATIONS VERSUS ZINC PHOSPHATE CEMENT

Material	Compressive Strength (psi)		
	at 7 minutes	at 30 minutes	at 24 hours
CaOH			
Hydrex*	500	700	1400
Dycal**	1100	1000	1100
ZnPO$_4$			
Tenacin**	1100	12,600	16,900

*Kerr Mfg. Co., Detroit, Mich.
**L.D. Caulk Co., Milford, Del.
Adapted from Chong et al. J.A.D.A., Jan. 1967.

and pulpotomy is required (Chapter 11), calcium hydroxide is deemed the material
of choice. Used over the exposed dental pulp or after coronal pulp amputation it
will stimulate continued odontoblastic activity and the possible formation of a
dentin bridge.[51]

In spite of the beneficial biologic properties of calcium hydroxide, zinc phosphate cement has been traditionally used as a base beneath amalgam and resin
restorations. Zinc phosphate cement has been considered superior because of its
high compressive strength, although its adverse effects on vital pulp tissue make it
the biologically inferior material. When calcium hydroxide bases are used it has
been recommended that they be overlaid with a stronger base of zinc phosphate
cement before inserting the amalgam restoration.

Commercial calcium hydroxide preparations which contain additives to increase their compressive strength may be used as the sole base underlying an
amalgam or other restoration. This change in therapeutic technique is possible
because, shortly after mixing, the compressive strength of these preparations,
although usually not as high as zinc phosphate cement, is high enough to prevent
displacement when amalgam is packed against them.

Table 9–4 presents the results of compressive strength tests made on cylindrical specimens of commercial calcium hydroxide products and evaluated against a
representative zinc phosphate cement at selected times after mixing.[14] Within 7
minutes after mixing, the commercial calcium hydroxide material (Dycal) is as
strong as the zinc phosphate cement.

It has already been mentioned that Chong and co-workers[14] have demonstrated that the minimum strength necessary for a base to support condensation
pressure is 100 to 170 psi. Thus, as seen in Table 9–4 both Dycal and Hydrex
possess sufficient compressive strength to support amalgam condensation. Chong
and co-workers packed amalgam into one- and two-surface cavity preparations in
extracted teeth. In the one-surface cavities the amalgam was packed against a 0.5
mm. thick calcium hydroxide base while in the two-surface cavities the base was
1 mm. thick. In no instance was the base found to be displaced by condensation
when ground sections of the teeth prepared through the restorations were examined microscopically.

Manipulation of the commercial preparations of calcium hydroxide is quite
easy. Small tubes of catalyst and base are usually used (Fig. 9–12) and the contents
are squeezed on a paper mixing pad in equal lengths. The paste is mixed thor-

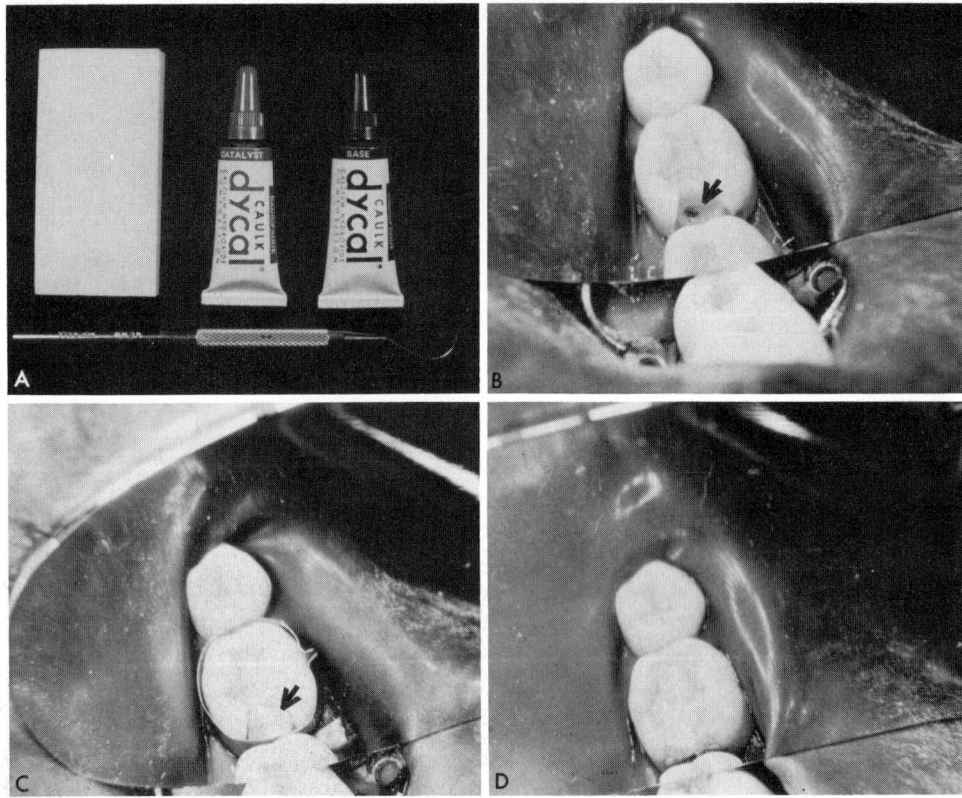

Figure 9–12   *A,* Example of a rapid setting calcium hydroxide proprietary material with a relatively high crushing strength. *B,* A small accidental pulp exposure in a primary tooth; an indication for direct pulp capping. *C,* The proprietary mix of calcium hydroxide has been applied to the exposure site and surrounding dentin. *D,* An amalgam restoration, prepared with a spherical alloy which requires less condensation pressure than conventional alloy, is placed over the hardened calcium hydroxide. (Courtesy of Dr. J. King.)

oughly with a specially designed instrument purchased from the manufacturer. The usual cement mixing spatula is not used because of the difficulty in removing the set calcium hydroxide. Using the same instrument the paste is flowed on the dentin floor of the cavity preparation. After approximately 2 minutes, when the material has set, excess is removed from the cavity walls with the tip of a sharp explorer.

CAVITY LINERS

One of the major shortcomings of all restorative materials is their inability to inhibit leakage of bacteria, moisture, and debris between the margin of the restoration and the tooth structure. Attempts to solve the leakage problem have resulted in the commercial development of a number of cavity liners or varnishes. These materials are used to line the walls and floor of the cavity preparation. The intended effect of the liner is to protect the pulp from the harmful effects of chemical agents derived from restorative materials that would otherwise penetrate the dentinal tubules, and also to prevent the ingress of oral contaminants at the cavosurface margins and thence through the dentin to the pulp. Cavity liners have also been advocated as thermal insulators.

The cavity liner usually consists of a resin or synthetic resin in an organic solvent such as acetone, chloroform, or ether. Other additives may include zinc oxide, calcium hydroxide, or polystyrene. The fluid cavity liner is painted on the walls and floor of the prepared cavity; the volatile solvent evaporates and leaves a thin protective coating.

Effect of Liners on Thermal Conductivity

It has usually been assumed that cavity liners impart a degree of thermal insulation when placed under metallic restorations and thus help prevent oral temperature changes from adversely affecting the dental pulp. However, in an *in vitro* study employing a commercial cavity liner, it was found that the liner did not possess any thermal insulative properties.[30] The results of this study cast doubt on the ability of cavity liners to protect the pulp from sudden thermal stimuli. The microscopic thickness of the coating generally applied to the prepared cavity also precludes the liner's functioning effectively as a thermal insulator under metallic restorations.

Effect of Liners on Marginal Leakage

As previously stated, all restorative materials in present usage exhibit marginal leakage to some degree. The ideal restorative material capable of forming a permanent bond with dental enamel and thus sealing the tooth-restoration interface has not yet been found. Amalgam restorations are unique, however, in that microleakage diminishes with time owing to a sealing of the cavosurface margin by products of corrosion.

Results of the effectiveness of cavity liners to prevent marginal leakage are variable. Several *in vitro* studies, using dyes and radioactive isotopes to demonstrate leakage, indicate that cavity liners placed beneath amalgam restorations and silicate cements can minimize leakage to a considerable extent. However, in these studies the effect of temperature variation, a common environmental factor in the oral cavity, was not investigated. When temperature variation was considered, it was found that leakage was reduced when a commercially available liner was used with silicate, but that it actually enhanced leakage when placed under an amalgam restoration. Furthermore, when placed beneath amalgam restorations inserted in primary molars in children, the liner failed to prevent ingress of bacteria through the margins to the cavity floor.[29] The adhesive bond between tooth structure and cavity liner is quickly lost, indicating that liners do not indefinitely eliminate marginal voids. In fact, coupled with factors of thermal expansion between the restoration, tooth, and liner, the placing of a liner at the cavosurface margins may result in a greater space at this site than if it is left unlined.

In the light of the present conflicting reports, more evaluation seems necessary before the cavity liners presently available can be judged effective in *sealing the margins* of restorations. Until that time, the use of these agents along the cavosurface margins of prepared cavities cannot be recommended.

Effect of Liners on Acid Penetration

The necessity to provide a protective barrier beneath zinc phosphate and silicate cements has been established. These materials are initially acidic and maintain an acid pH 24 hours or more after insertion. The leaching out of acid into underlying dentin can produce temporary or permanent damage to the dental pulp. The less dentin separating the pulp from the zinc phosphate or silicate cement, the greater will be the magnitude of the problem.

Cavity liners have been recommended to provide protection to the pulp from injurious agents, such as acid, present in dental restorative materials. The liner is painted over the dentin on the floor of the cavity in an attempt to seal the dentinal tubules and prevent ingress of the hydrogen ion toward the pulp. Studies have indicated that cavity liners are effective in this regard and will reduce the penetration of the hydrogen ion from the cement to the pulp. Since cavity liners harden into semipermeable membranes, they will not completely inhibit acid penetration; nevertheless, it is recommended that cavity liners be placed on the dentinal floor of the cavity preparation if a zinc phosphate cement base is to be used.

Application of the Liner

Philips[52] states that there are only minor differences between the brands of cavity liners available, and the operator should select "the product which can be most readily seen and which affords optimum flow and wetting of the tooth structure."

The liner is painted on the cavity floor using a thin bent-angled brush. Several applications should be made in an effort to impart a uniform layer to the floor of the cavity. If the bottled liner becomes too thick, it may be thinned with the appropriate solvent before application. Until further evidence indicates that cavity liners will provide an adequate marginal seal and in fact are not actually detrimental to the success of the restoration, the authors advise that cavity liners not be applied to the cavosurface margins. If the applicator brush should inadvertently touch these margins, the varnish should be removed with a slowly rotating fissure bur.

A cavity liner should not be placed under a resin restoration because the solvent may not be compatible with it. Instead the "primer" provided by the manufacturer of the resin product being used should be employed.

FISSURE SEALANTS

The occlusal pits and fissures of both primary and permanent teeth are the most caries susceptible tooth sites. In spite of the positive benefits of topical and systemic fluoride therapy, the least benefit is afforded the occlusal surfaces. Various attempts have been made to specifically prevent pit and fissure caries (see Chapter 24). These methods either were not successful or were not popularly accepted by the dental profession. Recently a technique has been developed of sealing occlusal pits and fissures to render them less caries susceptible. A layer of the sealant is applied over the occlusal surface isolating it from the oral microflora and their nutrients, thus preventing the initiation of dental decay.

Several clinical studies using different sealing agents have been reported. The initial clinical trials have used methyl-2-cyanoacrylate, an industrial adhesive, mixed with a powdered filler, which was applied to occlusal surfaces at 6 month or yearly intervals.[15, 50, 59, 60] With one exception,[50] these reports were favorable and reductions in occlusal caries of approximately 85 to 90 per cent were obtained. Although these studies demonstrated the effectiveness of the *technique* of fissure sealing, the methyl-2-cyanoacrylate was difficult to handle, was easily affected by changes in humidity, and had a limited shelf life. Furthermore, it was thought that frequent reapplication would be necessary for continued success.

Research by Dr. M. Buonocore at the Eastman Dental Center has led to the availability of a sealing agent* which has been reported to produce caries reductions of approximately 90 per cent or more in the occlusal surfaces of primary and permanent teeth.[9, 10, 42]

Chemically, the material is the reaction product of bisphenol and glycidyl methacrylate plus methyl methacrylate monomer and a catalyst, benzoin methyl ether. It is activated by ultraviolet light of 3600 Å wavelength. Buonocore reported that after a single application of this material to the occlusal surfaces of 200 teeth no occlusal caries developed over a one year observation period.[9] During the same time interval 42 of the 200 nontreated control teeth developed caries. This represented a caries reduction of 100 per cent. Two years after the material was applied 153 teeth were available for reevaluation.[10] Seventy eight per cent of the teeth still had sealant covering their occlusal surfaces and the reported caries reduction was 96 per cent. In an independent study, McCune and Cvar of the U.S. Public Health Service, testing the same material, reported that 9 months after application 90.2 per cent of treated teeth retained occlusal sealant and the caries reduction obtained was 88 per cent.[42] Table 9–5 summarizes the findings of these three reports and is the only clinical data published on this type of commercially available fissure sealant at this time.

Success of this technique depends upon the ability of the sealant to form a firm bond with enamel and to prevent penetration of bacteria at the interface between it and the occlusal surface. Prior to the application of the material a 50 per cent modified phosphoric acid solution is used to etch the occlusal surface. This produces small spaces in the enamel which allow tags of sealant as seen in Figure 9–13, to penetrate into the tooth structure to a depth of approximately 20 microns.[12, 26] It is believed that the tags extending into the tooth favor the clinical longevity of the material by enhancing bonding and by preserving the integrity of the sealant-tooth interface, thereby preventing the development of caries.

Method of Application

1. A non-carious tooth (or teeth) with deep occlusal grooves is selected (Fig. 9–14*A*). The surface to be treated is cleaned with an aqueous pumice slurry using a standard polishing brush.
2. The tooth is washed with a stream of water, isolated with cotton rolls, and thoroughly dried with a blast of warm compressed air.
3. The occlusal surface is "conditioned" by gently applying the phosphoric acid solution by means of a cotton pellet for approximately 60 seconds. The acid etch gives the treated enamel an opaque, dull appearance (Fig. 9–14*B*).

---

*Nuva-Seal and Nuva-Lite: L. D. Caulk Co., Milford, Delaware

TABLE 9–5   RESULTS OF CLINICAL TRIALS WITH AN ULTRAVIOLET
LIGHT CATALYZED FISSURE SEALANT

Investigator	Number of treated teeth	Time after application	Results	
			% of teeth retaining sealant	% caries reduction
Buonocore (J.A.D.A., 1970)	200	1 year	99.5	100
Buonocore (J.A.D.A., 1971)	153	2 years	78	96
McCune & Cvar (I.A.D.R. ABST., 1971)	1199	9 mos.	90.2	88

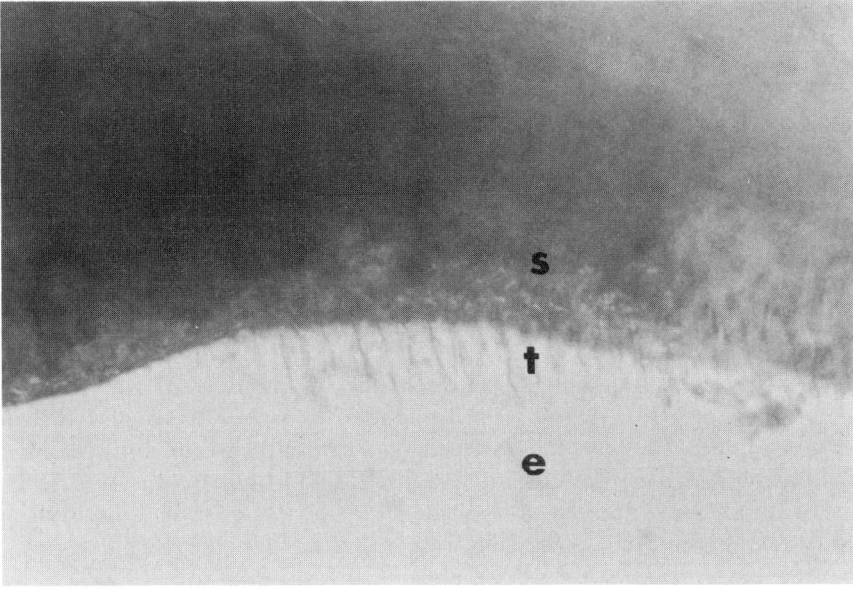

Figure 9–13 Microscopic appearance of sealant tags. The enamel (e) has been dissolved away to allow visualization of the tags (t) which extend from the sealant (s) into the enamel of the tooth.

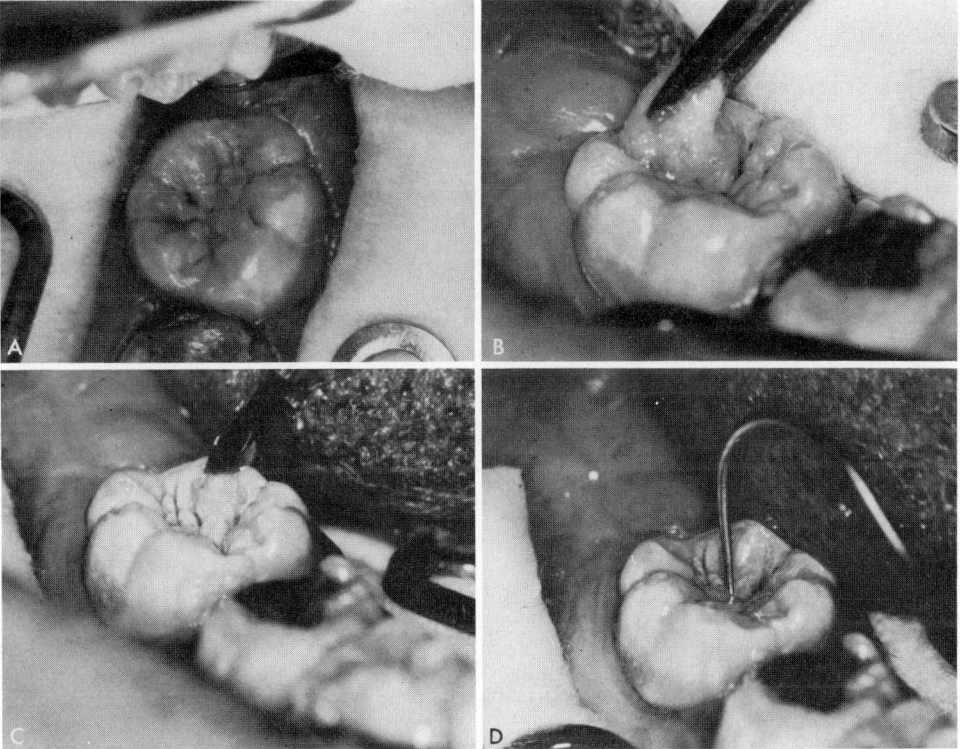

Figure 9–14 Fissure sealant technique using ultraviolet light catalyzed material (Nuva-Seal). *A*, Appearance of tooth to be treated. *B*, Application of phosphoric acid solution to occlusal surface. *C*, Application of sealant with brush to etched occlusal surface. *D*, Appearance of polymerized sealant after it has been exposed to ultraviolet light. (Courtesy of Dr. M. Buonocore.)

4. The tooth is thoroughly washed with a water spray, isolated with cotton rolls, and dried with compressed air.
5. The two liquid components of the sealant system are mixed together and painted on the prepared surface with a camel's-hair brush. The brush permits exact placement of the material over the pits and fissures (Fig. 9–14C).
6. Ultraviolet light from a proper ultraviolet light source is directed against the treated occlusal surface for approximately 30 seconds to allow for hardening of the material.
7. After hardening, the sealant surface should be checked for voids using the tip of a sharp explorer (Fig. 9–14D). If present these should be filled by reapplying a dab of adhesive and re-exposing to ultraviolet light.

The sealed teeth should be re-examined when the child returns for his usual 6 month recall examination. If material has been lost from the treated surfaces it should be reapplied using the same technique. The results of the clinical trials cited above, however, indicate that for most teeth reapplication should not be necessary for at least 1 or 2 years and that as long as the material is retained, occlusal caries will not develop. Primary molars should be sealed until they exfoliate, permanent bicuspids and molars at least until the child is in his late teens.

REFERENCES

1. Ambrose, E. R.: Pressure amalgamation. J. Canad. Dent. Assn., *28*:571–580, 1960.
2. Aponte, A. J., Hartsook, J. T., and Crowley, M. C.: Indirect pulp capping success verified. J. Dent. Child., *33*:164–166, 1966.
3. Barber, D. B., and Massler, M.: Penetration of isotopes through liners and bases under silicate cement restorations. J. A. D. A., *65*:786–796, 1962.
4. Bowen, R. L., Paffenbarger, G. C., and Millineaux, A. L.: A laboratory and clinical comparison of silicate cements and a direct-filling resin: A progress report. J. Prosth. Dent., *20*:426–437, 1968.
5. Braden, M.: Heat conduction in teeth and the effect of lining materials. J. Dent. Res., *43*:315–322, 1964.
6. Brannstrom, M., and Billberg, B.: Pulp changes beneath temporary fillings with Pharmatec and zinc oxide-eugenol, Odont. Rev., *18*:17–26, 1967.
7. Brauer, G., Simon, L., and Sangermano, L.: Improved zinc oxide–eugenol type cements. J. Dent. Res., *41*:1096-1102, 1962.
8. Brauer, G., White, E. E., and Mushonas, M. G.: The reaction of metal oxides with o-ethoxybenzoic acid and other chelating agents. J. Dent. Res., *37*:547–560, 1958.
9. Buonocore, M.: Adhesive sealing of pits and fissures for caries prevention, with use of ultraviolet light. J. A. D. A., *80*:324–330, 1970.
10. Buonocore, M.: Caries prevention in pits and fissures sealed with an adhesive resin polymerized by ultraviolet light: A two-year study of a single adhesive application. J. A. D. A., *82*:1090–1093, 1971.
11. Buonocore, M., Azevedo, N., and Dalton, E.: Evaluation of cavity liners for permeability and adhesion to dentin, New York Dent. J., *28*:239–244, 1962.
12. Buonocore, M., Matsui, A., and Gwinnett, A. J.: Penetration of resin dental materials into enamel with reference to bonding. Arch. Oral Biol., *13*:61–70, 1968.
13. Charbeneau, G. T.: An appraisal of finishing and polishing procedures for dental amalgam. J. Mich. Dent. Assn., *46*:135–138, 1964.
14. Chong, W. F., and Swartz, M. L., and Phillips, R. W.: Displacement of cement bases by amalgam restorations. J. A. D. A., *74*:97–102, 1967. ·
15. Cueto, E. I., and Buonocore, M.: Sealing of pits and fissures with an adhesive resin: Its use in caries prevention. J. A. D. A., *75*:121–128, 1967.
16. deFreitas, J. F.: The long-term solubility of silicate cement, Aust. Dent. J., *13*:129–134, 1968.
17. Delaney, J. M., and Seyler, A. E.: Hard-set calcium hydroxide as a sole base in pulp protection. J. Dent. Child., *33*:13–19, 1966.
18. Demaree, N. C., and Taylor, D. F.: Properties of dental amalgams made from spherical alloy particles. J. Dent. Res., *41*:890–906, 1962.

19. Doyle, W. A.: Operative dentistry. *In* Goldman, H. M., et al. (eds.), Current Therapy in Dentistry. 3rd ed., St. Louis, C. V. Mosby Co., 1968, pp. 843–844.

20. Dudding, N. J., Stookey, G. K., and Muhler, J. C.: Technique for the preparation and use of zirconium silicate as a cleaning and polishing agent. J. Indiana Dent. Assn., *44*:54–57, 1965.

21. Eames, W. B.: Preparation and condensation of amalgam with a low mercury-alloy ratio. J. A. D. A., *58*:78–83, 1959.

22. Eames, W. B., Mack, R. M., and Auvenshine, R. C.: Accuracy of mercury/alloy proportioning systems. J. A. D. A., *81*:137–141, 1970.

23. Eidelman, E., Finn, S. B., and Koulourides, T.: Remineralization of carious dentin treated with calcium hydroxide. J. Dent. Child., *32*:218–225, 1965.

24. Going, R. E., and Massler, M.: Influence of cavity liners under amalgam restorations on penetration by radioactive isotopes. J. Prosth. Dent., *11*:298–312, 1961.

25. Going, R. E., and Sawinski, V. J.: Microleakage of a new restorative material. J. A. D. A., *73*:107–115, 1966.

26. Gwinnett, A. J., and Matsui, A.: A study of enamel adhesives. The physical relationship between enamel and adhesive. Arch. Oral Biol. *12*:1615–1620, 1967.

27. Hallsworth, A. S., and Weatherall, J. A.: The microdistribution, uptake and loss of fluoride in human enamel. Caries Res., *3*:109–118, 1969.

28. Hargreaves, P., and Davies, E. H.: Physical properties of amalgam prepared from powder and tablet alloy. Brit. Dent. J., *117*:21–26, 1964.

29. Harrison, L. M.: Cavity varnishes shown ineffective. J. Dent. Child., *33*:174–179, 1966.

30. Hollenback, G. M., and Sullivan, M.: The thermal conductivity of restorative materials and cavity liners. J. S. Calif. Dent. Assn., *32*:208–213, 1964.

31. Kerkove, B. C., Jr., Herman, S. C., Klein, A. I., and McDonald, R. E.: A clinical and television densitometric evaluation of the indirect pulp capping technic. J. Dent. Child., *34*:192–201, 1967.

32. King, J. B., Crawford, J. J., and Lindahl, R. L.: Indirect pulp capping: A bacteriologic study of deep carious dentine in human teeth, Oral Surg., *20*:663–671, 1965.

33. Klein, A.: Association between deciduous dentin sclerosis and calcium hydroxide methyl cellulose base material, J. A. D. A., *63*:76–84, 1961.

34. Koran, A., and Asgar, K.: A comparison of dental amalgams made from a spherical alloy and from a comminuted alloy. J. A. D. A., *75*:912–917, 1967.

35. Laswell, H. R.: A prevalence study of secondary caries occurring in a young adult male population. IADR Program and Abstracts, Abst. 426, 45th annual meeting, March 1967, Washington, D.C.

36. Law, D. B., and Lewis, T. M.: The effect of calcium hydroxide on deep carious lesions. Oral Surg., *14*:1130–1137, 1961.

37. Lee, B. D., Phillips, R. W., and Swartz, M. L.: The influence of phosphoric acid etching on retention of acrylic resin to bovine enamel. J. A. D. A., *82*:1381–1386, 1971.

38. Lyll, J. S.: Base forming materials for restorations of silver amalgam. Aust. Dent. J., *5*:132–134, 1960.

39. Lyll, J. S., and Wing, G.: Proportioning of dental amalgam. Aust. Dent. J., *6*:127–129, 1961.

40. Macchi, R. L., and Craig, R. G.: Physical and mechanical properties of composite restorative materials. J. A. D. A., *78*:328–334, 1969.

41. Massler, M., and Mansukhani, N.: Testing liners under cements in vitro. J. Prosth. Dent., *10*:964–975, 1960.

42. McCune, R. J., and Cvar, J. F.: Pit and fissure sealants: Preliminary results. IADR Program and Abstracts, Abst. 745, 49th annual meeting, March 1971, Chicago, Illinois.

43. McCune, R. J., Cvar, J. F., and Ryge, G.: Clinical comparison of anterior and posterior restorative materials. IADR Program and Abstracts, Abst. 482, 47th annual meeting, March 1969, Houston, Texas.

44. Mizrah, E., and Smith, D. C.: Direct cementation of orthodontic brackets to dental enamel, an investigation using a polycarboxylate cement. Brit. Dent. J., *127*:371–375, 1969.

45. Mjor, I. A., Finn, S. B., and Quigley, M. B.: The effect of calcium hydroxide and amalgam on noncarious, vital dentine. Arch. Oral Biol., *3*:283–291, 1961.

46. Mohammed, Y. R., Van Huysen, G., and Boyd, D. A.: Filling base materials and the unexposed tooth pulp. J. Prosth. Dent., *11*:503–513, 1961.

47. Molnar, E. J.: Residual eugenol from zinc oxide-eugenol compounds. J. Dent. Res., *46*:645–649, 1967.

48. Nealon, F. H.: Acrylic restorations: operative non-pressure procedure. New York J. Dent., *22*:201–206, 1952.

49. Norman, R. D., Swartz, M. L., Phillips, R. W., and Raibley, J. W.: Direct pH determination of setting cements. 2. The effects of prolonged storage time, powder/liquid ratio, temperature, and dentin. J. Dent. Res., *45*:1214–1219, 1966.

50. Parkhouse, R. C., and Winter, G. B.: A fissure sealant containing methyl-2-cyanoacrylate as a caries preventive agent: a clinical evaluation. Brit. Dent. J., *130*:16–19, 1971.

51. Phaneuf, R. A., Frankl, S. N., and Ruben, M. P.: A comparative histological evaluation of three calcium hydroxide preparations on the human primary pulp. J. Dent. Child., *35*:61–76, 1968.

52. Phillips, R. W.: Cavity varnishes and bases. Dent. Clin. N. Amer., pp. 159–168, March, 1965.

53. Phillips, R. W.: Recent improvements in dental materials that the operative dentist should known. J. A. D. A., *73*:84–90, 1966.

54. Phillips, R. W.: Composite restorative materials. Report of Council on Dental Materials and Devices. J. A. D. A., *80*:357–358, 1970.

55. Phillips, R. W., and Love, D. R.: The effect of certain additive agents on the physical properties of zinc oxide-eugenol mixtures. J. Dent. Res. *40*:294–303, 1961.

56. Phillips, R. W., Swartz, M. L., and Norman, R. D.: Materials for the Practicing Dentist, St. Louis, C. V. Mosby Co, 1969.

57. Phillips, R. W., Swartz, M. L., and Rhodes, B.: An evaluation of a carboxylate adhesive cement. J. A. D. A., *81*:1353–1359, 1970.

58. Pinto, J., and Buonocore, M.: Effect of base and cavity liners on marginal leakage of filling materials. New York Dent. J., *29*:199–207, 1963.

59. Ripa, L. W., Buonocore, M., and Cueto, E.: Adhesive sealing of pits and fissures for caries prevention: Report of two-year study. IADR Program and Abstracts, Abst. 247, 44th annual meeting, March 1966, Miami Beach, Florida.

60. Ripa, L. W., and Cole, W. W.: Occlusal sealing and caries prevention: Results 12 months after a single application of adhesive resin. J. Dent. Res., *49*:171–173, 1970.

61. Rowe, A. H. R.: Reaction of the rat molar pulp to various materials. Brit. Dent. J., *122*:291–300, 1967.

62. Sawusch, R. H.: Dycal capping of exposed pulps in primary teeth. J. Dent. Children, *30*:141–149, 1963.

63. Sayegh, F. S.: Qualitative and quantitative evaluation of new dentin in pulp capped teeth. J. Dent. Child., *35*:7–19, 1968.

64. Seltzer, S.: The penetration of micro-organisms between the tooth and direct resin fillings. J. A. D. A., *51*:560–566, 1955.

65. Skinner, E. W., and Phillips, R. W.: The Science of Dental Materials. 6th ed., Philadelphia, W. B. Saunders Co., 1967.

66. Smirnow, M.: Conservative treatment of carious exposures. New York Dent. J., *35*:214–218, 1969.

67. Smith, D. C.: A new dental cement. Brit. Dent. J., *125*:381–384, 1968.

68. Smith, D. C.: Dental cements. Dent. Clin. N. Amer., pp. 3–31, January, 1971.

69. Stanford, J. W.: Dental materials. J. A. D. A., *72*:1461–1469, 1966.

70. Stanford, J. W.: The current status of restorative resins. Dent. Clin. N. Amer., pp. 57–66, January, 1971.

71. Swartz, M. L.: Dental cements and restorative resins, Dent. Clin. N. Amer., pp. 169–183, March, 1965.

72. Swartz, M. L., Niblack, B. F., Alter, E. A., Norman, R. D., and Phillips, R. W.: In vivo studies on the penetration of dentin by constituents of silicate cement, J. A. D. A.,*76*:573–578, 1968.

73. Swartz, M. L., and Phillips, R. W.: Residual mercury content of amalgam restorations and its influence on compressive strength. J. Dent. Res., *35*:458–466, 1956.

74. Swartz, M. L., and Phillips, R. W.: In vitro studies of the marginal leakage of restorative materials. J. A. D. A., *62*:141–151, 1961.

75. Swartz, M. L., and Phillips, R. W.: Influence of manipulative variables on the marginal adaptation of certain restorative materials. J. Prosth. Dent., *12*:172–181, 1962.

76. Swartz, M. L., Phillips, R. M., and Chamberlain, N.: Continued studies on the permeability of cavity liners. J. Dent. Res., *41*:66–74, 1962.

77. Sweeney, W. T., and Burns, C. L.: Effect of mercury-alloy ratio on the physical properties of amalgam. J. A. D. A., *73*:374–381, 1961.

78. Tani, Y., and Buonocore, M. G.: Marginal leakage and penetration of basic fuchsin dye in anterior restorative materials. J. A. D. A., *78*:542–548, 1969.

79. Truelove, E. L., Mitchell, D. F., and Phillips, R. W.: Biologic evaluation of carboxylate cement. J. Dent. Res., *50*:166, 1971.

80. Walcott, R. B., Jendresen, M. D., and Ryge, G.: Strength, dimensional change and adaptation of amalgam prepared with 1:1 ratio. J. A. D. A., *67*:375–381, 1963.

81. Wilson, A. D., and Batchelor, R. F.: Dental silicate cements. 3. Environment and durability. J. Dent. Res., *47*:115–120, 1968.

82. Wilson, C. J., and Ryge, G.: Clinical study of dental amalgam. J. A. D. A., *66*:763–771, 1963.

83. Wing, G.: Clinical use of spherical particle amalgams. Aust. Dent. J., *15*:185–192, 1970.

84. Wing, G.: Modern concepts for the amalgam restoration. Dent. Clin. N. Amer., pp. 43–56, January, 1971.

10

PULPAL TREATMENT OF PRIMARY TEETH

by THOMPSON M. LEWIS
and DAVID B. LAW

Preservation of the primary tooth whose pulp has been endangered by deep carious lesions or trauma is a major problem in caring for the teeth of children. For decades dental science has sought a successful method of treatment. Many techniques have been proposed. The practitioner will recognize familiar names such as direct pulp capping, indirect pulp capping, partial pulpotomy, pulpotomy, and pulpectomy. Different drugs and medicaments have been suggested to accompany these techniques, and varying degrees of success have been reported. Unfortunately, many of these techniques have been controversial and their results unpredictable.

The objective in pulp therapy by the dentist, however, has always been the same: the successful treatment of a cariously involved pulp so that the tooth can remain in the mouth in a nonpathologic, healthy condition and fulfill its role as a useful component of the primary dentition. It is apparent that the primary tooth which has been so preserved will not only fulfill its role in mastication, but will act as an excellent space maintainer for the permanent dentition. In addition, the factors of comfort, freedom from infection, speech, and prevention of aberrant habits such as tongue thrusting can be best controlled by retention of the primary tooth in the dental arch.

PHYSICAL STRUCTURE OF THE DENTAL PULP

Unlike the enamel, which is a relatively inert structure, the dental pulp contains elements which make it similar to other loose connective tissues in the body. Included in the pulp are blood vessels, lymph vessels, nerves, defense cells, ground substance, and fibroblasts. Another characteristic of the pulp, however, is the presence of odontoblasts necessary for the production of dentin.

201

Developmentally, the dental pulp emerges as the result of the dental lamina's promotion of the underlying mesoderm to form the dental papilla. Its shape is determined by the enamel organ. As this embryonic tissue matures, odontoblasts are formed which deposit dentin at the cusp tips. As the dental papilla matures, it creates dentin and moves apically, and the tissue becomes more cellular and vascular. With the establishment of more dentin, the sensory and autonomic vasomotor fibers assume their positions.

Each element in the structure of the dental pulp plays a significant role in the life and preservation of the tooth. The fibroblasts produce tropocollagen which in turn becomes collagen fibers. The ground substance bonds these fibers together. Its chemical action plays a significant role during inflammation. The odontoblasts from which dentin evolves create a cell cytoplasm that is evident not only in the pulp, but also in the dentin. Histologically, odontoblasts are seen as long cells with extensions which intermingle and become even more profuse as they approach the dentino-enamel junction. A direct connection is effected from the dentino-enamel junction to the pulp as is evidenced by the hypersensitivity encountered when first passing through the dentino-enamel junction while performing operative procedures. The pulp also contains undifferentiated mesenchymal cells which may develop into odontoblasts, histiocytes that act as phagocytes, and lymphoid wandering cells that function in antibody production. There is an intricate arrangement of arteries and veins in each dental pulp which in turn communicates with the rest of the body. Likewise, a lymphatic network functions similarly to that in other areas of the body. Autonomic and sensory nerves complete the elements which "unite" the tooth to the whole body. Through the autonomics' transmission of stimuli to the capillaries, increased vasodilation creates a pressure on the free nerve endings, or sensory nerves, and in turn a pain response is felt.

The dental pulp and its physiologic functions are similar in many ways to other parts of the body. Its individual characteristics, however, such as its close confinement by the structurally hard dentin, present a unique situation. The responsible clinician must have knowledge of the pulp's structure and be aware of his limitations of treatment in order to achieve optimum results in the treatment of diseased or traumatized teeth.

THE NEED FOR PULP THERAPY

A review of the anatomy of primary teeth readily explains the frequent need for pulp therapy in these teeth. Specifically, the enamel and dentin of the primary teeth are just half as thick as that in permanent teeth. The pulp, therefore, is correspondingly closer to the outer surface, and dental caries can effect a more rapid penetration. For example, the mesial pulpal horn of the maxillary first primary molar is about 1.8 mm. from the outer enamel surface, and in the mandibular first primary molar this same measurement is about 1.6 mm. The rapidity and ease with which dental caries can penetrate to the dental pulp necessitate that the dentist be familiar with good treatment procedures.

On first examination of the problem one might select endodontic therapy as the treatment of choice, particularly as Ingle[6] and others have reported success in nearly 95 per cent of the cases so treated. This approach to pulpal problems in primary teeth is undergoing a renewal in interest. Research is continuing in this field and may eventually resolve some of the problems. The difficulties in endodontic therapy are due to the unique anatomy of the primary tooth. The roots, particularly those of the molars, are long and slender and the canals narrow and flattened. Ancillary canals and the ever present resorption of root ends add to the problem of successful endodontic therapy in primary teeth.

What *is* a pulp exposure? An exposure of the dental pulp exists when the continuity of the dentin surrounding the pulp is broken by physical or bacterial means. A blow which breaks off part of the coronal portion of the tooth, too deep a penetration with rotary or hand instruments, and the invasion of dental caries are common causes of exposure of the dental pulp. Actually, in view of the fact that cytoplasmic processes extend from the dentino-enamel junction to the pulp, chemical or thermal insults can penetrate and injure the dental pulp. For purposes of clarification, however, pulp exposure is usually construed as direct destruction of the integrity of the dentin surrounding the pulp itself.

The first mention of a pulp treatment specifically for primary teeth was in 1872.[23] In a column titled, "Hints and Queries," the question, "What shall we do with deciduous teeth in which pulps are exposed?" was answered by A. A. in this manner:

> They should be treated in somewhat the same manner as the permanent teeth. A single application of the arsenical preparation in common use will so far destroy the vitality of the pulp in the crown so that it can be removed on the day after it is made. The pulp cavity and crown should then be filled. Either Hills' Stopping or osteoplastic may be used as the filling, but no attempts should be made to fill the roots. The parents of the child should be warned, however, that eventually periosteal inflammation may attack a tooth treated in this manner, and will probably result in alveolar abscess. After this takes place, no serious trouble will occur.

SELECTION OF TREATMENT

The basis for successful treatment of any disease is the proper diagnosis of the existing condition. Without this fundamental concept any pulp therapy procedure attempted is carried out blindly and any success is a matter of chance. It is recognized also that even with the present knowledge of the dental pulp, which has been gained through research, there exist many factors which cannot be controlled or readily assessed. For instance, excessive hemorrhage has been considered to be a sign of degenerative processes in the pulp.[11] How much a pulp must hemorrhage, however, for it to be considered excessive, has not been precisely resolved. Again, the penetration of caries and its bacteria into the pulp chamber can be superficial and slow enough to permit the defensive mechanisms to protect the pulp, but the actual depth and speed of penetration are clinically and radiographically unpredictable. Thus, the facts upon which one must base a diagnosis must be carefully selected before proceeding with any treatment.

Similarly, all treatments have certain limitations. As of the present time there is no established method of treatment even including full endodontic procedures which produces a 100 per cent success rate. In selecting treatment, many factors other than the condition of the dental pulp must be considered. These would include the length of time the tooth will be present in the mouth, the general health of the patient, the condition of the dentition, the type of restoration which will be employed to return the tooth to its most normal state, the use to which the tooth will be subjected, the time it takes to complete the operation, the cooperation that can be expected of the patient, and the cost of the treatment.

The presence of primary teeth in the usual sense must be considered transitory, although the occasional patient will best be served by retaining the primary tooth throughout life, as in the case of two missing mandibular second bicuspids. Therefore, a good diagnostic radiograph to show root length is necessary. In addition, there is needed an understanding by the dentist of the patient's age and the erupting status of the teeth. The patient's general health should be determined. A leukemic child, a hemophiliac, or one suffering from any form of blood dyscrasia would be considered a poor candidate for pulp therapy. Likewise, the child susceptible to bacteremias, such as the rheumatic fever patient who is susceptible to a bacterial endocarditis, is a poor risk. As previously stated, pulp therapy is never 100 per cent successful and a treatment failure might trigger a more serious systemic complication.

The condition of adjacent teeth and other teeth in the mouth should be verified. Very possibly several or many other teeth cannot be salvaged; and if an extensive prosthesis is indicated, it might be well to include the tooth under consideration in the prosthesis.

It is advisable to predetermine the future function of the involved tooth when making a decision concerning the feasibility of pulp therapy. If the tooth is to be used as an abutment for an extensive fixed prosthesis, it is necessary to weigh the possibility of success against the possibility of failure with loss of the appliance.

Cooperation of the patient is a must for any procedure in which sterility and care are needed. Oftentimes related to this is the length of time it takes to perform treatment. The child who requires general anesthesia each time treatment is necessary would be a poor risk for extensive pulp therapy involving long or multiple appointments. Last but not least, the cost of the treatment must be considered. As in the case of all nonemergency care, the cost should be thoroughly explored with the child's parent or the person responsible for his welfare before treatment is initiated.

CLINICAL AND RADIOGRAPHIC DIAGNOSIS

Prior to the actual initiation of pulp therapy in a primary tooth a thorough clinical and radiographic examination must be made. The clinical examination would naturally include a case history, using the classic format with appropriate alterations: i.e., *chief complaint* (CC), "What is the matter?" or "Why did you call for an appointment for your child?"; *present illness* (PI), "Does the tooth hurt now?" "Has it ever hurt you?" "Does it hurt when you drink cold water?" "Does it hurt when you chew?" Such questions may well determine whether one is dealing with a pulpitis or an apical periodontitis. Personal past history (PPH), "Is your child in good physical health at this time?" "Has he ever had any serious illnesses—diabetes, rheumatic fever, or the like?" "Is he allergic to any drugs?" will give indications as to the condition of his general health and any limitations on treatment.

Examination of the area is best started with an examination of the soft tissue. Any signs such as discoloration, a draining or quiescent fistula, or inflammation should cause serious doubts about proceeding with pulp therapy short of endodontics. Next, the tooth itself should be examined for clinical destruction of the crown and possible presence of a hypertrophied pulp. The tooth's mobility should be determined, which, if present, should warn one about a possibly necrotic pulp. Percussion of the tooth should follow, for if any sensitivity is registered by the patient, the probable periapical involvement should make one dubious of pulpal therapy success. A vitality test may be made, but the results obtained from primary teeth by this technique have been most unreliable.[12, 14]

Good radiographs are essential to complete the diagnosis subsequent to the choice of treatment and prognosis. Both periapical and bite-wing films are necessary. Through their use it is possible to acquire some idea as to the pulp's condition. For instance, should any form of internal resorption be present in the coronal or apical portions, it is unlikely that the pulp will respond well to treatment. Likewise, the radiograph might indicate periapical or bifurcation

Fig. 10–1

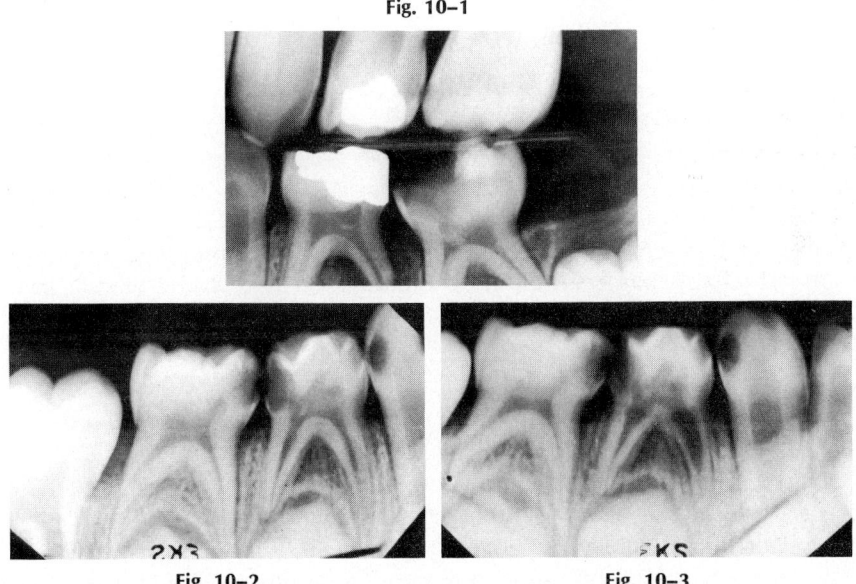

Fig. 10–2   **Fig. 10–3**

Figure 10–1 Mandibular primary molars and cuspid with deep carious lesions. In first primary molar note small calcific deposit in pulp chamber and beginning of internal resorption in mesial and distal roots. Pulp therapy is contraindicated.

Figure 10–2 Same teeth as in Figure 10–1, eight weeks later. Degeneration of first primary molar has rapidly increased as shown by larger area of internal resorption and signs of destruction in area of root bifurcation.

Figure 10–3 Bite-wing radiograph showing carious lesion penetrating pulp chamber that contains calcific mass near site of exposure. Prognosis for successful pulp therapy is poor.

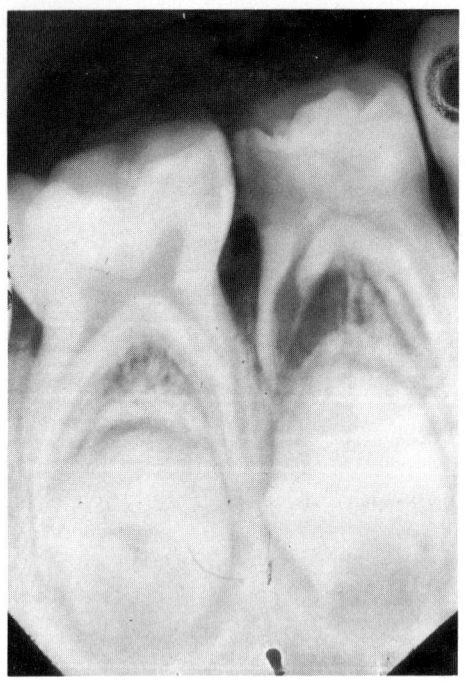

Figure 10–4 Periapical radiograph of mandibular first primary molar showing dental caries penetrating pulp, extensive calcific deposits, severe internal resorption of distal root, and periapical destruction. This tooth should be extracted. Bite-wing and periapical views are preferred when making a diagnosis or planning treatment.

involvement that suggests a degenerated pulp. The presence of calcified bodies, or pulp stones, has been reported to be evidence of pulpal degeneration (Figs. 10–1 to 10–4). Such an obvious finding as prematurely resorbed roots would negate pulp therapy.

In summary, wherever possible, it is desirable to evaluate as many diagnostic criteria as possible before proceeding with pulp therapy and particularly prior to any anesthesia. If the decision to perform pulp therapy has to be made after the tooth has been entered, reliance will have to be placed on radiographs and obvious clinical symptoms.

GENERAL PRINCIPLES OF TREATMENT

Certain procedures and techniques are applicable to all forms of treatment involving the dental pulp. First, a painless technique is essential. To accomplish this, adequate and profound anesthesia must be obtained. With the correct use of local anesthetic agents this can nearly always be achieved. Where pulpal involvement is suspected from the outset, sufficient anesthesia should be obtained at the beginning of treatment. Particularly when treating children, it seems undesirable to have to subject the patient to more injections.

In the mandibular arch, an inferior alveolar and a long buccal injection will give the desired results. The inferior alveolar injection will anesthetize all the mandibular teeth on that side of the mouth. The long buccal will obviate any discomfort from the application of the rubber dam clamp to the first permanent or second primary molar. The maxillary teeth are best anesthetized with subperiosteal injections on the buccal or labial *and lingual* (Fig. 10–5). Too frequently the lingual injection is omitted and minute nerve fibers remain sensitive, particularly those entering the lingual root of the maxillary molars.

Another invaluable adjunct in pulp therapy of primary teeth is the use of the rubber dam. This gives the operator a sterile field in which to operate by isolating the affected tooth or teeth, and also controls the inadvertent actions of the tongue and lips. It contributes to a sense of security as well as clearly reminding the child, whose attention may wander, that treatment is still in progress. It has long been the experience of those who routinely use local anesthesia and the rubber dam for operative dentistry on children that pulp therapy can be handled rapidly and effectively without undue stress upon the patient.

Cleanliness approaching sterile conditions should be followed at all times when operating within the pulp chamber. Following anesthesia and placement of the rubber dam, the hands should be scrubbed for 30 to 60 seconds, dried and rinsed with 70 per cent alcohol and allowed to air dry. Using presterilized (autoclave 121° C. at 15 lb. pressure for 15 minutes or dry heat 150° C. for 90 minutes) instruments, the dam and clamp too are decontaminated by rubbing for one minute with a gauze or cotton swab soaked in Zephiran. Burs and other cutting instruments should be sterilized, by previously described methods or by molten metal or glass beads, each time they are used on the same tooth. Strict adherence to aseptic techniques is of utmost importance if success is to be achieved.

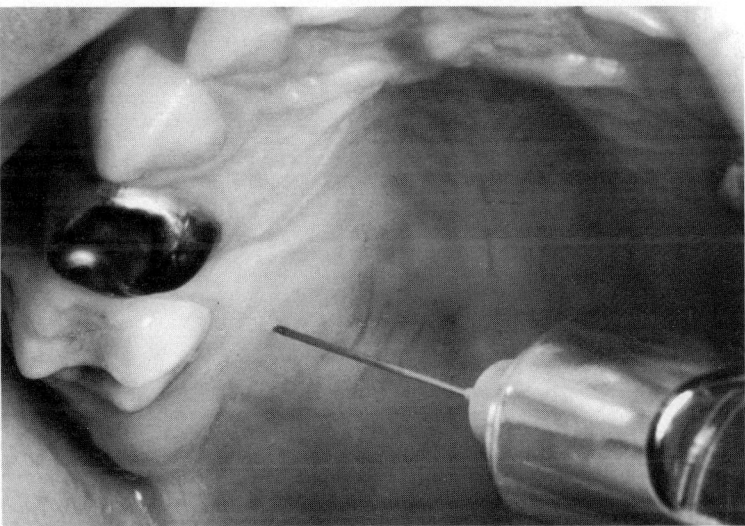

Figure 10–5 Lingual infiltration anesthesia is desirable for all maxillary teeth suspected of requiring pulp therapy. Such a precaution will obviate the need for secondary anesthetic injections and provide the greatest comfort to the patient.

PULP CAPPING

The simplest form of pulp therapy is pulp capping. As the name implies, it consists merely of placing a layer of protective material over the site of the exposed pulp prior to restoring the tooth. Many medicaments have been tried since Taft[20] (1860), Hunter[5] (1883), and others suggested the first pulp capping materials. Hunter recommended covering an exposure with a mixture of sorghum molasses and the droppings of the English sparrow and claimed a 98 per cent success rate.

Over the years materials such as lead, dicalcium phosphate, dentin chips, and formocresol have been tried, but calcium hydroxide has shown the most promise as the agent of choice in pulp capping.[13] The creation of new dentin in the area of the exposure and the subsequent healing or return to normal of the rest of the pulp is the desired objective.

Calcium hydroxide, first introduced by Teuscher and Zander[21] (1938) in the United States, is a drug which stimulates healing by encouraging the development of secondary dentin. It can, however, "overstimulate" or stimulate odontoclastic activity to such a degree that internal resorption of the dentin frequently occurs.

In the primary dentition, pulp capping is best carried out *only upon those teeth whose dental pulp has been exposed mechanically with cutting instruments during cavity preparation.* At times this is unavoidable as fine pulp horns may extend outwards in such a manner that they are located abnormally close to the surface and yet are of such small size as to be undetectable in the radiographs. In these cases there is minimal likelihood of bacterial invasion and no further operative procedures are necessary except for the cleansing of the exposed site with a cotton pellet saturated with hydrogen peroxide. This assumes, of course, that adequate anesthesia has been obtained and the rubber dam is in position. Under no circumstances should saliva be allowed to penetrate the cavity preparation or come into contact with the exposure site. There is usually little or no hemorrhage present.

Upon cleansing the area, a small amount (1 mm. thick) of calcium hydroxide is applied over the exposure. This is done either in dry powder form, it being carried to place by a spoon or amalgam carrier, or the powder may be mixed with sterile water to form a heavy paste that can be applied by a round ball burnisher or with an amalgam carrier. Inasmuch as calcium hydroxide does not set in a hard condition, a layer of zinc phosphate cement is then flowed over the capping material. This cement base is extended past the boundaries of the capping material in order to provide a sound base against which to pack the amalgam or other restorative material.

Although zinc phosphate can be highly irritating to the pulp, the layer of calcium hydroxide is sufficiently alkaline in nature to neutralize the acid of the cement. Likewise, the calcium hydroxide in contact with the pulp should stimulate odontoblastic activity for the development of secondary dentin.

Capping of the exposed pulp with calcium hydroxide is not recommended for teeth in which the capping site may be disturbed by restorative procedures. In many cases it is desirable to consider a full crown restoration in order to give maximum protection and the greatest opportunity for recovery.

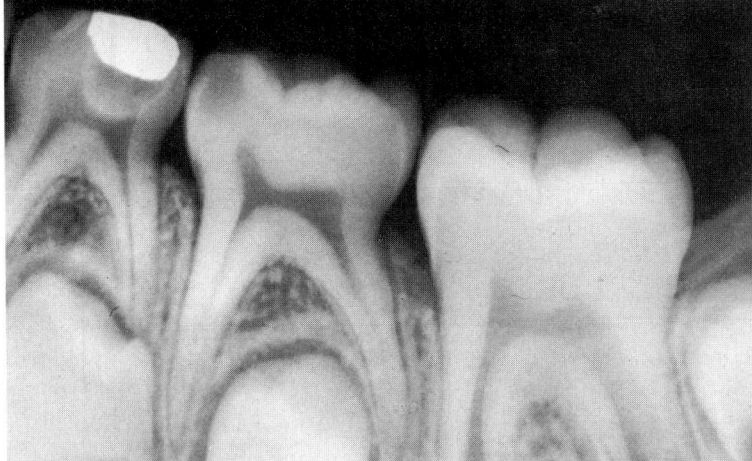

Figure 10-6 Radiograph of mandibular first primary molar six months after indirect pulp capping with calcium hydroxide. Temporary amalgam restoration and remaining caries will now be removed down to calcified, "healed" area, and a permanent restoration will be placed.

INDIRECT PULP CAPPING

Indirect pulp capping or the medication of carious material within the cavity adjacent to the anticipated exposure site has been attempted from time to time since 1866. In that year, Atkinson[2] reported leaving softened dentin over a vital pulp and soaking it with creosote. Often the dentin became hardened. This procedure utilizing calcium hydroxide is reported in more detail in the chapter on dental materials. Law and Lewis[10] reported a 76 per cent success on 38 primary teeth using this technique. In their study, teeth were selected which showed radiographic evidence of deep carious penetration of the dentin in close proximity to the pulp. Caries was partially removed to a depth that would avoid penetration of the pulp horn. A thick paste of calcium hydroxide and water was placed over the remaing caries and a restoration of amalgam placed directly over the calcium hydroxide. After six months, the amalgam and remaining caries were removed. In a significant number of cases no clinical exposure was then evident, and the underlying dentin was dense and hard (Fig. 10-6).

PULPOTOMY

PARTIAL PULPOTOMY

Partial pulpotomy or pulp curettage refers to the deliberate enlargement of a small carious exposure prior to the placement of a medication. Richardson,[16] Chatterton,[4] and others have reported on this procedure, but there is a lack of adequate histologic and clinical evidence to support its use. Advocates of partial pulpotomy have suggested that by eliminating only the infected material at the exposure site, surgical trauma to the pulp will be minimized and better healing will result. Unfortunately, the clinician cannot determine with any certainty the exact degree of bacterial penetration in the area of a carious exposure. Consequently, the complete coronal amputation is the treatment of choice even with small carious exposures in primary teeth.

PULPOTOMY WITH CALCIUM HYDROXIDE

Pulpotomy may be defined as the complete removal of the coronal portion of the dental pulp, followed by placement of a suitable dressing or medicament that will promote healing and preserve the vitality of the tooth. The importance of maintaining arch length in the primary dentition has long been recognized, and a healthy tooth is the best space maintainer. Efforts to conserve teeth by pulp amputation date back as far as 1886, when Witzel[24] described a method of pulpotomy. Teuscher and Zander[21] reported on the use of calcium hydroxide paste as a pulp dressing in pulpotomy of both primary and permanent teeth. Their histologic studies showed that in the successful cases the superficial portion of the pulp nearest the calcium hydroxide was first necrotized, a process accompanied by acute inflammatory changes in the immediate tissue beneath. After four weeks' time the acute inflammation subsided and was followed by development of a new odontoblastic layer at the wound site and eventually by a bridge of dentin. From a clinical standpoint the use of calcium hydroxide in pulpotomy has been most successful on young permanent teeth, especially traumatized incisors. The carious exposure on the primary tooth has not always reacted as favorably (Figs. 10–7 and 10–8). Law[8] reported 49 per cent success in a one year study of pulpotomy on primary teeth utilizing calcium hydroxide. Via,[22] in a two year study of calcium hydroxide pulpotomy on primary molars, found only 31 per cent success. Internal resorption with root destruction commonly follows this treatment, particularly in the primary tooth. This may be due to overstimulation of the undifferentiated cells of the pulp.

Procedure for Pulpotomy with Calcium Hydroxide

After securing adequate anesthesia, the rubber dam is applied and the exposed teeth and surrounding area cleansed with Zephiran solution or other suitable germicide. With a sterile 557 fissure bur with water coolant, the roof of the pulp chamber is exposed widely. Using a sterile sharp excavating spoon, the pulp is extirpated as nearly as possible in one piece. A clean amputation to the orifices of the canals is necessary. The pulp chamber may be irrigated and cleansed with sterile water and cotton. If hemorrhage persists, pressure from cotton pellets impregnated with calcium hydroxide will usually be sufficient to induce clotting. Unusual or persistent hemorrhage is frequently an indication of advanced degenerative changes, and the prognosis in such cases is poor. Following hemorrhage control of the radicular pulp tissue, a calcium hydroxide paste is placed over the amputated stumps. This paste may be prepared by mixing calcium hydroxide and sterile water, or a proprietary formulation may be used.

A cement base is now placed over the calcium hydroxide to seal the crown. This is usually of the zinc oxide and eugenol type. In most cases it is desirable to restore the tooth with a full coverage steel crown following pulpotomy, since the den-

Fig. 10–7.

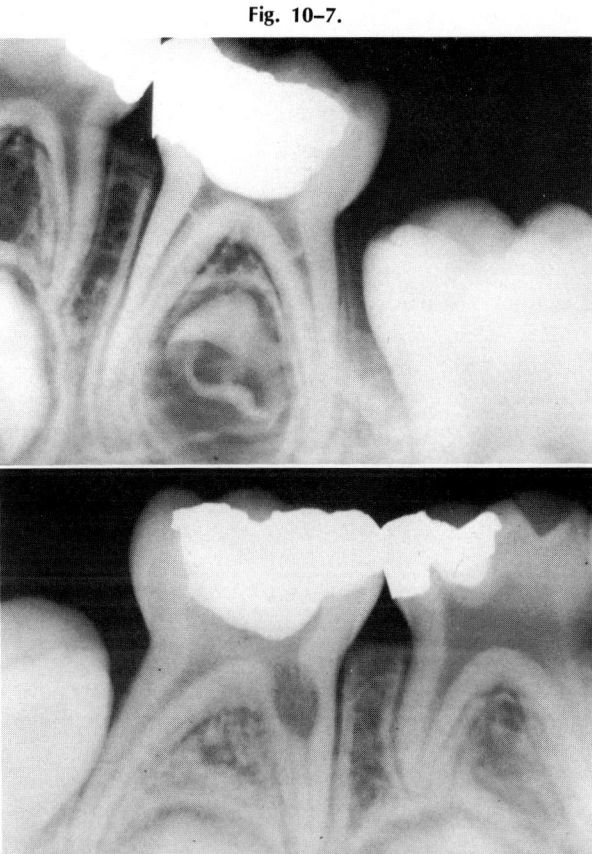

Fig. 10–8.

Figure 10–7 Successful calcium hydroxide pulpotomy showing dentin bridging in mesial and distal roots of mandibular second primary molar. The dentin bridge, though frequently radiographically seen following calcium hydroxide pulp therapy, is neither a criterion of nor necessary for a favorable prognosis.

Figure 10–8 Failure of a calcium hydroxide pulpotomy as shown by internal resorption of mesial root. Calcium hydroxide is radiolucent, thus the darkened area between the restoration and the area of resorption.

tin and enamel get brittle and dehydrated after this treatment. All patients who have undergone pulp therapy should be checked at periodic intervals to evaluate the health of the treated tooth. Absence of symptoms of pain or discomfort is no indication of success. Radiographs must be utilized to determine changes in periapical tissue or signs of internal resorption.

PULPOTOMY WITH FORMOCRESOL

In recent years there has been an increased use of formocresol as a substitute for calcium hydroxide when performing a pulpotomy on primary teeth. The drug itself—a combination of formaldehyde and tricresol in glycerin (19 per cent formaldehyde, 35 per cent tricresol, in a vehicle of ·15 per cent glycerin plus water) — has a protein binding effect in addition to being a strong bactericide. Originally, it was advocated as a disinfectant for root canals in endodontic treatment of permanent teeth. Later it was used by many clinicians as the medicament of choice in pulpotomy (Fig. 10–9). Sweet[19] pioneered in the clinical usage of formocresol in pulp therapy in primary teeth. He originally described it as a four appointment procedure following the initial pulp amputation, but it has gradually been modified until today it is usually performed as a one appointment operation. In some cases it may still be advisable to extend treatment over two appointments, especially where hemorrhage is difficult to control. Although advocated by many clinicians for a number of years, the use of formocresol was not supported by good histologic studies until the last decade. The action of this drug has now been investigated on the vital pulps of teeth of rats, dogs, and monkeys as well as humans. In all studies in which it has been compared to calcium hydroxide, formocresol has resulted in a higher success rate. In contrast to calcium hydroxide, formocresol does not usually induce formation of a calcified barrier or dentin bridge at the site of amputation (Figs. 10–10 and 10–11). It does create a zone of fixation, of varying depth, where it has been in contact with vital tissue. This zone is bacteria free and inert, resistant to autolysis, and it apparently acts as a deterrent to further microbial infiltration. The remaining pulp tissue in the root canal undergoes varying reactions from mild inflammation to fibroblastic proliferation. In some cases degenerative changes have been reported, of a mild degree. The pulp tissue below the zone of fixation remains vital following treatment with this drug, and in no instance is advanced internal resorption ever observed. This is one of the chief advantages of formocresol over

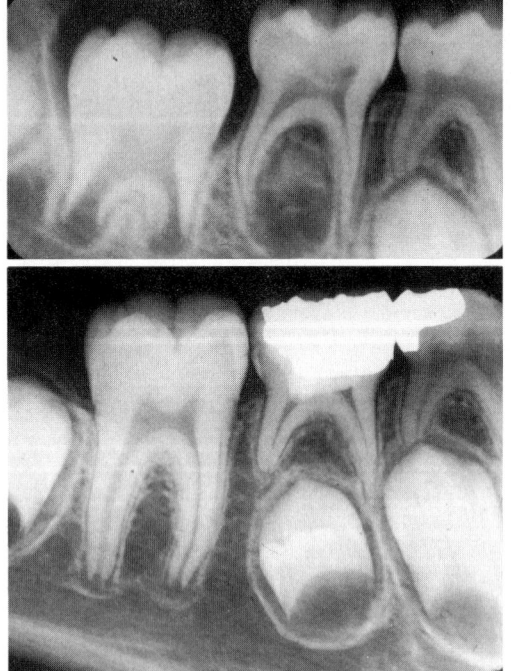

Figure 10–9 Primary second molar with large carious exposure treated by pulpotomy with formocresol. Over a period of four years this tooth has functioned as a healthy biological unit.

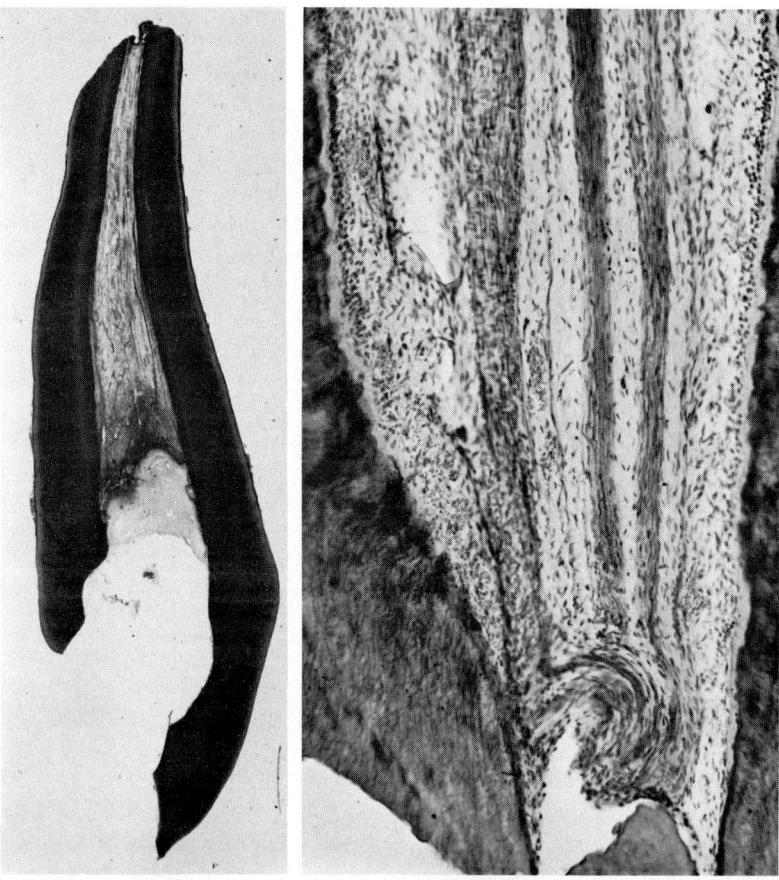

Fig. 10–10. | Fig. 10–11.

Figure 10–10 Histological section of normal primary cuspid four months after one step formocresol treatment. Darker staining area near amputation site is zone of fixation.

Figure 10–11 Apical portion of normal primary cuspid four months after one step formocresol treatment. Note extensive proliferation of fibroblasts and fibrous tissue.

calcium hydroxide. Many failures result from the latter's stimulation of formation of odontoclasts which destroy the root of the tooth internally.

Two studies on rhesus monkeys have been performed in which formocresol pulpotomies were done on both primary and permanent teeth according to the accepted clinical procedure for humans. Histologic sections of the jaws "in toto" failed to reveal any effect on succedaneous teeth, alveolar bone, or periapical tissues following the application of the drug. Spamer[18] made histologic sections of caries-free human primary cuspids which had undergone single appointment formocresol pulpotomies, employing a zinc oxide–eugenol cement base. Intially he observed an acute inflammatory reaction, succeeded by a chronic inflammatory response, proliferation of fibroblasts, increase in intercellular collagenous fibers, and frequently deposition of irregular (reparative) dentin. (See Table 10–1.)

Berger,[3] using a one appointment formocresol pulpotomy procedure, covered the pulp stumps of cariously exposed primary molars with a zinc oxide–eugenol

TABLE 10–1 HISTOLOGIC FINDINGS IN SINGLE APPOINTMENT FORMOCRESOL PULPOTOMY ON NORMAL PRIMARY CUSPIDS

24 Hours	7 Days	14 Days	1 Month	2 Months	4 Months	6 Months
Coronal Third Fibrin layer Layer erythrocytes Eosinophilic band Odontoblasts present in above layers Acellular zone Odontoblasts lost Intercellular edema Acute inflammatory cells Hyperemia	*Coronal Third* Fibrin layer Layer erythrocytes Eosinophilic band Odontoblasts present in above layers Acellular zone Odontoblasts lost Intercellular edema Acute and chronic inflammatory cells	*Coronal Third* Fibrin layer Layer erythrocytes Eosinophilic band Odontoblasts absent in above layers Acellular zone Odontoblasts lost Intercellular edema Acute and chronic inflammatory cells	*Coronal Third* Pulp tissue reactions similar to 14-day group with these gross exceptions: Increased inflammation Increased proliferation of fibroblasts in middle and apical thirds	*Entire Pulp* Fibrin layer Fibroblastic proliferation Increase in intercellular collagenous fibers Few blood vessels Chronic inflammation	*Coronal Third* Fibrin layer Increased chronic inflammation Fibroblastic proliferation Deposition of irregular (reparative) dentin	*Entire Pulp* Fibrin layers Deposition of irregular (reparative) den; especially in coronal third Vital pulp tissue throughout Increase in intercellular fibers
Middle Third Normal	*Middle Third* Normal	*Middle Third* Some inflammation Proliferation of fibroblasts			*Middle Third* Fibroblastic proliferation Increase in intercellular fibers Deposition of irregular dentin	
Apical Third Normal	*Apical Third* Normal	*Apical Third* Normal			*Apical Third* Fibroblastic proliferation Increase in intercellular fibers	

From Spamer, R. G., Master's thesis, University of Washington Library, 1965.

cement in which formocresol had been added (equal parts) to the eugenol liquid. This treatment was 97 per cent successful on the basis of radiographic evidence and 82 per cent successful on the basis of histologic evidence. His histologic findings showed the response of the pulp as follows:

1. At the site of amputation, a layer of superficial debris is observed, then a zone of fixation consisting of darker staining, compressed tissue with good cellular detail.

2. Below this area the pulp appears more acellular with the odontoblastic definition less well preserved.

3. Apical region shows minimal cellular change with a tendency for ingrowth of fibrous connective tissue.

Berger's experimental cases showed progressive ingrowth of connective tissue with entire replacement of the radicular pulp tissue.

Indications for Pulpotomy with Formocresol

This procedure is advocated for primary teeth only, since scientific studies of a clinical and histologic nature are lacking concerning the action of formocresol on permanent teeth.

Formocresol pulpotomy is indicated for all carious and accidental exposures on primary molars and incisors. It is the treatment of choice over pulp capping or partial pulpotomy, or pulpotomy with calcium hydroxide. In each instance the pulp must be demonstrably vital and free of suppuration or other evidence of necrosis. A history of spontaneous pain is usually considered an indication of advanced degeneration and a poor risk for pulpotomy. Likewise, radiographic signs of calcific globules seen in the pulp chamber are indicative of advanced degenerative change and a poor prognosis for healing. Quality and quantity of hemorrhage are difficult to assess clinically and should not be given major consideration. In general, the healthy pulp tends to bleed very little and clots quickly in contrast to the degenerating pulp, which often bleeds profusely and is difficult to check without coagulants. However, until further research more closely delineates the exact role of hemorrhage in prognosis of pulp therapy, other diagnostic criteria must be considered.

The decision to perform pulpotomy in a given case may be influenced by other factors. Children with a history of rheumatic fever probably are not good risks for any pulpal therapy because the possibility of pulpal necrosis and infection is always present. Sometimes in rampant caries cases involving numerous pulp exposures, the decision to extract or treat specific teeth must be based on an overall appraisal of the case including the type of space maintaining appliances to be constructed.

Procedure for Pulpotomy with Formocresol

Adequate and profound anesthesia must be secured in advance before operating on any primary tooth in which there is a possibility of pulp exposure. In the lower arch, the mandibular block injection is the procedure of choice. In the maxillary arch, infiltration is accomplished over the buccal roots and over the apex of the lingual root. A few drops of anesthetic solution are then deposited under the periosteum in the region of the apices of the buccal roots. This insures profound anesthesia for maxillary teeth. An excess of anesthetic solution should be avoided in subperiosteal injections.

The rubber dam should be used in all cases of pulpal therapy. After it is applied and properly adjusted, the tooth to be operated on and the surrounding area are cleared of superficial debris by wiping with a sponge liberally moistened with Zephiran chloride solution or similar germicide. Next, a small fissure bur in the air handpiece is used with water spray to open up the crown of the tooth and expose the coronal dentin. All caries and loose fragments of enamel should be eliminated prior to exposing the roof of the pulp chamber, in order to avoid unnecessary contamination of the operating field.

The roof of the pulp chamber is next removed. It is important to avoid plunging into the pulp cavity with the rotating bur. In some primary teeth, particularly the mandibular first molar, the floor of the pulp chamber is comparatively shallow and can be easily perforated. Removal of the coronal pulp tissue is accomplished by sterile spoon excavators. A clean amputation down to the orifices of the canals is required. A small pellet of cotton is now immersed in the formocresol solution, touched to absorbent gauze to remove excessive liquid, and placed in the pulp chamber (Figs. 10–12 and 10–13). After five minutes, the cotton is removed and a zinc oxide–eugenol cement used to seal the pulp cavity. The liquid for this cement should consist of equal parts of formocresol and eugenol. If hemorrhage is persistent, a pressure pack of sterile cotton should be placed against the root orifices. In some cases of persistent hemorrhage it may be advisable to use two appointments to complete the pulpotomy. In such event, the pack of cotton containing the formocresol is left in contact with the pulp and temporarily sealed with zinc oxide–eugenol cement. The tooth is reopened in three to five days, the cotton pledget is removed, and a base of zinc oxide–formocresol–eugenol cement is placed against the orifices of the canals.[9]

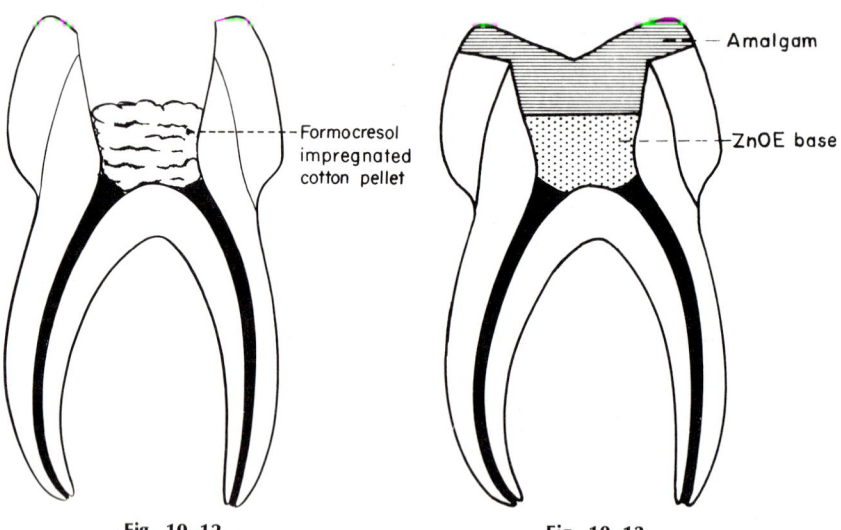

Formocresol impregnated cotton pellet

Amalgam

ZnOE base

Fig. 10–12.   **Fig. 10–13.**

Figure 10–12 The amputated coronal pulp is covered with formocresol for five minutes.

Figure 10–13 The completed restoration should cover the cusps. In many cases a steel crown may be used.

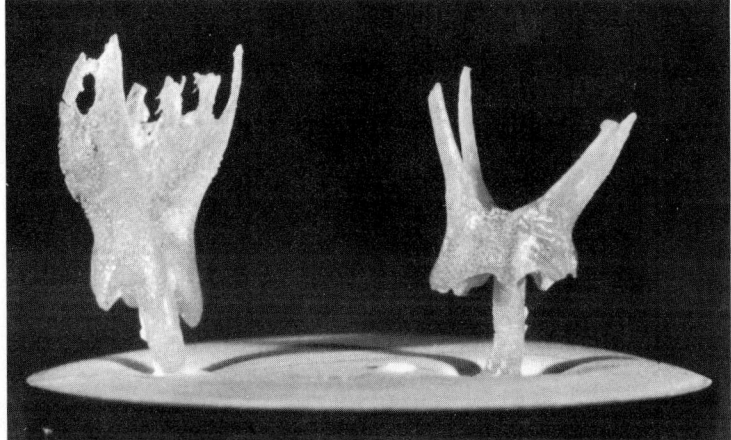

Figure 10–14 Plastic reproductions of pulps of primary molars. The root canals of the primary teeth are simple and uncomplicated in the first few years after eruption but become filled with secondary calcifications as the child grows older.

Restoration of the tooth by steel crowns is usually indicated after pulpotomy. This is done to minimize fracturing of cusps at a later date, a common occurrence in teeth that have undergone pulp treatment.

The parent should always be forewarned of the possibility of failure when vital pulp therapy has been performed on a child's tooth. It should be explained that periodic recalls will be necessary in order to evaluate the treated tooth, and that these will involve routine radiographs. In examining radiographs of teeth that have undergone pulp therapy, it is necessary to look for an intact lamina dura, absence of bony rarefaction at the bifurcation or in the periapical area, and a normal pulp chamber free of internal resorption. Other symptoms such as mobility, sensitivity to percussion, and history of pain or pressure can be of assistance. In many instances in which teeth have undergone pulp therapy that eventually failed, the prognosis for space maintenance is still far better than it would have been had the attempt not been made.

PULPECTOMY IN PRIMARY TEETH

Pulpectomy refers to the removal of all pulpal tissue from the tooth, including both coronal and root portions. Although the anatomy of the roots of the primary tooth may in some cases complicate these procedures, there is a renewed interest in the possibility of successfully retaining primary teeth in preference to the problems of long-term space maintenance. Andrew[1] and Rabinowitch[15] have long advocated pulpectomy in molars, as well as incisors, in cases of nonvital primary teeth. A greater understanding of the periapical tissues and their healing potential has reactivated the endodontic approach and the clinician should evaluate its advantages before removal of a primary tooth and placement of a space maintainer. Pulpectomy of nonvital primary teeth should be carefully considered, especially in the case of the second molar, when the first permanent molar is unerupted. It is hoped that new clinical research in this field will develop improved instrumentation and more practical methods of utilizing pulp canal sealants.

Anterior deciduous teeth are the most likely candidates for endodontic treatment. Being straight and single rooted for the most part, they frequently have root canals that are of sufficient size to be readily operated on (Figs. 10–15 and 10–16). It should be remembered, however, that primary teeth are noted for their many ancillary canals, and as such, the pulp chamber may not be completely extirpated or the canals subsequently filled.

For the technique of endodontic therapy in primary teeth, the reader is referred to one of the several texts[7, 17] in this field, for the actual procedure is very similar to that for permanent teeth. Several important points should be kept in mind, however, when performing endodontics on primary teeth. First, care should be observed not to penetrate past the apical ends of the tooth when reaming out the canal or canals. To do so might injure the permanent tooth bud which is developing. Second, a resorbable compound such as zinc oxide and eugenol paste should be used as the filling material. Silver points or gutta-percha should be avoided as they will not be resorbed and can act as irritants. Third, the filling material should be introduced into the canal with light pressure so that little, if any, is extruded through the apex of the root (Fig. 10–17). Fourth, apioectomy, the surgical removal of the root end of the tooth, should *not* be performed except in the absence of a developing permanent tooth.

Pulpectomy of nonvital or putrescent deciduous molars should be carefully considered and the plan evaluated in the light of the possibility of success, the number of appointments necessary, and the cost. As previously noted, some success

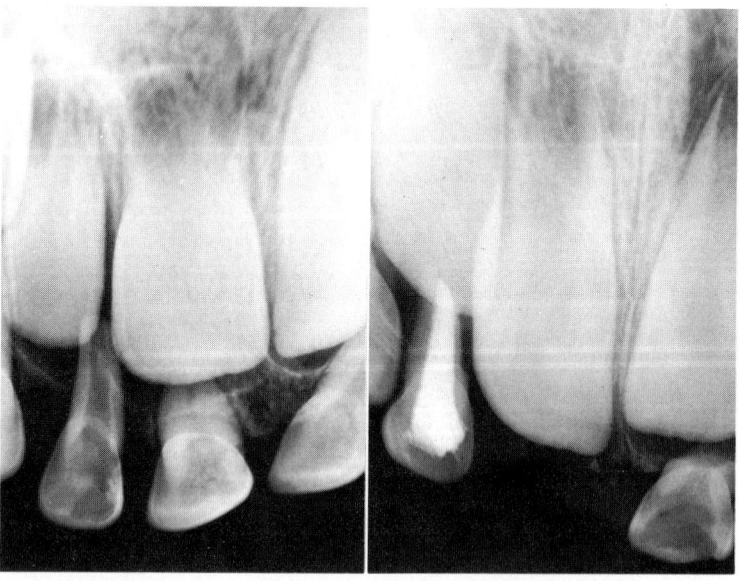

Fig. 10–15.   **Fig. 10–16.**

Figure 10–15 Maxillary primary lateral with cariously involved pulp.
Figure 10–16 Same tooth that successfully underwent endodontic therapy six months previously. Tooth will be exfoliated in normal manner.

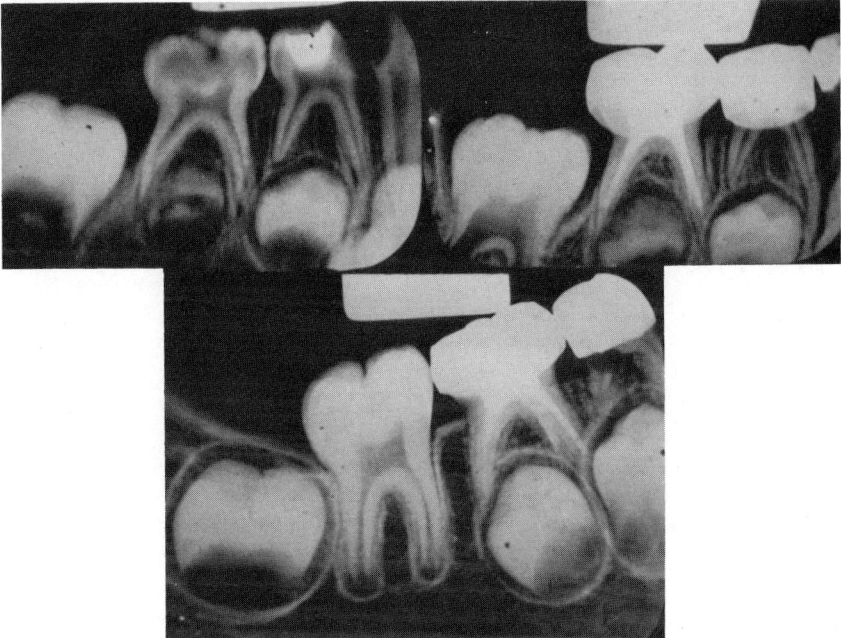

Figure 10–17 Radiograph of mandibular second primary molar in which endodontic therapy was successfully performed. Hedstrom files were used to open up the canals which were then filled with Oxpara paste. In this particular case, pulpectomy has obviated the need for placement of space maintaining appliances. (Courtesy of Dr. Paul Starkey.)

has been attained, but the narrow, tortuous ribbon-like canals make such a treatment tenuous at best. It is hoped that research in this field will prove encouraging.

YOUNG PERMANENT TEETH

In young permanent teeth, procedures similar to those used for primary teeth include indirect and direct pulp capping and pulpotomy with calcium hydroxide, either with water or in a proprietary preparation, as the material of choice. Indirect pulp capping in young permanent teeth is employed when caries encroaches upon but has not actually invaded the vital pulp as observed roentgenographically. Direct pulp capping is indicated when there is a small (less than 1 mm.) exposure of vital pulp tissue, especially when the exposure is the result of overzealous instrumentation rather than caries.

In young permanent teeth with incomplete root formation, when the state of the pulp is favorable, a pulpotomy is to be preferred to root canal fillings so that the roots may continue to form (Figs. 10–18 and 10–19). Continued root formation would suggest vital pupal tissue in this area. A pulpotomy, employing calcium hydroxide, is indicated when there is a large (greater than 1 mm.) exposure of *vital* pulp tissue. This includes a carious or mechanical exposure, or one associated with trauma and fracture of a young permanent anterior tooth (see Chapter 11.). The techniques for pulp capping and pulpotomy with calcium hydroxide have been discussed earlier in this chapter.

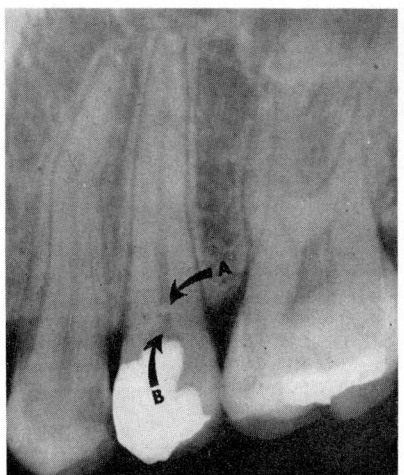 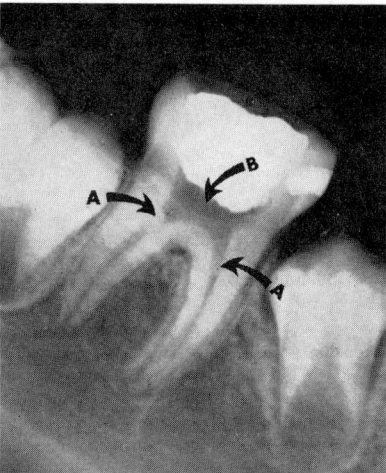

Fig. 10–18.   **Fig. 10–19.**

Figure 10–18 Roentgenographic evidence of healing following a pulpotomy. A dentin bridge is evident at A. The radiolucent zone at B represents the layer of calcium hydroxide placed over the amputated pulp.

Figure 10–19 The same type of healing in a molar following pulpotomy. In this case dentin bridges formed in both roots (A). Zone B again represents the layer of calcium hydroxide.

Since the root canals of young permanent posterior teeth do not exhibit the tortuosities and extensive branching typical of primary molars, they are amenable to routine pulpectomy procedures. Formocresol treatment, therefore, is not indicated for use in the permanent dentition. Furthermore, the formocresol pulpotomy technique is not recommended for young permanent teeth because of possible fixation of the tissues at the apical end and discontinuance of root formation.

If endodontic procedures are required for young permanent teeth, especially anterior teeth, some modification of the standard technique is required in order to obtain a proper seal where a wide and perhaps funnel-shaped apex exists. In attempting endodontic filling of a wide open canal, required techniques should be followed, such as provision for a sterile field, adequate access to the pulpal area, proper debridement and irrigation of the canals, sterilization of the canals and their proper sealing. Young permanent incisors having a blunderbuss type of apex can be prepared with No. 7 to No. 12 files or reamers. If the file is not large enough to contact all surfaces at once, filing can be done from wall to wall until complete.

In filling the canal, if the largest size gutta-percha cones are not large enough, it may be necessary to hand roll a point by placing several points together tip to butt. By repeated gentle warming and rolling between two glass slabs, one can fuse the points to the desired size. The cone can be cut to fit the apical opening as determined clinically and radiographically. The point is cemented into place, and additional points are condensed laterally when necessary to complete the filling.

In cases in which a young permanent tooth has undergone pulpal devitalization and necrosis prior to normal development of the apical tip area, it may be possible to stimulate sufficient growth through *root induction* procedures to achieve apex completion (Figs. 10–20, 10–21, 10–22). The canal is first thoroughly cleaned

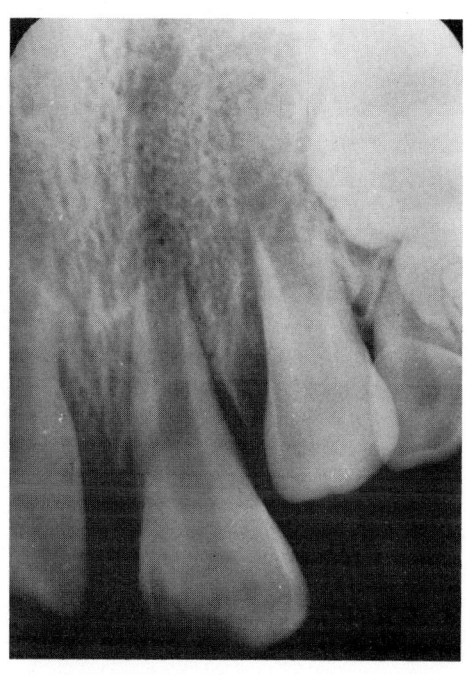

Figure 10–20 Nonvital central incisor in an 8-year-old boy. The tooth was opened, treated, and a Ca(OH)$_2$–CMCP paste inserted. (From Steiner, J. C., Dow, P. R., and Cathey, G. M.: Inducing root end closure of non-vital permanent teeth. J. Dent. Child., *35*:47, 1968.)

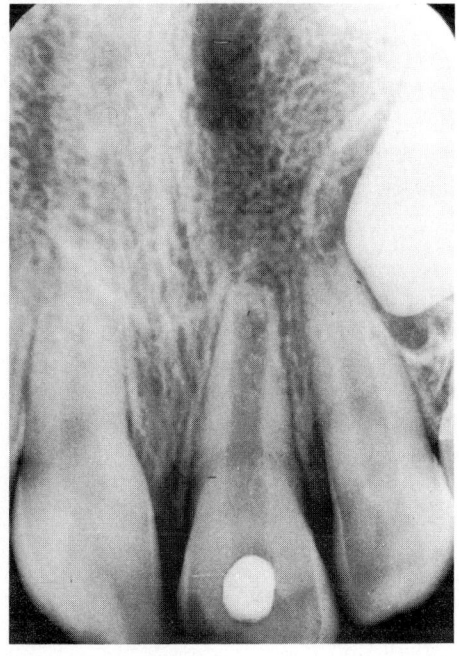

Figure 10–21 Same tooth 13 months later. Note completion of foramen and apical area. (From Steiner, J. C., Dow, P. R., and Cathey, G. M.: Inducing root end closure of non-vital permanent teeth. J. Dent. Child., *35*:47, 1968.)

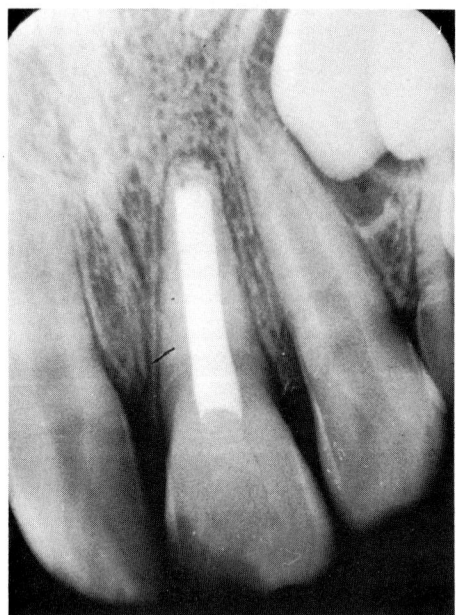

Figure 10–22 The tooth has been reopened, paste removed, and the canal filled with gutta percha. (From Steiner, J. C., Dow, P. R., and Cathey, G. M.: Inducing root end closure of non-vital permanent teeth. J. Dent. Child., *35*: 47, 1968.)

and filed to about one-half its length, and a dressing of CMCP placed for about one week's time. At the second appointment the remainder of the canal is debrided, care being taken to avoid the apical area, if possible staying approximately 3 mm. short of the apex. After cleaning and drying the canal, a paste of CMCP and calcium hydroxide U.S.P. is inserted. Overfilling is preferable to underfilling as any excess will be resorbed by the periapical tissues. A suitable restoration should then be placed to seal the canal and the tooth observed at six-month intervals. If successful, the apex will gradually wall itself off, forming a root-end closure. It is then possible to re-enter the canal, remove the paste, and place a conventional endodontic filling. If no closure occurs after six months, the tooth should be re-entered, the old paste removed, and new material inserted.

REFERENCES

1. Andrew, P.: The treatment of infected pulps in deciduous teeth. Brit. D.J., *98*:122–126, 1955.
2. Atkinson, W. H.: The preservation of exposed dental pulps. D. Cosmos, *7*:425–428, 1865-1866.
3. Berger, J. E.: Pulpal therapy for primary teeth. J. Michigan State D.A., *46*:33–40, 1964.
4. Chatterton, D. B.: Pulp curettage. J. S. California D. A., *17*:30, Sept. 1950.
5. Hunter, F. A.: Capping pulps. D. Items of Interest, *5*:352, 1883.
6. Ingle, J. I.: Endodontics. Philadelphia, Lea & Febiger, p. 54, 1965.
7. Ibid., pp. 78–232.
8. Law, D. B.: An evaluation of vital pulpotomy technic. J. Dent. Child., *23*:40, 1956.
9. Law, D. B., and Lewis, T. M.: Formocresol pulpotomy in deciduous teeth. J.A.D.A., *69*:601–607, 1964.
10. Law, D. B., and Lewis, T. M.: The effect of calcium hydroxide on deep carious lesions. Oral Surg., Oral Med. & Oral Path., *14*: No. 9, 1130–1137, 1961.
11. McDonald, R. E.: Diagnostic aids and vital pulp therapy for deciduous teeth. J.A.D.A., *53*:14–22, 1956.
12. Ibid.

13. Nyborg, H.: Healing processes in the pulp on capping. Acta Odont. Scandinavica, *13*:Suppl. 16, 1955.
14. O'Toole, T. J.: A study of electrical stimulation of primary anterior teeth. Master's thesis, University of Washington, 1962.
15. Rabinowitch, B. Z.: Pulp management in primary teeth. Oral Surg., Oral Med. & Oral Path., *6*:542–550, April, 1953; 671–676, May, 1953.
16. Richardson, J.: Treatment of exposed nerves. D. Cosmos, *2*:366–368, 1860.
17. Sommer, R., Ostrander, F., and Crowley, M.: Clinical Endodontics. 2nd ed. Philadelphia, W. B. Saunders Co., 1960.
18. Spamer, R. G.: The formocresol pulpotomy: A histological study of a single application of formocresol on the dental pulps of human primary teeth. Master's thesis, University of Washington, 1965.
19. Sweet, C. A.: Procedure for treatment of exposed and pulpless deciduous teeth. J.A.D.A., *17*:1150–1153, 1930.
20. Taft, J.: Exposed or wounded pulps. D. Cosmos, *2*:118, 1860.
21. Teuscher, G., and Zander, H.: Preliminary report on pulpotomy. Northwestern Univ. D. Bull., *39*:4, 1938.
22. Via, W. F., Jr.: Evaluation of deciduous molars treated by pulpotomy and calcium hydroxide. J.A.D.A., *50*:34, 1955.
23. What shall we do with deciduous teeth in which the pulps are exposed? "Hints and Queries." D. Cosmos, *14*:225, 1872.
24. Witzel, A.: Compendium der Pathologie und Therapie der Pulpakrankheiten. Berlin, [1886] (cited by Levine, 1934).

11

THE CARE OF INJURIES TO THE ANTERIOR TEETH OF CHILDREN

by LOUIS W. RIPA
and SIDNEY B. FINN

There is perhaps no single dental disturbance that has greater psychological impact on both the parent and the child than the loss or fracture of a child's anterior teeth, especially if the injury affects the permanent dentition and involves the loss of extensive tooth structure. The majority of fractures and displacements result from simple accidents and involve little more than local oral tissues. Minor falls, accidents while participating in sports, or childish pranks which were not intended to harm produce the greatest number of fractures and displacements in children. From these seemingly benign accidents, the child's facial appearance may become so altered as to make an attractive child appear unattractive. Aside from the pain and discomfort of the injury, the child's changed appearance may make him the target for teasing and even ridicule by other children, for children can be unintentionally cruel.

Every dentist who treats children must be well prepared to meet these emergencies. It is incumbent upon the dentist to preserve the vitality of injured teeth whenever possible and to restore them skillfully to their original appearance, without producing additional trauma or endangering the integrity of the teeth. The wanton extraction of injured teeth without careful consideration of the possibility of saving them has no place in good dental practice. With present day restorative materials fractured teeth can usually be restored to an acceptable functional and esthetic state.

Since time is such an important consideration in the treatment of fractures or displacements, every effort should be made to see the patient in the office immediately. Even if it means delaying a scheduled appointment, the injured child should be given preference and emergency treatment should be rendered. By prompt handling of the case, further irritation to the pulp can be prevented, avulsed teeth can be replanted with a higher percentage of success, and displaced teeth can be repositioned with greater ease. In general, a more favorable result can be anticipated.

PREVALENCE OF INJURIES TO ANTERIOR TEETH

The exact number of children who sustain injuries to their teeth each year is unknown; however, the incidence, judged by the number of such injuries seen in clinics and private dental offices, must be high. Korns[30] observed that, within a two-year period, 221 (54.14 per cent) of 408 private patients, 6 years of age or younger, presented with an injury to one or more primary anterior teeth.

Ellis and Davey[15] reported that of 4251 secondary school children in a large city, 4.2 per cent had fractured anterior teeth. Marcus[37] and Gutz,[21] however, in separate studies, reported considerably larger frequencies of 16 and 20 per cent respectively. The latter frequencies were derived from dental clinic observations of children seen on a regular basis and therefore are more likely to represent the coronal fracture frequency of a group of children receiving regular dental care in a private office.

The teeth most frequently involved in a traumatic episode are the maxillary central incisors. Boys are more prone to sustain a fracture of a permanent anterior tooth than girls, the ratio being approximately 2:1.[18] As seen in Figure 11–1, children aged 9 and 10 appear to be the most susceptible group for sustaining this type of injury in the permanent dentition.

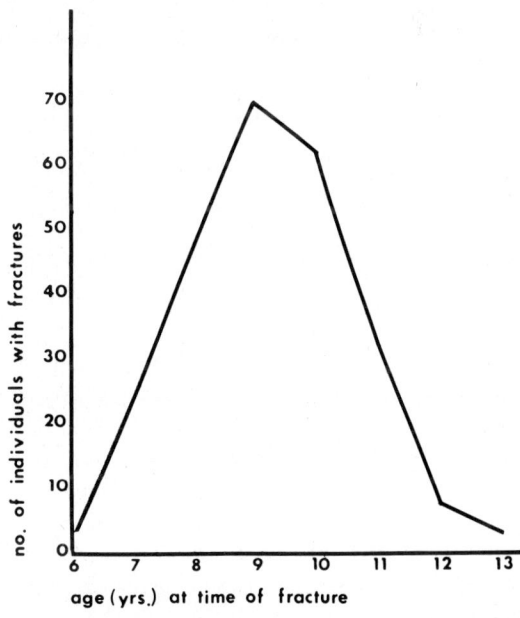

Figure 11–1 Distribution of coronal fractures in permanent incisors relative to age of injury. Based upon a sample of 1166 children treated in a dental school clinic between ages 6 and 13. (After Gutz, D., J. Dent. Child., 38, 1971.)

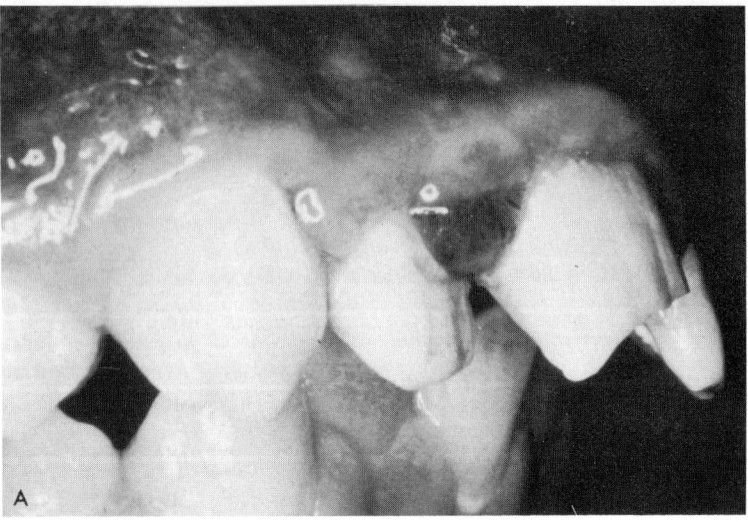

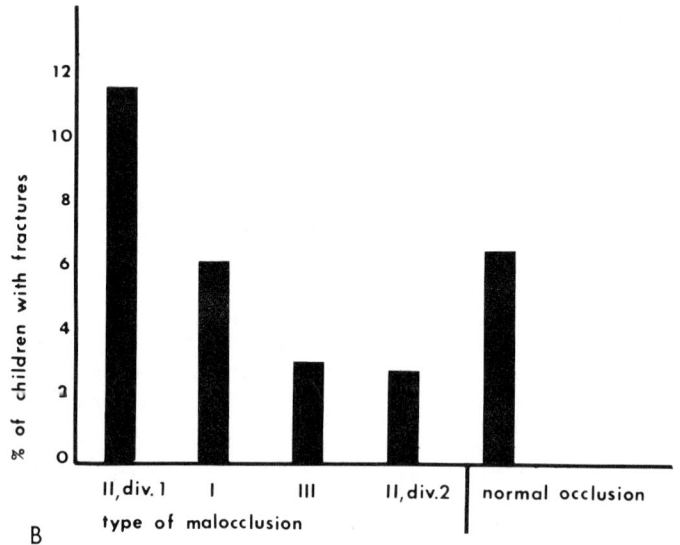

Figure 11–2 *A,* Characteristic procumbent maxillary incisor teeth of child with an "accident prone profile." Note the fracture of the maxillary permanent central incisor. (Courtesy of Dr. G. Habansky.) *B,* Percentage of children with "normal" occlusion and with each of Angle's classes of malocclusion who sustained a fracture to the incisor teeth. (Fractures involving only the enamel not included). (After McEwen, J. D., and McHugh, W. D., Trans. Europ. Ortho. Soc., 1969.)

The dental profession recognizes the existence of an "accident prone profile" characterized by children with protruding anterior teeth representing either Class I, type 2 or Class II, Division I malocclusions (Fig. 11–2*A*). Twice as many children with this accident prone profile sustain injury to the anterior permanent teeth compared with children with any other type of occlusion (Fig. 11–2*B*). McEwen and McHugh[39] found that as overjet increased, the incidence of fractured maxillary incisors increased. They estimated that in boys with 1 mm. or less overjet the chance of fracture was 1 in 25; however, in the most susceptible group, boys with 10 mm.

or more overjet, there was one chance in four of sustaining a fracture before age 13.

CLASSIFICATION OF INJURIES TO ANTERIOR TEETH

The classification of injuries to the anterior teeth should be standardized so that when a definite type of injury is referred to by classification it is recognized by everyone. Ellis and Davey[15] have succeeded in classifying all injuries simply and clearly. Their classification is as follows:

Class 1
Simple fracture of the crown—involving little or no dentin (Fig. 11–3*A*).
Class 2
Extensive fracture of the crown—involving considerable dentin, but not the dental pulp (Fig. 11–3*B*).
Class 3
Extensive fracture of the crown—involving considerable dentin and exposing the dental pulp (Fig. 11–3*C*).
Class 4
The traumatized tooth which becomes nonvital—with or without loss of crown structure.
Class 5
Teeth lost as result of trauma.

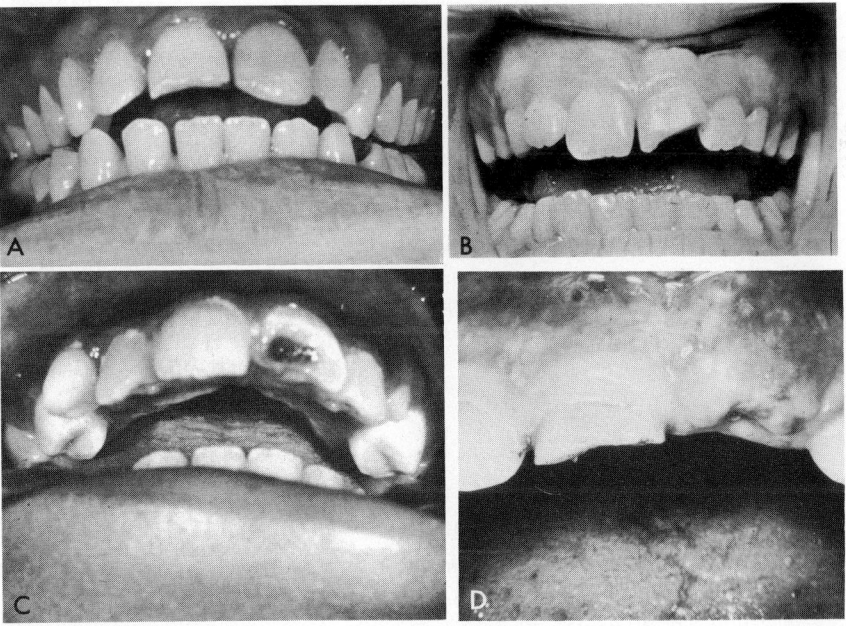

Figure 11–3   Types of coronal fractures. *A,* Simple fracture involving little or no dentin (Class 1). *B,* Fracture involving enamel and dentin but not exposing pulp (Class 2). *C,* Fracture in which the pulp is exposed (Class 3). *D,* Fracture of the crown *en masse* (Class 8). (Figs. *A* and *C,* courtesy of Dr. L. Abelardo; Fig. *B,* courtesy of Dr. R. Kracke; Fig. *D,* courtesy of Dr. W. Houck.)

Class 6
Fracture of the root—with or without loss of crown structure.
Class 7
Displacement of a tooth—without fracture of crown or root.
Class 8
Fracture of the crown en masse and its replacement (Fig. 11–3*D*).
Traumatic injuries to primary teeth are considered separate from those of the permanent teeth because of the different treatment criteria and techniques.

HISTORY AND CLINICAL EXAMINATION

Since injuries to the teeth should be treated as soon after they occur as possible, much time can be saved in taking a preliminary history and in the clinical examination if a routine procedure is followed. It is recommended that printed sheets appropriate for this purpose be available in the office when emergencies present themselves. Figure 11–4 is an example of the type of form that may be used. Since the injury may involve insurance claims, especially if the accident has occurred in a school or other public area, it behooves the dentist to secure all pertinent data.

The examination should consist of the following:

1. *Visual observation* to determine the type and extent of the injury: whether teeth are displaced or avulsed; whether teeth are fractured with or without pulpal exposure; whether there is laceration, swelling or hemorrhage of the soft tissue.
2. *Roentgenography* to reveal root fractures and to give additional pertinent information such as: the proximity of the coronal fracture to the pulp, the stage of development of the root apex, possible injury to adjacent and occluding teeth, presence of other pathosis in the area, and for comparison with future roentgenograms. Periapical roentgenograms of the opposing teeth should also be taken.
3. *Manipulation* to determine the mobility or relative firmness of the injured teeth.
4. *Vitality tests* with a vitalometer or cold and heat to determine the relative response of involved teeth. These methods have traditionally been used as aids in establishing a plan of treatment. However, correlated clinical and histologic studies, described below, have failed to establish a consistent relationship between the biologic condition of the pulp and the observed clinical responses to these tests. The results of "vitality tests" at the initial examination should be recorded and used principally as a standard of comparison with tests made at recall visits and with tests made of adjacent teeth.
5. *Percussion* should be used since sensitivity to tapping may indicate injury to the periodontal membrane and other supporting structures.

The prognosis of the injured tooth will depend heavily on the histologic condition of the pulp. Is it vital or necrotic, moderately or severely inflamed, and so forth? To determine the condition of the pulp, the dentist evaluates the evidence obtained from the history and clinical examination, specifically the patient's subjective complaints and the response of the tooth to vitality tests and percussion. Combined clinical and microscopic studies, however, have indicated the poor correlation between clinical signs and symptoms and the histologic appearance of the

TOOTH INJURY FORM

Date of Examination_____

Patient's Name_____   Age_____

Address_____   Phone no._____

Parents_____

History of Injury

Date of injury_____

Time of injury_____

Place of injury_____

How injury occurred_____

_____

Previous history of injury   yes_____   no_____

    if yes, describe_____

_____

<table>
<tr><td>

Signs

Teeth involved_____

Type of fracture_____

Pulp exposed_____

Mobility_____

Displacement_____

Color_____

Radiographic_____

</td><td>

Symptoms

Pain on mastication   yes_____   no_____

Reaction to percussion   yes_____   no_____

Reaction to heat   yes_____   no_____

Reaction to cold   yes_____   no_____

Vitalometer reading

</td></tr>
</table>

$$\frac{7 \quad 8 \quad\quad 9 \quad 10}{26 \quad 25 \quad\; 24 \quad 23}$$

Emergency treatment_____

_____

Follow-up examination_____

_____

Figure 11–4.

pulp. Mitchell and Tarplee,[43] for instance, noted that 26 permanent teeth, histologically evaluated as having coronal pulpitis, gave highly variable responses to thermal and percussion tests prior to their extraction. In a later study, Hasler and Mitchell[24] microscopically evaluated the pulps of 47 extracted permanent teeth and found some degree of pulpitis in 27 of them. Despite the histological diagnosis of pulpitis, none of the 27 teeth were painful prior to extraction, 5 were negative to percussion, 10 were negative to heat, 5 were negative to cold, and 5 gave the same response to the electric pulp tester as apparently sound control teeth. In a separate study, Johnson and co-workers[29] found that of 35 extracted teeth, histologically shown to be "completely necrotic," 15 gave a false positive response to the electric pulp tester prior to extraction.

TABLE 11–1   RESPONSE TO THE ELECTRIC PULP TESTER OF ANTERIOR TEETH
                    LOOSENED BY MECHANICAL INJURY*

Root Development at Time of Injury	Vitality Immediately After Injury	Vitality at Follow-Up Examination	
Complete	17 vital	15 vital	2 nonvital
	31 nonvital	8 vital	23 nonvital
Incomplete	22 vital	20 vital	2 nonvital
	37 nonvital	20 vital	17 nonvital

*The teeth were tested immediately after injury and in follow-up examinations over a period of one to six years. Teeth which originally tested vital but became nonvital usually did so within the first two months; conversely, teeth which were originally nonvital and subsequently gave a vital response usually did so in one month. In several cases, however, as much as 10 to 13 months was required before a change in response was observed. After Skieller, V.: Acta Odont. Scandinavica, *18*, 1960.

Skieller[52] emphasized that electrical pulp testing of mechanically loosened teeth *immediately after injury* is not a reliable criterion for assessing vitality. He found that of 39 teeth that tested positive (vital) immediately after injury, four gave a negative (nonvital) response in follow-up examinations. Conversely, of 68 teeth that originally tested negative, 28 teeth tested positive in the follow-up examination (Table 11–1). It is recommended, therefore, that the results of the history and initial clinical examinations be interpreted with discretion when evaluating the pulpal condition of a recently traumatized tooth, and a negative response to the pulp tester should not be regarded as prima facie evidence of loss of vitality.

TREATMENT OF CORONAL FRACTURES

FRACTURES INVOLVING ONLY THE ENAMEL

Fractures involving only the enamel are either a chipping out of the central portion of the incisal edge of the tooth or the much more common fracture of an incisal-proximal angle. The great danger in these apparently benign fractures lies in underestimating the possible deleterious effects of concussion on the pulp. If the patient is seen soon after the accident, the fractured edge can be covered with a commercial adhesive to protect the pulp from additional irritation. If the fracture is of long standing when first observed by the dentist and the pulp is vital and asymptomatic, no palliative or protective covering may be necessary.

If the tooth has been recently fractured, the patient should be scheduled for a follow-up examination in six to eight weeks. At this appointment periapical roentgenograms are taken and any color change in the tooth recorded. Discoloration of a traumatized permanent tooth is usually an indication of loss of pulpal vitality. Vitality tests should be performed at this time and compared with those taken at the initial examination. The results of these later tests are more reliable than those taken immediately after the injury. The parents must be advised at the initial visit that the tooth may become nonvital and require root canal therapy.

For fractures in which minimal tooth substance is lost a good cosmetic result can often be obtained by reshaping the incisal edge with a diamond wheel, in which case no restoration would be necessary. The anatomically similar tooth in the adjacent quadrant can be rounded off similarly to obtain a symmetrical appearance. Grinding the incisal edge should be undertaken only after one is reasonably certain that the pulp has fully recovered from the impact of the injury.

FRACTURES INVOLVING THE ENAMEL AND DENTIN, WITH NO PULP EXPOSURE

These fractures may be horizontal, involving the entire incisal surface, or they may be diagonal, in which case a large portion of the incisal-proximal angle may be lost.

As in every case of injury, after the complete history is carefully studied and results of the clinical examination are evaluated, emergency treatment is undertaken. Although in this category of fracture the pulpal tissue is not visibly exposed, emergency treatment is necessary to protect the already traumatized pulp from further insult from excessive thermal, bacterial, and chemical stimuli and to hasten the formation of a layer of secondary dentin in the fractured area. Many dentinal fractures, especially of the horizontal type, may be so close to the pulp that a pink color will be visible through the thin dentin of the pulpal wall. In the diagonal type fracture involving an incisal-proximal angle, a minute opening into the pulp chamber often occurs, but it may be so small as to defy detection. In any case, a protective and dentin-stimulating layer of calcium hydroxide is placed over the dentin at the fracture line. A hard-setting commercial calcium hydroxide preparation should be used, which will not be displaced into the pulp if a minute exposure is present, as a temporary restoration is being seated.

To insure that the calcium hydroxide dressing is retained until the pulp has retreated from the proximity of the fracture and adequate layer of secondary dentin has formed, a suitable temporary retainer must be employed. A commercial adhesive, an orthodontic band, a celluloid crown form filled with a composite restorative material, or a stainless steel crown can be utilized for this purpose.

Adhesive Sealing

After the dentin is coated with a layer of calcium hydroxide the fracture site may be sealed with a commercial adhesive. Figure 11–5 illustrates this procedure using a commercial adhesive that employs ultraviolet light to activate polymerization.

The adhesive sealing technique is rapid and requires no cutting of tooth structure. Although it does not restore tooth form the material itself is not cosmetically detracting.

Orthodontic Band

Either a preformed orthodontic band or a custom made band may be used to retain the calcium hydroxide preparation. If a custom made band is desired, a stainless steel strip, approximately 1¼ inches long, is adapted to the teeth with finger pressure, the free edges being positioned lingually. The two lengths of the band are brought together on the lingual by crimping with a How pliers. Without

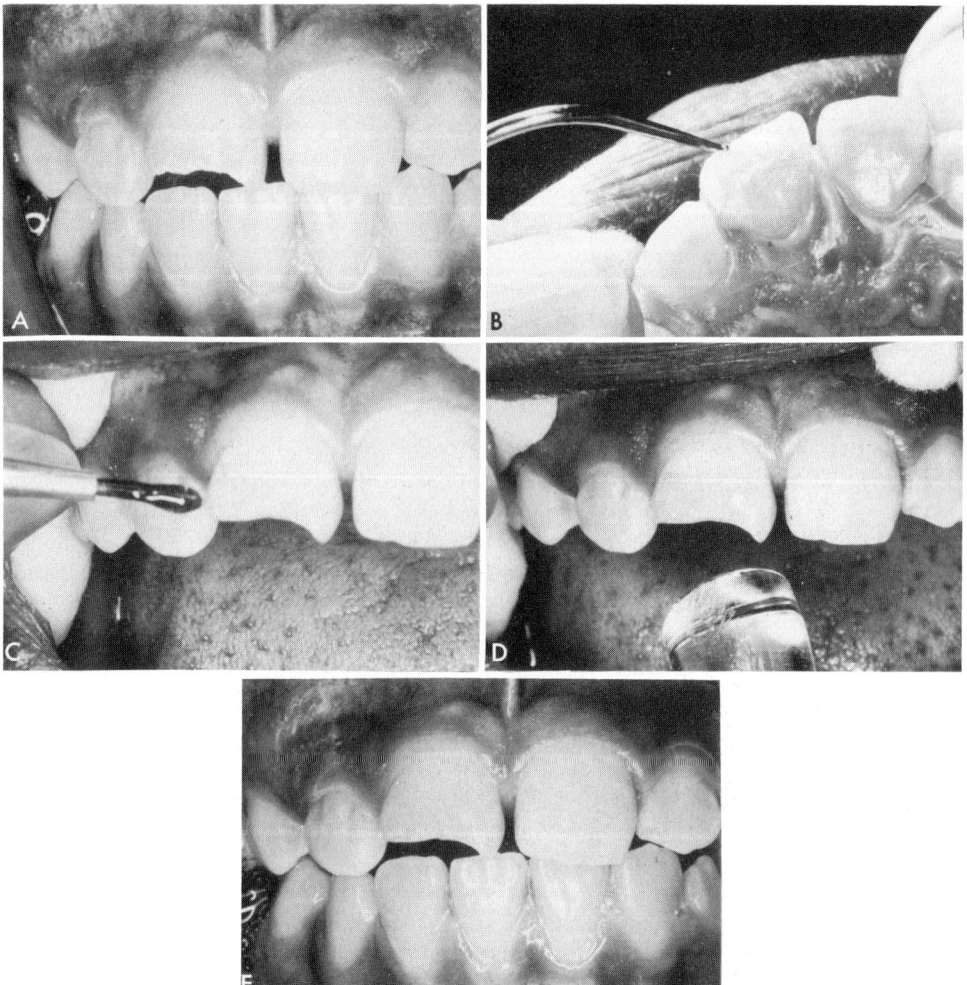

Figure 11–5   Adhesive sealing of a class 2 fracture. *A,* Maxillary central incisor with a fracture of the enamel and dentin but with no pulp exposed. *B,* A proprietary calcium hydroxide preparation is layered over the exposed dentin. *C,* Liquid adhesive is applied by brush to the fracture site and painted over approximately 2 mm. of labial and lingual enamel adjacent to the fracture. The enamel which received the adhesive was first conditioned by etching for 1 minute with a 50 per cent phosphoric acid solution, washing, and thoroughly drying with the air syringe. *D,* Ultraviolet light, directed by a quartz rod, is applied for approximately 30–45 seconds to harden the adhesive. *E,* Because the hardened adhesive is transparent it provides protection without itself being unsightly. Tooth form, however, is not restored. (Courtesy of Dr. C. Whitmer.)

loosening the pliers, the band is removed from the tooth. The band is spot welded and the excess material is cut off to within 1 mm. of the band. The band is reseated on the tooth, and the 1 mm. tag is bent against the band and burnished. The band is removed from the tooth and the burnished tag is spot welded. The band is contoured, using No. 137 pliers, reseated with a band pusher, and checked for retention and occlusion. Additional protection for the palliative dressing may be obtained by covering the incisal edge with a stainless steel strip spot welded to the labial and lingual aspect of the band. After the tooth is lightly pumiced, the band is cemented with a commercial zinc oxide-eugenol, ethoxy benzoic acid cement. The band encloses the fracture site and the cement covers and protects the layer of calcium hydroxide (Fig. 11–6).

Although the orthodontic band is an excellent device for retention of the palliative dressing, it has the serious disadvantage of being unesthetic, especially when used on a permanent maxillary incisor.

Celluloid Crown

A celluloid crown form is selected using the corresponding tooth in the adjacent quadrant as a guide for correct size and shape. The gingival margin is trimmed carefully with a curved scissors to fit approximately 1 mm. below the free gingival margin. Two holes are placed in the incisal third of the lingual surface as escape hatches for trapped air and excess composite resin.

The composite material is mixed according to the manufacturer's directions and placed in the crown form with a plastic instrument in small increments to prevent entrapment of air. The crown form and contents are slowly and gently seated on the tooth, taking care to prevent dislodgment of the calcium hydroxide covering the exposed dentin and to allow trapped air to escape. The crown is held

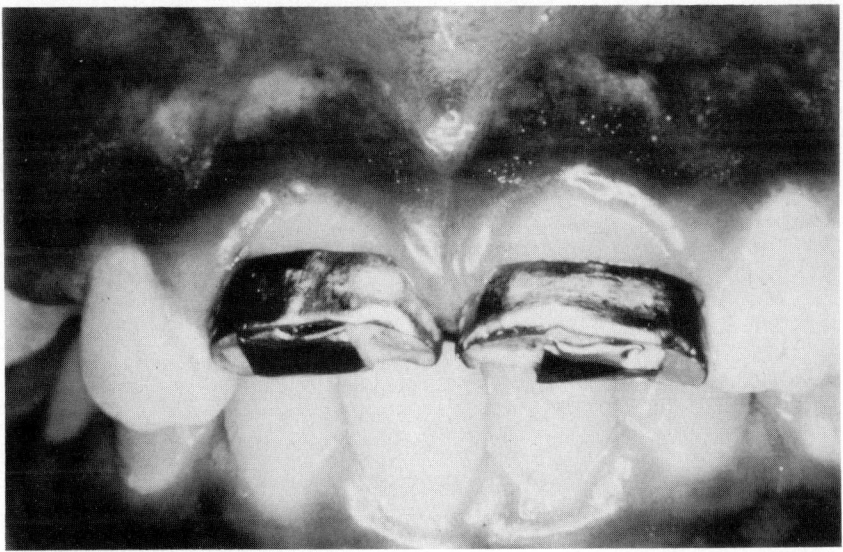

Figure 11–6 Orthodontic bands as temporary restorations following class 2 fractures of both maxillary central incisors. Note the strip of band material that covers the fractured incisal edge providing additional protection. (Courtesy of Dr. G. Rosen.)

in place for 3 to 5 minutes until the material has set. When polymerization is complete any excess resin is trimmed from the lingual holes and cervical margins. The crown form is removed by slicing the lingual aspect with a scalpel and peeling off the split celluloid form. The bite is carefully checked to determine the amount of clearance. Final trimming and polishing are accomplished with abrasive disks and white pointed finishing stones (Fig. 11–7A,B,C).

Stainless Steel Crown

A stainless steel crown may be easily trimmed, contoured, and adapted to a fractured anterior tooth. Generally, with the exception of eliminating proximal contact and removing a small amount of enamel in the incisal and cingulum areas, no preparation of the tooth is required. Handling of the crown is no different than when it is used to restore a cariously involved tooth and is described elsewhere in the text (see Chapter 8). Since esthetics is often a consideration, a "window" can be cut in the labial surface of the crown and filled with a composite material of suitable shade after the crown is cemented (Fig. 11–8). Of the three types of temporary restorations, the steel crown provides maximum protection and retention, and, if tooth preparation is minimal, is the temporary restoration of choice.

The temporary restoration should remain in place for at least eight weeks, which is regarded from clinical observation as the critical period for the pulp to return to normal. After this waiting period, if no untoward effects are evident, the temporary restoration, be it band, celluloid crown, or stainless steel crown, may be removed and the pulp tested for continued vitality. If the tooth appears normal

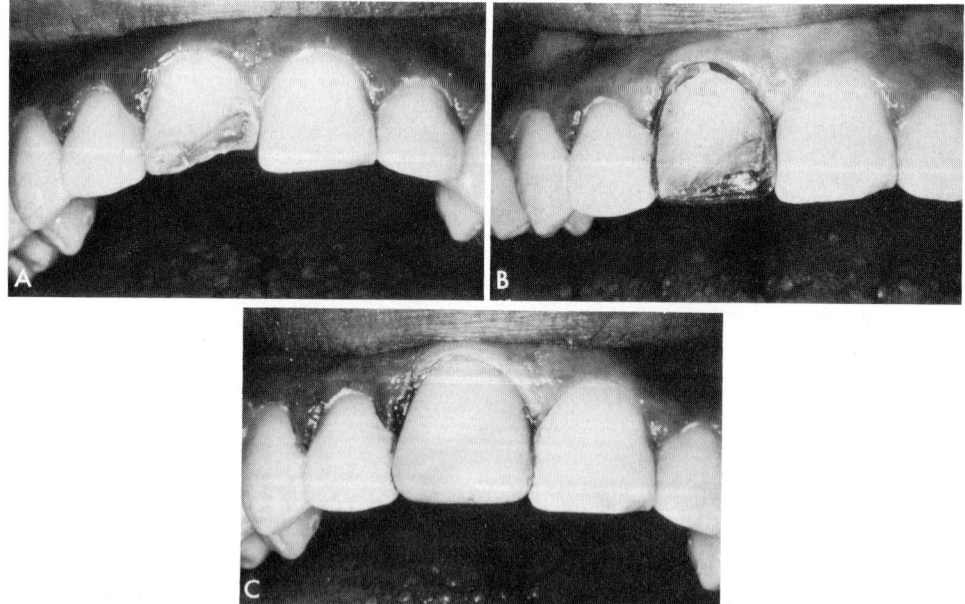

Figure 11–7 Use of celluloid crown form to temporarily restore a fractured incisor. *A,* Class 2 fracture of the maxillary central incisor. *B,* Fitting the celluloid crown. *C,* Restoration of the injured tooth using a composite resin. (Courtesy of Dr. C. Brenner.)

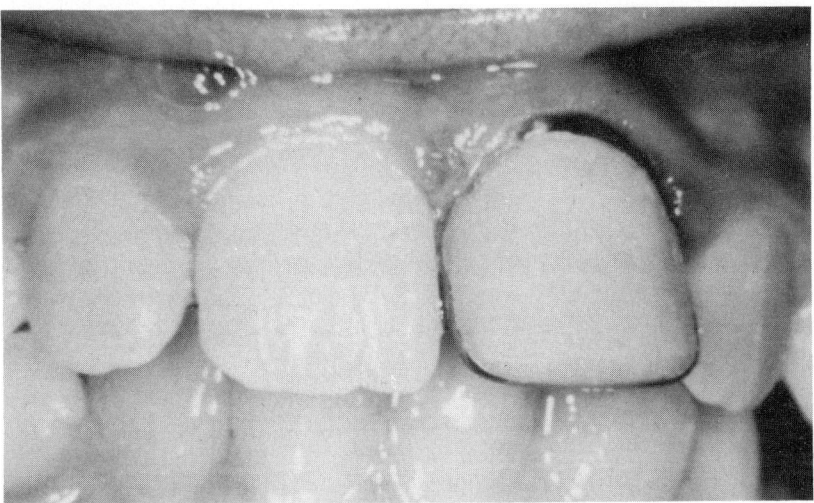

Figure 11–8 A stainless steel crown with a labial "window" filled with composite material used to temporarily restore a fractured permanent maxillary central incisor.

both clinically and roentgenographically, an intermediate or temporary-permanent restoration is placed. This is to be retained until the child is old enough to have a permanent restoration placed, such as a porcelain jacket crown.

FRACTURES INVOLVING THE PULP

If a coronal fracture includes a pulpal exposure, every effort must be made to retain the vitality of the pulp. An exposed pulp is a contaminated pulp. It is imperative that immediate emergency treatment be instituted to minimize bacterial contamination, thus favoring a better prognosis for the case. There are four courses of treatment open to the dentist: (1) pulp capping, (2) pulpotomy, (3) pulpectomy with or without apicoectomy, and (4) extraction of the tooth. The choice of procedure depends greatly upon the extent of the exposure, the condition of the pulp itself and extent of development of the apical foramen, and the extent of injury to the root and supporting tissues. Secondary conditions such as the general appearance of the oral cavity and the patient's interest and cooperation must be considered in deciding the advisability of pulp therapy and the type to be used.

Pulp capping can be employed if the exposure is minimal and not over 24 hours in duration. The fracture may be close to the pulp horn with pink showing through a thin dentin wall, or only the very tip of the mesial or distal pulp horn may be exposed to the oral fluids. When a small tip of the pulp horn is exposed, the tissue should appear clinically healthy and vital. The presence of a wide, incompletely formed apex is an additional factor in favor of this treatment.

Local anesthesia is administered and the tooth is isolated with a rubber dam. Pulp capping is accomplished by gently teasing a commercial calcium hydroxide preparation of relatively high crushing strength over the exposed pulpal tissue and surrounding dentin walls. Chong and co-workers[10] have demonstrated that the early (7 minute) crushing strength of Dycal, a commercial calcium hydroxide preparation, is similar to that of zinc phosphate cement, hence a secondary cement layer is not necessary. An orthodontic band, celluloid crown form containing a composite resin, or, preferably, a stainless steel crown is placed, as previously described, to protect the calcium hydroxide dressing and exposure site.

It must be stressed that pulp capping may be employed only on those teeth with minute, very recent exposures in which the pulp appears healthy despite the trauma it sustained. In clinical practice, pulp capping is sometimes chosen because it is the least time consuming of the possible therapeutic treatments and, therefore, is assumed to be the simplest; however, the sequela of selection on the basis of expediency often is degeneration of the pulp capped tooth with pulpectomy the ultimate recourse.

Pulpotomy is indicated when there is moderate hemorrhage with a relatively large pulp exposure, and the patient is seen within 72 hours. An incisor with a wide apex and incomplete root formation is considered a good candidate for this technique because of the better recuperative powers of the young pulp and because of the difficulty in attempting conventional endodontic procedures.

Local anesthesia should be administered and the tooth isolated with a rubber dam. The entire pulp chamber is exposed, using a bur revolving in a high speed handpiece. Amputation of the coronal pulpal tissue is accomplished with a sterile round bur rotating counter clockwise in a slow speed handpiece or with a sterile sharp spoon excavator. After hemorrhage has been controlled a layer of calcium hydroxide is placed over the pulp stump and a commercial zinc oxide and eugenol preparation is applied over this. A protective temporary restoration is then placed.

There are several calcium hydroxide preparations currently available. Phaneuf and associates[47] evaluated three — Dycal,* Hydrex,** and Pulpdent Paste*** — for their effect on human *primary* pulp tissue following pulpotomy under a stringently aseptic technique. Pulpdent Paste was found to produce early pulp organization and to stimulate dentinal bridge formation at the amputation site most frequently. Dycal produced an inconsistent pulpal response with slower, irregular bridge formation, and Hydrex produced no bridge formation within the 28 to 107 day postoperative observation period. Clinically and radiographically, however, all treatments were considered successful. These findings indicate that other agents included in a proprietary calcium hydroxide formulation may influence the pulp's response to therapy and, consequently, make the dentist's choice of therapeutic agent more difficult.

At subsequent appointments the traumatized tooth which has been pulp-capped or upon which a pulpotomy has been performed should be clinically examined and radiographed. The criteria for judging the success of treatment include an asymptomatic clinical course, continued normal apical development, and the absence of internal resorption, external resorption, and periapical infection.[7] Radiographic evidence of bridging has often been regarded as clinical evidence of success. However, interpretation of a clinical radiograph may lead to a false impression since a complete or incomplete bridge can produce the same radiographic

---

*Dycal, L. D. Caulk Co., Milford, Del.
**Hydrex, Kerr Manufacturing Co., Romulus, Mich.
***Pulpdent Paste, Pulpdent Corp., Brookline, Mass.

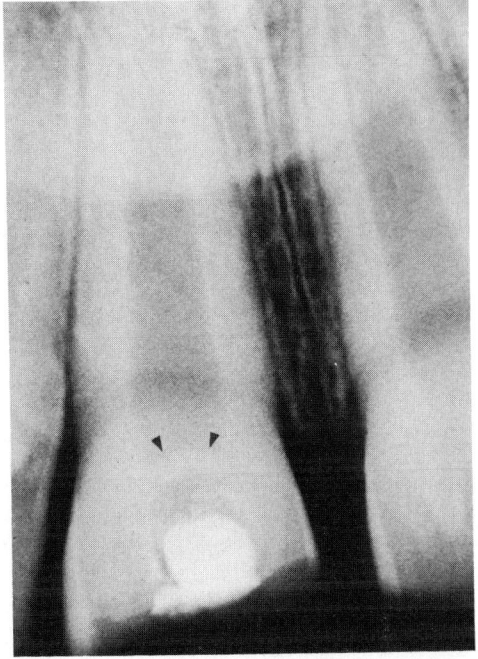

Figure 11–9 A maxillary central incisor treated by pulpotomy following a class 3 coronal fracture. Note the dentinal bridge that has formed. Since a radiograph is a two-dimensional representation, it is impossible to determine if the bridge is imperforate.

image[53] (Fig. 11–9). Since the stimulation of calcific repair is not necessary for the survival of the pulp in a healthy state,[47] bridging may be regarded as a desirable but not necessary criterion of success.

After approximately six months, a restoration of intermediate duration may be constructed if the tooth remains vital and symptomatic.

At future recall appointments the treated tooth should continue to be monitored clinically and radiographically. Some reports have indicated that although initially there may be a high success rate with the pulpotomy technique, after two to three years a calcification of the pulp canals tends to occur.[22, 46] Contrary to this observation, Bodenham[8] reported that six pulpotomized teeth in five patients which were followed for eight to 16 years did not develop calcification or pulp necrosis. Publication of continued long-term evaluations of pulpotomized teeth is necessary before definitive conclusions can be drawn concerning the ultimate prognosis of this treatment. In the meantime, the dentist who elects to use this technique should carefully evaluate his postoperative radiographs for a developing constriction of the pulp canal.

Pulpectomy, the complete removal of the pulp, is indicated if the pulp is degenerated, putrescent, or of questionable vitality. If the exposure is of longer than 72 hours' duration, the pulp is generally infected beyond recovery and pulpectomy is indicated.

A fractured tooth with a completely developed root apex is amenable to the usual endodontic procedures of biomechanical instrumentation and root filling. The treatment of traumatized young anterior teeth with an incompletely developed, wide apical foramen, however, requires special procedures in order to effect a complete apical seal. Techniques for successful filling of teeth with incomplete apical development have included (1) reverse spreading of gutta percha cones and

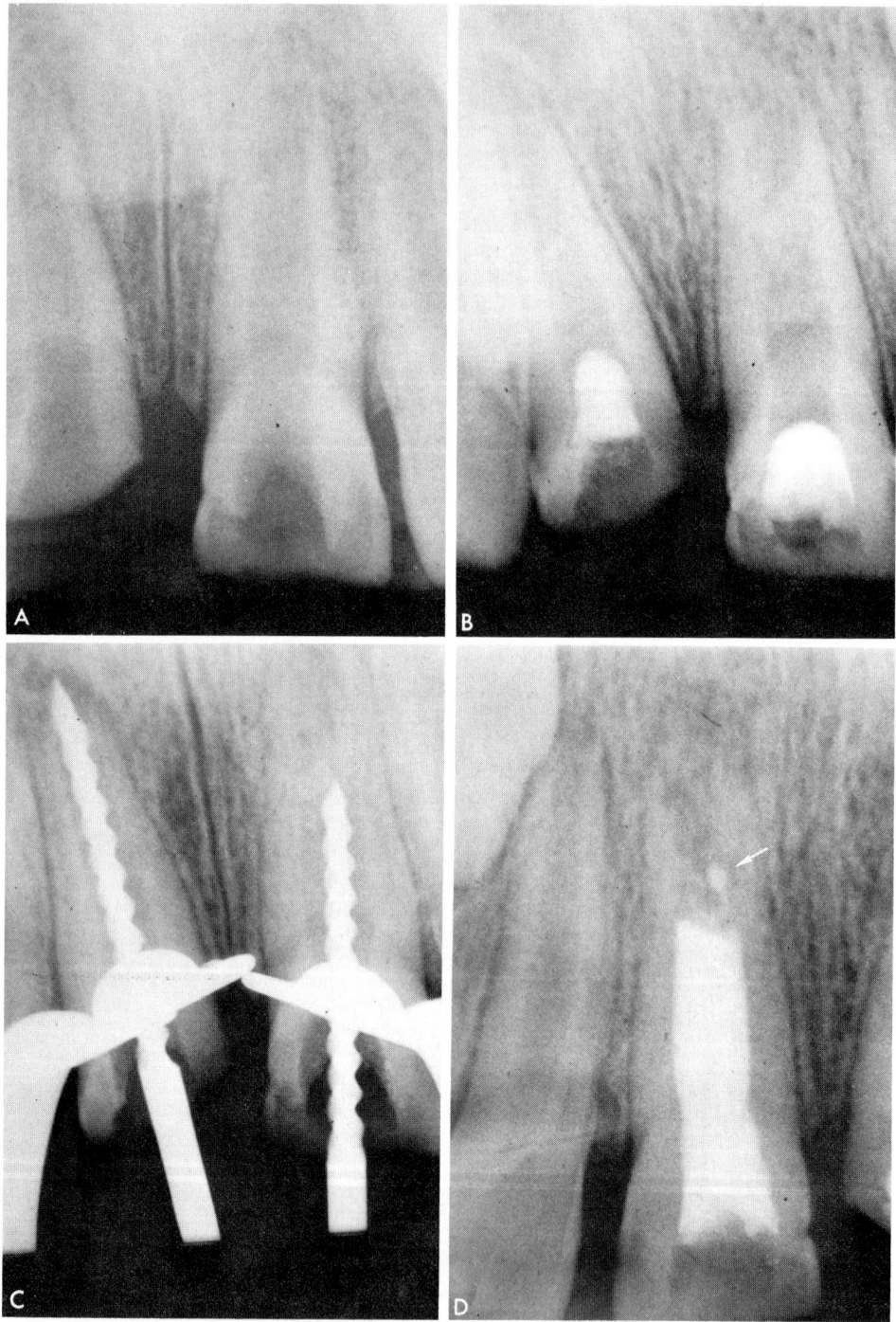

Figure 11–10   Treatment of fractured anterior teeth by pulpectomy and stimulation of continued apex development. *A*, Preoperative radiograph demonstrating extent of the fractures. *B*, Pulpectomies have been performed and a paste of calcium hydroxide and p-chlorophenol (not visible in the radiograph) has been packed in the canals and sealed at the coronal openings. *C*, Testing for apical obstruction. In this case one incisor demonstrated formation of a calcific bridge coronal to the apex, while the other remained negotiable. *D*, The calcific bridge permitted a lateral condensation filling technique using gutta percha points. Note the radiopaque plume of root canal cement indicating the presence of a small opening in the calcific bridge. (Courtesy of Dr. W. Houck.)

(2) root filling coupled with surgical intervention (apicoectomy) and retrograde amalgam.

A third alternative procedure has recently been described for the treatment of immature teeth with wide root apices.[17, 32, 40, 55] This procedure allows apical development to continue in *nonvital* permanent teeth until the root end is sufficiently constricted to allow conventional endodontic procedures. It involves three steps: First, the canal is biomechanically cleaned and enlarged to the apex. Second, a thick paste of a resorbable material, such as a mixture of calcium hydroxide and camphorated-p-chlorophenol, is packed into the canal flush with the apex of the tooth and temporarily sealed. Third, the postoperative course is followed until closure of the apex is demonstrated radiographically. When sufficient closure has occurred the medicating paste is removed and a gutta percha filling is placed in the standard manner (Fig. 11–10*A,B,C,D*). The successful stimulation of apical development enables the root canal to be filled by standard endodontic procedures. This avoids the technique of reverse spreading which is mechanically difficult, and surgical intervention, which can be psychologically traumatizing to the young patient. The reader is referred to the outline in Figure 11–11 for a more complete description of this technique.

Extraction of the tooth is the indicated procedure when the conditions for survival of the tooth are not favorable.

MASSIVE FRACTURE OF THE CROWN

Occasionally a tooth may be fractured horizontally near the cemento-enamel junction. If the line of cleavage is such that restoration of the tooth is impossible, extraction is indicated.

Figure 11–11   Procedure for continued apex development.

FIRST APPOINTMENT
1. Anesthetize tooth, isolate with rubber dam, and swab field with 70% alcohol.
2. Make access opening into pulp chamber.
3. Determine length of apex radiographically with file introduced into canal.
4. Remove necrotic material with file and reamers. Irrigate with alternate solutions of hydrogen peroxide and sodium hypochlorite. Dry the canal, using sterile paper points and wisps of cotton wrapped around the end of a file or reamer.
5. Pack a thick paste of calcium hydroxide and camphorated p-chlorophenol into the canal. Use an endodontic plugger to push the paste to, but not past, the root apex.
6. Cover paste filling with a cotton pellet, followed by zinc oxide-eugenol and then zinc phosphate cement.

SECOND APPOINTMENT (3 to 6 months after first appointment)
1. Radiograph treated tooth to determine if apical closure is occurring.
2. If apex has not closed sufficiently, repeat procedure outlined in first appointment and recall in 3 to 6 months.
3. If apex appears developed, remove filling material, insert file and verify apical constriction by encountering a definite stop.
4. Take radiograph with file in place to redetermine new length.
5. Fill canal using lateral condensation of gutta percha cones. Seal coronal access opening with composite resin material.

(After Frank, A. L., J. A. D. A., 72, 1966.)

Because the clinical crown in a child is short, a fracture near the cemento-enamel junction may be several millimeters below the free gingival margin. Since within a few years the gingiva will reach the level of the cemento-enamel junction, the tooth should be treated if possible. A gingivectomy is performed first to expose sufficient tooth structure to allow for proper endodontic procedures. It may be necessary to remove a small amount of bone as well. A pulpectomy is then done, and the apical third of the root is filled. A cast gold core is cemented into the root and a porcelain jacket crown or porcelain veneer full gold crown is cemented over this (Figs. 11–12A,B,C and D).

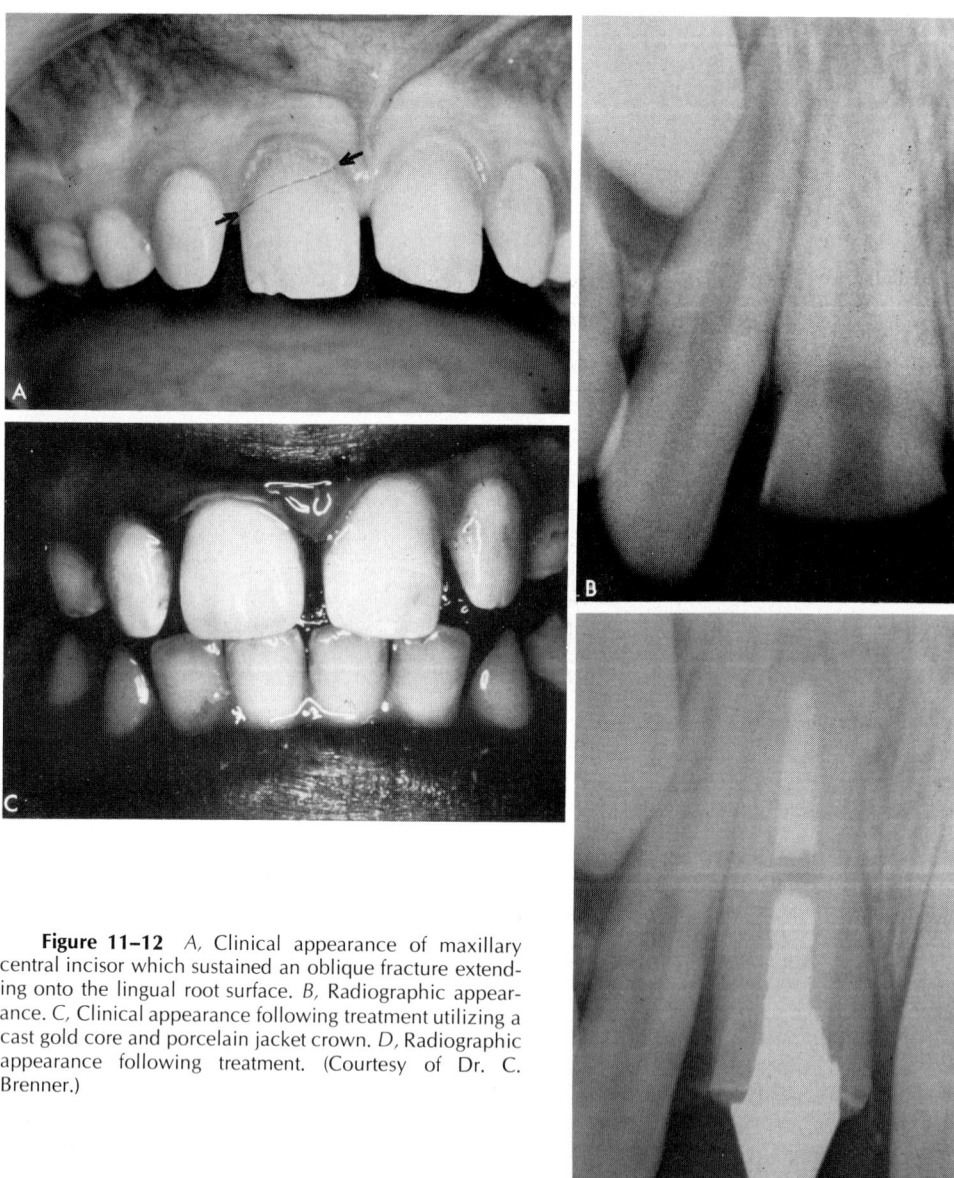

Figure 11–12 A, Clinical appearance of maxillary central incisor which sustained an oblique fracture extending onto the lingual root surface. B, Radiographic appearance. C, Clinical appearance following treatment utilizing a cast gold core and porcelain jacket crown. D, Radiographic appearance following treatment. (Courtesy of Dr. C. Brenner.)

TEMPORARY-PERMANENT RESTORATIONS

The requirements for a temporary-permanent restoration used in the treatment of fractured anterior teeth, according to Law,[31] are the following:

1. The preparation must be such that it will not endanger the pulp.
2. It should be durable and functional.
3. It should not increase the mesiodistal width of the original tooth or the labiolingual dimension.
4. It should be as esthetic as possible.

There are several kinds of restorations that can be made to serve for an intermediate time period; these include:

1. A composite resin restoration using a retentive wire.
2. A porcelain veneer full gold crown.
3. A modified cast three-quarter crown.
4. A processed acrylic jacket.
5. Reinforced core and crown.

A porcelain jacket crown is contraindicated as a temporary-permanent restoration because of the gross removal of tooth structure required for this type of preparation. Since fractured incisors occur most frequently in pre-teenage children, the added trauma of the cutting procedure on a large and already shocked pulp may cause irreversible damage. Although stainless steel crowns have been recommended and are used as temporary-permanent restorations, the authors feel that replacements are available that are more esthetic and more compatible with the gingival tissues. The use of stainless steel crowns should be limited to the temporary restoration.

In the following sections the technique for restoring fractured anterior teeth with pins and composite resin or with a reinforced core and crown will be described in detail. Since standard crown and bridge texts[42] include excellent descriptions for the technique of construction of three-quarter crowns, porcelain veneer crowns, and acrylic crowns the discussion of these restorations will be limited to their application in the treatment of fractured anterior teeth in children.

Pin-Retained Composite Restorations

Pin-retained composite resin restorations are placed at one sitting and are esthetically satisfactory. Although they are not as durable as cast gold restorations, they have the advantages of being more economical and of requiring minimal reduction of tooth tissue. These restorations can be utilized in class 2 fracture cases and in class 3 cases in which pulp capping has been performed. Before placing the restoration, a period of approximately 8 weeks following injury should elapse during which time the pulp has been protected by a calcium hydroxide medicating layer and suitable temporary restoration.

The pins are placed in holes drilled in the dentin and serve to retain the composite restoration, since no other form of mechanical locking is used. There are three types of pins commercially available:

1. *Cemented stainless steel pins* — The holes in which the pins are placed are .002 to .003 inch wider than the pins themselves and zinc phosphate cement is required to hold them in their position.

2. *Friction-lock pins* — This type of pin is driven into holes which are .001 inch narrower than the pin. Retention is obtained by the resiliency of the dentin which provides a friction lock.

3. *Self-threading pins* — Using a special contra-angle handpiece or a manual threading device, the pins are screwed into dentin in holes that are .002 to .004 inch narrower than they are.

Table 11–2 presents the diameters of the pins available under the three systems and the spiral drill sizes which are recommended by the respective manufacturers.

While the technique that is adopted rests with the individual operator, each pin system has its own advantages and disadvantages. Laboratory tests have demonstrated that the self-threading pins are the most retentive and require a maximum dentin depth of 2 to 3 millimeters.[12, 44] Friction-lock pins are intermediate in retention, and cemented pins are least retentive. Other tests have shown that craze lines occur in tooth structure with the self-threading or friction-lock systems since the pins are forced into holes which are smaller in diameter than the pins.[11] Crazing is not presumed to occur with the cemented pins. While the development of craze lines is not desirable, it is not known what effect they have on the ultimate clinical success of the restoration or on the life of the tooth itself. The technique using cemented pins is described below; however, with appropriate modifications the procedure may be used with any of the three systems.[28, 54]

PIN TECHNIQUE

Preparation of the Tooth

1. Loose enamel rods or an external bevel along the line of fracture are removed with garnet discs. The remaining cavosurface margin of the fracture is left as rough as possible to aid in retention of the restoration.

2. Two holes are drilled approximately 2 mm. into the dentin, using the smallest drill size compatible with the pin diameter being used (see Table 11–2).

TABLE 11–2   SPECIFICATIONS OF COMMON PIN SYSTEMS

Pin Type	Pin Diameter (inches)	Drill Diameter (inches)	Manufacturer
Cemented	0.018	0.021	E. A. Beck, Anaheim, Calif.
	0.022	0.024	K & R Dental Prod., Blue Island, Ill.; Star, Philadelphia, Penn.
	0.025	0.027	Star, Philadelphia, Penn.
Friction-Lock	0.022	0.021	Unitek, Monrovia, Calif.
Self-Threading	0.023	0.021	(Minum) Whaledent, Brooklyn, N. Y.
	0.031	0.027	(Regular) Whaledent, Brooklyn, N. Y.

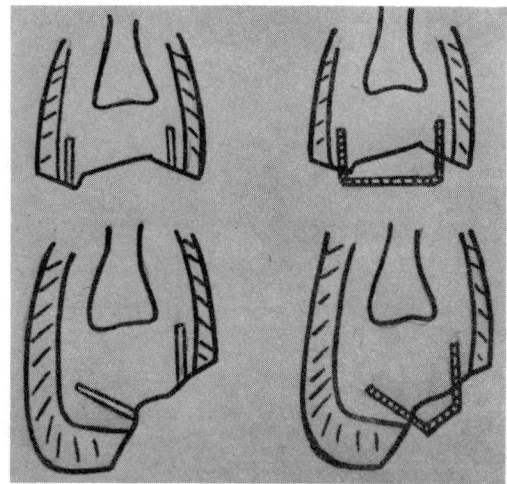

Figure 11–13 Restoration of fractured incisor corner or edge using cemented pins.

The .021-inch drill and .018-inch pin diameter are recommended. Before drilling the holes, radiographs of the fractured tooth must be judiciously studied to determine the size and relative position of the pulp chamber and pulp horns. If the fracture is horizontal, involving both incisal angles, the holes are placed mesial and distal to the pulp chamber. If the fracture is diagonal, involving one incisal angle only, one hole is drilled to the side of the pulp chamber while the other is drilled approximately halfway between the pulp horn and incisal edge (Fig. 11–13). The holes are positioned so that the pins will be at least 1 mm. from the labial surface in order for the pin to be masked by the labial thickness of the restorative material.

3. If a .021-inch drill is used, an .018-inch wire is bent to form a staple which will fit into the prepared holes and lie at least 1 mm. below the incisal edge (Fig. 11–13).

4. Using a lentulo spiral drill, white zinc phosphate cement is carried into the prepared holes.

5. The pin is pushed into the cement and positioned so that it will lie at least 1 mm. from the labial surface and 1 mm. from the incisal edge. The same cement is used as a mask to coat the labial surface of the wire.

Protection of the Pulp

6. After the cement has hardened, the excess is removed and calcium hydroxide is layered over the dentin.

Placement of the Restoration

7. Depending upon the operator's choice of restorative material, the restoration is either built up around the staple-shaped pin using the Nealon or brush technique (Fig. 11–14), or it is placed in bulk. If the latter method is chosen, a properly contoured plastic crown form will serve as a matrix to seat the freshly mixed resin. A hole, to serve as an escape hatch for excess material and air, is punched in the lingual of the crown form with an explorer tip. Material is placed in the form and also around the pin. The filled crown is pushed into position and held until the material has hardened. The celluloid matrix is then removed by slitting it along the lingual surface.

8. Trimming and polishing is accomplished with a curved #12 scalpel blade, discs, and finishing stones.

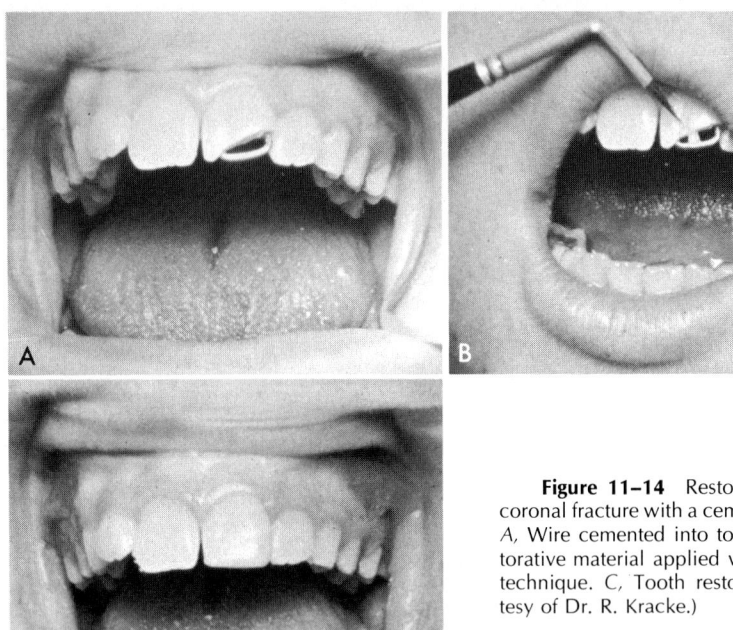

Figure 11–14 Restoration of a coronal fracture with a cemented wire. A, Wire cemented into tooth. B, Restorative material applied with Nealon technique. C, Tooth restored. (Courtesy of Dr. R. Kracke.)

Repair of Restoration

9. If the restoration wears or discolors it is a simple matter to remove the outer layer from the labial surface with a stone and place a new layer of the proper shade to restore esthetics.

Reinforced Core and Crown

After a Class III fracture has been successfully treated by pulpotomy, the temporary restoration may be replaced by a more permanent one. Since the accident that caused the pulp exposure often results in the loss of an extensive coronal portion of the tooth, a jacket crown is usually indicated. If the remaining coronal tooth structure is insufficient to support a crown, it may have to be built up or reinforced or both.

The core upon which the jacket crown will ultimately rest may be built with pins and amalgam, as described by Markley,[38] or with a resin reinforced with an orthodontic tube as described by Starkey.[54] The latter method is more versatile, since the fabricated post and core is easier to remove if a pulpectomy is required at a later date. The following is a modification of the Starkey technique.

Technique

1. Remove the temporary restoration and most of the medicating agent that was previously placed in the pulp chamber. Leave the deepest layer of calcium hydroxide intact. Place a protective zinc phosphate cement base over this.

2. Cut a piece of hollow orthodontic tubing (usually .036-inch diameter) so that its one end rests on the cement base and the other end is within the confines of the proposed coronal core. With a No. 1/2 round bur rotating in a high speed handpiece make several perforations in the tube.

3. Lute the tube to the cement base with a small bit of zinc phosphate cement.

4. Mix a high crushing strength composite material and quickly place it in an applicator tube. Force the material around and into the orthodontic tube. The same mix is used to build a bulk of material along the fracture site.

5. After polymerization the tooth and core are prepared in the usual manner to receive a jacket crown.

6. A jacket crown is constructed and cemented to place on the prepared tooth and core (Fig. 11–15).

Porcelain Veneer Full Gold Crown

From the standpoint of esthetics and durability the porcelain veneer full gold crown is a very satisfactory restoration (Fig. 11–16). It is recommended in children when some pulpal recession has occurred in the vital tooth and the gingival tissue level is not unduly coronal.

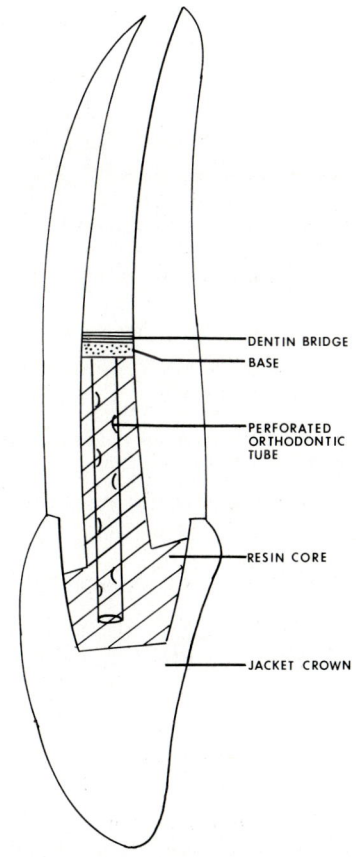

Figure 11–15 Reinforced resin core-jacket crown combination restoring a previously pulpotomized tooth that had been extensively fractured.

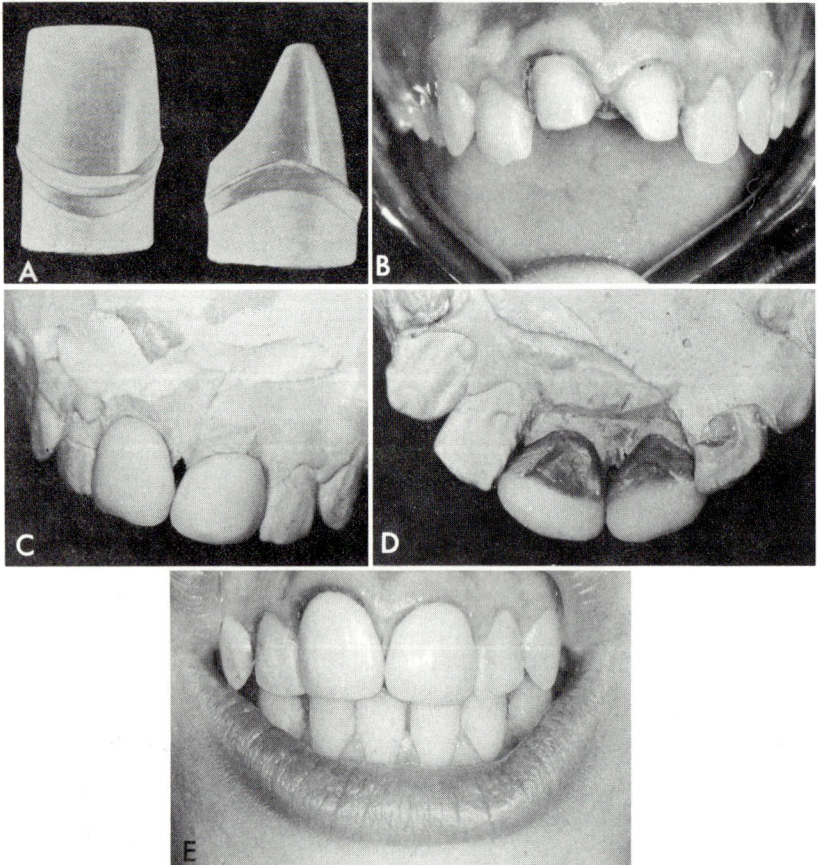

Figure 11–16 A porcelain veneer full gold crown. *A,* Models showing preparation of the teeth. (Courtesy of Dr. E. Warnick and J. Dent. Child.) *B,* Teeth prepared as illustrated in *A*. *C,* Cast gold crowns with porcelain baked on labial surface (unglazed). *D,* Porcelain extends over incisal edge onto lingual surface. *E,* The finished crowns cemented on the teeth.

With high speed techniques and sufficient water coolant, excess trauma to the pulp can be avoided. The limiting factor in the use of this restoration is the size of the pulp in the young patient. If the pulp is too large, adequate labial reduction to accommodate sufficient bulk of porcelain on the labial is difficult to attain.

Modified Three-Quarter Crown

If the lost tooth structure includes more than one third of the area of the crown, a modified three-quarter gold crown can be constructed (Fig. 11–17) as a temporary-permanent restoration until a porcelain jacket crown can be made when the child is older. Gold three-quarter crowns have the advantages of requiring a minimal removal of tooth structure and, because the labial-gingival area is not involved in the preparation, of not being esthetically affected by the continued eruption of the tooth. The three-quarter crown has the disadvantage of being less esthetic than a porcelain veneer full gold crown since some gold will usually be visible in the interproximal and incisal areas and the labial "window" area tends to discolor.

Full Acrylic Crown

Full acrylic crowns may be employed as temporary-permanent restorations. Like porcelain veneer full gold crowns, the cervical margins of the acrylic crowns may become exposed as the gingival level changes. There is a tendency on the part of some dentists and dental laboratories to fabricate crowns that are overly bulky. As long as this tendency is avoided, acrylic crowns make esthetic, serviceable restorations.

SUMMARY: TREATMENT OF CORONAL FRACTURES

The treatment of crown fractures in which the pulp remains vital is summarized in Figure 11–18. If it is decided that the tooth is not to be extracted or the pulp extirpated, treatment will usually consist of three phases. First is an emergency phase in which the traumatized pulp is protected from further insult

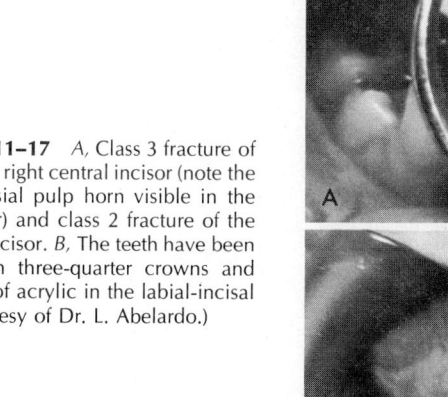
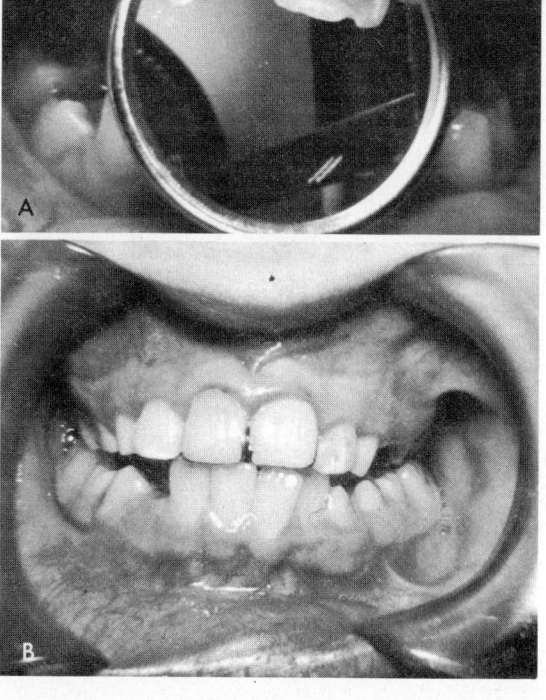

Figure 11–17 *A,* Class 3 fracture of the maxillary right central incisor (note the exposed mesial pulp horn visible in the dental mirror) and class 2 fracture of the left central incisor. *B,* The teeth have been restored with three-quarter crowns and "windows" of acrylic in the labial-incisal areas. (Courtesy of Dr. L. Abelardo.)

AN OUTLINE FOR THE TREATMENT OF CORONAL FRACTURES IN VITAL TEETH

Type of Fracture	Emergency Phase	Intermediate Phase	Permanent Phase
I. Enamel only	→Adhesive coverage		→Cosmetic grinding *or* resin with acid pretreatment
II. Enamel and dentin	→Ca(OH)₂ protective layer plus orthodontic band *or* stainless steel crown *or* resin and celluloid crown form *or* adhesive coverage	→Pin retained composite resin *or* cast ¾ crown *or* processed acrylic jacket crown *or* porcelain veneer full gold crown	→Porcelain jacket crown *or* porcelain fused to gold crown
III., VIII. Enamel, dentin, and pulp	→Pulp capping using Ca(OH)₂ plus orthodontic band *or* Stainless steel crown *or* resin and celluloid crown form		
	→Pulpotomy using Ca(OH)₂ plus orthodontic band *or* stainless steel crown *or* resin and celluloid crown form	→Possible reinforced core plus acrylic jacket crown	→May require pulpectomy
	→Pulpectomy		→Cast gold core and crown
	→Extraction	→Removable partial denture	→Fixed bridge

Figure 11–18

and a temporary restoration is placed. The temporary restoration serves mainly to protect the pulpal dressing. Esthetics is not a primary consideration at this time. The second phase of treatment begins at least eight weeks after the initial injury. If there are no signs of pulpal degeneration, a more esthetic intermediate restoration may now be constructed. The type of intermediate restoration will be determined by the extent of the fracture, the relative size and maturity of the pulp, and the degree of eruption of the tooth.

The third phase consists of placing the so-called "permanent" restoration. It was recommended that a "permanent" restoration, such as a porcelain jacket crown, not be placed until age 14 or 16 when the pulp has receded sufficiently and the incisor tooth has undergone most of its eruption. The authors feel this is an arbitrary and archaic approach. The dentist should decide when to initiate this phase of treatment based on the circumstances of the individual case. Besides the age of the patient, such factors as sex, amount of physical activity, and degree of social contact should be considered. With modern high speed and washed field techniques, it is possible to begin this phase of therapy *before* the teen-age period if the dentist feels it is indicated.

If the pulp becomes nonvital as a result of injury, a pulpectomy must be done if the tooth is to be retained. The technique of continued apical development in immature pulpectomized teeth has been discussed and seems an excellent mode of therapy in the young patient.

If the tooth is fractured to a degree that it cannot be properly restored, extraction will be necessary.

TREATMENT OF CONCUSSION

The treatment of tooth injury associated with coronal fracture has already been discussed. Concussion, however, can occur without producing a loss of tooth structure. Such accidents frequently are not seen by the dentist at the time of the accident since no apparent damage is visible. Yet, from these seemingly minor accidents pulpal or periodontal changes may ensue which produce symptoms requiring the services of a dentist.

A direct blow received by a tooth usually results in the compression of the root of the tooth against the wall of the socket. The associated injury to the periodontium may make the tooth painful for several days, and the patient may feel that the tooth is elongated. Radiographically, there may be a thickening of the periodontal space (Fig. 11–19). Injury to the periodontal ligament in trauma cases is not uncommon. Magnusson and Holm[36] reviewed the dental records of 237 Swedish school children who presented to a dental clinic for treatment because of a traumatic tooth injury. Of 460 involved teeth, 249 were diagnosed as having sustained a periodontal injury.

Concussion can also affect the blood supply to the tooth. The force of the blow may completely sever the apical blood vessels or may produce an apical edema and/or hematoma which might occlude the pulpal blood vessels as they enter the tooth. Rupture of the blood vessels within the pulp chamber can also occur, in which case there is discoloration of the tooth due to extravasation of red blood cells into the dental hard tissues. Any of these occurrences can result in pulpitis and eventual pulp necrosis. The risk of pulpal complications, however, is less if the injury occurs

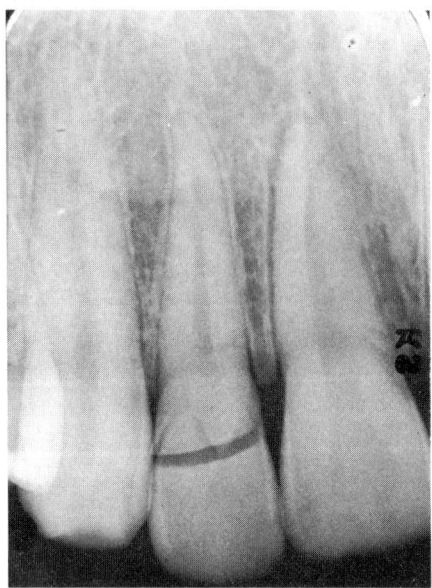

Figure 11–19 The force of the blow has caused injury to the periodontal membrane of the central incisor, accompanied by edema. The lateral incisor reveals a fractured crown.

in a tooth with a root that is still growing and in which there is a wide apical foramen.

The emergency treatment for concussion is actually treatment of the periodontitis and any pulpitis. In treating periodontitis, an effort should be made to relieve the bite by either slightly grinding the opposing teeth or constructing a splint which will open the bite slightly in the anterior region of the mouth. The patient should be instructed not to use the tooth in biting or chewing and to avoid other forms of trauma. The pulpitis can be treated by instructing the child to avoid any and all irritation to the pulp, such as traumatic bite and extremes of temperature. If the pain from the tooth is severe, analgesics should be prescribed.

In an extremely painful pulpitis it may be necessary to open the pulp chamber and allow for drainage. Subsequent treatment should consist of removal of the pulp and filling of the root canal by an acceptable technique.

Concussion can result in necrosis of the pulp without the patient feeling symptoms. Only a combination of diagnostic techniques can detect this development. Radiographs may reveal a periapical radiolucency. Clinical examination may show the tooth to be discolored or it may fail to respond to vitality tests. Two precautions, however, should be observed. Discoloration by itself is insufficient evidence for doing root canal therapy, and lack of response to pulp testing within the first months after injury is unreliable. Since MacDonald[35] has shown that the pulps of teeth which have become nonvital as the result of injury usually are infected, the same rules of sterility should apply to the endodontic treatment of these teeth that are followed in cases where exposed and infected pulp tissue was initially present.

TREATMENT OF FRACTURED ROOTS

Most root fractures occur in teeth with roots that are fully formed and are embedded in well matured alveolar bone. Fractures may occur in the cervical third, middle third (Fig. 11–20), or apical third of the root. The least frequent, and also the most difficult to treat, are the fractures that occur in the cervical third.

The fracture site will appear radiolucent on radiographic examination and a diagnosis is made based upon the finding of a radiolucent line disrupting the normal continuity of the root. Hargreaves and Craig[23] have stressed that the diagnostic quality of the radiograph in cases of root fracture will depend upon the angulation of the x-ray beam relative to the fracture and the plane of the fracture itself. By cutting the roots of extracted teeth in various planes they simulated different root fractures. They then reassembled the segments, oriented the teeth in different planes relative to the central ray of their x-ray tube, and demonstrated that when the central ray does not pass directly through the plane of fracture, the radiolucent image of the fracture site may be obscured (Fig. 11–21). If, for instance, the root is fractured obliquely in a labio-palatal direction, the fracture site may not be detected radiographically. In actual clinical cases where a question of root fracture exists, Hargreaves and Craig suggest that radiographs be taken at several angulations in order to view the suspected tooth root from different perspectives.

Treatment of root fracture involves (1) reduction of the displaced tooth and apposition of the fractured parts, (2) immobilization, and (3) close observation for pathologic changes in the injured tooth or surrounding apical region.

When a patient presents with a fractured root, the segments may be in close proximity or they may be separated. If they are apart, effort should be made to bring the ends into close apposition by digital manipulation of the crown segment under local anesthesia. A more favorable outcome is assured if these segments are in close contact. Following reduction, the injured tooth must be immobilized for a period sufficient to allow healing. This may be months, or even years. The patient should be placed on prophylactic antibiotic coverage for one week. With the absence of infection and the stabilization of the fragments, prognosis of middle third and apical third root fractures is very good. Prognosis of cervical third fractures is

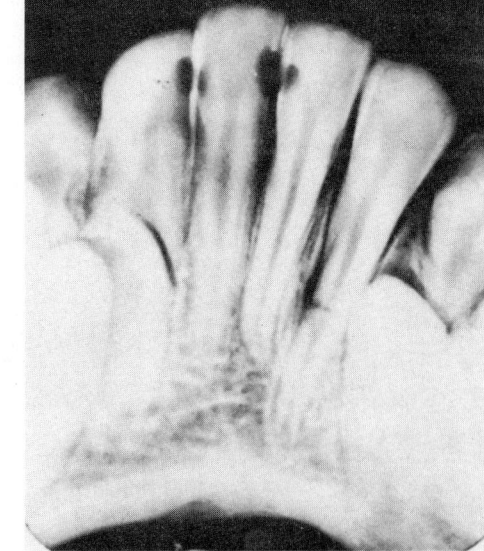

Figure 11–20 Fracture at middle third of root.

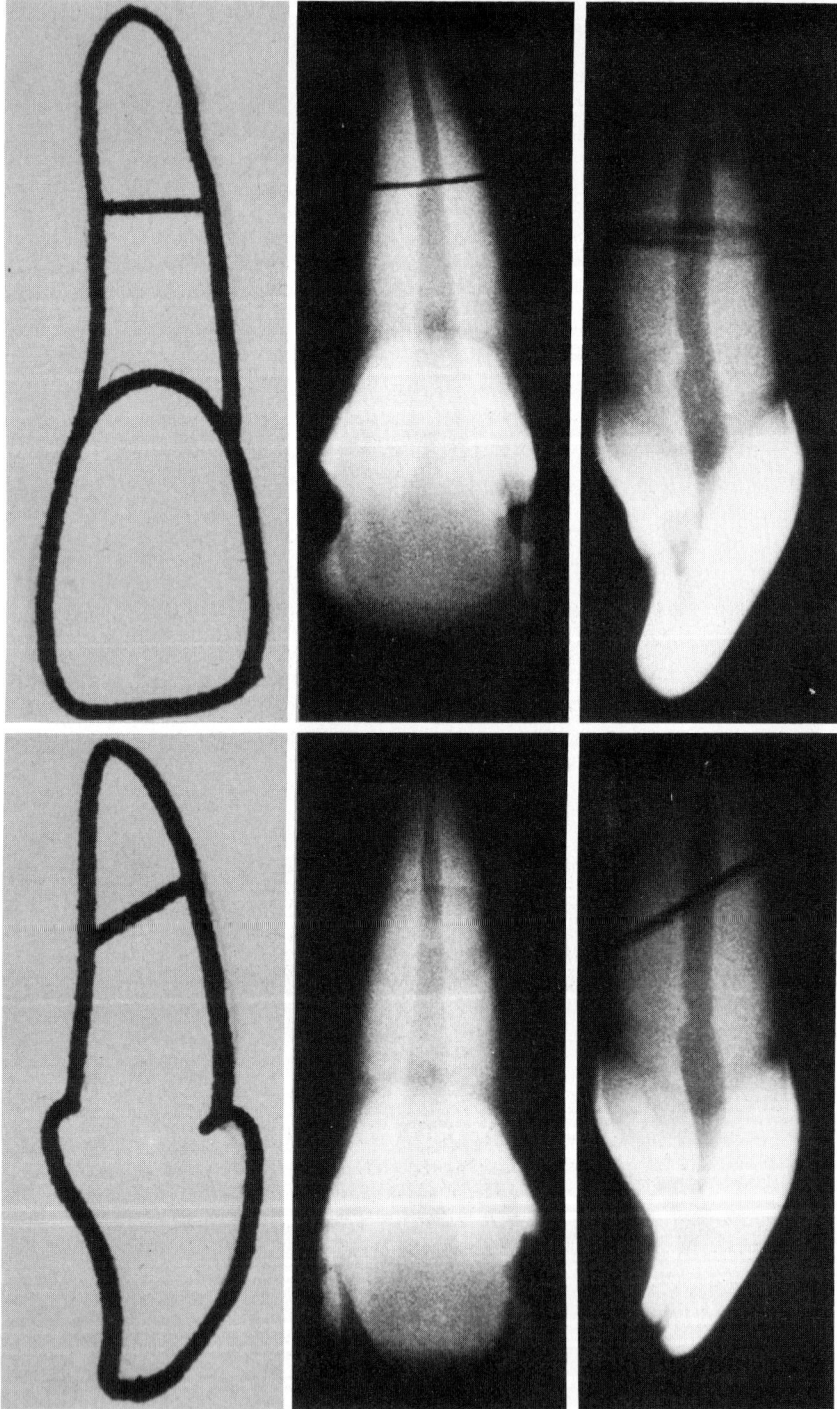

Figure 11–21   The effect of the path of the central ray and the plane of fracture on the radiographic image. Two extracted teeth were sectioned to simulate root fractures. One tooth (top row) was cut perpendicular to the long axis of the tooth, the other (bottom row) was cut obliquely in a labiopalatal direction. Each tooth was reassembled and radiographed from the labial direction and from the proximal. Note the different radiographic images of the "fracture sites." (After the technique of Hargreaves and Craig [ref. 23].)

poor because of the difficulty of stabilizing the crown segment and because of the ease with which bacteria from the gingival crevice and saliva can infect the fracture area. Andreasen and Hjørting-Hansen[5] have reported that minimal coronal displacement, optimal reduction, and immediate fixation are all factors conducive to a favorable prognosis. The patient's systemic health and oral conditions will also influence healing.

If pathologic changes occur during the period of immobilization a decision must be made as to whether the tooth should be retained. Under such circumstances, retention will necessitate root canal therapy in the principal segment. The apical segment may be left alone, filled with an extension of the root filling from the principal segment, or surgically removed (apicoectomy).

The methods of root healing have been described by Andreasen[2] and by Michanowicz and co-workers.[41] Michanowicz and co-workers believe that the integrity of the periodontal ligament is the essential requirement for root healing to occur, while the presence of a vital pulp is not necessary. Andreasen[2] has described three categories of root repair, based upon histologic and radiographic criteria:

1. Healing of the fractured area with dentin, surrounded by cementum and cementoid. Radiographically, the fracture line is discernible but the segments are in close contact. The margins of the segments are rounded. Clinically the teeth are firm and give a normal or slightly decreased response to vitality tests.

2. Healing of the fracture area by a filling-in of connective tissue. Radiographically a radiolucent narrow band separates the segments, the margins of which are rounded (Fig. 11–22). Clinically the teeth are firm and usually give a normal response to vitality tests.

3. Healing of the fracture area by interposition of bone and connective tissue. Radiographically bone can be seen between the segments. Clinically the teeth are normal.

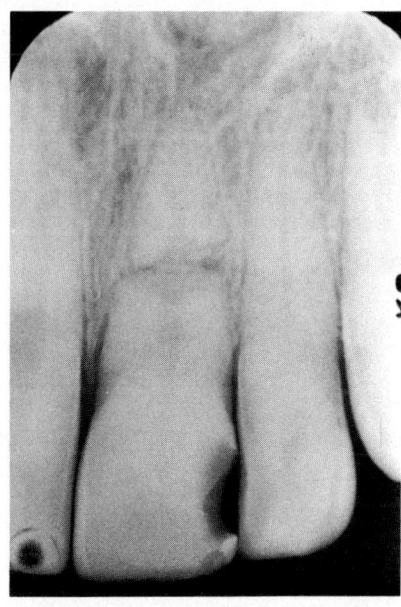

Figure 11–22 Line of old fracture undergoing healing is recognized by the rounded margins of the fracture ends.

Histologic studies have shown that if granulation tissue is interspersed between the root segments healing does not occur. Instead, there is a widening of the fracture line. Clinically a fistula may be present and the teeth are mobile and nonvital. Radiographically the bone associated with the fracture is radiolucent. These cases are considered failures.

STABILIZING APPLIANCES IN ROOT FRACTURES

Wiring

A 15 cm. length of .020 stainless steel wire can be used to ligate an injured incisor tooth to the adjacent incisor teeth and canines (Fig. 11–23B). The wire is wiped with a sterilizing solution and the end is cut on a bevel so that it can pass through tissue if necessary. The wire is placed along the labial aspect of the anterior teeth. One end rests several millimeters beyond the distal surface of the canine tooth. The other end is passed from labial to lingual through the interproximal space between the opposite canine and adjacent bicuspid. This end is passed around the lingual aspect of the canine, into the mesial interproximal space, and emerges under the labial wire. It is then bent above the labial wire and back to the lingual aspect through the same interproximal space. This process is repeated for each anterior tooth until it passes between the cuspid and first bicuspid in the adjacent quadrant. Each time the wire emerges labially, it is pulled taut with a needle holder; a cleoid-discoid is used to position the wire apical to the height of contour on the lingual side of the teeth.

When the segment has been wired, the two ends are crossed approximately 10 millimeters away from the canine tooth. The crossed ends are clamped with the needle holder and twisted clockwise until the twist almost contacts the tooth. The free end is then trimmed and turned into the interproximal embrasure.

The wires may be reinforced with acrylic for better stabilization (Fig. 11–23C).

Wiring to Surgical Arch Bars

Surgical arch bars may be employed for stabilization when one or several teeth are fractured (Fig. 11–23A). The bar is wired to supporting teeth, then wire is looped about the individual fractured teeth and tied to the horizontal arch bar. Although this method may be used for fractured roots, it has wider application in immobilizing avulsed or partially displaced teeth.

Band and Wire Splint

The tooth to be splinted and the adjacent teeth on both sides are fitted with bands. An .030 inch or .036 inch orthodontic wire is adapted to the labial aspect of the bands. The bands are removed and the wire soldered or spot welded to the bands. If the fractured tooth is too sensitive for banding, the adjacent teeth are banded and two bars, one on the labial and one on the lingual aspect, are soldered or spot welded to the bands around the adjacent teeth.

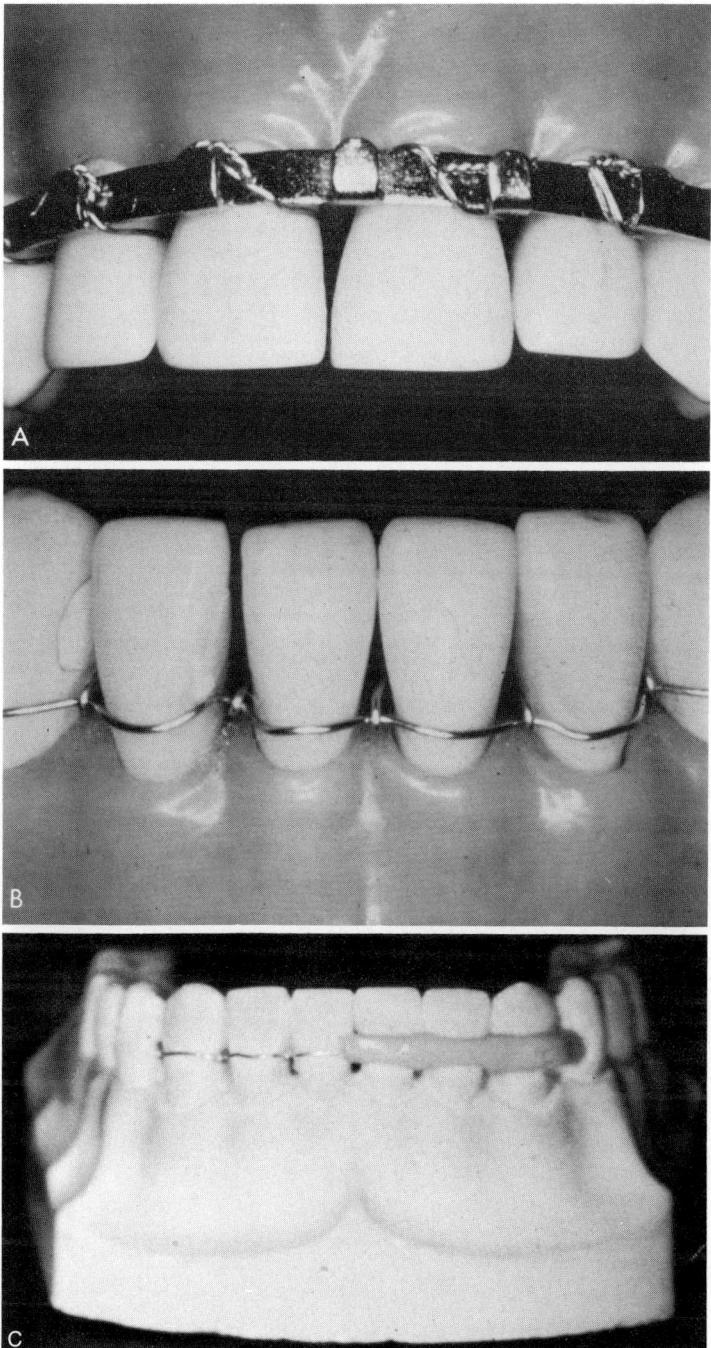

Figure 11–23 Stabilizing techniques. *A,* Surgical arch bar wired to teeth. *B,* Multiple wiring. *C,* Acrylic painted over wire and into embrasures for better stabilization.

Acrylic Splint

An acrylic splint may be made to cover the necessary teeth by taking an impression and then, by either the sprinkle or brushing technique building up the acrylic on the model. The splint should cover the incisal two-thirds of the labial surfaces of the teeth, extend over the incisal edges, and continue for 3 or 4 millimeters cervically along the lingual surfaces. After trimming and polishing, the splint is cemented in place. The acrylic splint may be modified to open the bite and thus relieve the biting force on the traumatized teeth.

TREATMENT OF DISPLACED TEETH

Displacement of permanent teeth, with or without loss of tooth structure, covers a wide variety of involvements from simple looseness to actual positional change, with various degrees of severity in each category. In this section displacement shall refer to labial, lingual, or lateral displacement, intrusion, or partial extrusion; avulsion will be considered in the next section.

In treating loosened teeth or those displaced in a lateral or labiolingual direction, every effort should be made to reduce the displacement and realign the teeth in their former position as soon as possible. If the displacement is not too great and the patient is seen soon after the accident, reduction can be effected in some cases without anesthesia by placing a gauze sponge over the displaced teeth and manipulating them into position, using adjacent sound teeth as a guide. If the displacement is considerable and painful to touch, reduction can be accomplished under local anesthesia or nitrous oxide-oxygen analgesia or both. In all tooth reductions one must be sure that the tooth alignment is normal and that there is no bite interference. Warm applications may be used to reduce any attendant discomfort, and the patient should be splinted for from 4 to 12 weeks depending on the character of the displacement, using any of the various splints already described.

If teeth are extruded they should be manipulated gently back into their sockets and splinted (Fig. 11–24).

Permanent anterior teeth that are intruded should be permitted to re-erupt. Generally, no splinting is necessary, but the teeth should be carefully watched for signs of pulp necrosis. An intruded tooth is generally driven firmly into the socket. The dentist should be cautioned against trying to bring an extensively intruded tooth back to the occlusal plane. By so doing death of the pulp may be produced by severing the blood supply to the tooth.

The prognosis and ultimate survival of the pulp depend on many variables of which the stage of root formation is one of importance. In cases of loose teeth with incomplete root formation, Skieller[52] has found that more pulps give a vital response immediately following the trauma and more cases continue to retain vitality, indicating a better recuperative capacity of the pulp (see Table 11–1). As previously indicated, pulpal responses immediately after injury cannot be relied upon to assess the vitality of a traumatized tooth accurately. Repeated pulp testing of displaced teeth over a period of months is certainly indicated. When intrusion or extrusion occurs, the pulp tends to undergo more severe damage. Thus, there is a larger percentage of nonvital pulps resulting and a greater chance of cessation of root formation. An additional sequela may be root resorption. Radiographic evi-

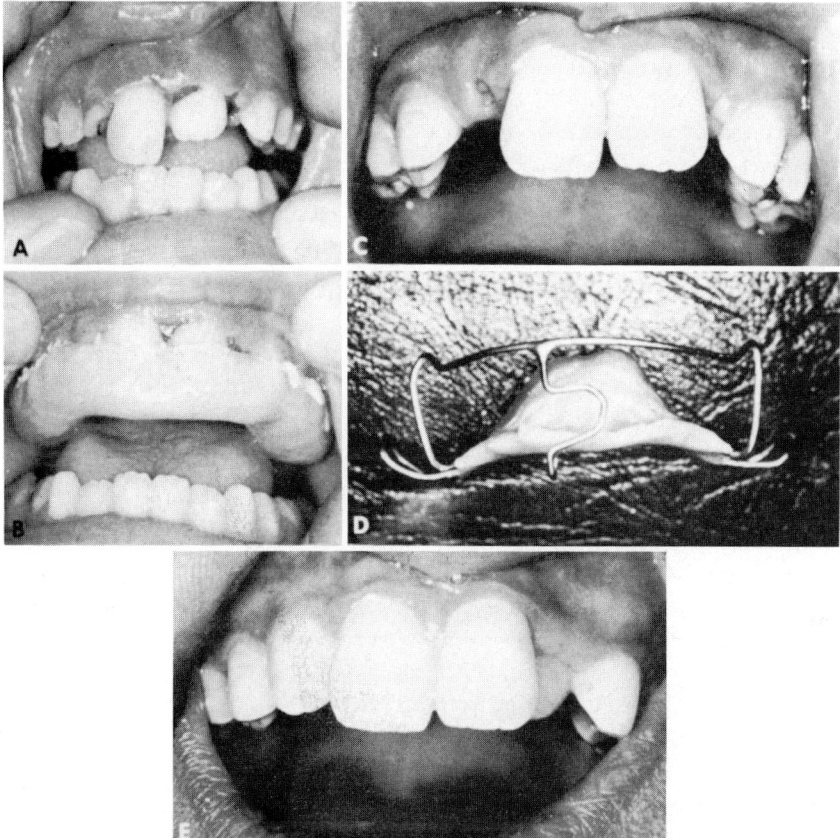

Figure 11–24 Treatment of a displaced tooth by immediate repositioning and subsequent orthodontic intrusion. *A,* Displacement by extrusion of permanent central incisor. *B,* Full occlusal acrylic splint constructed to open bite and stabilize tooth. *C,* Splint removed with tooth slightly elongated. *D,* Hawley-type appliance to continue intrusion; a benign spring was utilized to exert necessary force. *E,* Tooth repositioned where slight incisal edge grinding will eliminate any difference.

dence of internal or external root resorption is an indication for pulpectomy in the affected tooth. Lack of a positive response to the vitalometer several months after injury is also an indication for institution of pulpectomy procedures; however, a negative response to electric pulp testing immediately after displacement is by itself an insufficient reason for electing to do a root canal procedure.

TREATMENT OF TOOTH LOSS

An individual may lose one or several anterior teeth through a variety of different trauma-related causes. The tooth may be completely avulsed at the time of injury, an unfavorable crown or root fracture may necessitate extraction, or the tooth may succumb to internal or external root resorption or extensive periapical pathosis. Depending upon the individual circumstances, treatment will involve replantation or the construction of prosthodontic replacements for the missing tooth members.

REPLANTATION

In cases of avulsion, the teeth should be replanted in their sockets and immobilized as soon as possible. If replantation can occur within the first few minutes of the accident, it may not be necessary to fill the root canal as there is a possibility of revascularization of the blood supply to the pulp and also reattachment of the fibers of the periodontal membrane.

Observations were made by Andreasen and Hjørting-Hansen[3, 4] on 110 human replanted teeth. They concluded that the length of time the avulsed tooth is out of the mouth before replantation has a significant effect on the success of treatment. These investigators reported that when the tooth was out of its socket for 30 minutes or less, replantation was successful in 90 per cent of the cases based upon absence of root resorption and other pathology. When the extra-oral period was 30 to 90 minutes, replantation was successful in 43 per cent of the cases. When teeth were replanted after 90 minutes, the success rate dropped to only 7 per cent. Inflammatory external resorption of the root and periapical pathology were the principal causes of failure of therapy and tooth loss.

If the tooth is received immediately, it may be gently washed and immediately replanted and splinted, deferring endodontics until when and if it is indicated (Fig. 11–25). Before insertion, the root surface should be gently cleaned and large tissue remnants clinging to the surface should be removed. In order for reattachment to occur, it is believed by some that fragments of the periodontal ligament must remain attached to the avulsed tooth.[20] Hence, harsh scrubbing procedures should be avoided.

In many cases, by the time the dentist receives the tooth the pulp will be nonvital, and before replantation it is necessary to open into the pulp chamber, remove

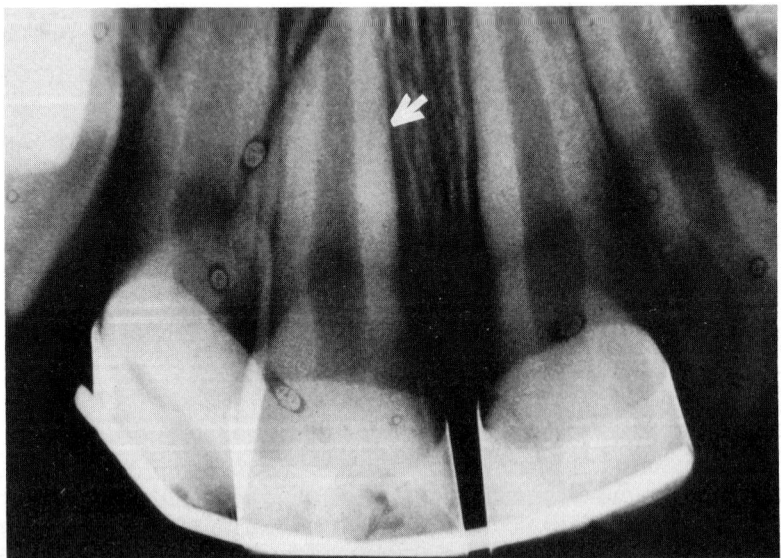

Figure 11–25 Immobilization of an avulsed permanent maxillary incisor using a soldered band and wire splint. Because the tooth was received immediately, endodontics was deferred. (Courtesy of Dr. J. Barenie.)

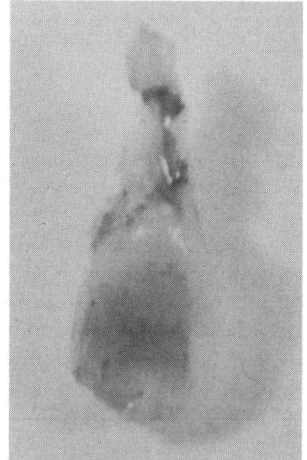

Figure 11–26 Appearance of a maxillary central incisor removed approximately 6 years after replantation. Note the extensive resorption of the root that finally caused the case to fail.

the pulp, and aseptically fill the canal. If the apices are wide the canal can be filled from the apical end using a gutta percha filling. The outside of the root should be gently cleaned and loose tissue removed. Before insertion it may be necessary to curette the alveolar socket; then the tooth is replanted. The tooth must be stabilized until it is firm in the socket.

Prognosis of these cases is extremely uncertain. Healing with establishment of a normal periodontal ligament may occur, in which circumstances the case is considered successful. Replacement resorption may occur in which there is a disappearance of the periodontal space, progressive resorption of the root and a filling in of the resorptive areas with bone. Such teeth are immobile but ankylosed. The cosmetic problem that ankylosis creates can be corrected with a jacket crown. Unsuccessful cases are those that undergo inflammatory resorption wherein the root is externally resorbed and no bony replacement occurs (Fig. 11–26). Occasionally, root canal therapy may halt the external resorption but usually the tooth is lost.

PROSTHODONTIC REPLACEMENT

A permanent anterior tooth, lost due to the direct effects of a traumatic episode or because it failed to respond to therapy requires a prosthodontic replacement. The replacement should be esthetic, function in speech and mastication, and prevent tipping of adjacent teeth.

In the young patient, a removable temporary appliance is constructed and worn until all permanent anterior teeth have erupted, alveolar bone changes have decreased, and the pulp chambers have receded to allow preparation for fixed replacements.

In constructing the temporary appliance, consideration must be given to those areas in which teeth are soon to erupt, and provision must be made either for leaving the areas of eruption outside the area of the denture or for easy removal of the part of the denture in the area of tooth eruption. If teeth are permitted to erupt beneath a denture, rapid decalcification may occur, especially if the teeth are not brushed frequently.

The removable appliance may be constructed of acrylic, or acrylic and metal. The choice of material will depend upon the desired permanence, the intended function, and the design of the appliance.

TRAUMA TO THE PRIMARY TEETH

As in the permanent dentition, the primary teeth most often traumatized are the maxillary central incisors. These teeth erupt between 6 and 9 months of age and normally remain until exfoliation occurs at about age 7. The frequency of injuries to the primary dentition increases as the child gains independence and mobility, yet lacks proper coordination and judgment; thus Schrieber[49] found that the majority of injuries to primary teeth occur between 1 1/2 to 2 1/2 years of age.

Ellis and Davey [15] consider injuries to the primary teeth in one group; nevertheless, all the various types of injuries seen in the permanent dentition can occur in the primary dentition. There is a difference, however, in the prevalence of the various types of injuries and there are modifications in treatment. Displacement, rather than fracture, appears to be the more common injury. This may be ascribed to the plasticity of the alveolar bone in the young child, which yields more readily to an apically propelled tooth. The denser alveolar bone of the older child stabilizes the permanent tooth and renders it more susceptible to fracture.

Because of the proximity of the developing succedaneous tooth, definitive treatment of a traumatized primary tooth should be instituted as soon as possible (Fig. 11–27). The effect on the underlying permanent tooth, according to Hawes,[25] will depend upon the "state of development of the permanent tooth, the nature and extent of the injury to the primary tooth, and the duration of the injury to the primary tooth."

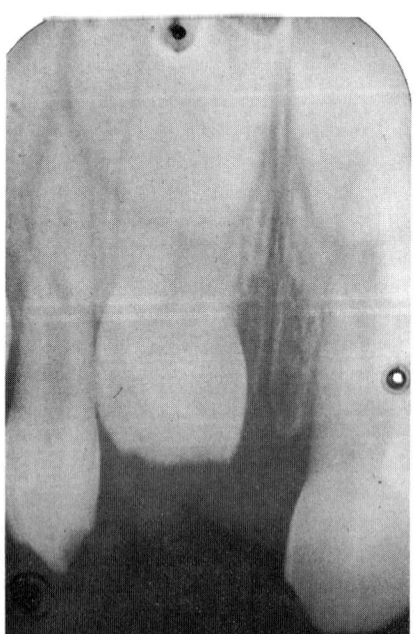

Figure 11–27   Marked intrusion of a primary central incisor. Immediate removal of the tooth is indicated.

CORONAL FRACTURES

Coronal fractures which involve only the enamel or a small amount of enamel and dentin are seen infrequently on an emergency basis. Parents are seldom concerned about such seemingly minor accidents, especially when there is no associated soft tissue involvement. When such fractures do present, they should receive the same treatment as has been described for similar fractures in the permanent dentition. Fractures which expose vital pulp tissue will, however, require immediate emergency therapy.

Vital exposed pulps in primary teeth should be treated by pulpotomy if cooperation of the patient can be secured. When the apex of the tooth is not fully developed, the same procedure is employed as described for a pulpotomy employing calcium hydroxide in an immature permanent tooth. If root formation is complete at the time of injury, a formocresol pulpotomy may be done or the dentist may elect to do a pulpectomy. If the latter procedure is chosen, the canal should be reamed and filed, irrigated with alternate solutions of sodium hypochlorite and hydrogen peroxide and filled with resorbable paste such as zinc oxide and eugenol. Preferably, this should all be accomplished during one appointment. Pulpectomy is the treatment of choice when the pulps are nonvital (Fig. 11–28).

After pulp therapy has been accomplished and presuming that sufficient retention can be secured, one of the following types of restorations can be placed: (1)

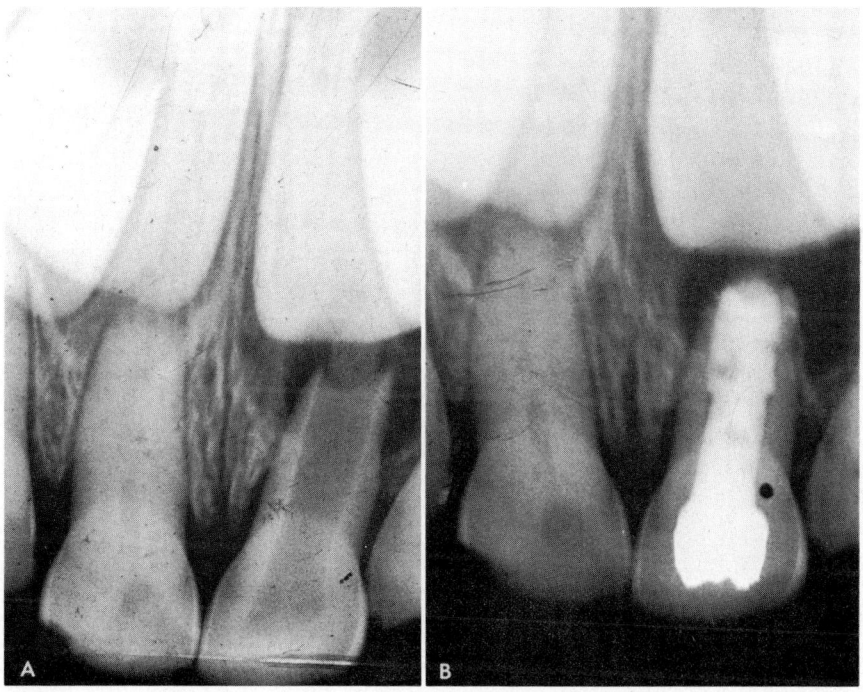

Figure 11–28 *A,* Periapical rarefaction is associated with a primary maxillary central incisor which sustained a traumatic injury resulting in pulp necrosis. Notice that the adjacent maxillary central incisor, whose incisal-proximal angle was fractured during the same accident, remains vital. *B,* An x-ray taken immediately after a pulpectomy was performed and the root canal was filled with a resorbable zinc oxide and eugenol paste. (Courtesy of Dr. R. Kracke.)

a stainless steel crown, with or without a labial window; (2) a fabricated acrylic jacket crown, utilizing a celluloid form, or (3) a preformed polycarbonate crown.

Stainless Steel Crown

Preparation of the tooth and adaptation of the crown employs the same technique used for restoring permanent anterior teeth. Because of their smaller size, manipulation of the primary crown forms is more difficult than that of the permanent forms.

Fabricated Acrylic Jacket Crown

Sherman and co-workers[51] have described an acrylic jacket crown for fractured primary incisors which can be fabricated in one appointment. The crown's primary indication is esthetic; however, it cannot be used on teeth so small or extensively fractured that there is insufficient tooth structure to ensure adequate retention, nor can it be used in patients with a deep overbite and small overjet or in patients who brux their teeth. The technique is as follows:

1. A celluloid crown form of the same mesiodistal width as the tooth to be treated is trimmed approximately 1 to 2 mm. longer than the normal clinical length of the crown. If the fracture precludes proper measuring of the injured tooth, the morphologically similar tooth in the adjacent quadrant may be measured.

2. The incisal edge of the tooth is reduced by approximately 2 mm. All axial surfaces are prepared as for an acrylic jacket crown except the lingual. A shoulder is extended well below the free gingival margin on the labial, mesial, and distal surfaces, but only 0.5 mm. on the lingual. The mesial and distal surfaces should be nearly parallel. A thin tapered fissure bur (69L) is used to prepare the tooth.

3. With a No. 1/4 round bur, the mesial, distal, and labial surfaces are undercut at the shoulder.

4. The crown form is tried on the prepared tooth. It should fit below the shoulder on the mesial, distal, and labial surfaces, but will not fit on the lingual.

5. Hemorrhage is controlled by packing hemostatic cord into the gingival crevice.

6. The prepared tooth is lubricated with petroleum jelly.

7. The crown form is filled with the appropriate shade of acrylic. Small additions of powder and liquid should be made to prevent bubbles from forming. The crown form is held for about one minute until the surface "frosts" and then it is seated firmly on the lubricated tooth. The labial margin of the crown form should approximate the labial shoulder of the tooth when properly seated.

8. The crown is held stationary for two to three minutes with firm finger pressure, and then it is carefully removed from the tooth. At this stage the acrylic is still pliant enough to pull away from the undercuts.

9. The crown is placed in a glass of warm water for 10 to 15 minutes. When removed, the acrylic will be hard. There will be an excess ledge of rolled acrylic on the lingual. This should be trimmed away and all margins should be trimmed back, flush with the gingival shoulder. After the proper gingival margins have been established, the celluloid crown form is removed, using a scalpel blade, and the margins are carefully buffed with fine pumice on a rag wheel held in the straight handpiece.

10. The crown is placed on the tooth. If seating is impossible because of the undercut, the ridge of acrylic in the undercut area is trimmed until proper seating can be accomplished. The crown is then removed and prepared for cementation. If zinc phosphate cement is to be used, the tooth should first be coated with cavity varnish.

11. The acrylic crown is cemented into place using the appropriate shade of zinc phosphate cement.

Preformed Polycarbonate Crown

Preformed polycarbonate crowns are commercially available for primary anterior teeth. The fractured primary tooth may be prepared as just described, the crown trimmed and cemented to place with zinc phosphate cement.

ROOT FRACTURES

In case of root fracture, an uncommon occurrence in primary teeth, extraction of the tooth is generally indicated. If an attempt is made to retain the tooth the pulp should not be exposed, and it must be possible to obtain satisfactory stabilization by splinting.

Occasionally old root fractures are diagnosed following a routine radiographic survey. If the tooth is asymptomatic and there is no pathology detectable the tooth should be left untreated. The presence of the fracture should be recorded and the tooth be periodically assessed.

DISPLACEMENTS

Among the partial displacements, intrusion is the more prevalent in the upper arch. These displacements are generally produced by the impact of falling on objects, a common accident of infancy and early childhood. In the lower arch, displacement lingually is prevalent for the same reason. A period of watchful waiting is indicated. Even though little of the crown is showing, there is a tendency for these teeth to re-erupt in six to eight weeks. If, however, the intruded tooth is pressing upon the permanent tooth bud or there is a likelihood of damaging the developing permanent crown, the area should be anesthetized and the primary tooth should be gently manipulated into proper alignment with finger pressure. Fixation of the traumatized primary tooth is difficult to accomplish with ligature wires, especially if the primary cuspids have not yet erupted. The tooth can be immobilized, however, by cementing an immediate acrylic splint. An impression of the affected tooth and adjacent teeth is taken with self-curing acrylic. This is used as a splint. It is trimmed on all surfaces and contoured to the gingival margin of the tooth without encroaching on the free gingival margin. The splint is cemented with a commercial zinc oxide and eugenol preparation and retained in position for six to eight weeks. Splinting in the primary dentition usually is not a very satisfactory procedure because the morphology of the primary teeth is not conducive to good retention.

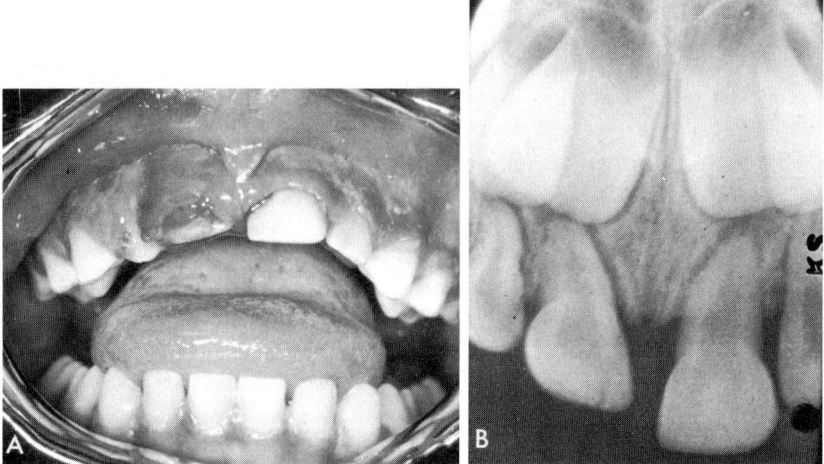

Figure 11–29   Primary incisor intruded. *A,* Considerable edema and hemorrhage increased the appearance of extreme intrusion. *B,* Roentgenogram reveals only a minor degree of intrusion.

If there is attendant swelling of the soft tissues around the intruded tooth, the degree of impaction always appears greater than it really is (Fig. 11–29).

Displacement by extrusion is not common in the primary dentition. When extrusion is present, according to Ellis and Davey,[15] it is generally due to root fracture and the resultant extrusion of the coronal segment.

If the displaced tooth becomes nonvital, a pulpectomy may be performed. Appropriate adjuncts may be used as necessary to secure patient cooperation. It is preferable to retain the primary tooth rather than to create a situation in which the child is required to wear an artificial replacement for a number of years.

AVULSION

Replantation in cases of avulsed primary teeth is a questionable procedure. Because of the morphology of the primary teeth, stabilization with wires or other splints is difficult. The very young patient, furthermore, may have too few teeth to make splinting feasible. In the older child, normal physiologic root resorption may have already begun, making replantation less indicated from a practical standpoint.

When an anterior primary tooth is lost due to traumatic avulsion or it must be extracted because of extensive fracture or periapical pathosis, the dentist must always consider the problem of space management. Three factors should be evaluated when deciding whether an anterior space maintainer should be inserted, viz., the age of the patient at the time of tooth loss, the type of primary dentition, and the number of missing teeth. Any one or a combination of the following circumstances warrants the placement of an anterior space maintainer: (1) loss of an anterior tooth in a very young child (4 years or younger), (2) loss of an anterior tooth in a patient with a Baume type II (crowded) primary dentition, (3) loss of multiple adjacent anterior teeth. The space maintainer may be fixed, in which case the second primary molars are banded and artificial teeth are attached to a lingual arch wire (.040 inch) with acrylic resin (Fig. 11–30), or a removable acrylic space main-

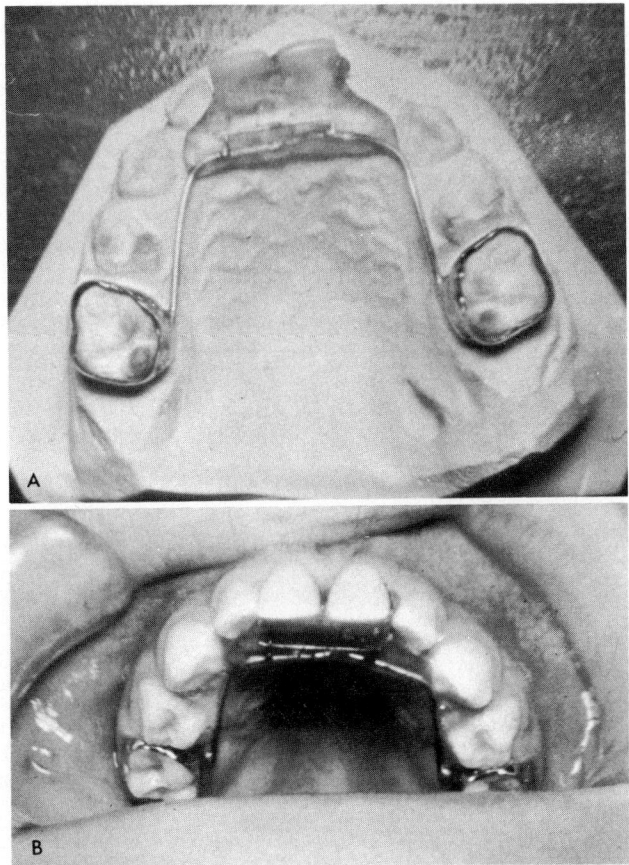

Figure 11–30 *A,* Fixed space maintainer replacing two lost maxillary primary central incisors. The second primary molars are banded, and the artificial teeth are joined by acrylic to a soldered lingual arch bar. *B,* The appliance cemented in the mouth. (Courtesy of Dr. R. Kracke.)

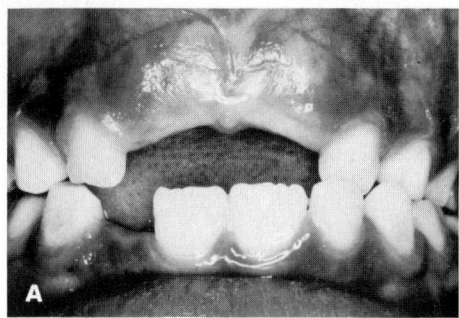

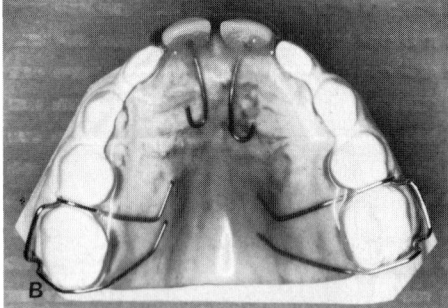
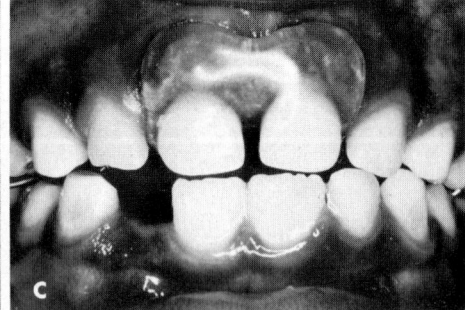

Figure 11–31 Replacement of avulsed primary teeth with a maxillary acrylic denture. *A,* Missing maxillary right and left primary central incisors. *B,* An acrylic appliance was constructed to satisfy function and esthetics and serve as a space maintainer. Retention was obtained by clasping the maxillary second primary molars. The primary denture teeth can be purchased commercially. *C,* The appliance in the mouth. (Courtesy of Dr. C. Brenner.)

tainer may be constructed (Fig. 11–31), Scures[50] suggests the construction of a porcelain fused to gold anterior bridge to replace a missing primary incisor. Both porcelain and gold are well tolerated by the gingival tissues; however, the cost of this essentially temporary appliance may make it prohibitive to many dental patients. The authors prefer a removable acrylic space maintainer. An acrylic appliance restoring the lost tooth has good appearance, restores function, maintains the space, and is usually accepted by the patient. The principal disadvantage of this type of maintainer is its susceptibility to loss or breakage by the young patient.

PREVENTION OF TOOTH INJURIES

There are two positive approaches to prevention of injuries to the permanent dentition:
1. Orthodontic correction of the trauma-prone profile.
2. The use of mouth protectors in contact sports.

ORTHODONTIC CORRECTION

It has been stated earlier in this chapter that as overjet increases the propensity to incur a fracture of the anterior teeth increases concomitantly. As can be seen in Table 11–3, while the child with a 1 to 5 mm. overjet has one chance in 18 of sustaining an anterior tooth injury, the child with an overjet of 10 mm. or more has one chance in six. The child, especially if he is a boy between the ages of 9 and 10, with a Class II, Division 1 malocclusion is literally on a "collision course" regarding permanent tooth injury.

Recognition of this trauma-prone profile and its correction constitutes a sound preventive approach.

MOUTH PROTECTORS

The National Alliance Football Rules Committee, in January, 1961, adopted a rule making the wearing of mouth protectors in football and hockey mandatory for all high school and college boys under their jurisdiction.* This rule went into effect in September, 1962, and affects the majority of the schools in the United States. In 1968, the American Dental Association's Bureau of Dental Health Education published a progress report on the effects of this rule.[1] A survey of several states showed that with the use of face guards and mouth protectors the number of dental injuries decreased significantly. In Iowa, for instance, before a protective device was required, the high school association reported an average of 125 dental injuries due to football. When face guards and some mouth protectors were made mandatory the average dropped to 73. When both face guards *and* mouth protectors were mandatory the average was only 30 injuries. This is a significant figure since it is based upon approximately 20,000 players.

Although the protective benefits from the use of mouth protectors alone cannot be separated from the combined use of the face guard and mouth protector, the value of the latter in reducing tooth injuries can at least be implied. There is also the impression, supported both by case histories[56] and laboratory data,[27] that mouth protectors may also be effective in reducing the incidence of cranial concussion.

There are three general types of mouth protectors available: (1) stock or ready-made, (2) those formed directly in the mouth, and (3) custom made from a cast of the maxillary dental arch. Each of these three types has its own advantages and disadvantages, and the superiority of one type over the other in preventing injuries has never been evaluated under field conditions, although evaluations have been

---

*All schools that are members of the National Federation of State High School Athletic Associations, the Junior College Athletic Association, and the National Association of Inter-Collegiate Athletics are under the jurisdiction of the National Football Rules Committee.

TABLE 11–3   THE PROBABILITY OF CHILDREN WITH VARIOUS DEGREES OF OVERJET SUSTAINING A FRACTURE OF A MAXILLARY CENTRAL INCISOR*

Overjet	Boys	Girls	All Children
<1 mm.	1:25	1:55	1:34
1–5 mm.	1:13	1:27	1:18
6–9 mm.	1:7	1:11	1:8
10 + mm.	1:4	1:10	1:6

*From McEwen and McHugh, Europ. Ortho. Society Rep. Congs. 1969 (ref. 39).

made using treated stone casts.[19] Whether information obtained under laboratory testing conditions can be extrapolated to the field or "in-use" situation is debatable.

The following is a description for the construction of a custom made mouth guard using a thermoplastic polyvinyl resin.

An impression of the upper arch is taken and a cast is poured in the usual manner. The vestibular area is trimmed to permit ready access to the mucobuccal fold region. The base of the cast is trimmed so that the palatal portion has a maximum thickness of 1/4 inch; greater thickness decreases the efficiency of the vacuum technique to be employed.

The proposed periphery of the protector is inscribed on the cast (Fig. 11–32A). A line 1/4 inch cervical to the gingival margin of the teeth is drawn around the palate. On the facial aspect of the cast a line is drawn 1/8 inch short of the mucobuccal fold and frenum attachment. The two lines are connected in the tuberosity area. The facial and palatal outline are beaded with a No. 4 round bur (Fig. 11–32B), and the entire cast is sprayed with a separating medium.

Polyvinyl resin is available in sheets and requires the use of a heating and vacuum apparatus for mouthguard construction.* The polyvinyl sheet is softened by heating coils and is impressed on the prepared cast by suction (Fig. 11–32C). After the polyvinyl sheet is adapted to the cast, the vacuum is discontinued and the adapted mouthguard is allowed to cool.

The adapted mouthguard is removed from the cast and trimmed along the beaded margin with scissors. The margins are buffed gently with a dry rag wheel. Sharp edges created by trimming or cloudy areas caused by buffing may be removed by careful flaming with an alcohol torch. If a name is to be placed in the mouthguard it is typed on a piece of lens paper and sealed against the protector

---

*Omnivac II vacuum adapter, Omnidental Corp., Harrisburg, Pennsylvania.

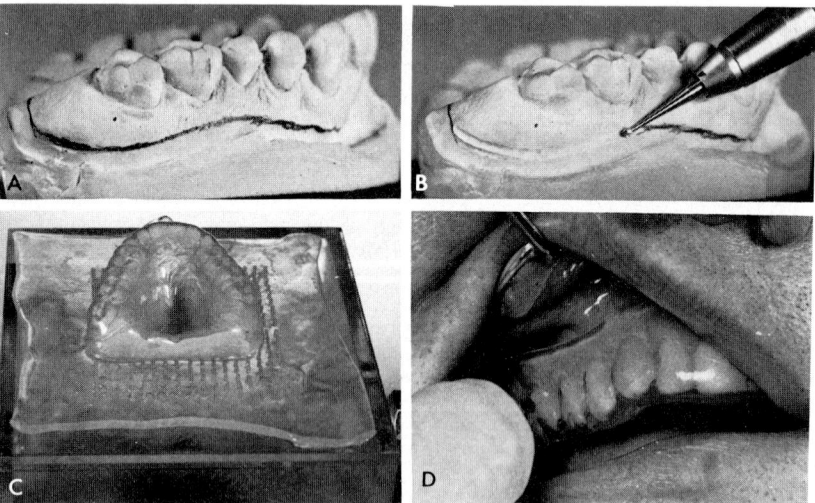

Figure 11–32   *A,* The outline of the mouth protector drawn on the cast. *B,* Inscribing the line with a No. 4 round bur to produce a bead on the finished mouth protector. *C,* A softened sheet of vinyl resin is drawn over the cast by vacuum. *D,* The finished mouthguard is checked in the mouth by the dentist. (Courtesy of Drs. P. J. Wehner and D. Henderson.[57])

while it is on the cast, using a piece of scrap polyvinyl and a hot flat bladed metal instrument. The area is subsequently flamed.

The mouth protector is inspected on the cast and in the mouth for accuracy of fit and proper extension of borders (Fig. 11–32D). Occlusal interferences are corrected by carefully flaming the offending area and allowing the athlete to close on the softened material.

The polyvinyl mouth protector is washed with soap and water after each use and air dried. Before being placed in the mouth, it is moistened with water.

Acknowledgment

The authors wish to thank Dr. J. Barenie for his critical reading of the manuscript of this chapter.

REFERENCES

1. American Association for Health, Physical Education and Recreation and the American Dental Association: Report of Joint Committee on Mouth Protectors, 1960.
2. Andreasen, J. O.: Treatment of fractured and avulsed teeth. J. Dent. Child., *38*:29–31, passim. 45–48, 1971.
3. Andreasen, J. O., and Hjørting-Hansen, E.: Replantation of teeth. I. Radiographic and clinical study of 110 human teeth replanted after accidental loss. Acta Odont. Scand., *24*:263–286, 1966.
4. Andreasen, J. O., and Hjørting-Hansen, E.: Replantation of teeth. II. Histological study of 22 replanted anterior teeth in humans. Acta Odont. Scand., *24*:287–306, 1966.
5. Andreasen, J. O., and Hjørting-Hansen, E.: Intraalveolar root fractures: Radiographic and histologic study of 50 cases. J. Oral Surg., *25*:414–426, 1967.
6. Andrews, R. G.: Emergency treatment of injured permanent anterior teeth. Dent. Clin. N. Amer., pp. 703–710, November, 1965.
7. Bennett, D. T.: Traumatized anterior teeth. Brit. Dent. J., *115*:309–311, 346–348, 392–396, 432–435, 487–489, 1963; *116*:7–9, 52–54, 96–98, 1954.
8. Bodenham, R. S.: The prognosis for vital pulpotomy of traumatized permanent incisors. Dent. Pract. and Dent. Rec., *17*:327–330, 1967.
9. Bruszt, P.: Secondary eruption of teeth intruded into the maxilla by a blow. Oral Surg., Oral Med., & Oral Path., *11*:146–149, 1958.
10. Chong, W. F., Swartz, M. L., and Phillips, R. W.: Displacement of cement bases by amalgam restorations. J.A.D.A., *74*:97–102, 1967.
11. Dilts, W. E., Welk, D. A., Laswell, H. R., and George, L.: Crazing of tooth structure associated with placement of pins for amalgam restorations. J.A.D.A., *81*:387–391, 1970.
12. Dilts, W. E., Welk, D. A., and Stovall, J.: Retentive properties of pin materials in pin-retained silver amalgam restorations. J.A.D.A., *77*:1085–1089, 1968.
13. Dow, P. R., and Lewis, T. M.: Pulp management for the immature fractured anterior tooth. J. Canad. D. A., *26*:5–9, 1960.
14. Eichenbaum, I. W.: A correlation of traumatized anterior teeth to occlusion. J. Dent. Child., *30*:229–236, 4th quart., 1963.
15. Ellis, R. G., and Davey, K. W.: The Classification and Treatment of Injuries to the Teeth of Children. 5th ed., Year Book Medical Publishers, Inc., Chicago, 1970.
16. Feldman, G., Solomon, C., and Notaro, P. J.: Endodontic management of traumatized teeth. Oral Surg., Oral Med., & Oral Path., *21*:100–112, 1966.
17. Frank, A. L.: Therapy for the divergent pulpless tooth by continued apical formation. J.A.D.A., *72*:87–93, 1966.
18. Gelbier, S.: Injured anterior teeth in children: a preliminary discussion. Brit. Dent. J., *123*:331–335, 1967.
19. Godwin, W. C., and Craig, R. G.: Stress transmitted through mouth protectors. J.A.D.A., *77*:1316–1320, 1968.
20. Groper, J. N., and Bernick, S.: Histological study of the periodontium following replantation of teeth in the dog. J. Dent. Child., *37*:25–35, 1970.
21. Gutz, D. P.: Fractured permanent incisors in a clinic population. J. Dent. Child., *38*:94–95, passim. 99, 121, 1971.
22. Hallett, G. E. M., and Porteous, J. R.: Fractured incisors treated by vital pulpotomy. A report of 100 consecutive cases. Brit. Dent. J., *115*:279–287, 1963.

23. Hargreaves, J. A., and Craig, J. W.: The Management of Traumatised Anterior Teeth of Children. London, E. & S. Livingstone, 1970.
24. Hasler, J. F., and Mitchell, D. F.: Painful pulpitis. J.A.D.A., *81*:671–677, 1970.
25. Hawes, R. R.: Traumatized primary teeth. Dent. Clin. N. Amer., pp. 391–404, July, 1966.
26. Heintz, W. D.: Mouth protectors: a progress report, Bureau of Dental Health Education. J.A.D.A., *77*:632–636, 1968.
27. Hickey, J. C., Morris, A. L., Carlson, L. D., and Seward, T. E.: The relation of mouth protectors to cranial pressure and deformation. J.A.D.A., *74*:735–740, 1967.
28. Johnson, D. F.: Anterior tooth fracture repair using Addent 12. Dent. Dig., *74*:340–342, 1968.
29. Johnson, R. H., Dachi, S. F., and Haley, J. V.: Pulpal hyperemia—a correlation of clinical and histologic data from 706 teeth. J.A.D.A., *81*:108–117, 1970.
30. Korns, R. D.: The incidence of accidental injury to primary anterior teeth. J. Dent. Child., *27*:244, 3rd quart., 1960 (Abstract).
31. Law, D. B.: Prevention and treatment of traumatized permanent anterior teeth. Dent. Clin. N. Amer., pp. 615–629, November, 1961.
32. Law, D. B., Lewis, T. M., and Davis, J. M.: An Atlas of Pedodontics. Philadelphia, W. B. Saunders Co., 1969, pp. 204–205.
33. Lawrence, K. E.: Restoration of fractured anterior teeth for the young patient. North-West Dent., *44*:269–273, 1965.
34. Lewis, T. E.: Incidence of fractured anterior teeth as related to their protrusion. Angle Orthodont., *29*:128–131, 1959.
35. MacDonald, J. B., Hare, G. C., and Wood, A. W. S.: The bacteriologic status of the pulp chambers in intact teeth found to be nonvital following trauma. Oral Surg., Oral Med., & Oral Path., *10*:318–322, 1957.
36. Magnusson, B., and Holm, A-K.: Traumatized permanent teeth in children—a follow-up. I. Pulpal complications and root resorption. Svensk. Tandlak. T., *62*:61–70, 1969.
37. Marcus, M.: Delinquency and coronal fractures of anterior teeth. J. Dent. Res., *30*:513–514, 1951.
38. Markley, M. R.: Pin-retained and pin-reinforced amalgam. J.A.D.A., *73*:1295–1300, 1966.
39. McEwen, J. D., and McHugh, W. D.: Predisposing factors associated with fractured incisor teeth. Europ. Ortho. Society Rep. Congr., pp. 343–351, 1969.
40. Michanowicz, J. P., and Michanowicz, A. E.: A conservative approach and procedure to fill an incompletely formed root using calcium hydroxide as an adjunct. J. Dent. Child., *34*:42–47, 1967.
41. Michanowicz, A. E., Michanowicz, J. P., and Abou-Rass, M.: Cementogenic repair of root fractures. J.A.D.A., *82*:569–579, 1971.
42. Miller, C. J.: Inlays, Crowns, and Bridges. An Atlas of Clinical Procedures. Philadelphia, W. B. Saunders Co., 1963.
43. Mitchell, D. F., and Tarplee, R. E.: Painful pulpitis, a clinical and microscopic study. Oral Surg., Oral Med., & Oral Path., *13*:1360–1370, 1960.
44. Moffa, J. P., Razzano, M. R., and Doyle, M. G.: Pins—a comparison of their retentive properties. J.A.D.A., *78*:529–535, 1969.
45. Olsen, N. H.: The family dentist and injured teeth in children. Practical Dent. Monographs, pp. 3–29, September, 1964.
46. Patterson, S. S.: Pulp calcification due to operative procedures—pulpotomy. Int. Dent. J., *17*:490–505, 1967.
47. Phaneuf, R. A., Frankl, S. N., and Ruben, M. P.: A comparative histological evaluation of three calcium hydroxide preparations on the human primary pulp. J. Dent. Child., *35*:61–76, 1968.
48. Rabinowitch, B. Z.: Replantation of teeth and management of root fracture. Dent. Clin. N. Amer., pp. 555–568, July, 1962.
49. Schreiber, C. K.: Effect of trauma on the anterior deciduous teeth. Brit. Dent. J., *106*:340–343, 1959.
50. Scures, C. C.: Porcelain baked to gold in pedodontics. J. Dent. Child, *30*:9–12, 1st quart., 1963.
51. Sherman, G., Bugg, J. L., and Carruth, K. R.: Restoration of primary incisors with acrylic jacket crowns—one appointment procedure. J. Dent. Child., *33*:182–185, 1966.
52. Skieller, V.: Teeth loosened after mechanical injuries. Acta Odont. Scand., *18*:171–181, 1960.
53. Spedding, R. H., Mitchell, D. F., and McDonald, R. E.: Formocresol and calcium hydroxide therapy. J. Dent. Res., *44*:1023–1034, 1965.
54. Starkey, P.: The use of self-curing resin in the restoration of young fractured permanent anterior teeth. J. Dent. Child., *34*:15–29, 1967.
55. Steiner, J. C., Dow, P. R., and Cathey, G. M.: Inducing root end closure of non-vital permanent teeth. J. Dent. Child., *35*:47–54, 1968.
56. Stenger, J. M., Lawson, E. A., Wright, J. M., and Ricketts, J.: Mouth guards: protection against shock to head, neck, and teeth. J.A.D.A., *69*:273–281, 1964.
57. Wehner, P. J., and Henderson, D.: Maximum prevention and preservation: An achievement of intraoral mouth protectors. Dent. Clin. N. Amer., pp. 493–498, July, 1965.
58. Warnick, M. E.: The use of porcelain fused-to-gold in the restoration of fractured young permanent teeth. J. Dent. Child., *29*:3–8, 1st quart., 1962.

12

REMOVABLE PARTIAL DENTURES FOR CHILDREN

by SATISH R. RAO

The purpose of this discussion is to introduce and acquaint the dentist with the concept of management of premature tooth loss in children with the aid of removable partial dentures. Premature tooth loss in children may consist of single or multiple, primary or permanent, and anterior or posterior units of the dentition. This tooth loss may be due to either trauma or caries and in some cases to congenital absence.

Irrespective of the cause, premature loss of teeth in children results in a loss of structural balance, functional efficiency, and esthetic harmony. Psychologic trauma is another consequence of premature tooth loss in children, especially when primary maxillary anterior teeth are involved.

A review of literature as well as personal clinical experience indicates that removable partial dentures are tolerated well by children and can be used successfully to prevent and restore the consequences of premature tooth loss.

SPECIFIC EFFECTS OF PREMATURE TOOTH LOSS

Premature tooth loss may lead to certain specific effects. These are:
1. Changes in dental arch length and occlusion.
2. Misarticulation of consonants in speech.
3. Development of deleterious oral habits.
4. Psychological trauma.

CHANGES IN DENTAL ARCH LENGTH AND OCCLUSION

It is well known that premature loss of primary teeth leads to a disruption of the integrity of the dental arches and occlusion. Improper management of this problem can lead to closure of spaces and malpositioning of succedaneous teeth in anterior as well as posterior segments of the dental arches (Figs. 12–1, 12–2, and 12–3).

MISARTICULATION OF CONSONANTS IN SPEECH

Concern has been expressed about the effect of premature tooth loss upon the development of speech, especially the articulation of consonant sounds, (s), (z), (v), (f). Speech pathologists[1,6] who have studied the relationship between missing teeth and selected consonant sounds conclude that statistically significant dif-

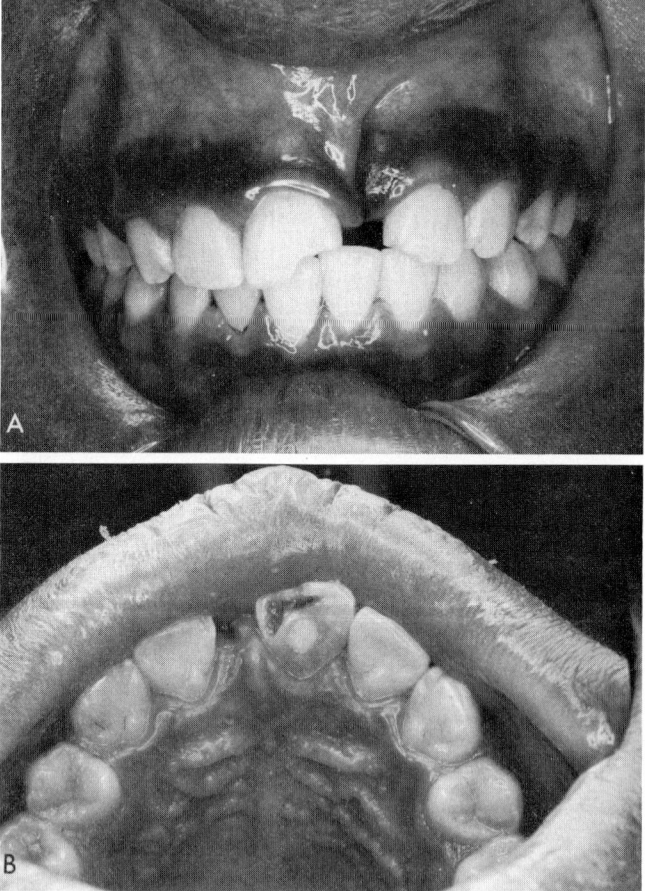

Figure 12–1. *A,* Labial and *B,* palatal views of an 11-year-old patient showing closure of space following loss of the maxillary permanent central incisor. (Courtesy of Dr. William Bailey III).

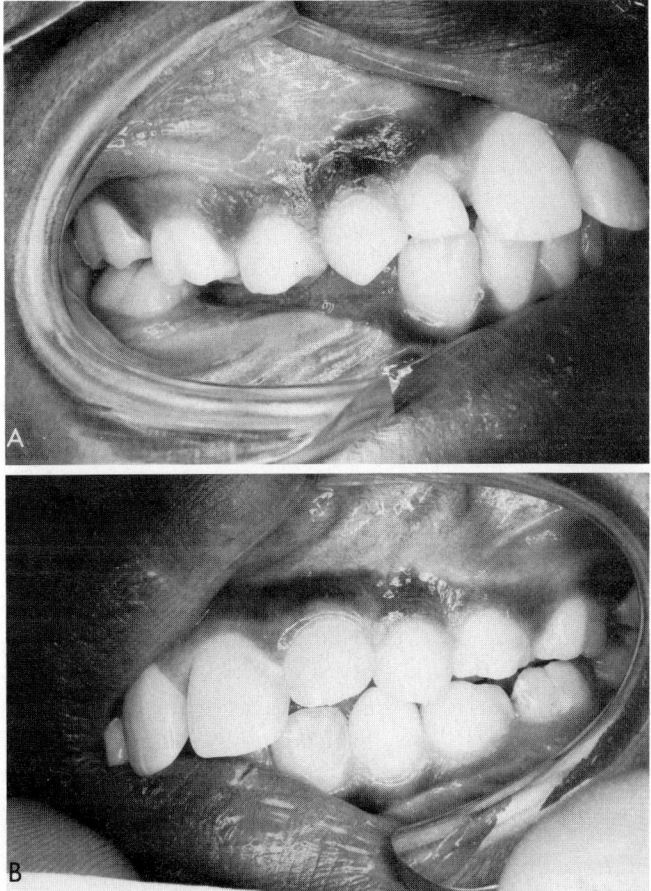

Figure 12–2   Over-eruption of maxillary posterior teeth following premature loss of the mandibular teeth on the patient's right side *(A)* as compared with the normal left side *(B)*.

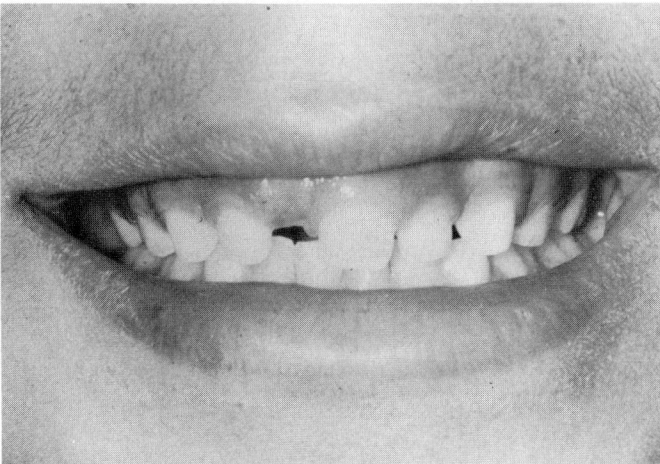

Figure 12–3   Closure of space following loss of maxillary primary central incisor due to trauma.

ferences exist in articulation between groups, with and without missing incisors. (See Chapter 26.) However, other findings indicate that the condition of teeth is a crucial factor in the correct development of articulation only in the case of a few children. In general, missing and defective incisors do not usually interfere with the correct articulation of the consonants studied. If speech problems are suspected, the dentist should promptly refer the patient to a speech pathologist for a thorough diagnosis.

DEVELOPMENT OF DELETERIOUS ORAL HABITS

Premature loss of anterior as well as posterior primary teeth may invite exploration by the tongue of the space created. Persistence of this behavior after the eruption of succedaneous teeth may lead to malpositioning of the teeth due to the excessive pressure by the tongue (Fig.12–4).

PSYCHOLOGICAL TRAUMA

Premature loss of primary teeth, especially the anterior teeth, is often the cause of considerable embarrassment to children, particularly girls. Psychological trauma may be due to unintentional, yet unkind, remarks by friends or relatives. In a society in which children spend a considerable amount of their time watching television, it may not be too uncommon for children with missing teeth to compare their personal appearance with that of their television peer group. This comparison, added to unkind remarks from friends or relatives, may lead children to develop feelings of inadequacy regarding their personal appearance.

INDICATIONS

Generally, removable partial dentures are indicated when prevention and restoration of the consequences of premature loss of primary teeth are necessary. Specifically, partial dentures are indicated when:

1. There is premature loss of primary molars, and space maintenance, and when restoration of masticatory function is important.

2. Radiographic examination shows that the time interval between the loss of primary teeth and the eruption of succedaneous teeth is greater than six months.

3. Primary anterior teeth are lost as a result of trauma.

4. Young permanent teeth are lost as a result of trauma.

5. Teeth are missing due to congenital absence, i.e., partial anodontia in ectodermal dysplasia.

6. Esthetics is a major consideration (Fig. 12–5). Concern is often expressed regarding the age at which partial dentures can be used by children. They have been used successfully in patients as young as two to three years of age. Lindahl[4] recommends a mental age of $2\frac{1}{2}$ years as a prerequisite for removable partial dentures used in children.

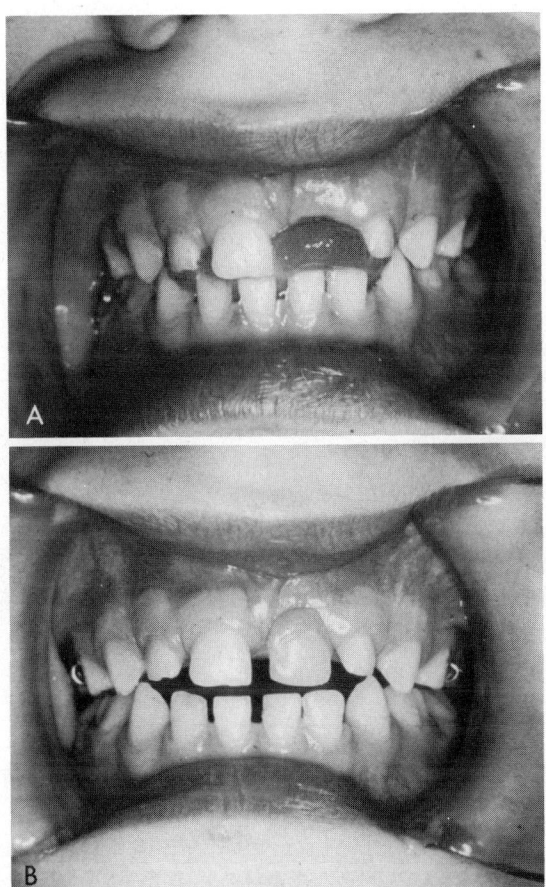

Figure 12–4. *A,* Exploration of space created by the tongue after the traumatic loss of the maxillary primary central incisor. *B,* Same patient treated with a partial denture to restore the tooth loss and possibly aid in the prevention of a persistent harmful oral habit. (*A* and *B,* courtesy of Dr. James King.)

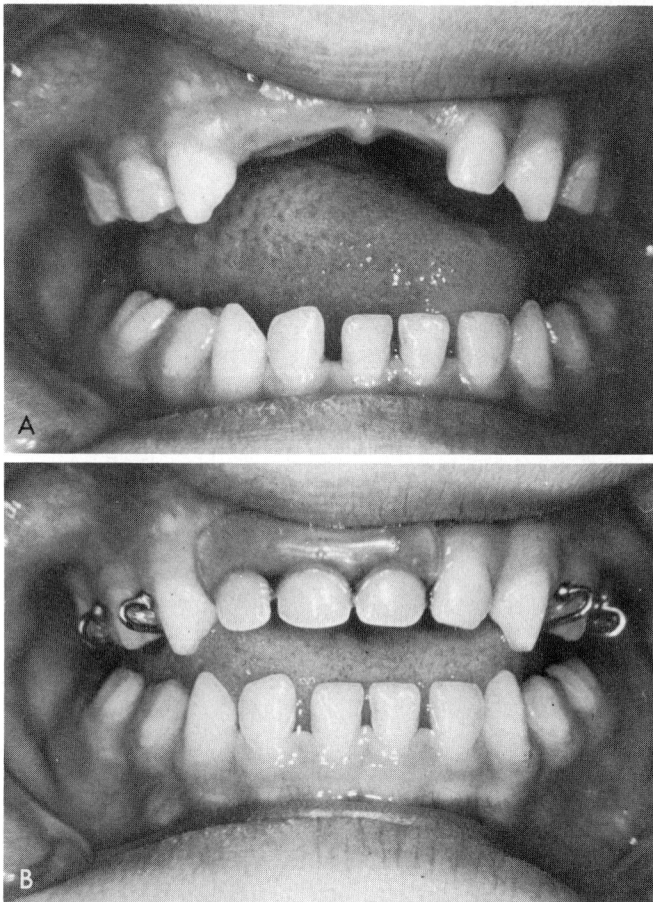

Figure 12–5. *A,* Premature multiple tooth loss. *B,* Restoration of the tooth loss by an esthetically pleasing partial denture. (*A* and *B,* courtesy of Dr. James King.)

(Fig. 12–5 continues on the opposite page.)

EXAMINATION, DIAGNOSIS AND TREATMENT PLANNING

Clinical examination of the child is carried out in the usual manner; however, the radiographic examination needs particular attention. Ideally, a panoramic radiograph would be desirable, so that one could visualize the different stages of development at which the various succedaneous teeth are at that particular point in time. This information can help the operator to predict the approximate time, and perhaps sequence, of eruption of the succedaneous teeth and also decide whether a particular patient presents the indications for a removable partial denture.

If the clinical findings and radiographic examination show that the indications for a removable partial denture exist, then the operator can proceed to design, construct, and insert one. The stage of treatment planning at which partial dentures are inserted will vary in accordance with the different needs of the various patients. However, restoration of at least the abutment teeth must be completed prior to insertion of the partial denture.

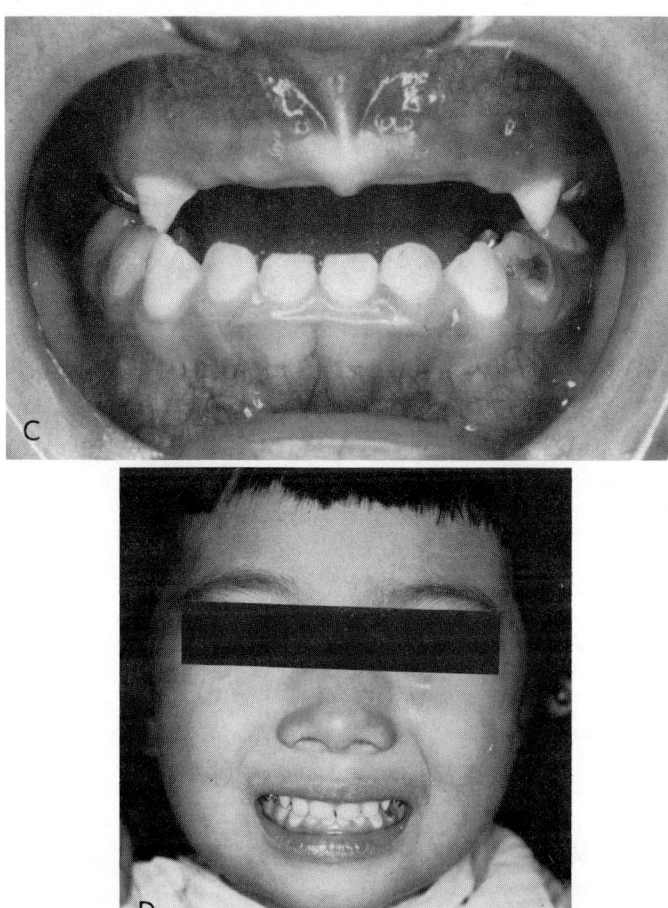

Figure 12–5 (Continued) *C,* Premature multiple loss of primary incisors in a 5-year-old child. *D,* Subsequent restoration with an esthetically pleasing partial denture. (*C* and *D,* courtesy of Dr. W. Alton.)

IDEAL REQUIREMENTS FOR REMOVABLE PARTIAL DENTURES FOR CHILDREN

An acceptable prosthetic device, in order to meet the needs for which it was designed, must usually satisfy some requirements. Listed below are some of the requirements:

1. It should restore or improve masticatory function.
2. It should restore or improve esthetics.
3. It should restore or improve facial contours.
4. It should not interfere with the normal growth of the dental arches.
5. Its bulk should not be an impediment to good speech.
6. Its design should allow the patient to insert and remove it easily.
7. Its design should permit easy adjustments, alterations and repairs.
8. It should be cleaned easily.
9. Its design should require minimal or no preparation of the abutment teeth.

Although the above requirements are quite specific and ideal in a sense, the operator should try to satisfy as many of these as possible. The means by which the operator can satisfy these requirements for a removable partial denture in differing situations will depend upon the operator's desire and ability to be innovative during unusual situations.

DESIGN FOR REMOVABLE PARTIAL DENTURES IN CHILDREN

The design for any acceptable removable partial denture should satisfy accepted basic principles of partial denture design in general. This design should be further influenced by the needs a particular appliance must meet. In children two very important considerations are the duration for which the partial dentures will be worn and the changing nature of the dental arches.

An important principle of design that every removable partial denture must try to meet is the inclusion of the means for tooth and tissue support of the denture. Lack of this principle in design can cause soft tissue pathosis with prolonged use (Fig. 12–6).

Ideally, any appliance should be designed at the chairside with the patient present, along with the study models and radiographs. Although this procedure may be inconvenient, it will ensure that all relevant existing factors have been taken into consideration and it may prevent expensive and time-consuming alterations after fabrication of the denture.

TYPES OF REMOVABLE PARTIAL DENTURES

Removable partial dentures have been grouped into different types according to the nature of their parts. They may be listed as the following types.

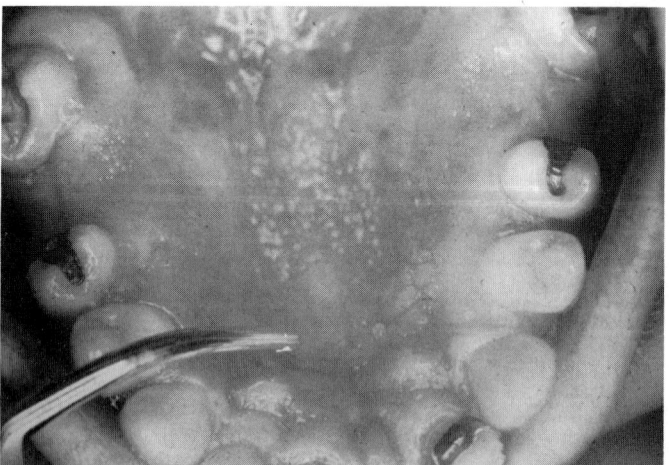

Figure 12–6. Tip of a blunt dental explorer in contact with the soft hyperplastic palatal mucosa. This patient had worn an acrylic partial denture without any clasps for a period of five years.

Maxillary Dentures

1. Acrylic.
2. Acrylic with wrought wire clasps.
3. Acrylic with cast metal clasps.
4. Acrylic saddles with cast metal framework.

Mandibular Dentures

1. Acrylic.
2. Acrylic with wrought wire clasps.
3. Acrylic with lingual bar and wrought wire clasps.
4. Acrylic with cast metal clasps containing occlusal rests.
5. Wrought wire clasps soldered to a lingual bar with acrylic saddles.
6. Cast metal framework and clasps with acrylic saddles.

However, the majority of clinical situations can be met satisfactorily by a removable partial denture consisting of an acrylic denture base, wrought wire clasp, and artificial teeth. When prolonged use is anticipated, the cast chrome-cobalt alloy framework may be considered.

PARTS OF A REMOVABLE PARTIAL DENTURE

Usually a removable partial denture for children consists of the following parts.

1. The denture base.
2. Clasps.
3. Artificial teeth.

The Denture Base

The denture base for most partial dentures is made of acrylic resin, although in some cases it may consist of metal alone or metal and acrylic resin. It provides a means for fixation of the clasps and artificial teeth. The denture base should be light and have sufficient strength to meet its functional needs. When acrylic resin alone is used it should be approximately 2 to 3 mm. thick so that portions of the clasps embedded into the denture base will be covered.

Clasps

Clasps are used to provide adequate fixation or retention of the denture base. They provide tooth support to the denture base and complement the tissue support it receives from the soft tissues.

Clasps may be either cast or wrought. Wrought wire clasps are ordinarily used in partial dentures for children. They may be constructed from 0.028 inch thick, round stainless steel wire and usually engage two or more external surfaces of the abutment tooth.

Different types of clasps may be used for different situations. Some commonly used wrought clasps for partial dentures in children are the Adams clasp, the ball

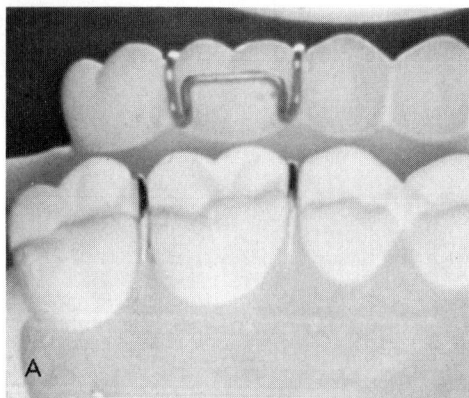
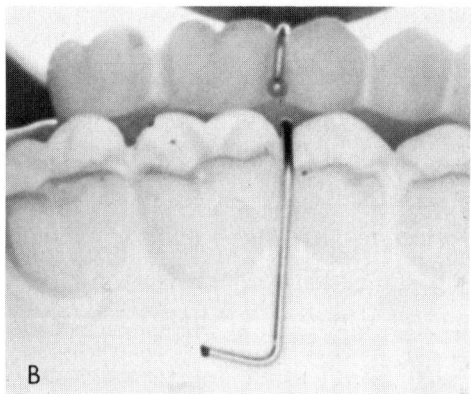
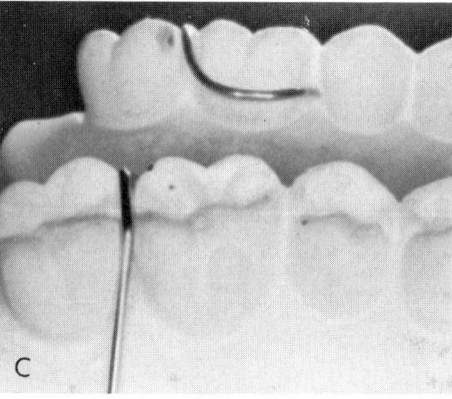

Figure 12–7. The different kinds of wrought clasps which may be used with removable partial dentures for children: *A,* Adams clasp; *B,* ball clasp; *C,* circumferential clasp. (Courtesy of Dr. James Palmer.)

clasp, and the circumferential clasp (Fig. 12–7). Of these, the Adams clasp is very versatile and is used primarily on posterior teeth. Because it clasps the mesiobuccal and distobuccal areas of the molars, it can be used to obtain retention from young permanent molars that have not fully erupted. Semi-preformed Adams clasps can be commercially obtained. Cast clasps of varying designs can be made to order upon prescription from the dentist by the commercial dental laboratories.

Occasionally, occlusal rests are used along with wrought wire as well as cast metal clasps, especially when the first permanent molars are used as abutment teeth for prolonged periods. Lindahl[4] has suggested that the rest may be placed in the central fossa using a lingual approach or placing the rest on the mesiocclusal portion of the tooth. He has also reported that failure to use occlusal rests on permanent molars may lead to settling of the dentures in the second primary molar area, causing mesial tipping of the permanent molars.

Artificial Teeth

In recent years artificial teeth for the primary dentition have become available: however, it may be occasionally necessary for the dentist to fabricate the teeth.

One suggested method is to use alginate impressions of study models of other children of approximately the same age, as molds. Into these molds an appropriately shaded mix of white cold curing acrylic resin is poured to obtain the required artificial primary teeth. Occasionally, for posterior segments of both mandibular and maxillary partial dentures, the occlusal half of preformed stainless steel crowns may be embedded in the denture base as suitable substitutes for artificial teeth (Fig. 12–8).

PROCEDURES FOR CONSTRUCTING REMOVABLE PARTIAL DENTURES FOR CHILDREN

Previous to the insertion of the partial denture the following steps are carried out.

Selection of Impression Trays

A variety of impression trays in sizes suitable for children are commercially available and can be used in many situations. After selecting the appropriate tray or trays, the edge of the rim of the tray should be beaded with beading or rope wax. This procedure cushions the edge of the rim to provide comfort to the patient and also helps to secure the alginate material to the tray.

Impression Material

The impression material of choice is alginate. Either the regular setting or fast setting type may be used; manufacturers' instructions regarding water:powder ratios must be followed in order to obtain a superior result.

Management of the Gag Reflex

It is generally a good practice to ask patients to rinse their mouths with a mouthwash so that any accumulated mucus may be removed. If the history or the obser-

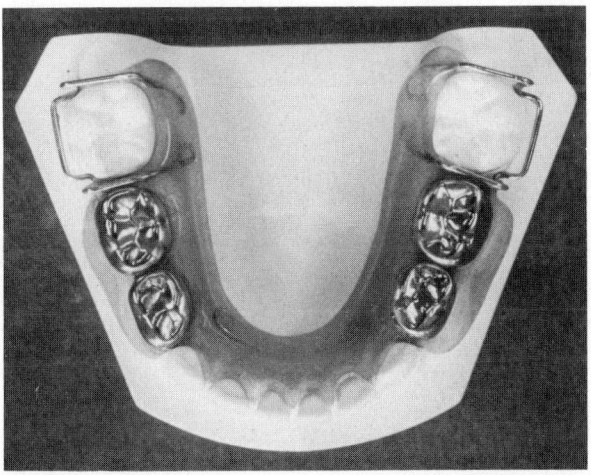

Figure 12–8. Model of mandibular acrylic partial denture using preformed stainless steel crowns as a substitute for artificial primary molars.

vations made during selection of the tray suggest that the patient may gag, the operator should take suitable measures either to prevent the gagging or to control it.

Gagging can be prevented in younger children by asking the patient to rinse with warm water containing some flavored surface anesthetic agent prior to the impression procedure, by asking the patient to breathe rapidly, or by distracting his attention with any other suitable procedure until the impression is completed. It is also wise to be prepared with a cuspidor or emesis basin and high speed evacuation equipment in case the patient vomits.

Maxillary and Mandibular Impressions

These are obtained in the usual manner. However, discomfort to the patient may be prevented, especially while obtaining the maxillary impression, by introducing the tray in the oblique sagittal plane and seating it in an upward and backward direction so that the excess impression material will overflow anteriorly instead of running down the patient's throat (Fig. 12–9).

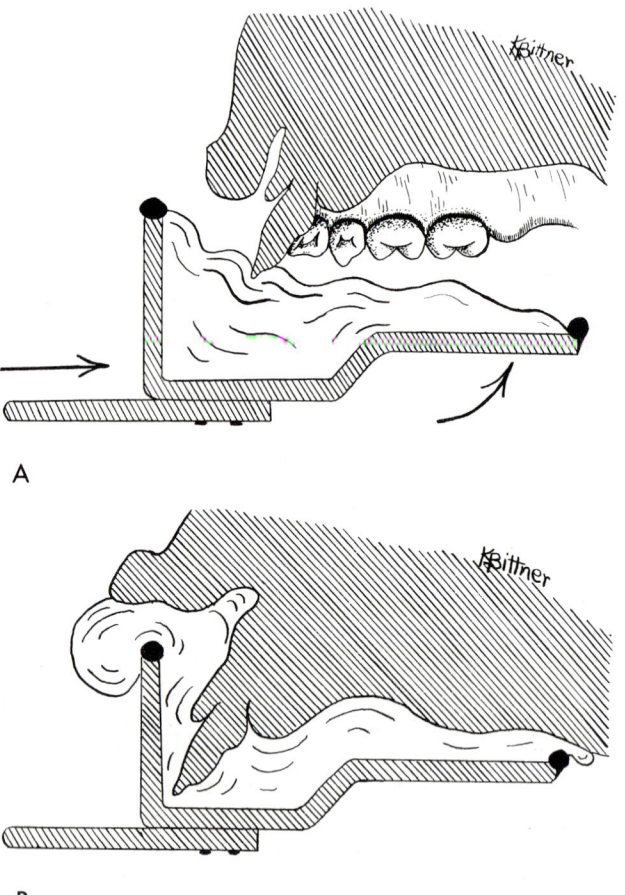

A

B

Figure 12–9   Schematic diagrams showing that if the maxillary impression tray is seated in an upward and backward direction the excessive impression material will overflow anteriorly.

After completion, the impressions should be inspected carefully. Any excess mucus or blood should be carefully rinsed off prior to pouring up the impression.

Bite Registration

A centric bite registration is necessary in order to establish an accurate relationship between the maxillary and mandibular models prior to mounting them on the articulator. This is obtained by asking the patient to close in centric occlusion on a prewarmed and softened bite registration wax wafer. For some young children who have a tendency to approximate their incisors in an edge to edge relationship when asked to close, it may be necessary for the dentist or the assistant to demonstrate to the child how to occlude the teeth in centric occlusion. The bite registration record should be inspected carefully and, if it is satisfactory, set aside along with the working models.

WORKING MODELS

The working model should be cast in artificial stone so that its surface will not be abraded by the metallic components of the partial denture. Once the working model is completed, the dentist can fabricate the partial denture himself or he can send the working model to a commercial dental laboratory.

If the model is sent to a commercial laboratory, the dentist should carefully prescribe the requirements and outline the desired design on it.

SPECIAL CONSIDERATIONS FOR THE MAXILLARY AND MANDIBULAR PARTIAL DENTURES

1. For the maxillary partial denture, the acrylic base should provide full palatal coverage.

2. If buccal or labial flanges are used, these should be relatively short and should match the color of the surrounding soft tissues.

3. It has been suggested that if clasps are used around primary cuspids, they should be removed at the appropriate time to allow the cuspids to drift laterally and distally to accommodate the erupting permanent incisors.

4. For the mandibular partial denture, an acrylic base will be suitable in most cases, though if prolonged use is anticipated, it is wise to use a metal framework or a wrought lingual bar. This lingual bar should be adapted about 2 mm. away from the soft tissue, so that it will accommodate the developmental changes in the dental arch when succedaneous teeth start erupting.

5. If prolonged use is anticipated, occlusal rests should be placed on the permanent molars. If the rest is placed in the central fossa, it should not interfere with the opposing cusp during closure.

6. When necessary, the appliance should be fabricated before extraction of the teeth and used as immediate partial dentures as well as immediate space maintainers.

INSERTION OF THE PARTIAL DENTURES

The appointment for insertion of the partial dentures should also be used to provide information and instruction to the patient and the parent regarding the insertion, removal, and home care of the partial dentures and the abutment teeth. After the dentist has finished inserting and adjusting the partial dentures, using a suitable mirror, he should show the patient the proper way to insert and remove them. To ensure that the patient can accomplish this procedure, he or she is asked to demonstrate the insertion and removal of the denture in the presence of the parent. The parent and the child should be impressed about the precision necessary in the construction of the denture so that they should not casually misplace or break it.

INSTRUCTIONS TO THE PATIENT AND THE PARENT

1. The patient is instructed to remove the partial denture during athletic activities such as swimming or contact sports. The parent is requested to provide the patient with a small plastic box for storage of the appliance during such periods. It is recommended that a mouthguard be worn during participation in contact sports.

2. The partial denture should be removed at night and stored in a glass of water. It should be cleaned every day either with denture cleanser or by brushing the denture with denture cleaning pastes.

3. The parent is shown the abutment teeth and instructed to check them frequently with disclosing tablets or a cotton swab stick dipped in food coloring to aid in the identification and removal of plaque.

4. If the denture does not fit or causes irritation, the parent should be asked to call the dentist and inform him.

5. The patient and the parent are informed in an appropriate manner that abuse of the partial denture leading to breakage or loss will result in prolongation of the treatment and extra expenditure.

6. The dentist should provide the parent and the patient with a written copy of instructions for the use and home care of partial dentures. A note should be made in the patient's chart indicating that written instructions were provided.

ADVANTAGES OF REMOVABLE PARTIAL DENTURES FOR CHILDREN

1. The partial dentures may be left in the patient's mouth with minimal supervision.

2. Should any problems arise, the patient or the parent can always remove the denture.

3. Good home-care of both the denture and the remaining teeth is easier to accomplish.

DISADVANTAGES OF REMOVABLE PARTIAL DENTURES IN CHILDREN

1. Lack of cooperation by the patient and the parent can negate the value of the treatment.

CONCLUSION

The dentist and the pedodontist have the responsibility of making the period of transition from the primary dentition through the mixed dentition to the permanent dentition as smooth and uneventful as possible. The ability to use removable partial dentures for children in an appropriate manner provides them with one more adjunct to fulfill their responsibility adequately.

REFERENCES

1. Bankson, N. W., and Byrne, M. C.: The relationship between missing teeth and selected consonant sounds. J. Speech Hearing Dis., *27*:341–348, 1962.
2. Brauer, J. C. et al: Dentistry for Children. 5th ed. New York, McGraw-Hill Book Co., Inc., Blakiston Division, pp. 509–529.
3. Law, D. B., et al. An Atlas of Pedodontics. Philadelphia, W. B. Saunders Co., 1969. pp. 249–267.
4. Lindahl, R. L.: Denture techniques suitable for growing arches. Dent. Clin. N. Amer., Nov. 1961, pp. 649–660.
5. McDonald, R. E.: Dentistry for the Child and the Adolescent. St. Louis, C. V. Mosby Co., 1969, pp. 341–343.
6. Snow, K.: Articulation proficiency in relation to certain dental abnormalities. J. Speech Hearing Dis., *26*:209–212, 1961.

13

PERIODONTAL DISEASES IN CHILDREN

by GILBERT J. PARFITT

INTRODUCTION

The term "periodontal disease" has been associated with the terminal stages of the disease: tooth loss, deep pockets, pus formation, and severe bone loss. During these degenerative stages methods of treatment are seldom effective. This had led to the common assumption that periodontal disease is a degenerative disease of later life and that little can be done about it. But periodontal disease is a slow, progressive disease which extends over many years and the early stages are extremely common in children. It is true that periodontal degeneration is unusual in children, but a few cases do occur. In these cases periodontal disease has progressed rapidly from the early stages to the terminal stages. In the past only these few cases have been recognized as periodontal disease, and the vast majority of children who present a marginal gingivitis of variable degree have been considered normal.

Periodontal disease occurs at any age, and is usually an extremely slow process, the early stages of which are common before puberty. Unless these early stages are eliminated, degenerative periodontal disease is inevitable in later years.

In childhood, therefore, periodontal disease has already begun; it is most important to recognize it and to treat it.

THE NORMAL GINGIVAE IN CHILDHOOD

The gingivae in children should be a pale pink color resembling the color of the skin of the face rather than that of the lips, and should be firmly bound to the

286

alveolar bone. The primary teeth have short bulbous crowns and the contact point is nearer to the occlusal surface than in the permanent teeth. The gingivae in the primary dentition, therefore, are closer to the occlusal surfaces of the teeth, and the papillae are squat, bulky, and completely fill the interproximal space.

The pale pink color of the normal uninflamed gingivae is due to the preponderance of connective tissues over blood vessels. These vessels, although too small to be seen by the naked eye, when magnified × 10 are clearly visible through the epithelium. The epithelial surface is soft and velvety with many surface irregularities which, when more pronounced, are described as "stippling." Stippling may be seen on the gums of children at the age of three years, but at this age there are only a few discrete umbilical elevations on the epithelial surface. By the age of ten, when some of the permanent teeth are in position, the gingivae in some children show stippling in a band ⅛ inch wide, extending from close to the free gingival margin and papilla as far as the attached mucosa. Stippling is not limited to the attached mucosa.

The free margin of the gingivae extends to the bulge of the crown of the tooth which in the primary teeth is nearly as accentuated as in carnivores. The crown of the tooth and the buccal or lingual gingiva form an almost unbroken surface to food as it passes from the hard masticatory surfaces of the teeth to the soft reflecting tissues.

The gingival crevice in the primary dentition extends 1 mm. or less beneath the bulge of the tooth. It is a narrow trough bounded by the tooth on one side and an ample bulk of tough, resilient gingival tissue on the other. The epithelial surface of the crevice, as well as that of the gingiva and oral mucosa, grows continuously, desquamates freely and heals rapidly. The whole dental unit in the child is adapted to vigorous function, and the gingival tissues, though close to the masticatory surfaces of the teeth, are protected from damage by the shape of the crowns.

The permanent teeth are not as bulbous as the primary teeth. The papillae are narrow and less bulky, and both the papilla and the margin are situated farther from the occlusal surfaces of the teeth (Fig. 13–1). The gingival crevice surrounding a permanent tooth is deeper and is not supported by as great a bulk of tissue; in fact, some marginal gingivae around permanent teeth are so thin that an explorer point introduced into the crevice is visible through them.

Throughout childhood, changes in the jaw occur owing to growth and development. Spaces appear between the teeth as a result of appositional alveolar bone growth, and may be seen as early as 3½ years. Food shows little tendency to pack in these spaces if the marginal ridge of a tooth is intact, and this spacing of the teeth is not associated with gingivitis.

A period of up to two years elapses between the shedding of the primary teeth and the eruption of the permanent successors. Before the gum is punctured, the tissues are thinned over the rising cusps of the teeth; after the teeth appear in the mouth, and while the teeth are erupting into final position, the marginal gingivae are thickened and have a protuberant rolled edge. Active reorganization of connective tissue fibers takes place within them, and appears as a slight hyperemia but never approaches the color of an inflammation associated with bacterial infection. This should not be confused with a gingivitis of bacterial origin.

Between the ages of 5 and 12 years, 20 primary teeth are shed and 24 permanent teeth erupt. Although the order of eruption of the teeth is generally maintained, the upper and lower and the right and left members of any one type of

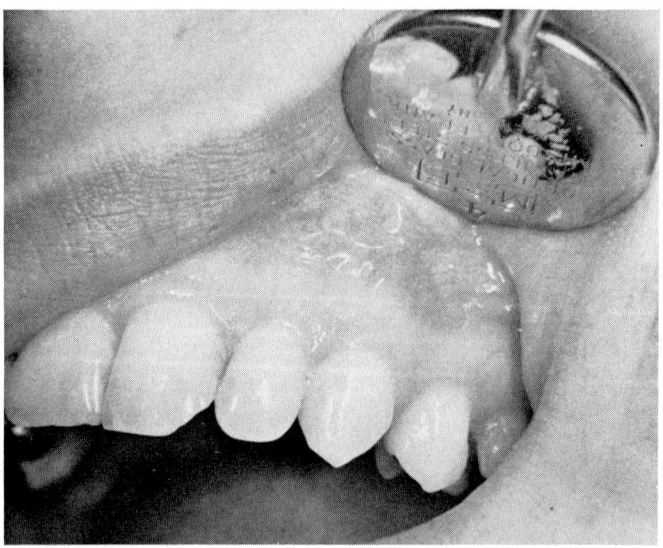

Figure 13–1   The normal gingival contour surrounding fully erupted permanent teeth. Note the pointed papillae, the thin gingival margin, and the width of the attached mucosa.

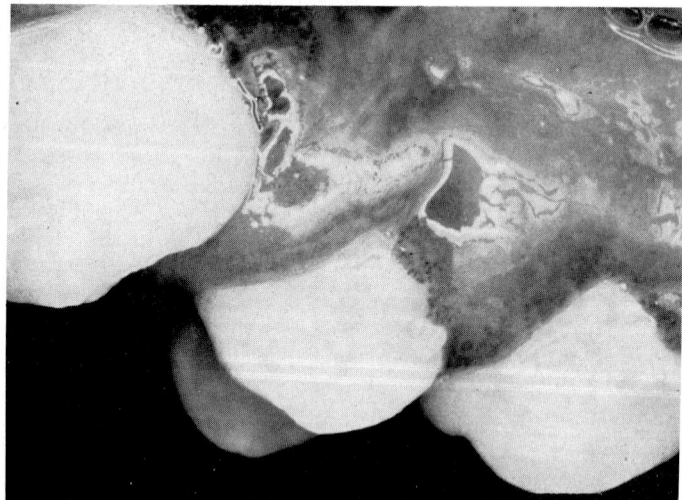

Figure 13–2   Gingivitis around two erupting premolars. Gingivitis is also present about fully erupted teeth in the same mouth and is not associated with tooth eruption. Note the dilated and engorged capillary vessels in the gingival margin.

tooth do not erupt simultaneously. For instance, eighteen months may elapse before all four first permanent molars appear in the mouth, and six to twelve months after that before they come into occlusion.

The process of eruption of teeth through previously uninflamed gingivae produces very little local reaction (Fig. 13–2). The wound produced by the exfoliation of a primary tooth heals in a matter of hours and rarely becomes infected. It is also most unusual for the gingivae to become infected at the site of tooth eruption. When this does happen the gums appear edematous and intensely painful, and may be accompanied by a fever. In thousands of children examined repeatedly by the author few instances of gingivitis due to eruption of the teeth have been observed. The statement by many authors that eruption of the teeth is a common cause of gingivitis in children has not been substantiated. Rarely, a displaced tooth erupts beyond the area of attached mucosa. When this occurs, eruption of the tooth is delayed, and the tissues overlying the submerged cusps are freely movable and may become traumatized and inflamed. Infection rarely happens during eruption of a tooth, and a fever in a child should not lightly be attributed to tooth eruption. The fact that some tooth is likely to be in an active stage of eruption at any time during childhood has been a great convenience to those who wish to give some label to a fever of which they do not know the origin.

THE NATURE OF GINGIVITIS

When the gingival tissue becomes inflamed, hyperemia is first noted. The pale peach-pink color changes to blood-red, owing to the dilatation of capillaries, so the blood content of these tissues is enormously increased. In areas of ulceration where the epithelium is lost, the color is even more vivid. This hyperemia is associated with edema; the gingivae become enlarged and the surface appears shiny, wet, and tense (Fig. 13–3). As the papillae and the free gingival margins are not bound as closely to the alveolar bone as is the adjacent attached mucosa, a disproportionate amount of swelling is possible in these tissues (Fig. 13–4). The papilla is bounded each side by the adjacent teeth, the crest of the alveolar bone beneath, and the contact point of the teeth above, thus swelling can only occur buccally and lingually. The papilla also contains a greater bulk of tissue than the gingival margin, and with edema and inflammation, appears as a cherry-red nodule protruding between the teeth. Swelling of the gingival margin over the bulbous portion of the crown of the tooth not only causes a deepening of the natural crevice into a pocket, but also produces a ledge which inevitably collects debris.

In some areas of inflammation the tissues degenerate to expose the root of the tooth. If this should occur in one discrete area, such as the buccal surface of an incisal tooth, and the area of degeneration is narrow, the edematous papillae approach one another across the front of the tooth and leave a narrow cleft between them. Such a cleft is called a "Stillman's cleft," and passes down to the root surface. The area of degeneration may be wider and almost the full width of the root may be exposed (Fig. 13–5); such a process may extend almost to the apex of the tooth.

Where irritation and inflammation of the attached mucosa are of long standing, an excessive amount of connective tissue may be formed, and the gingivae become rough, fibrous and greatly enlarged.

Fig. 13-3.

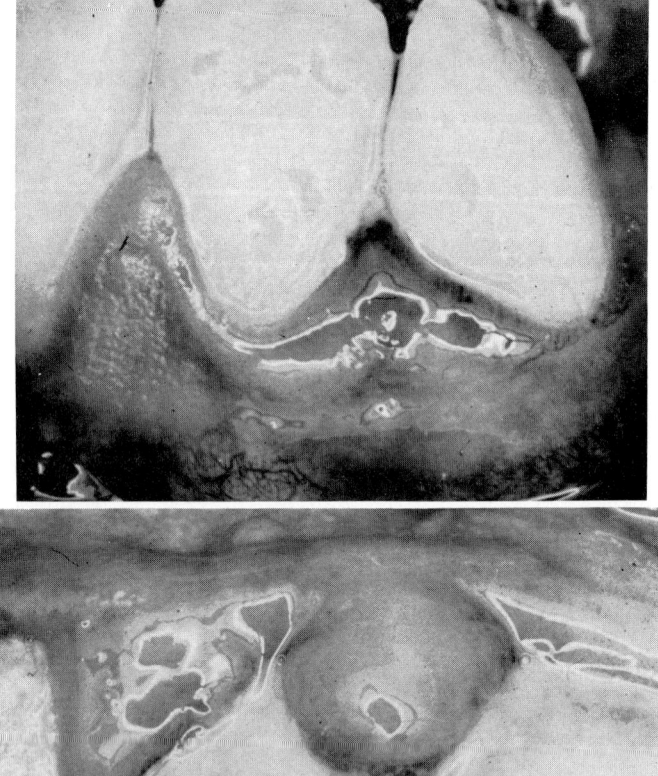

Fig. 13-4.

Figure 13-3 Marginal gingivitis. Note the prominent papilla, accentuated marginal roll and stippling between the central and lateral teeth, the ulceration, intensity of color, and dilated blood vessels at the marginal rim, the collection of debris between the lateral and canine, and replacement of stippling by a shiny, tense, wet surface.

Figure 13-4 Marginal gingivitis demonstrating edema and enlargement of papillae and marginal rim. The papillae appear as cherry red nodules protruding between the teeth. The approaching papillae across the surface of the tooth are one form of Stillman's cleft.

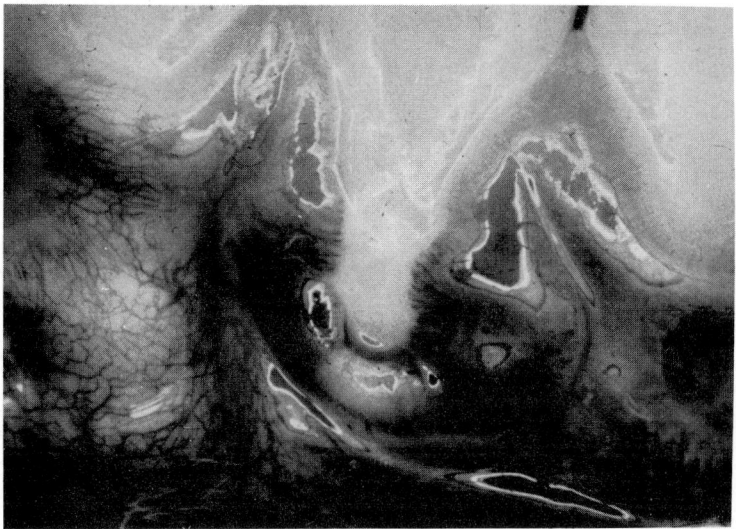

Figure 13–5 Wide- dumbbell-shaped, localized recession due to buccal eruption and displacement of the tooth, and toothbrush trauma of the soft tissues over the prominent root. Note the blood vessels in the oral mucosa, attached mucosa, and marginal rim, and the highly inflamed area.

INDEX OF GINGIVITIS

The prevalence of disease is expressed as the number of individuals in a group suffering from disease, the individual being the unit involved. The incidence of a disease is the number of attacks or sites of attack the individual suffers from the disease. In expressing severity, the intensity of inflammation or extent to which tissues are involved is considered and the units used are arbitrary degrees, such as *very mild, mild, moderate* and *severe*.

Schour and Massler introduced a method of assessing gingivitis by observing the condition of each gingival unit surrounding a tooth and divided each gingival unit into three anatomic parts: the papilla, P; the marginal gingiva, M; and the attached gingiva, A. The index is known as the "PMA index" and consists of a summation of the inflamed areas of the mouth. Schour and Massler attempted a form of severity rating based on the degree of extension of inflammation from the papillae through margin to attached mucosa. A fourth *most severe* grade was added, based on the intensity of inflammation, where gross swelling, ulceration, etc., was present. In the first three grades the intensity of inflammation is only necessary for a diagnosis to be made. Other degrees of severity of inflammation have been described and many indices have been evolved. Some indices also include degeneration of bone or pocket formation. Many indices thereby become complicated. It is felt that each tissue is capable of being involved to a different degree and should be assessed separately.

PREVALENCE, INCIDENCE AND SEVERITY OF GINGIVITIS IN CHILDREN

If a detectable hyperemia is taken as the criterion of gingivitis, the prevalence of gingivitis is found to be below 5 per cent at the age of 3 years, 50 per cent at the age of 6 years, with a peak of 90 per cent at 11 years. Between 11 and 17 years the level falls slightly between 80 and 90 per cent.

Five degrees of severity of gingivitis can be described as follows: *None*, where there is no clinical evidence of inflammation; *very mild*, where there is a detectable hyperemia in papilla, margin or attached mucosa; *mild*, where there is also loss of stippling, redness, swelling or bleeding on pressure; *moderate*, where the severity is such that blood appears on a toothbrush and where sensitivity or tenderness is present (at this level the parent or child is generally aware of the condition); *severe*, where there is severe hyperemia and obvious swelling, when hemorrhage occurs spontaneously or on the slightest touch of food or toothbrush. These categories can be reduced to four by merging the *very mild* and *mild* cases into one group, but subdivision into seven, eight, or ten grades has been found inaccurate, as the clinical grades are not clear cut, and reproducibility is poor.

Severity of gingivitis also increases with age but somewhat differently in the two sexes. In girls severity increases to a peak at 10½ years and falls for the next three or four years, leveling off by the age of 16. In boys the severity peak occurs between the ages of 13 and 13½ years. After this age the severity declines in a pattern similar to that found in girls, taking into consideration the three year age difference. Above the age of 12 years the number of children suffering from gingivitis remains approximately the same, but the severity of gingivitis diminishes considerably until the age of at least 17 years, when it again increases.

In one particular group of boys the severity of gingivitis was as follows:

	AGE 7½	AGE 13½
None	45%	3%
Very mild	41%	42%
Mild	9%	31%
Moderate	5%	10%
Severe	0%	14%

In serial examinations of children it is found that the same individuals for five years and more demonstrate the most severe degrees of gingivitis. It is believed that this condition continues into adult life and that the periodontal disease seen in adults was already present in early life. Treatment of periodontal disease before a great deal of damage has occurred is of great importance and periodontal disease in children should be considered a serious matter.

INVOLVEMENT OF THE DEEPER TISSUES

The presence of pockets of 3 mm. or more in depth has been described by McIntosh in over 70 per cent of children between the ages of 6 and 11 years. Most of these pockets were situated interproximally.

Where hyperplasia of the gingivae is present or where the tooth is not fully erupted, a cleft of over 3 mm. in depth may not necessarily indicate that the attachment to the tooth has receded apically (Fig. 13–6), but where pocket formation due to recession is observed, destruction of periodontal tissues must have taken place.

As the tooth migrates through the bone and erupts into occlusion, the alveolar bone re-forms the socket and the bone grows with the changing tooth position. The

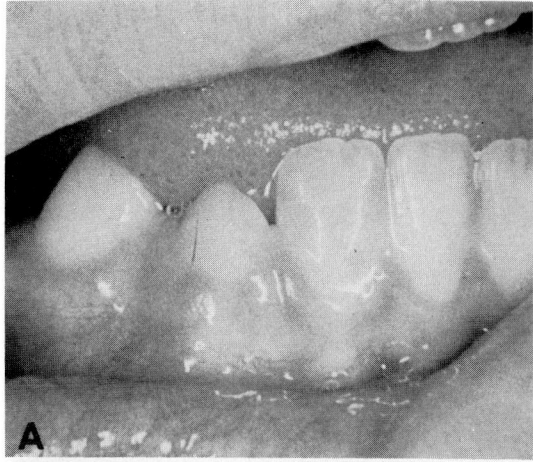

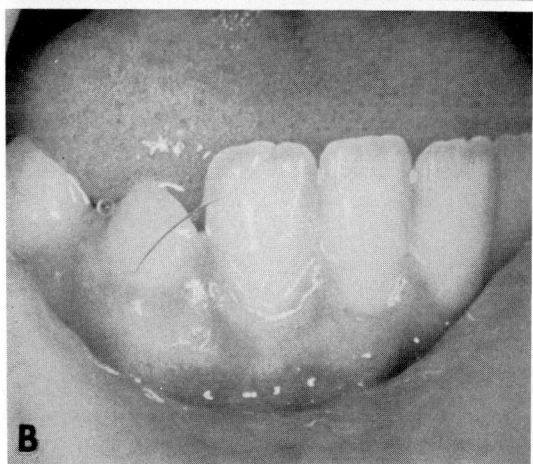

Figure 13–6 *A,* A hair impacted in the gingival crevice of the erupting lower canine. The crevice extends 4 mm. below the gingival margin. No instrumentation has taken place. *B,* The hair removed, demonstrating the depth of the undisturbed gingival crevice of the erupting lower canine. The presence of a high epithelial attachment has not been confirmed.

level of alveolar bone around a newly erupted tooth in occlusion is 1 mm. below the cemento-enamel junction. When the alveolar margin of the bone level recedes apically but remains parallel to the occlusal plane, the process is described as horizontal bone absorption. Vertical bone absorption is the destruction and loss of the bony wall of the socket and consequent enlargement of the socket which is accompanied by an increase in the mobility of the tooth. In this condition the bone loss is parallel to the root of the tooth and is at an angle to the occlusal plane of the teeth. The alveolar margin between two teeth, however, under some physiologic conditions assumes an angle, particularly in erupting teeth or where teeth are tilted. If the teeth are tilted forward, the mesial surface is depressed and the distal surface is elevated above the general level of the alveolar border. Consequently, the bone between the cemento-enamel junction of one tooth and the next makes an angle with the occlusal plane, but this is not indicative of disease.

Alveolar bone grows rapidly throughout childhood, and localized areas of extremely rapid bone absorption and formation accompany the shedding and eruption of teeth. Very little haversian bone is present in the child's jaw, but it appears in increasing amounts in young adults. The bone of the child's jaw, therefore, is highly vascular and is actively growing, which may account for the rapid healing and unusual occurrence of bone absorption due to periodontal infection. At this age there is complete recovery from even severe inflammatory conditions, whereas in older individuals irreversible changes take place early. On rare occasions, however, localized bone absorption occurs in children with loss of support of the teeth, particularly around the first permanent molars. Such cases have been described from the age of eight upwards.

CAUSES OF GINGIVITIS

LOCAL IRRITANTS

Although systemic factors and general health profoundly modify the reaction of the tissues to local irritation, gingivitis at all age groups is primarily caused by local conditions. The gingivae and mucous membrane of the mouth are constantly receiving physical trauma. Mechanical irritation is received during the mastication of food and movement of tongue, lips and cheeks; and from alternate wetting by saliva and drying in air. Chemical irritation occurs from condiments and from the acidity and alkalinity of foods, and bacterial irritation arises from the products manufactured by the high concentration of bacteria in infected masses which collect about the teeth.

Physical Properties of Food

The gingivae are scrubbed and kept free from debris by mastication of food, which brushes past the papilla and margin at every chewing motion. A child's tissues are perfectly adapted to this heavy function by their position, contour, and structure. Heavy fibers bind the gingivae to bone or approximate them to the necks of the teeth, deep rete pegs assure the firm attachment of epithelium to corium, and the epithelium is constantly being replaced by growth and desquamation. However, irritation above that which is tolerated by the tissues often occurs in the child's mouth. Adherence of debris about the teeth is the most common cause (Fig. 13–7). The factors which contribute to it are numerous and include the physical properties of food, the effectiveness of the occlusion of the teeth, the vigor of chewing and the flow of saliva.

The physical nature of food is an important factor. When groups of children are examined, one finds some remarkably clean mouths soon after the end of the meal, whereas in some voluminous plaques and debris remain about their teeth. Such a finding is associated with diet and is often not due to a difference in oral hygiene practice. The preparation of food is of more importance than the nature of food. The type which leaves the most debris about the teeth is a soft, mushy, semiliquid mixture which calls for a minimal amount of chewing. Included in this group are the crisp or even hard refined starchy foods which become an extremely sticky mass in the mouth on admixture with saliva. Such foods are impossible to chew vigorously, but they invite mouthing until softened by saliva or liquid food. Following this, the pasty mass is swallowed, leaving much of it about the teeth, the buccal sulcus or even in a high vaulted palate. Some overfed children, forced by anxious parents to take more than they want, park the unwanted food in the buccal sulcus or the palate.

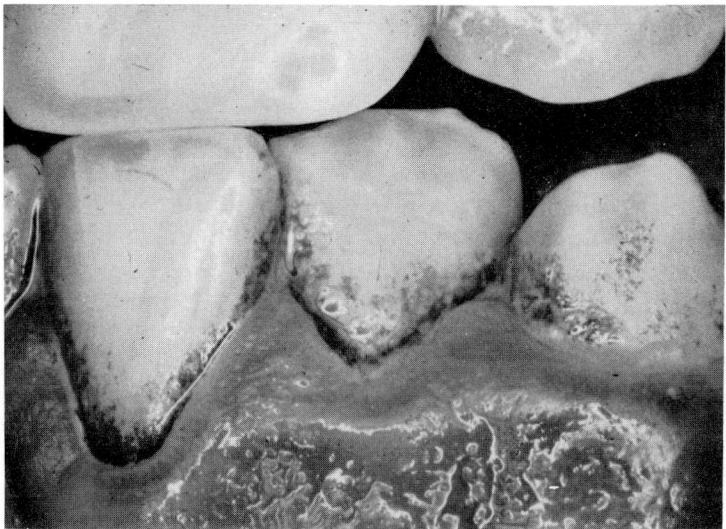

Figure 13–7 Typical pattern made by the collection of debris about the teeth. Debris consists of bacteria, living and dead, desquamated epithelial cells, mucus and other substances from saliva and bacteria, and particles of food immediately after a meal, which soon become liquefied or otherwise altered.

Although in unhygienic mouths, numerous areas of stagnation occur, few become the site of dental caries each year; but in every area where plaque collects adjacent to the gum, the gingivae show some degree of inflammation.

A type of food that cleans the teeth and mouth most effectively is fibrous food which demands chewing, such as unground meat, fish, crisp fresh raw vegetables and fruits. Such foods should not be followed by sticky mixtures.

ORAL HYGIENE

Children seldom wash in play and seldom clean their teeth. Oral hygiene has to be stimulated, supervised, and the end result examined, for it to be effective. It is not easy to clean the teeth. Particularly sticky, adherent bacterial masses in the less accessible areas are difficult to remove. Rough and vigorous scrubbing hurts the gums and the child refuses to continue. Gentle movement of the toothbrush may be ineffective in that it is time consuming, thus trying the child's patience.

The conscientious cleaning of the teeth may not be completely effective in removing all the damaging material. Demonstration of such ineffectiveness may dishearten the child and result in less cooperation and interest. It is difficult for the child to understand what cleaning the teeth is for, as the teeth look clean. The use of disclosing rinses and tablets to stain the debris is helpful in that the adherent material is made visible; thus tooth brushing may be continued until the unsightly stain is removed.

There is no question that a regime of oral hygiene improves gingival health, but supervised oral hygiene has to be carried out for the cleaning to be effective, and such effectiveness only lasts while supervision is maintained. Little improvement in gingival health remains six or even three months after the end of the dental health program, as children revert to previous habits.

A continuous program of oral hygiene is necessary, and this requires enthusiastic care and interest by the dentist, weekly lectures and demonstrations in school, and understanding and trained parents who supervise tooth cleaning daily. The child may not have the manual dexterity required to clean his own teeth, and the patience and effort required on the part of the parents to teach and encourage the child may be more than the parent is able to give. This extra duty may be neglected for the sake of peace in the family and, in effect, may be beyond the intention or capability of the parent to carry out.

Food Impaction

Teeth in good occlusion are self-cleansing, whereas teeth crowded together or tilted become the site of food impaction and plaque formation. Gingivitis is so common about these teeth that malalignment of teeth and the improper gingival contour which this entails may even be considered of more importance than the physical nature of the foods eaten. Spaces between teeth do not become sites of food impaction unless the crest of the papilla is far from the occlusal or cutting surfaces of the teeth and the approximal tooth surfaces are flat and featureless. Both of these conditions are common in adults, but spaced primary teeth are cleansed by the mastication of food, for their interproximal surfaces are bulbous and the crests of the papillae almost reach the occlusal plane.

Interproximal food impaction also depends on the shape of the occlusal surface of the tooth. Where the marginal ridge is present and pronounced and the contact points or bulges of the tooth are high, food does not lodge, and if some fibers or portions of leafy vegetable become impacted between the teeth and remain after the end of the meal, they soon become dislodged. Where, however, the marginal ridge and interproximal surfaces of the teeth have become destroyed and have not been replaced by correctly contoured restorations, or where the marginal ridges of the two adjacent teeth are on different occlusal levels, food becomes increasingly impacted between the teeth until the soft tissues are pushed aside and the alveolar bone is absorbed. Replacement of lost tooth structure and correct contouring of restorations is, therefore, an important periodontal treatment.

The opposing cusp of a tooth in an area of food impaction is often blamed for the condition. The cusps which should articulate with the fossae inside the marginal ridge, and with the marginal ridge itself in protrusive and lateral movements, are now unopposed, and food impacts between the teeth that have become multilated. These unopposed cusps are often called "plunger cusps" and are savagely removed with little effect. The correct procedure is to restore the opposing ridges and contact points, as well as to reshape the opposing occlusal surfaces. When such a cusp is removed no amount of restoration can restore function, and however carefully the marginal ridges and contact points of the teeth are shaped, if they are not opposed by an occluding tooth and not restored to function, food impaction will occur.

Trauma to the Soft Tissues

In addition to the localized areas of degeneration of both soft and hard tissues between two adjacent teeth due to the trauma of food impaction, localized areas of recession occur on the buccal and lingual surfaces of the teeth. This type of

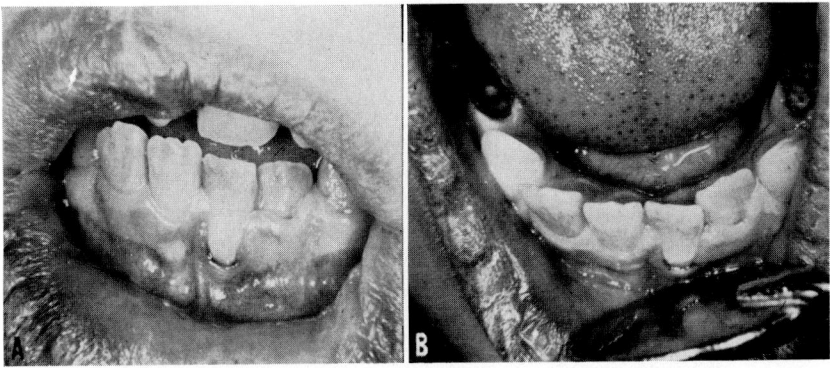

Figure 13–8 *A,* Localized recession on the lower left incisor. Tooth is not in traumatic occlusion. Note the levels and conditions of the gingival margins of all four incisors. *B,* Localized recession on the lower left incisor. Note that the tooth is rotated and buccally displaced.

degeneration is particularly common on the buccal surfaces of the lower incisors and may extend to the apex of the tooth.

This condition has been attributed to traumatic occlusion, but in most cases the involved tooth does not show signs of trauma, and some do not even come into functional occlusion. Most of these teeth erupt outside the dental arch (Fig. 13–8), and the sequence of events is (a) eruption of the tooth buccally (or lingually), in which case both the alveolar bone and gingivae over the erupting tooth root are thin or stand at a more apical level than adjacent teeth in the arch; (b) frictional trauma of lips, cheeks, tongue, food, and toothbrush against the soft tissues stretched thin over the outstanding root, causing degeneration and apical recession; (c) collection of debris and calculus at the lowered gingival margin, which recedes progressively farther from the coronal area cleansed by the turmoil of mastication; (d) involvement of a frenum attachment causing a sudden increase in the detachment of tissues (Figs. 13–9 and 13–10).

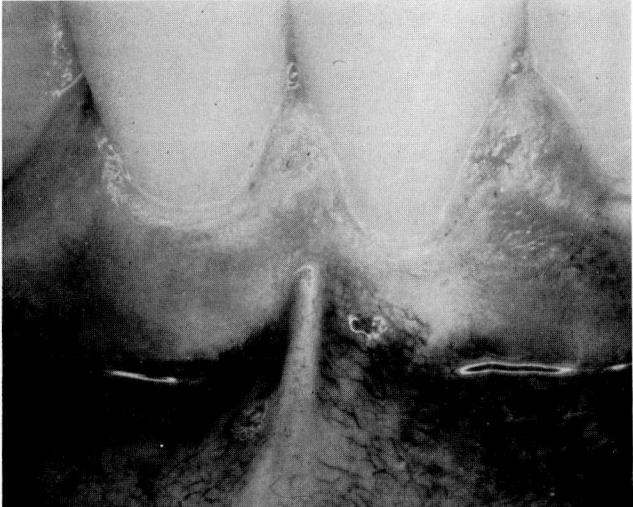

Figure 13–9 Normal frenum attachment below attached gingiva. Note normal width of attached gingiva on right lower incisor and recession and narrow attached gingiva on left incisor.

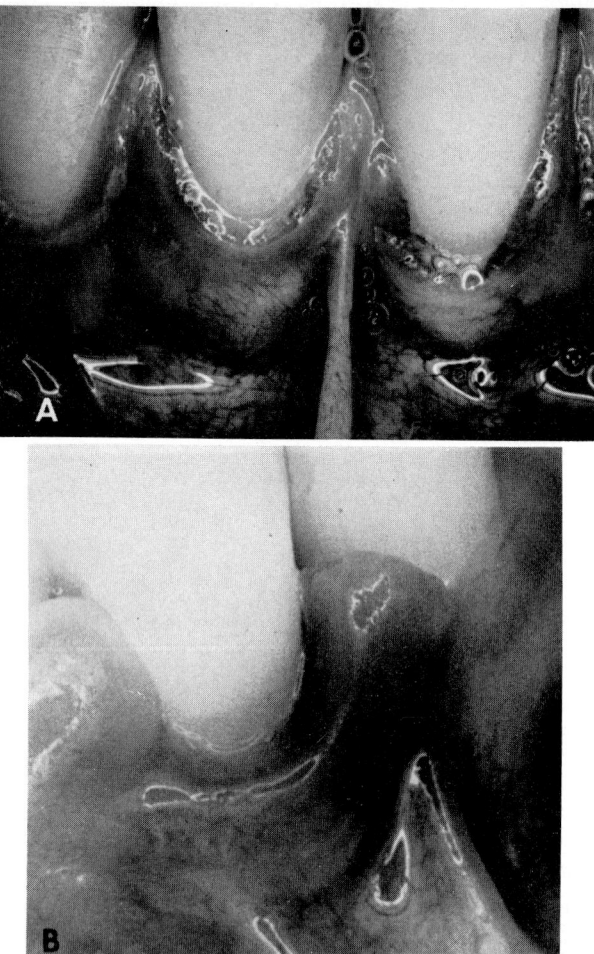

Figure 13–10 *A,* Gingival inflammation, and recession approaching the attachment of the lower labial frenum. Note that the level of the gingival margin on the left central incisor is below the level of the frenum attachment. *B,* Gingival recession involving attachment of lower labial frenum. Note that the papilla is dislodged from its position between the teeth by tension on the frenum.

Trauma caused by improper use of the toothbrush may be found on correctly aligned teeth. Lateral scrubbing causes contusion of the exposed surfaces of the interdental papillae and a wide dumbbell-shaped recession of tissues over the root (Fig. 13–5); vertical scrubbing causes painful narrow clefts which cut the gingival margin to the root of the tooth.

The Effective Occlusion of the Teeth

Vigorous chewing of food is impossible if the teeth do not come into effective occlusion, and correction of tilted and malaligned teeth by orthodontic means is followed by a marked improvement in the gingival condition. The ideal situation is, therefore, one in which the gingivae come close to the occlusal surface of the teeth, in good functional occlusion in a child who vigorously chews the correct type of food.

Children with open bites, edge to edge occlusion, or considerable protrusion of the upper teeth, in fact, any discrepancy of the upper and lower arches, will be found to have debris about the teeth and some form of gingivitis. A factor contributing to the collection of material on the buccal surfaces of upper incisor teeth is the immobility of a short upper lip, particularly where the upper teeth protrude.

The vigor with which a child chews his food also affects cleanliness of the mouth. One child will suck food and swallow it with as little expenditure of energy as possible, whereas another will chew food for an excessive period of time, and between meals will work tongue, lips and cheeks continually.

Mouth Breathing

While actual breathing through the mouth and not through the nose is uncommon except during periods of nasal catarrh, many children are labeled as mouth breathers because they hold their lips apart for long periods of time, apparently closing their mouths only to swallow (Fig. 13–11). In some children protrusion of the upper teeth makes closure of the lips impossible. In others no obvious obstruction is present, and no obvious reason for holding the lips apart is apparent, but it may be the result of habit, posture, inadequate tissue or poor muscle tonus. Children will often hold their mouths open while watching something intently, but few actually breathe through the mouth. The gingivae, however, become air-dried, and the constant wetting and drying constitutes an irritation to the gingival tissues.

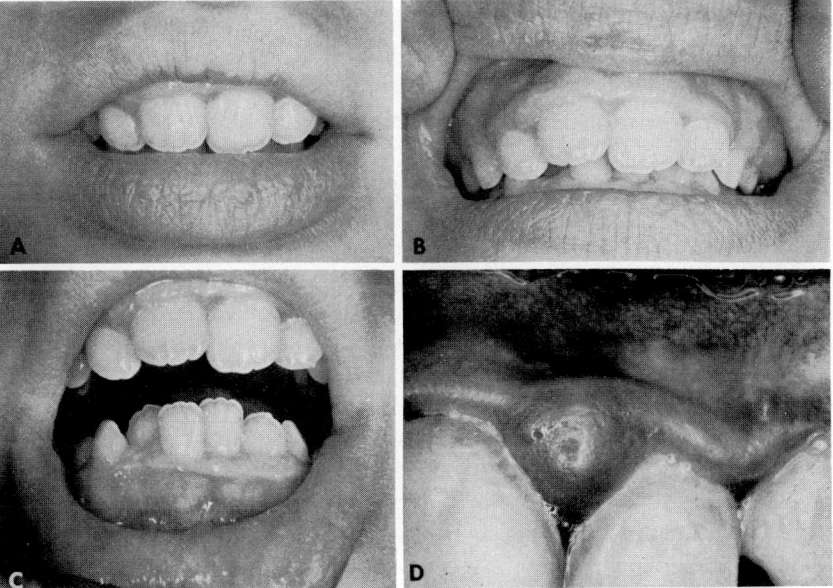

Figure 13–11   *A,* Child with lips apart habit. Patient is not a mouth breather but breathes normally through the nose. *B,* Upper lip elevated to show gingival enlargement in exposed areas between the continuously parted lips. *C,* Lower lip retracted to show the gingival enlargement associated with continuous exposure of the gingiva to air drying. Note that although the mouth is open and the lower lip retracted, the upper gingivae are still exposed. *D,* Close-up of gingival enlargement involving margin and papilla.

Saliva about the exposed gingivae becomes viscous, debris collects on the gingivae as well as on the surfaces of the teeth, and the bacterial population becomes enormously increased. In true mouth breathers the tongue and palate are air-dried in addition, whereas in the children who only hold their lips apart the palate remains normally wet, and no gingivitis is present on the lingual and palatal aspects of the teeth but is localized on the buccal aspect of the exposed teeth.

Treatment for true mouth breathers is to remove the cause of nasal obstruction, but the pseudo-mouth breathers, who also often sleep with their mouths open, can be assisted by an oral screen worn at night. These are extremely comfortable and efficient appliances, and are not only well tolerated but replace the comfort obtained by sucking blankets, thumbs, and toys. (See Chapter 17.)

Irritation Caused by Bacterial Activity

The mouth swarms with bacteria living a precarious existence on the surface of the tongue, mucous membranes, and teeth. They are extremely adherent to the tooth surfaces but are continually being washed away and swallowed during the mastication of food and flow of saliva, assisted by the movement of the lips, cheeks and tongue. But with each replenishment of food about the teeth at the end of a meal, another source of food is available to the remaining bacteria, which multiply accordingly. Carbohydrate food debris is fermented by the appropriate bacteria, which are always present in the mouth. Numerous types and strains of bacteria are present, all capable of utilizing some stage of carbohydrate fermentation in their metabolism. Starches are broken down by the enzymes of bacterial digestion, through sugars to the final acid waste product. Similarly, proteins are putrefied and fats are denatured, stage by stage, by these bacterial scavengers which render solid food particles to liquids which become diluted and eliminated from the mouth. These organisms, therefore, perform a valuable hygienic function in ridding the teeth of particles of food. Teeth and tissues are remarkably resistant to these bacterial products, but where excess acid is formed on the tooth surface the tooth suffers, and where massive accumulations are present about the tissues with the production of adhesive dextran-like materials, the constant presence of bacterial products and by-products causes an inflammation. Bacteria capable of digesting any type of food which may lodge about the teeth are always present in the mouth, and digestion of debris upon the tissue surface is only one step removed from the digestion of debilitated and damaged gingival tissue itself. Bacteria capable of producing collagenase, hyaluronidase, and other protein-destructive enzymes can be isolated from healthy gingivae and particularly so from ulcerated and diseased areas. Their presence in diseased tissues may well indicate that these organisms are taking part in the destructive processes, but it does not necessarily mean that such organisms are the primary cause of the disease or that the gingivitis in the particular instance in which they were recorded is an infective or a contagious condition. However, debris from about the teeth is highly irritating to the tissues. Redness and swelling occurs at the site of an injection in experimental animals even after the organisms have been destroyed by heat, and inflammation of the mucous membrane of the inner surface of the lips or cheeks opposite an area of gingivitis is commonly seen. In addition, on removal of the debris from the tooth surface both the acute gingivitis in the immediate area and the inflammation of the opponent cheek subside within hours.

Where tissues have become damaged by agents other than bacteria, such as trauma to gum tissue, herpetic ulcerations or drugs, or where tissues are debilitated by severe general disease, an infection by the common mouth organisms may ensue and a more or less severe necrosis of tissues may occur. In such areas of localized necrosis one or another form of fusiform bacillus and spirochetes abound, and these organisms can be demonstrated deep in the tissues even among the bone trabeculae. In addition, cocci and vibrios are easily identified, and recently other organisms have been described. Each bacterium recognized has in turn been named as the cause of such conditions; but most, if not all, of these organisms are present in the healthy mouth, although not in such concentrations.

Among the innumerable organisms in the mouth are opportunists which attack debilitated tissues, and by their attack cause further destruction and inflammation. Acute ulcerative stomatitis is most unusual in children; when it occurs, an underlying herpetic stomatitis should be suspected. Where no local factor is obvious, serious blood dyscrasias or serious general disease should be considered.

The usual type of gingivitis encountered is a marginal gingivitis. Temporary removal of bacteria by antibiotics or bactericidal substances may relieve the immediate inflammatory condition, but it is of little more than academic interest, for improvement is temporary and the drug may directly or indirectly cause irritation to the child's tissues. Local treatment consists of an efficient oral hygiene regime and permanent elimination of debris retention areas by orthodontic or other means, so that the bacterial population decreases to a level that can be tolerated by the tissues. Children exhibiting gingivitis due to some general debility should immediately be referred to a physician for treatment.

Stains on the Teeth

The collection of debris on the tooth surfaces, particularly at the gingival margin, consists of bacteria and epithelial cells. It is usually a dirty white color and is called materia alba. In some areas it may be voluminous, but in others it is so slight that it might pass unnoticed unless stained by a disclosing dye of some contrasting color. This material may become stained in the mouth and present one of several distinct colors — green, brown, yellow, orange, or black. Leung found that 80 per cent of children living in institutions had some degree of staining on their teeth; in many of them more than one color was present. The author also found a high incidence of stains on the teeth in institutionalized children, but few cases were found in 15,000 Caucasian, Negro, and North American Indian school children.

Green stain is most common. It occurs mainly on the labial surface of the incisors and canines in both the upper and lower jaws and is more common in boys than in girls. Few cases indeed are reported in adults, but the reason for its occurrence in children is unknown. The color varies from dark olive green to bright green. The stain is not voluminous. It is relatively difficult to remove, and in many instances decalcification of the tooth surface is found immediately beneath the stain.

The second most common stain is brown. In contrast to the green stain, it occurs on the posterior teeth and can be removed with scalers but not readily with the toothbrush. Although it may cover much of the tooth surface, it often presents as a narrow continuous line or a series of dots. This line follows the contour of the gingival margin but is separated from it by an unstained band of tooth surface 1 to 2 mm. wide. This stained line has been called the "mesenteric line," and both Pickerill and Shourie found it to be associated with a lowered caries incidence. However, other surveys find no such correlation, and in many instances the stain occurs on teeth when active caries is present.

Black, yellow, and orange stains are uncommon. Leung found each of these was present between 2 and 5 per cent of his group of children, but in school children the incidence is nearer 0.1 per cent. Yellow and orange stained material is more voluminous than the other stains and is readily removed. In one remote Indian village three school children had brilliant orange-red material, but it was limited to one or two teeth. No particular food was found to be responsible. Stains originating from food color all the teeth, and every child taking this food is affected to some degree.

All these stains are probably of bacterial origin, but although many organisms produce stains of varying color, none are definitely associated with a particular color of stain. All stains are unsightly, and all stained material is believed to be potentially irritating to the gingival margin or damaging to the tooth surface. Stains should be removed and the tooth surface polished. Bleaching the stained material and leaving it in situ is indefensible.

Calculus

Calculus is responsible for a great deal of the gingivitis and deeper periodontitis seen in the adult, a fact which can readily be demonstrated by the subsidence of inflammation upon the removal of the offending deposit. However, even in the adult the deposit of calculus is not the primary cause of periodontal disease, but is a subsidiary process. In children calculus formation is more common than generally realized. It may be seen covering the entire crowns of the teeth where dental caries has made mastication of food too painful to be carried out on one side of the mouth. Debris collects over the crowns of the unused teeth and becomes calcified. In approximately 5 per cent of children between the ages of 10 and 12, calculus forms on the lingual surface of the lower incisors and on the buccal surface of the upper molars. This is the same pattern that occurs in adults, but the deposit is seldom so heavy. Gingivitis is present in these areas, but the commonest site of gingivitis in a child is not the same as in an adult; instead, it is on the upper labial segment, an area which is least liable to form calculus. Gingivitis in a child is not usually caused by calculus; and gingivitis may be present for many years in a child before any sign of supra- or subgingival calculus occurs. Moreover, the most inflamed area within the child's mouth is often not the site of calculus formation. The role of calculus as the primary cause of gingivitis must, therefore, be questioned, but its effect on the continuance of inflammation is common knowledge. In localized areas of recession, calculus is commonly observed in children. In such areas the gingiva has receded far from the cleansing areas of mastication, and debris collects in the cleft or pouch formed and becomes calcified. This produces a secondary source of irritation, for not only is the highly infected mass of calculus an immovable harbor of harmful bacteria emanating toxins, but its rough, pumice-like surface causes physical irritation.

Traumatic Forces on the Teeth

Acute occlusal trauma produced by a high restoration or a tilting tooth is not unusual in children; but the condition tends to correct itself rapidly, so that the symptoms of chronic occlusal trauma seen in adults are unusual in children. The bone supporting the teeth is continually being re-formed by the growth of the alveolus, which grows nearly 1 cm. in height between the ages of 4 and 12 years. Forces applied to the teeth during this formative period produce movement of the teeth by suppression or slight deflection of growth. Also, the degree of instantaneous movement of the tooth in its socket with the forces of mastication during the eruptive and formative stages of development is much greater than in the completely formed and occluding teeth of an adult. This is true in both the axial and lateral directions. This may be a further reason why trauma from occlusion is rarely seen in the child. In some instances during formation the normal movement is so great that it is visible. If the parent should notice it, he may be reassured of the normality of the condition. Even depression of a tooth below the occlusal plane of other growing teeth can easily be brought about by retarded growth. In adults, bone destruction must precede movement of a tooth, but in the child movement of a tooth may be merely a deflection of growth. This fact is extensively utilized in orthodontic practice.

GENERAL FACTORS

Tissue response to bacterial, chemical or physical irritants is profoundly altered by systemic conditions. Tissue cells rely on a constant supply of materials for their metabolism. These include hormones, vitamins and minerals, as well as nutrients and oxygen. An alteration in the level of any of these substances may be the cause of severe local disturbance. Local irritations which are tolerated or which produce only a mild reaction under normal circumstances , may give rise to severe inflammation and destruction if the cells are denied the materials they require for repair. Normal healthy tissues have ample reserves, so that heavy function and local damage produce an unnoticeable reaction, but where deficiencies are present even light functional stresses may cause considerable local reaction followed by degenerative changes.

High Fever

During a period of high fever, because of a general disturbance such as one of the exanthematous fevers, a gingivitis frequently occurs. The sick child does not make the normal cleansing mouth movements and does not take the usual food but lies listlessly taking semiliquids. In this condition the saliva is scanty and debris consisting of a mixture of food and saliva accumulates in the mouth. The bacterial flora becomes enormously increased and a gingivitis follows.

Alterations in Hormone Levels

During major changes in the hormone levels, the gingivae together with other mucous membranes are observed to undergo a change. A desquamative gingivitis is associated with the menopause, and a hyperplasia with pregnancy. Changes in the level of the sex hormones during puberty may affect the gingivae. It is suggestive that the peak incidence of gingivitis is two to three years earlier in girls than in boys, and that the peaks occur at approximately the age of puberty; an improvement in gingival health follows this stage. Local factors have been suggested as the cause of this difference of gingivitis between the sexes, such as the difference in the time of tooth eruption. But the teeth erupt four years before the peak incidences of gingivitis occur in the incisal region; moreover, the difference in the time of eruption between boys and girls is only six months. The greater interest in hygienic habits among girls has also been claimed as the reason why girls have a lower incidence of gingivitis at the age of 14 and above, but the girls have passed their peak incidence of gingivitis at this age by three and a half years, whereas the boys are experiencing their peak or have just passed it. The same argument must explain why girls have a greater incidence of gingivitis before the age at which the boys experience their peak period.

Another possible sex difference after the age of puberty is that fibrous hyperplasia in the incisal region is more common in boys than in girls, whereas a marginal gingivitis characterized by hyperemia and thinning of the epithelium and hemorrhage is more common in girls.

Vitamin Deficiencies

When experimental animals are deprived of any one of the vitamins, severe generalized symptoms are observed. They lose weight, become extremely debilitated, suffer from severe gastrointestinal disturbances, and before death display varying degrees of gingivitis. But because experimental animals that are dying from a vitamin deficiency suffer a gingivitis, it does not mean that 90 per cent of the normal healthy children in this country who present some degree of gingivitis also have an insufficient vitamin intake.

Of all the vitamins, vitamin C (ascorbic acid) is the one most likely to affect the periodontal tissues, for it is essential in the production of connective tissue fibers. Experimental deficiency causes a decrease in the fiber content of periodontal tissues, owing to inhibition of the normal replacement. In scurvy the gingivae become detached, hemorrhages occur in the tissues and the disease is often accompanied by acute inflammation. Deficiency of vitamin C alone, however, does not produce a gingivitis; local irritation is also necessary to initiate the inflammatory reaction. A plentiful supply of vitamin C is available in present day food stores, and if a child is given a normal balanced diet, no extra supplement should be necessary. However, some children, either by their own choice or because of family food habits, are denied vitamin C, for they do not eat the foods which contain it. Thus, amidst plenty, true cases of vitamin C deficiency can be found. To produce symptoms of gingivitis in healthy individuals an acute deficiency of vitamin C is required, and many other symptoms also appear. Children suffering from a vitamin deficiency because of an inadequate diet probably are also suffering from a deficiency of many other substances, and treatment with one of the refined vitamin preparations alone is unlikely to cure the complaint.

The usual case of gingivitis seen in everyday practice is not likely to be due to a vitamin deficiency, but in some cases massive doses of vitamin C, vitamin A or vitamin B will produce temporary improvement. Such therapy has a place in the treatment of periodontal disease, but it cannot replace the main treatment or eliminate the main cause of gingivitis which is of local origin. An unbalanced diet should be corrected; anemias and other general disturbances must be diagnosed and treated; but in addition, local treatment must be even more thorough in a debilitated patient than is necessary in a normal, healthy individual.

Vitamin B therapy is a useful adjunct in the treatment of hormonal imbalance. All the vitamin B complex should be administered, for if an excessive dose of only one member of the complex is given, a deficiency of another member of the complex may be produced. Ziskin demonstrated that artificially induced pregnancy-type tumors in animals could be aborted by administration of vitamin B at the same time that the hormones were given, and clinically dramatic improvements can sometimes be obtained. The type which is most amenable to this treatment is the proliferative hyperemic gingivitis with a tendency to bleed, which is found in girls between the ages of 12 and 20 years. Such vitamin therapy should not be prolonged but should be given over a period of not more than four weeks, and the patient must be carefully observed for any reaction to the excessive doses.

In acute generalized gingivitis, vitamin A therapy has been accompanied by dramatic improvement but the success of such empirical treatment does not demonstrate that the individual is suffering from a gingivitis due to a lack of one or another of the vitamins.

Drugs

With the present level of education, the prolonged administration of drugs to children is less common, and acute poisoning from such substances as teething powders has almost disappeared. However, Dilantin sodium is given for epilepsy over a prolonged period and may produce a gingival hyperplasia in 50 per cent of the persons using it. In some cases the gingivae become enlarged to such an extent that the entire crowns of the teeth become covered with a bulky, fibrous mass. A gingivitis due to excessive plaque formation is commonly superimposed. Such cases are rare in private practice, but every clinic has examples of this condition. Gingivectomy may be necessary where the tissues are tough, bulky and fibrous, but where the tissues are somewhat hyperemic, removal of the excess tissue can be carried out by simple packs or by chemical cauterization such as with potassium hydroxide. If strict oral hygiene is carried out, recurrence is not inevitable. Where possible, the cooperation of the physician should be sought and an alternative drug used.

Oral Manifestations of Specific Diseases

A sick child is more liable to gingivitis, for the factors which contribute to the normal hygiene of the mouth are in abeyance. The movements of the lips and tongue are less active, the less detergent foods are chosen, the saliva is scanty and mouth breathing may take place. Such gingivitis is common to all sickness, but in addition some diseases have particular oral manifestations associated with them.

The diseases with characteristic oral symptoms commonly met with in childhood are measles, scarlet fever, herpes, and occasionally chickenpox. In the exanthematous fevers the oral mucosa or skin may show characteristic eruptions, in which case the diagnosis is easy. Herpes, however, may occur without vesicle formation and appear as an acute painful gingivitis, the diagnosis of which can only be tentative until vesicles appear. The treatment is to cleanse the debris from about the teeth with hydrogen peroxide or sodium bicarbonate mouth washes, followed by careful oral hygiene. Antibiotics and bactericidal agents are not indicated, but in the more severe cases topical anesthesia may be resorted to before meals to allow eating.

Skin eruption due to drugs and allergies may also be encountered, and many rarer conditions have specific oral symptoms.

General Principles of Treatment of Periodontal Conditions in Children

The vast majority of cases of gingival inflammation are caused by the collection of highly infected debris on the surface of the tooth in the ledge formed by the gingival margin. All the factors which contribute to collection of material on the tooth surface must be reduced or eliminated. The commonest causes are malalignment of teeth, malocclusion, open mouth position, dental caries and poor oral hygiene. When a frenum is involved in gingival recession, the frenum should be removed. When the gingival contour, because of malalignment of teeth, hypertrophy of the gingival tissues, or deep pocket formation, is such that debris collects at the gingival margin, surgical intervention may be necessary and gingivectomy or one of its associated operations should be performed. In severe cases, where reaction to treatment is poor, or in any case of doubt, systemic factors should be suspected and the general medical condition investigated promptly. In these cases local therapy should not be neglected because systemic treatment is being given, but should be even more scrupulously carried out — not vigorously, but effectively, gently and persistently.

On occasion children have difficulty using a toothbrush. The procedure is often omitted when parents are not around, or is so perfunctory that debris remains. Patience and understanding are required to teach the child how to brush the teeth, and the shape, size, and stiffness of the brush may be modified to suit the particular child's needs. When gingivitis is present a soft bristle brush should be used. The two methods preeminently suitable for children with gingivitis, particularly if soreness is present, are Dr. Bass's method, which is a tapping motion with a very soft brush against the teeth and gingivae similar to the movement used in brush stenciling, and the reciprocating automatic toothbrush (to and fro motion) used with a soft brush.

Alternative methods of oral hygiene should also be considered, such as the hardwood point. This should be used in a sweeping motion, the same movement used to manicure the nail cuticle. This method is particularly useful for the removal of debris from the gingival crevice. It is more efficient than the toothbrush for cleaning this area and does no damage to the gingival margin. Where the gingival margins are irregular, such as in an area of localized recession, this method is ideal. A holder can be obtained for prophylactic wood points which enables cleaning of the lingual, palatal, and distal surfaces of the teeth. The soft wood point, useful in older patients for cleaning between the teeth, is of little value in the child's mouth.

In the child there is a narrow interproximal space inaccessible to the bristles of the toothbrush. For these areas dental floss may be used, but the procedure is often painful, too difficult for the child to perform, and inefficient. Many children, however, are able to pull a rubber band between the teeth. This procedure removes debris from the interproximal areas efficiently, as the stretched rubber band adapts to the shape of the interproximal space and causes no damage to the gingival tissues. Wool thread is the most efficient method for cleaning interproximal areas. The only drawback to its use is that some wool fibers often remain between the teeth and have to be removed with silk floss. A hard rubber point inserted in the handle of the toothbrush or in a separate holder can also be manipulated by a child and is most helpful in cleaning between the teeth and in cleaning the tooth at the level of the gingival margin.

* * * * *

Periodontal disease is usually the result of a long-standing inflammation, rather than the result of an acute disorder. It is associated with the formation of calculus, which is almost universally present in the mouths of individuals over the age of 30. For these reasons periodontal disease is generally considered to be a disease of middle age, but the onset of periodontal disease occurs in childhood, and only the dramatic end results are seen in later life.

When gross loss of the periodontal tissue has taken place as a result of long-standing disease, treatment is unlikely to cure the condition. The time to give treatment is before irreversible destruction has taken place. When it is realized that 90 per cent of children have some degree of gingivitis before the age of 12, it is obvious that periodontal disease in children deserves the greatest attention.

REFERENCES

1. Akhter, H.: The incidence of periodontal diseases in the Punjab. Pakistan D. Rev., 5:109–110, 1955. D. Abs., 1:3, 134–135, 1956.
2. Alldritt, W. A. S.: Some consideration of the aetiology and treatment of gingivitis with particular reference to children. Dental Health, 5:65–70, 1966.
3. Armenio, G., Branzi, A., and Zerosi, C.: Periodontal (parodontal) diseases: Aetiology and pathology. Internat. D. J., 7:2, 284–315, 1957.
4. Baden, T. E.: Gingivitis in Negro school children. N.Y. J. Den., 36:46–48, 1966.
5. Baer, P. N.: Periodontal disease in children and adolescents: A clinical study. J.A.D.A., 55:5, 629–634, 1957.
6. Benjamin, E. M., Russell, A. L., and Smiley, R. D.: Periodontal disease in rural children of 25 Indiana counties. J. Periodont., 28:4, 294–298, 1957.
7. Binstock, M. L., Lindahl, R. L., Noonan, M. A., Sydow, P. F., Williams, H. T., and Cody, W. E.: Diseases of the oral soft and supporting tissues of children (Review of literature by study group presented to Am. Acad. Pedodont.). J. Dent. Child., 25:3, 169–176, 1958.
8. Bratthal, D., Koch, G. M., and Tynelius, G. M.: Comparison of 3 methods of teaching oral hygiene to school children. J. Dent. Educ., 34:98–104, 1970.
9. Brauer, John C.: Periodontic problems in the child patient. J. Periodont., 11:1, 7–13, 1940.
10. Brucker, Marcu: Gingivitis and Vincent's infection in children. J. Dent. Child. 23:2, 116–134, 1956.
11. Butler, J. H.: The familial pattern of juvenile periodontitis. (Periodontosis). J. Periodont., 40: 114–117, 1969.
12. Cohen, M. M.: Periodontal disturbances in childhood. D. Radiog. & Photog., 30:3, 41–45, 1957.
13. Cohen, M. M., and Green, L. B.: Brookline, Massachusetts, pre-school dental survey. J. D. Res., 33:5, 654–655, 1954.
14. Edlan, A.: The prevention of inflammatory damage to the periodontium in children. Int. Dent. J., 17:329–338, 1967.
15. Greene, J. C.: Periodontal disease in India: Report of an epidemiological study. J. D. Res., 39:2, 302–312, 1960.
16. James, P. M. C.: The prevalence of gingivitis in schoolchildren. Dental Health, 5:71–75, 1966.
17. Jasper, E. A.: Periodontal therapy in a general practice. J.A.D.A., 58:4, 41–49, 1959.
18. Jimenez, M. L., Ramos, J., Garrington, G., and Baer, P. N.: The familial occurrence of acute necrotizing gingivitis in children in Colombia, South America. J. Periodont., 40:414–416, 1969.
19. Kelsten, L. B.: Periodontal and soft tissue diseases in children. J. D. Med., 10:2, 67–76, 1955.
20. King, J. D.: Gingival disease in Dundee. D. Record, 65:1, 9–16, 1945.
21. King, J. D., Francklyn, A. B., and Allen, I.: Gingival disease in Gibraltar evacuee children. Lancet, 1:16, 495–498, 1944.
22. Koch, G., and Lindhe, J.: The effect of supervised oral hygiene on the gingiva of children. J. Periodont. Res., 2:64–69, 1967.

23. Leung, S. W.: Naturally occurring stains on the teeth of children. J.A.D.A., *41*:191–197, 1950.

24. Lindhe, J., and Koch, G.: The effect of supervised oral hygiene on the gingiva of children. J. Periodont. Res., *2*:215–220, 1967.

25. Lindhe, J., and Koch, G.: The effect of supervised oral hygiene on the gingiva of children. Progression and inhibition of gingivitis. J. Periodont. Res., *1*:260–267, 1966.

26. Lindhe, J., Koch, G., and Mansson, U.: The effect of supervised oral hygiene on the gingiva of children. Effect of mouth rinsings. J. Periodont. Res. *1*:268–275, 1966.

27. Love, W. C.: An assessment of the knowledge and the practice of oral health by selected school children in Kalamazoo, Michigan. J. Pub. Health, *28*:153–166, 1968.

28. McIntosh, W. G.: Gingival and periodontal diseases of children. J. Periodont., *25*:2, 99–104, 1954.

29. Marshall-Day, C. D., Stephens, R. G., and Quigley, L. R., Jr.: Periodontal disease: Prevalence and incidence. J. Periodont., *26*:3, 185–203, 1955.

30. Marthaler, T. M., and Schroeder, H. E.: DMF-experience in children with and without supra-gingival calculus on lower front teeth. Helv. Odont. Acta, *10*:120–130, 1966.

31. Massler, M.: Co-report: Periodontal disease in children. Internat. D. J., *8*:2, 323–326, 1958.

32. Massler, M., and Schour, I.: P-M-A index of gingivitis. J. D. Res., *28*:6, 634, 1949.

33. Mehta, F. S., Sanjana, M. K., Scroff, B. C., and Doctor, R. H.: Prevalence of periodontal (parodontal) disease. 5. Epidemiology in Indian child population in relation to the socio-economic status. Internat. D. J., *6*:1, 31–40, 1956.

34. Murray, J. J.: Gingivitis in 15-year-old children from high-fluoride and low-fluoride areas. Arch. Oral. Biol., *14*:951–959, 1969.

35. Nord, C. E., Frostell, G., and Söder, P. O: A comparison between proteolytic enzymes in dental plaque material from children and adults. Sven. Tandlak. Tidskr., *62*:3–6, 1969.

36. Nord, C. E. and Söder, P. O: Proteolytic activity of dental plaque material from children with healthy and diseased gingiva. Sven. Tandlak. Tidskr., *61*:587–593, 1968.

37. Parfitt, G. J.: Cleansing the subgingival space. J. Periodont., *34*:133–139, 1963.

38. Parfitt, G. J., and Mjör, I. A.: A clinical evaluation of the local gingival recession in children. J. Dent. Child., *31*:3, 257–262, 1964.

39. Pickerill, H. P.: The Prevention of Dental Caries and Oral Sepsis. New York, Paul B. Hoeber, 1924, p. 263.

40. Pindborg, J. J., Bhat, M., Devanath, K. R., Narayana, H. R., and Ramachandra, S.: Occurrence of acute necrotizing gingivitis in South Indian children. J. Periodont., *37*:14–19, 1966.

41. Pindborg, J. J., Bhat, M., and Roed-Petersen, B.: Oral changes in South Indian children with severe protein deficiency. J. Periodont., *38*:218–221, 1967.

42. Powell, R. N., and Alexander, A. G.: The treatment of periodontal disease. 12. Periodontal disease in childhood. Brit. Dent. J., *120*:351–353, 1966.

43. Sanjana, M. K., Mehta, F. S., Doctor, R. H., and Shroff, B. C.: D.M.F. in permanent teeth and generalized periodontal disease amongst Indian male children and their correlation. J. All India D. A., *29*:9, 183–189, 1957.

44. Sanjana, M. K., Mehta, F. S., Doctor, R. H., and Shroff, B. C.: A follow-up study of the gingival aspects of periodontal disease and the local factors involved in its aetiology amongst a group of school children in India. J. All India D. A., *31*:4, 55–62, 1959.

45. Schour, I., and Massler, M.: Gingival disease in postwar Italy (1945): I. Prevalence of gingivitis in various age groups. J.A.D.A., *35*:7, 475–482, 1947.

46. Sheiman, A.: The epidemiology of chronic periodontal disease in Western Nigerian schoolchildren. J. Periodont. Res., *3*:257–267, 1968.

47. Shourie, K. L.: The cause and prevalence of periodontal disease. J. All India D. A., *28*:11, 219–228, 1956.

48. Sinclair, V., and Goose, D. H.: The periodontal condition of grammar school children in Cheshire. Brit. Dent. J., *121*:420–423, 1966.

49. Stahl, D. G., and Goldman, H. M.: The incidence of gingivitis among a sample of Massachusetts school children. Oral Surg., Oral Med. & Oral Path., *6*:6, 707–715, 1953.

50. Stoner, J. E., and Prophet, A. S.: Early periodontal disease in children and young adults. Dent. Prac. Dent. Rec., *20*:173–176, 1970.

51. Thomas, B. O. A.: The child patient as a future periodontal problem. J.A.D.A., *35*:11, 763–774, 1947.

52. Westerholm, N., and Vennstrom, B.: A study of the frequency of plaque formation in Finnish schoolchildren. J. Periodont., *2*:81, 1967.

53. Williams, N. B., Parfitt, G. J., and Richards, M. D.: A preliminary study of microbial smears as an aid in diagnosis of gingival health. J. Periodont., *35*:197–201, 1964.

54. Williford, J. W., Johns, C., Muhler, J. C., and Stookey, G. K.: Report of a study demonstrating improved oral health through education. J. Dent. Child., *34*:183–189, 1967.

55. Zappler, S. E.: Periodontal disease in children. J.A.D.A., *37*:3, 333–345, 1948.

56. Ziskin, D. E., Blackberg, S. N., and Stout, A.: The gingivae during pregnancy. Surg., Gynec. & Obst., *57*:6, 719–726, 1933.

14

FACE DEVELOPMENT AND TOOTH ERUPTION

by H. PERRY HITCHCOCK

Oftentimes parents will ask the dentist why certain conditions exist in their child's mouth. If something is obviously different about that mouth as compared to other children's mouths, or to the child's mouth at an earlier age, the dentist has to give a reasonable explanation. To say, "It is nothing," will not suffice but will leave with the parents the impression that the dentist is ignorant of the nature of the condition which is "something" to them. It is essential to have an explanation based on a knowledge of growth and development and of the variations seen in the changing child.

This chapter will include nothing about the embryology of the face, and will confine itself to the so-called normal situation (using the word "normal" as a group yardstick with which to measure the individual against the background of his own type). There is a type normal and an individual normal. We can here consider only the type normal. It will be necessary for the reader himself to classify the variations he sees in the individual as either within the range of type or individual normal, or as abnormal. One of the aims of this chapter is to assist in making that decision.

FACE DEVELOPMENT

There are many bones of the face, but our attention will naturally be centered on the maxillae and their associated palatine bones, and the mandible. One must not forget, however, that they are but part of the complete face.

309

LIMITS OF THE FACE

For our purposes, the upper limit of the face is at a point which corresponds to the bony landmark, the nasion. This is at the junction of the nasal and frontal bones (Fig. 14–1).

The lower limit anteriorly corresponds to a chin point, the bony landmark being the gnathion or the menton. The menton is behind and below the gnathion. The pogonion is the anterior-most point on the bony chin prominence.

The ear canal is a convenient posterior landmark, and the posterior upper limit (of our limited face) is a point called the porion, which on the skull is at the top of the ear canal.

The posterior lower limit is in the region of the junction of the horizontal ramus and the ascending ramus. This point is called the gonion, hence the name "gonial angle."

THE MAXILLAE AND PALATINE BONES

The upper jaw is composed of the maxillae in association with the palatine bones. Surface additions to bones make them increase in size. Resorption is important in keeping the shape of bones and in reducing the bulk of bones where bony tissue is not needed.

In the maxillae, certain sutures are the sites of prolific growth. In profile, the slant of the frontomaxillary and the zygomaticomaxillary sutures indicates that growth at these places would give a forward and downward positioning to the

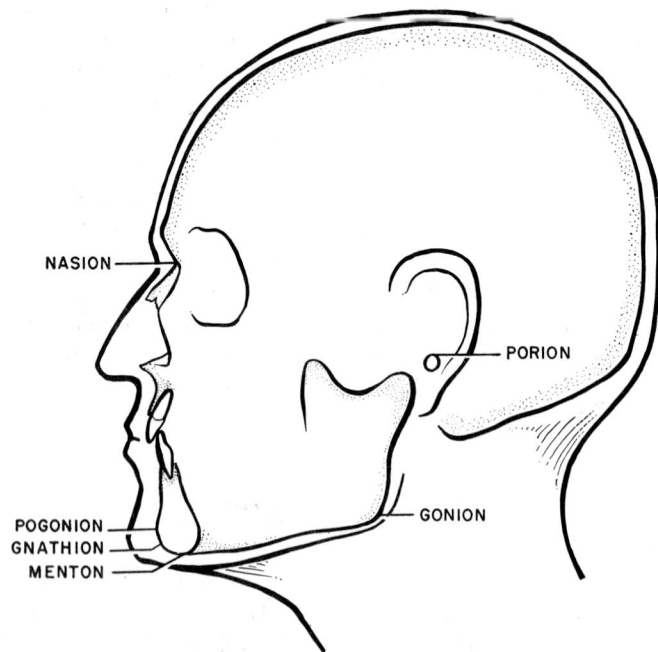

Figure 14–1   Arbitrary bony landmarks bounding the face.

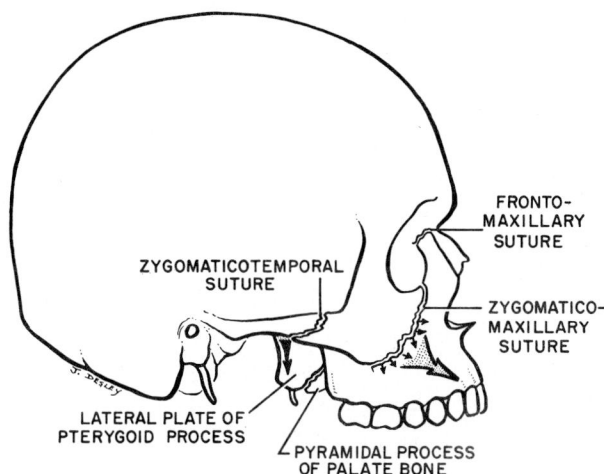

Figure 14–2 Downward growth of the pterygoid process of the sphenoid bone. Anteroposterior contribution in the zygomatic arch.

whole maxilla. Loosely speaking, growth takes place in a direction perpendicular to the suture line, which is itself, however, not straight (Fig. 14–2).

The sphenoid bone, which is not strictly a part of our limited face, articulates by means of sutures with all of the bones of the cranium and most of the bones of the face.[13] The pterygoid processes of the sphenoid bone are in close relationship to the tuberosity of the maxilla. Many writers have stated that the tuberosity butts up against the pterygoid process, which it may well do in adult life. While the child is growing, however, the tuberosity does not make contact with the pterygoid process, but is lateral to it and separated from it by means of the pyramidal process of the palatine bone.

The pyramidal process has been shown to be a site of much resorption in order for the palatine bone to extend from orbital portion to pyramidal portion.

After the first year of life, the pterygoid processes are not positioned forward (in relation to a registration point somewhere in the sphenoid bone). Rather, they grow only downward (Fig. 14–2).

Therefore, growth at the tuberosity is reflected forward from the pterygoid process of the sphenoid and the pyramidal process of the palatine bone, and finds expression in forward positioning of the maxilla.

The alveolar process is the site of constant bone growth, including additions and resorption. Considering its contents, the infratemporal surface of the maxilla may be considered a bent-up portion of the alveolar process until the third molar erupts.

The oral surface of the hard palate comprises two main bones, the paired maxillae, including the premaxillae, and the paired palatine bones.

In the palate there are two main sutures, the median palatine suture and the transverse palatine suture. The median palatine suture closes at an early age. Additions are made, however, on either side of the transverse palatine suture. Experiments indicate that no additions are made to the posterior rim of the hard palate after early childhood.

Surface apposition has been reported on the oral surface of the palate, or on the nasal surface, depending on the investigator and the monkeys investigated.[6, 9]

The palate is never extremely thick; therefore it follows that while bone is being deposited on the nasal surface, it is being resorbed on the oral surface or vice versa.

Surface additions to the alveolar process contribute to width. Authors are agreed on one thing at least; the greatest dimension of the face at birth is width. During postnatal life, it is this dimension that increases the least; it has the shortest distance to go. During rapid growth, the alveolar process of yesterday may become part of the main base of the maxilla tomorrow.

While additions are being made to the surface and at the alveolar process and certain sutures of the maxilla, resorption results in the formation of the maxillary sinuses. Nature is thrifty to the extent that no more bony tissue than is needed is kept in a bone. Hollowing out of the maxilla (and sometimes of the zygomatic bone's maxillary process) is in keeping with the principle of strength without bulk.

THE ZYGOMATIC BONE

The zygomatic bone contributes to the depth of the face by growing at the zygomaticomaxillary suture and the zygomaticotemporal suture (Fig. 14–2). It contributes to the width of the face by surface additions on the lateral surface and by resorption on its medial surface.[7]

GROWTH OF THE MANDIBLE

Some of the best research on growth of the mandible was done nearly two hundred years ago by John Hunter. He observed that in young children the ascending ramus rose almost directly behind the second primary molar; yet by the time the person became an adult, room had been made for three additional molars. He was able to show that bone is added to the posterior aspect of the ascending ramus and that bone is resorbed from the anterior border at a slower rate. This gives increased length to the horizontal ramus, and increased depth anteroposteriorly to the ascending ramus (Fig. 14–3).

The mandible is an interesting bone in that it originally develops directly from membranous tissue. Sometime after the bone is formed, isolated areas of cartilage cells and cartilage appear. These areas are at the head of the condyle, the coronoid process and the angle. By birth, the condylar cartilage is the only one that remains and it persists indefinitely.

The cartilage at the head of the condyle, unlike that of other joint surfaces, is covered by fibrous tissue. Additional cartilage can be developed from the fibrous tissue. Deeper toward the neck of the condyle, the cartilage becomes calcified, and is then able to be replaced by bone.

No mitoses or daughter cells have been seen in the normal condylar head after birth, so it does not grow interstitially, according to our present knowledge. This point, however, is still controversial.[11, 12]

Growth at the head of the condyle adds to the height of the face and also to the depth, depending on the obtuseness of the gonial angle. If the gonial angle were a right angle, then growth at the head of the condyle would contribute only to height of the face (Fig. 14–4).

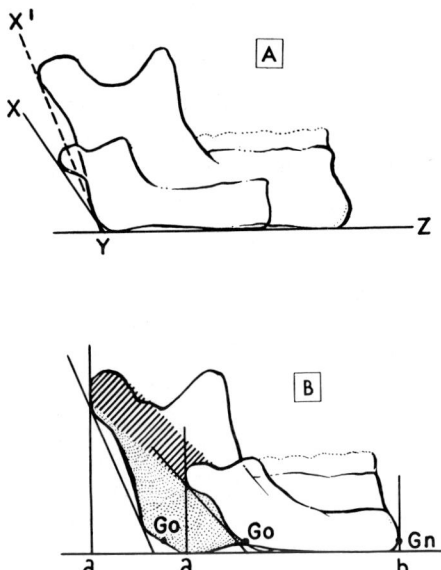

Figure 14–3 *A,* Superposition of the diagrammatic outline of an infantile and an adult mandible. The condylar angle *xyz* of the child decreases to *x′yz* of the adult. *B,* Outline of an infantile and an adult mandible superposed on the gnathion to show the increments of the ramus due to cartilaginous condylar growth (hatched) and appositional bone growth (stippled). (After Weinmann et al.: The Temporomandibular Joint, Charles C Thomas.)

Concomitantly with increase in the width of the skull (and therefore with separation of the two glenoid fossae), the condyles are oriented in a more lateral position. Because the horizontal processes of the mandible diverge from anterior to posterior, any additions at the posterior of the ascending rami increase the width of the lower face in that area.

HEREDITY AND FUNCTION

Ordinarily, the face will not grow beyond the limits of a preconceived genetic pattern. Yet we know that in certain diseases such as Paget's disease of bone and in

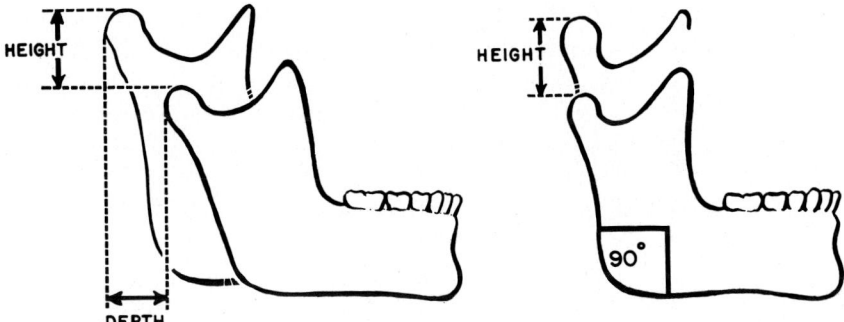

Figure 14–4 Growth at the condyle contributes to depth and height of the mandible when the gonial angle is obtuse.

acromegaly, normal limits are exceeded. Muscular stimulation through use cannot be totally disregarded as an aid to growth. Experimental rats on a hard diet have larger areas of muscle attachment than do their litter mates on a soft diet.[9]

The preceding paragraph touches lightly on a definite difference of opinion concerning the roles of function and heredity in postnatal growth. Both schools have experimental evidence for their views. Until more conclusive evidence is forthcoming one can only agree that a lot can be said for both sides.

FACIAL GROWTH AS A UNIT

We have discussed growth of some individual bones of the face. In studying growth of the face as a unit, the use of standardized roentgen cephalometry has been extensively employed by such men as Broadbent, Brodie, and their co-workers. From the study of successive roentgenograms taken at different ages on the same normal children, a definite *average* pattern of growth can be recognized. However, individuals may vary considerably from the typal average without being considered abnormal.

The works of Broadbent and Brodie have been incorporated in most modern textbooks in orthodontics, so only a brief recapitulation will be included here, for the sake of completeness.

Using a registration point in the vicinity of the sphenoid bone, Broadbent[3] showed with serial roentgenograms the following movements of skull landmarks:

The nasion moves forward and upward, the anterior nasal spine moves downward and forward.

The chin moves downward and forward. The gonion moves downward and backward. The pterygomaxillary fissure and the posterior nasal spine move straight downward. The floor of the nose, or hard palate, moves down parallel to its preceding state. The occlusal plane and lower border of the mandible move downward to a plane nearly parallel to their preceding positions (see Fig. 14–5).

Brodie,[5] using serial roentgenograms, divided the face into three areas: nasal area, upper alveolar and dental area, and lower dental and mandibular area.

Superposing the cranial base lines from sella turcica to nasion, at the sella turcica Brodie was able to show the nose being positioned forward, in a manner nearly parallel to the preceding stages (Fig. 14–6A). The palate, represented by a line connecting the anterior nasal spine and the posterior nasal spine, moves downward nearly parallel to its preceding positions (Fig. 14–6A). In less than half of the cases studied, the anterior nasal spine moved downward slightly faster than the posterior nasal spine. Rarely the posterior nasal spine moves downward at a faster rate. The posterior nasal spine moves almost straight downward. The anterior nasal spine moves downward and forward (Fig. 14–6A).

Superposing the palate lines on the posterior nasal spine, Brodie showed the occlusal plane descending in a nearly parallel manner (Fig. 14–6B). In less than half of the cases the posterior part of the occlusal plane comes down farther than the anterior part.

The upper central incisal edges move forward at a faster rate than the anterior nasal spine until occlusion is established. From then until 8 years of age, the line

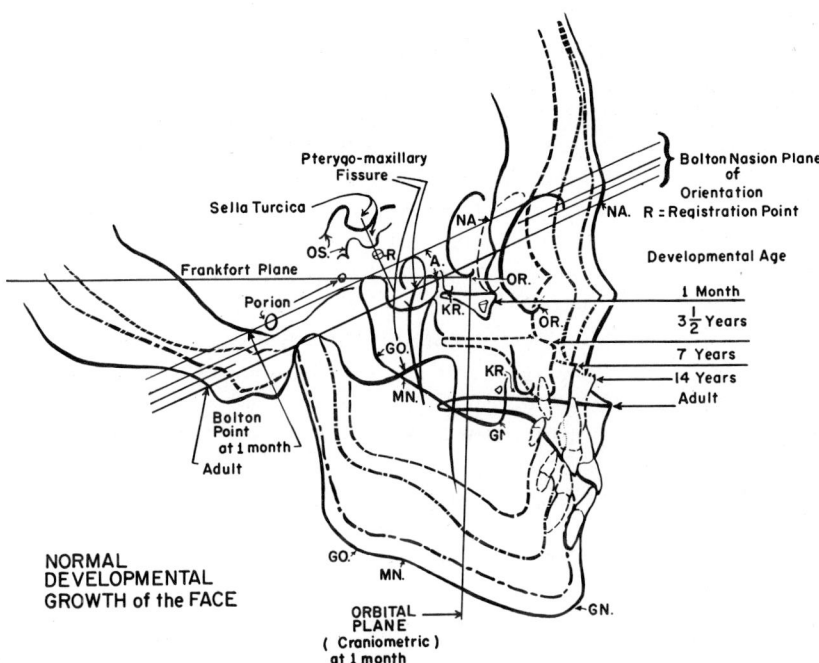

Figure 14–5   Profile of facial growth in the average normal child. (After Broadbent: Angle Orthodont., 7, 1937.)

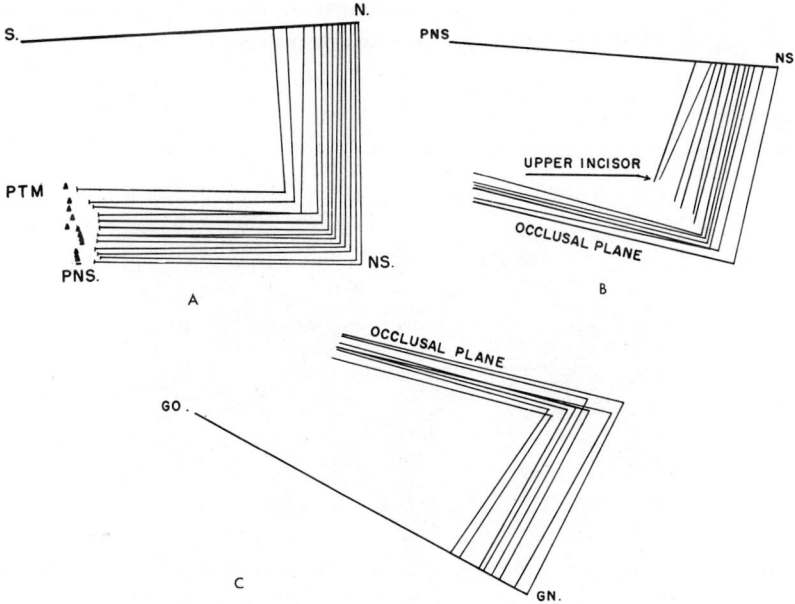

Figure 14–6   A, Composite pattern of growth of nasal area of twenty-one white males from the third month to the eighth year of life. B, Composite pattern of growth of upper alveolar and dental region of twenty-one white males from the third month to the eighth year of life. C, Composite pattern of growth of mandible from 2¹/₂ years to 7 years of life. (From Brodie: Am. J Anat., 68, 1941.)

from the anterior nasal spine to the incisal edge moves forward parallel to preceding stages (Fig. 14–6B).

Placing serial pictures of the mandible over one another on the lower border of the mandible at the gonion, Brodie showed that the growth and positioning upward of the occlusal plane were nearly parallel, and that the chin moved forward at a slightly faster rate than the incisal edges of the lower centrals (Fig. 14–6C).

Particularly in later growth stages, between 7 and 17 years, the posterior end of the horizontal ramus (the region of the gonion) may descend at a faster rate than the chin, but this occurred in less than 50 per cent of the cases. The majority of cases showed the mandibular plane descending parallel to its preceding stages.

In changing from child to adolescent to adult, the incisors assume a variety of inclinations to the occlusal plane or mandibular border. Also, the limits of upper and lower alveolar processes lag behind the total profile of the face in the later age groupings.

During growth, the porion point may move downward and backward, directly downward, or directly backward.

An exciting use of metallic implants in humans was published in 1955 by Dr. Arne Björk.[2] He showed five cases, exhibiting different growth patterns. His work intensifies the impression that in each individual growth and development have different manifestations.

Three or four vitallium pins, 2 mm. long, were placed in each jaw (Fig. 14–7). The indicators do not shift except when they do not enter the bone properly or are caught in the eruption path of the teeth. Also, as a result of resorption of the nasal floor, implants in the vicinity may end up in the floor of the nose.

Analysis of generalized growth was carried out by measurements from a line connecting the sella turcica to the nasion, and from a line perpendicular to it. Actual growth within the maxilla and mandible was shown by superimposing the x-ray images of the metallic implants after the two year period.

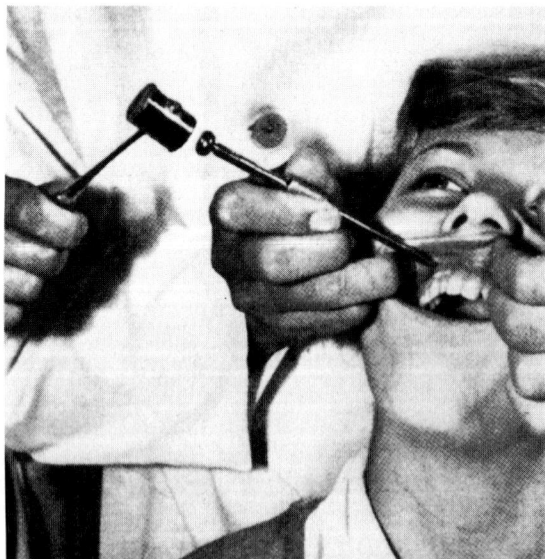

Figure 14–7 Method of placing vitallium implants. (Björk: Acta Odont. Scandinavica, *13,* 1955.)

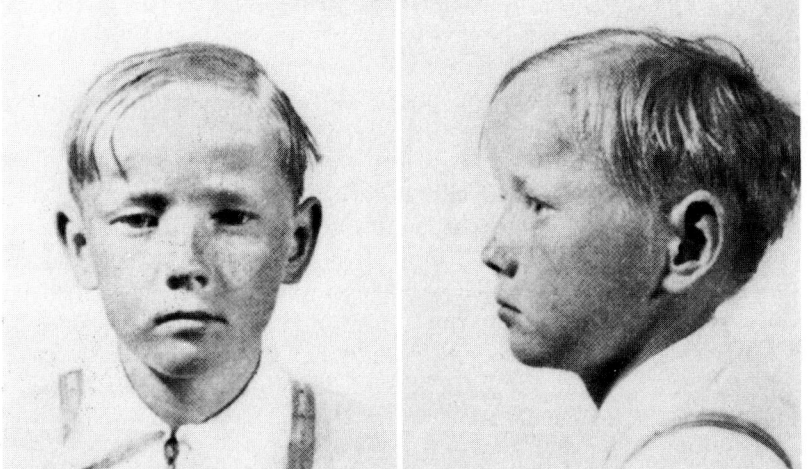

Figure 14–8   Face of a boy with normal occlusion. (Björk: Acta Odont. Scandinavica, *13*, 1955, p. 248.)

A study of two of Björk's cases should emphasize the important implications of this method.

His case, 2627g (Fig. 14–8), is that of a boy having normal occlusion. Figure 14–9 shows the tracings of the x-rays taken exactly two years apart, using the cranial base superposition. Metallic implants 1 and 2 in the maxilla moved down 3 mm. and forward 2 mm. Metallic implants in the mandible take different paths. Implant 3 moved forward 2.5 mm. and down 5 mm. Implant 4 moved 4.5 mm. down and 3.5 mm. forward, and implant 5 moved 4 mm. forward and 4mm. downward. Notice that when the x-ray tracings are superposed on the cranial base,

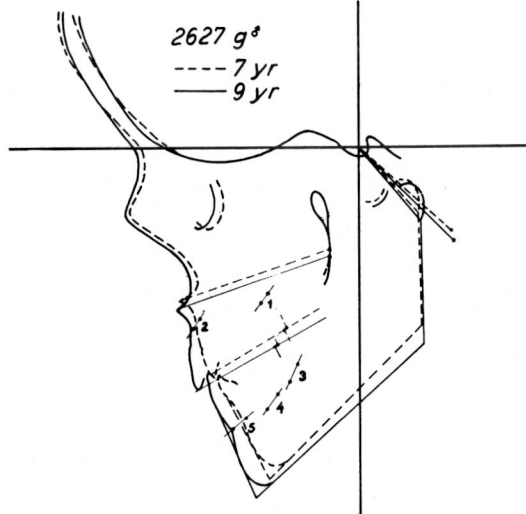

Figure 14–9   Tracings two years apart, using cranial base superimposition. (Björk: Acta Odont. Scandinavica, *13*, 1955.)

nasion to sella turcica, the following viewpoint is obtained: the orbit has moved forward and the nasal floor has descended nearly parallel to its preceding stage; the occlusal plane and mandibular plane have descended more in back than in front. The different directions taken by the mandibular implants indicate a rotation of the mandible during the two year growth.

If attention is shifted now to the tracings superposed on the metallic implant images (Fig. 14–10), we get an entirely different idea about growth in the maxilla and mandible. Björk points out that the lowering of the maxilla is mainly due to growth at the sutures in this case (3 mm. at the frontomaxillary suture). There is very little resorption of the nasal floor during the two year period. "The orbit has retained its position vertically in the facial diagram, due to periosteal growth despite of marked sutural lowering of the maxilla."[2] There has been actual resorption in the area of the anterior nasal spine. Significant growth appears in the tuberosity (2.5 mm.) and the alveolar border is lowered by 1.5 mm. of appositional growth in the first molar area.

In the mandible, resorption has taken place in the anterior alveolar process above the chin, although 2 mm. of appositional growth has been added to the superior alveolar border. There is slight surface apposition, anteriorly, at the lower border of the mandible, and more marked resorption in the gonial angle area. Growth of the condyle has been nearly vertical, with added bone at the posterior border of the ascending ramus, except at the area of the neck, where modeling resorption has taken place. There was no resorption at the anterior border of the ascending ramus during the two year period in this particular case. The path of eruption of the teeth is nearly vertical to the occlusal plane.

Another case (Björk 5574g) (Fig. 14–11) shows an entirely different pattern of growth. Four indicators were placed in each jaw. Forward movement of the maxillary implants, as shown in Figure 14–12, amounted to 2.5 mm. Vertical movement was only 0.5 mm. as measured from the cranial base line.

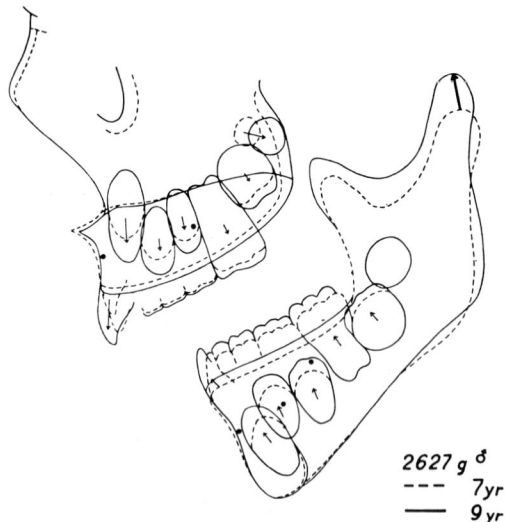

2627 g ♂
- - - 7 yr
——— 9 yr

Figure 14–10 Tracings two years apart, using metallic implant superimposition. (Björk: Acta Odont. Scandinavica, *13*, 1955.)

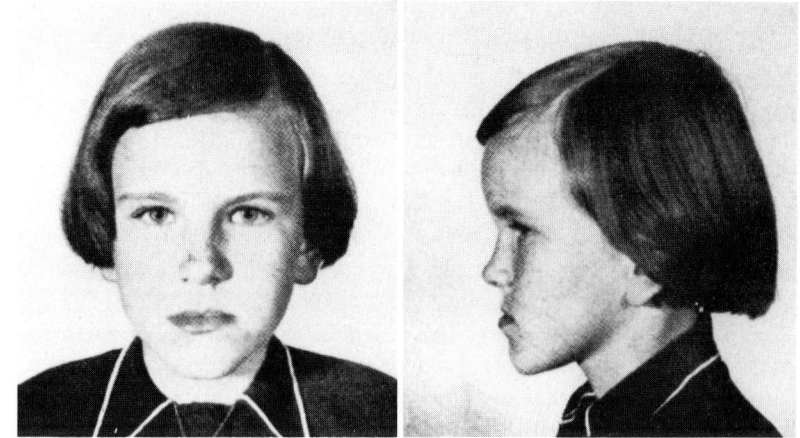

Figure 14–11 Face of a girl with malocclusion. (Björk: Acta Odont. Scandinavica, *13*, 1955.)

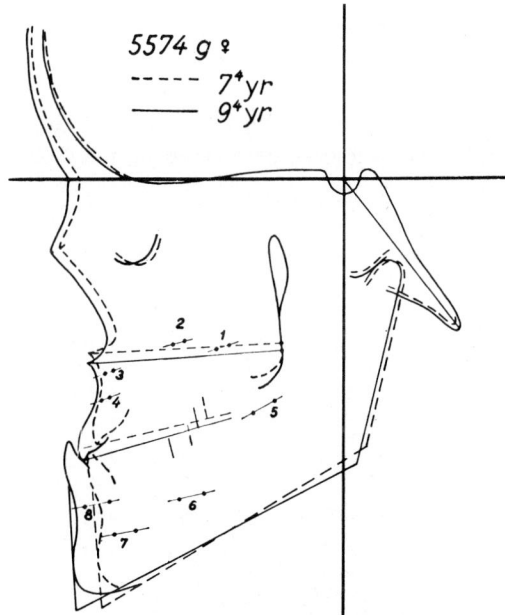

Figure 14–12 Tracings two years apart, using cranial base superimposition. (Björk: Acta Odont. Scandinavica, *13*, 1955.)

Metallic implants in the mandible took different paths. Implant 5 moved forward 5.5 mm. and down only 2.5 mm. Implant 6 moved forward 6 mm. and down 2 mm. Implants 7 and 8 moved forward 7 mm. and down 1 mm.

This view also shows that the mandible has been displaced forward as evidenced by the forward position of the condyle and the forward position of the posterior border of the ascending ramus. The mandibular plane has tipped up anteriorly and down posteriorly. The forward positioning of the maxilla has been much less than that of the mandible. In this case also the different directions and distances taken by the mandibular implants imply a rotation of the mandible during the two year growth.

Superposing metallic implants in the maxilla (Fig. 14–13) shows some differences between these two patients. Comparisons of the position of the orbit and the frontonasal suture as an indication of frontomaxillary sutural growth indicate very little sutural growth in this case and very little orbital floor appositional growth. The nasal floor, on the other hand, has been positioned downward because of resorption. There has also been resorption of the anterior nasal spine. Tooth eruption in the maxilla of this case shows a downward and anterior direction.

In the mandible, condylar growth is seen to have occurred rearward, but with little increase in height. Note that there has been resorption of the anterior border of the ascending ramus along with deposition on the posterior border. In contrast to the first case, bone has been added to the lower border, posteriorly. There has been resorption of the anterior alveolus above the chin. The path of eruption of most of the mandibular teeth seems to be upward and backward. One exception to this is the movement of the third molar, which is seen to be migrating *downward* into the body of the mandible.

Of course it can be argued that in this case anterior mandibular growth is obvi-

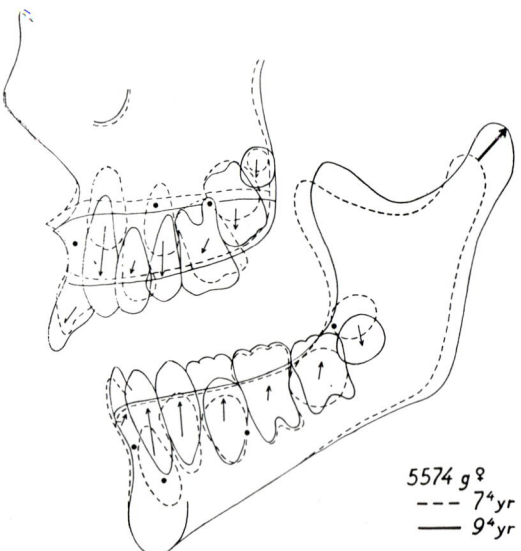

5574 g ♀
--- 7⁴yr
—— 9⁴yr

Figure 14–13 Tracings two years apart, using metallic implant superimposition. (Björk: Acta Odont. Scandinavica, *13*, 1955.)

ous without the aid of cephalometrics or metallic implants. In the case of the boy with normal occlusion, however, certain changes have taken place which would not have been suspected if metallic implants had not been used.

The possibility exists that many assumptions of stability in facial growth patterns need to be reconsidered in the light shed by these adventuresome experiments on individual humans.

TOOTH ERUPTION

The teeth themselves are of great importance in contributing to the shape of the face.

SEQUENCE OF ERUPTION

The usual eruption sequence in the primary dentition is as follows: "First the central incisors, followed in order by the lateral incisors, first molars, canines and second molars. Mandibular teeth usually precede the maxillary teeth."[2]

This sequence is not always followed, and the author has seen a case in which the maxillary lateral incisor was the first primary tooth to erupt. In another case, the maxillary primary laterals came in before the mandibular primary laterals.

Time of eruption is usually stated as 6 months of age for the maxillary primary centrals, 7 to 8 months for the mandibular primary laterals, and 8 or 9 months for the maxillary primary laterals. At about 1 year, the first primary molars erupt. At around 16 months, the primary cuspids appear. Two years is usually given as the age for the second primary molars to erupt.

It would seem that the sequence of tooth eruption has more bearing on proper development of the dental arch than the actual time of eruption. Three or four months either way would not necessarily mean that a child is abnormal in his eruption time schedule; it is not unusual for a child to be born with one or more teeth erupted.

The first permanent tooth to erupt is usually the mandibular first permanent molar, at about 6 years, but often the permanent central incisor may come in at the same time or even before it. The mandibular lateral incisors may erupt before any of the permanent maxillary teeth.

Then the maxillary first permanent molar erupts at age 6 to 7 years, followed by the maxillary central incisor at 7 to 8 years. The maxillary permanent lateral incisors erupt between the ages of 8 and 9.

The mandibular canine usually erupts at about 9 to 11 years, followed by the first premolar, second premolar, and second molar.

In the maxillary arch, there is usually a difference in the eruption sequence: The maxillary first premolar erupts between 10 and 11 years of age, before the maxillary canine at 11 to 12 years of age. Then the maxillary second premolar comes in, either at the same time as the canine or after it. The "12 year molar," or second molar, is supposed to come in at 12 years of age. *Variations from this pattern may be a factor in producing certain types of malocclusion.*

ERUPTION AND ARCH DEVELOPMENT

The preceding statements about tooth eruption are rather sterile facts. To get a more fruitful picture, certain modifications in tooth position and arch size will be dealt with in detail as they pertain to growth and development of the face.

At age 1 year, when the first primary molar erupts, the permanent cuspids begin calcifying between the roots of the first primary molars. As the primary teeth erupt toward the line of occlusion, the permanent incisors and cuspids migrate forward at a greater rate than the primary teeth themselves. So, by 2½ years of age, the first bicuspids are beginning to calcify between the roots of the first primary molars, the site of previous calcification of the permanent cuspid. Thus, as the primary teeth erupt and the jaws grow, more space is left apically for the developing permanent teeth.[3]

One of the most challenging concepts of tooth eruption and arch development was emphasized in published form in 1950 by Louis J. Baume, of the University of California.[1]

He observed that primary dental arches occur as two types: either there are spaces between the teeth or there are no spaces. Very often two consistent diastemata occur in the spaced type of primary dentition, one between the mandibular primary canine and first primary molar, and the other between the maxillary lateral primary incisor and the maxillary primary canine (Fig. 14–14). (These diastemata are present in the mouths of all other primates. Hence, when they occur in humans, they are referred to as the primate spaces.)

Spaces do not develop in arches previously closed during the completed primary dentition. One arch may have spaces and the other not. Closed arches are narrower than spaced ones. The primary dental arches, once formed and with second primary molars in occlusion, show no increase either in width or in length. Slight shortening of arches may take place as a result of forward movement of second primary molars or as a result of interproximal caries. Vertical growth of alveolar processes does take place and anteroposterior growth of the jaws also takes place, manifesting itself in retromolar space for the future permanent molars.

The relationship of the maxillary primary canine to the mandibular primary canine remains constant throughout the period of the completed primary dentition. In a few cases the distal surface of the mandibular second primary molar will be mesial to the distal surface of the maxillary second primary molar. When this is the case, the mandibular and maxillary first permanent molars can erupt directly into normal occlusion at this early age (Fig. 14–15A).

Ordinarily, however, the first permanent molars erupt in an end to end position (Fig. 14–15B). If the mandibular arch contains a primate space, the erupting first permanent molar will cause the second primary molar and the first primary

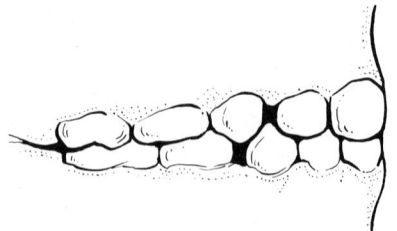

Figure 14–14   Primate spaces between maxillary primary lateral incisor and primary cuspid, and between mandibular primary canine and mandibular first primary molar. (After Baume: J. D. Res., 29, 1950.)

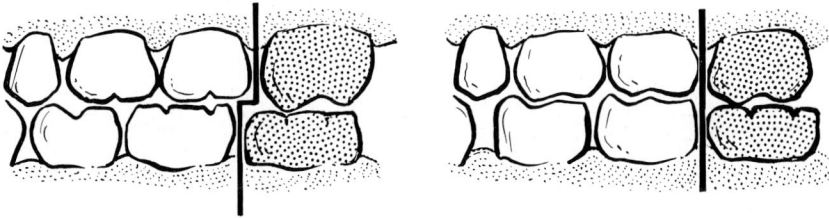

Figure 14–15 *A,* Permanent molars erupting directly into normal occlusion. *B,* Permanent molars erupting in an end to end relation.

molar to move forward, obliterating the diastema between the lower primary cuspid and the first primary molar and allowing the maxillary molar to erupt directly into normal occlusion (Fig. 14–16).

If, on the other hand, there should be no space in the mandibular primary arch, the maxillary and mandibular molars will usually maintain an end to end relationship until the mandibular second primary molar is replaced by the smaller mandibular second premolar. This occurs much later, of course, and then allows the late mesial shift of the mandibular first permanent molar into normal occlusion with the maxillary molar.

A poor combination is to have no spaces in the mandibular arch, a maxillary arch with spaces between the teeth, and the distal surface of the maxillary second primary molar mesial to the distal surface of the mandibular second primary molar. Then when the permanent first molars erupt, they will immediately be in distoclusion (Fig. 14–17). Even if the distal surfaces of the second primary molars are in a straight line, but the maxillary permanent molar erupts before the mandibular molar, the space in the upper arch will be closed by mesial migration of the

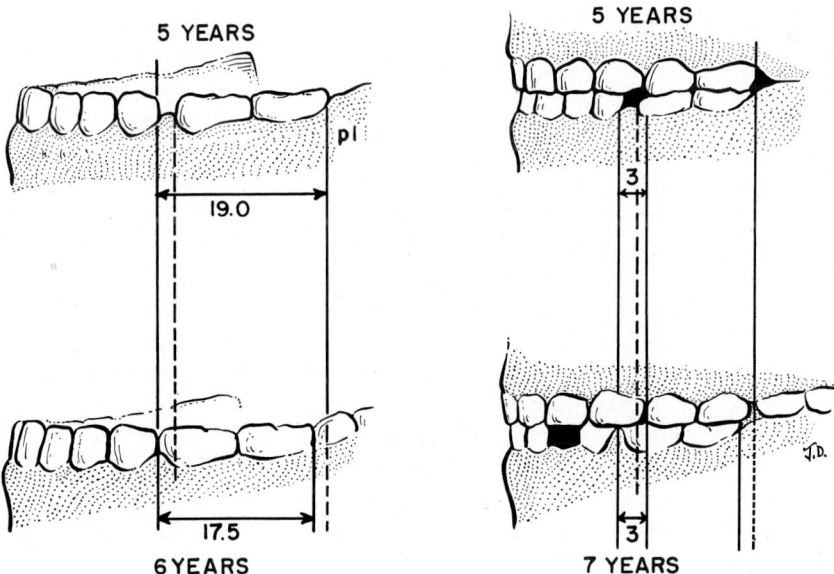

Figure 14–16 Maxillary molar erupts into normal occlusion, *after* the mandibular first permanent molar migrates mesially to obliterate the mandibular diastema between the primary first molar and cuspid. (After Baume: J. D. Res., *29,* 1950.)

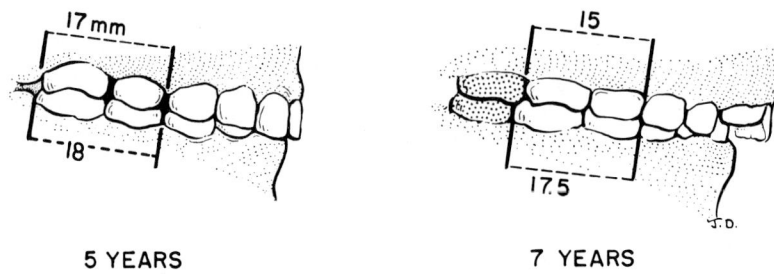

5 YEARS   **7 YEARS**

Figure 14–17 Development of distal occlusion when maxillary first permanent molar erupts prior to mandibular first permanent molar. Maxillary diastemata are obliterated by mesial movement of maxillary first permanent molar.

maxillary molars. When the mandibular permanent molars erupt they cannot move mesially because there is no space in the primary part of the arch. The result is distoclusion of the permanent molars.

It has been stated above that there is little or no change in dimension of the primary arches during the completed primary dentition. On a time basis, this is from 3½ years to 6 years, on the average. From a physiologic standpoint, this is during the time when the primary teeth and only the primary teeth are visible in function in the oral cavity. We have already seen that with eruption of permanent molars, there may be a shortening of the arch if spaces are available to be closed up by the forward influence of the permanent molars.

What happens when the permanent incisors erupt? With the eruption of the lower permanent incisors, a widening of the arches takes place.

Arches that were closed during the primary dentition widen more in the canine region than do arches that were previously spaced (Table 14–1).

Between the primary second molars there is an increase in width, but it is not as great as in the canine region, nor as great in previously closed arches.

Sometimes the arch widens even though there is enough spacing between the primary incisors originally to accommodate the larger permanent incisors. This would indicate a *genetic* or *phylogenetic impulse,* rather than simply the presence of teeth alone. Sometimes this increased spacing is closed up eventually; other times it remains permanently open.

Before any of the maxillary primary teeth are shed, sometimes enough intercanine increase occurs in the mandibular arch to institute a widening of the maxillary arch. Then the maxillary primary anteriors will exhibit a spacing. Here is an *instance of direct cause and effect,* rather than just concomitance.

With the eruption of the permanent maxillary incisors, there is a widening of the maxillary arches, both in the canine region and in the molar region. Here again, the greater width increase appears in arches that were previously closed during the completed primary dentition.

In Baume's study, the average intercanine increase in the mandibular arches amounted to 2.27 mm. in previously spaced arches and to 2.5 mm. in previously closed arches (Table 14–1). The average intercanine increase in the maxillary arches amounted to 2.5 mm. in the previously spaced arches and to 3.2 mm. in the previously closed arches (Table 14–2).

Yet, in spite of the greater growth of previously closed arches, in almost half of the cases studied there was not enough room to align the permanent incisors prop-

TABLE 14–1 AVERAGE INCREASE IN WIDTH OF THE MANDIBULAR DENTAL ARCHES DURING AND AFTER ERUPTION OF PERMANENT INCISORS

| Type | Stage | No. Cases | Intercanine Width | | | | Distance M_2-M_2 | | | |
| | | | Present Studies | | Korkhaus | | Present Studies | | Korkhaus | |
			Min.-Max. Variation, mm.	Average Increase, mm.	No. Cases	Average Increase, mm.	No. Cases	Average Increase, mm.	No. Cases	Average Increase, mm.
I	1–2	15		0.5	2	1.25	15	0.3	2	0.75
	1–3	24	0.3/0	2.27	2	2.0	23	1.7	2	1.75
II	1–2	5		1.2	3	1.2	4	1.0	3	0.2
	1–3	15	0/5.0	2.5	16	2.4	10	1.0	10	0.75

Type I: primary dentitions with spacing. Type II: primary dentitions without spaces. Stage 1: deciduous dentition is completed. Stage 2: first permanent incisors have erupted. Stage 3: all permanent incisors have erupted. From Baume: J. D. Res., 29, 1950.

TABLE 14–2 AVERAGE INCREASE IN WIDTH OF MAXILLARY DENTAL ARCHES DURING AND AFTER ERUPTION OF UPPER PERMANENT INCISORS

| Type | Stage | No. Cases | Intercanine Width | | | | Distance M_2-M_2 | | | |
| | | | Present Studies | | Korkhaus | | Present Studies | | Korkhaus | |
			Min.-Max. Variation, mm.	Average Increase, mm.	No. Cases	Average Increase, mm.	No. Cases	Average Increase, mm.	No. Cases	Average Increase, mm.
I	1–2	11		1.4	4	2.3	13	0.5	4	0.37
	1–3	24	0/4.0	2.5	2	3.0	19	1.5	2	2.0
II	1–2	3		1.5	15	2.1	5	0.7	19	0.6
	1–3	12	0/6.5	3.2	12	3.7	8	1.6	16	1.5

erly. Not only was there lack of room but often the original position of the tooth buds, either in lingual version or in torsiversion, had a bearing on the final malposition in the arch.

The increased size of the permanent incisors as compared to the primary incisors indicated that the limited lateral expansion is not enough to provide adequate room.

Baume measured the increase in forward extension of the upper and lower arches. It has already been observed that if there is space, the primary molars will migrate forward on eruption of the permanent molars. The primary canines, however, maintain their anteroposterior relationship. Therefore, the forward extension of the anterior section of the arches was measured forward from the distal aspect of the canine (Fig. 14–18).

The average forward extension in the lower arches was 1.3 mm. and in the upper arches 2.2 mm., after eruption of the permanent incisors (Table 14–3).

Maximal forward extensions amounted to 3 mm. in the lower and 4 mm. in the

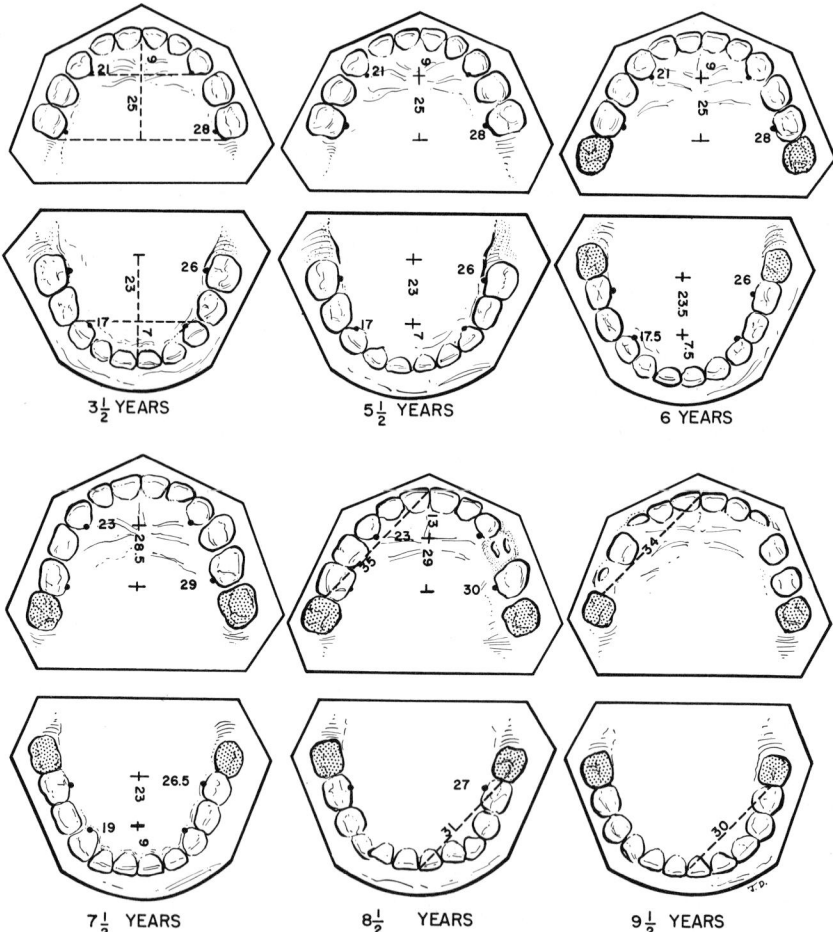

Figure 14–18 Development of occlusion, showing lateral growth as the incisors erupt, and forward extension of the anterior segments, greater in the maxilla than in the mandible. (After Baume: J. D. Res., *29,* 1950.)

TABLE 14–3 AVERAGE FORWARD EXTENSION OF FRONTAL PORTION OF ARCHES DURING AND AFTER ERUPTION OF PERMANENT INCISORS*

Type	Stage	Lower Arch			Upper Arch		
		No. Cases	Min.-Max. Variation, mm.	Average Increase, mm.	No. Cases	Min.-Max. Variation, mm.	Average Increase, mm.
I	1–3	26	0/3.0	1.3	36	−0.5/4.0	2.2
II	1–3	16	−0.5/3.0	1.3	12	0/4.0	2.2
I & II	1–2	16		0.5	7		1.5
	1–3	42	−0.5/3.0	1.3	48	−0.5/4.0	2.2

*Increase of the frontal arch length from a line connecting the two distal contact points of the primary canines to the prosthion or infradentale.

Type I: primary dentitions with spacing. Type II: primary dentitions without spaces. Stage 1: deciduous dentition is completed. Stage 2: first permanent incisors have erupted. Stage 3: all permanent incisors have erupted.

From Baume: J. D. Res., 29, 1950.

upper. There is no correlation between the forward growth of the anterior sections and previously closed or previously spaced arches.

The average amount of forward extension in the maxillary arch is greater by 1 mm. than in the mandibular arch. This is not due to greater labiolingual dimension of maxillary incisors as compared to mandibular incisors in transferring from the primary to the permanent teeth. It is possibly another reflection of the phylogenetically reduced mandible in man!

The average forward positioning of the upper anterior segment is greater than the lower. Yet, individual differences between upper and lower forward growth in specific cases indicate that sometimes the mandibular arch can exhibit a greater forward extension than the maxillary arch. Once again, it is important to exercise discretion when applying a statistical average to an individual case!

The difference in maxillary anterior forward growth and mandibular anterior forward growth has an effect on the amount of incisal overbite which develops during the mixed dentition.

Generally speaking, incisal overbites increase in going from the primary dentition to the mixed dentition. But, when the amount of forward extension of the anterior sections of both arches is equal, then the degree of overbite in the mixed dentition will be the same as in the primary dentition (see Fig. 14–19). In some cases, the forward extension of the mandibular anterior section may be greater than that in the maxilla. If this happens, the degree of incisal overbite will be less in the mixed dentition than in the primary dentition.

The amount of overbite in the permanent dentition is a result of the above factors, plus the eruption of the permanent canines and premolars. The mandibular permanent canine usually erupts before the maxillary permanent canine, and before the loss of the mandibular second primary molar. Room for the larger permanent mandibular canine may be made by a further forward extension of the lower anterior segment (Fig. 14–20).

In the upper arch, the permanent canine usually erupts after the first premolar and after loss of the second primary molar. Here the larger permanent canine makes room for itself by moving the first premolar distally into the space left by the lost second primary molar. This space is larger than is needed by the second premolar.

Complicated adjustments are often needed to provide proper accommodations for all of the teeth, and sometimes the results are not achieved. Thus, tooth eruption sequence plays a very important role in the establishment of the normal dental arch!

Sometimes the complicated adjustments produce transient disharmonies which dentists and parents view as abnormalities. Possibly the most frequent cause for misunderstanding of development occurs in the anterior maxillary region during and after the eruption of the maxillary lateral incisors. The sequence of events and the cause for misunderstanding are most lucidly shown by Broadbent's cephalometric studies.[3, 4]

The period from eruption of the lateral incisors to the eruption of the canine is termed by Broadbent as the "ugly duckling" stage. It is an apt term, implying an unesthetic metamorphosis leading to an esthetic result (Fig. 14–21). During this period, parents become worried. A space may develop between the maxillary central crowns. The lateral crowns may flare. Frenums are often sacrificed in an effort to remove the cause of the space between the centrals.

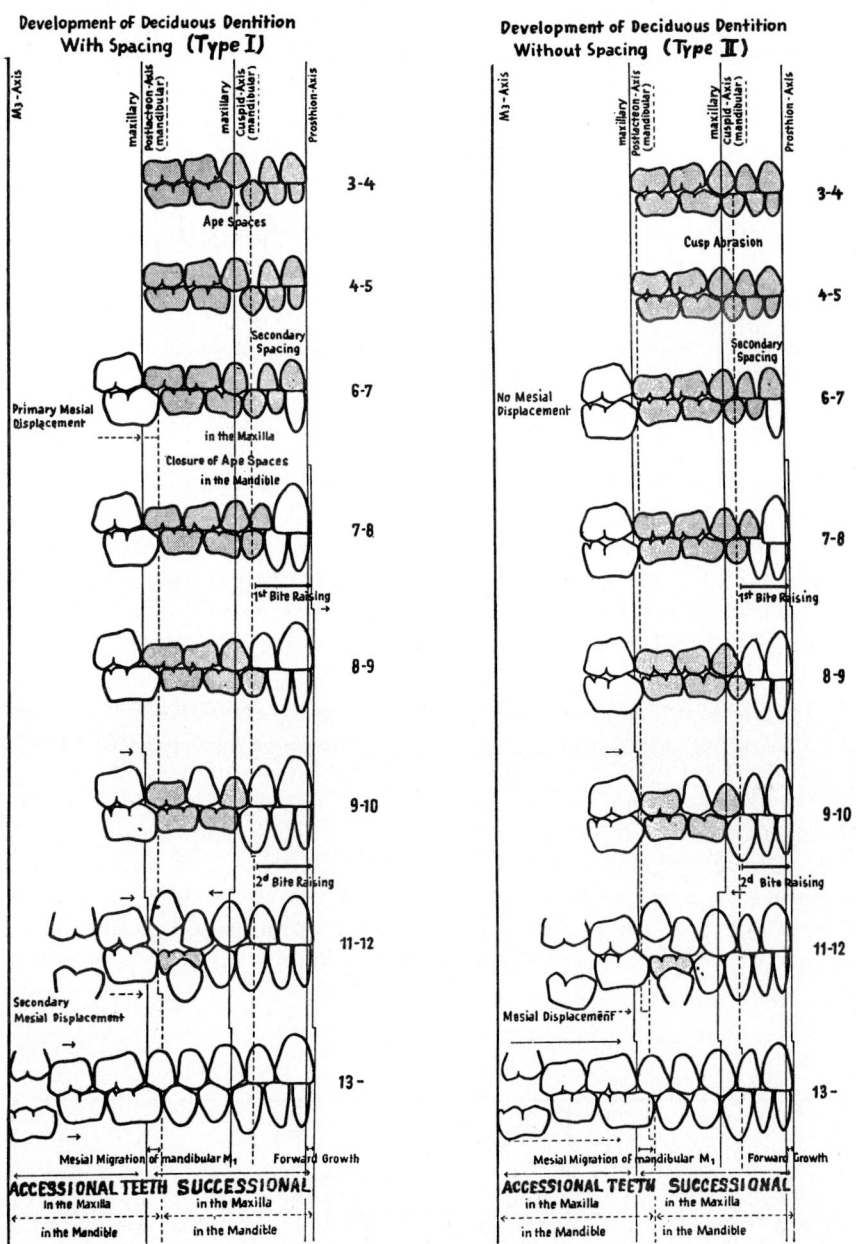

Figure 14–19 Illustration of the physiologic tooth migration in the sagittal plane, the result of a biometric survey on 60 series of development. (Courtesy of Baume: J. D. Res., 29, 1950.)

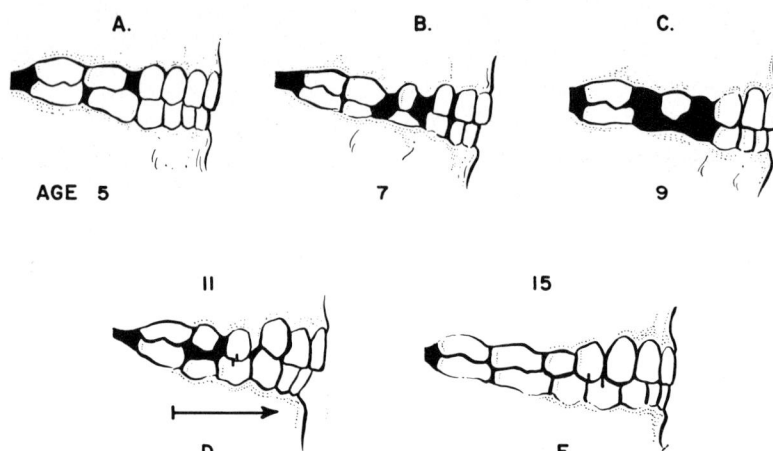

Figure 14–20 Forward extension of mandibular anterior segment allows room for permanent canine and premolars, leading to a normal occlusion in the permanent dentition. (After Baume: J. D. Res., 29, 1950.)

Actually, the crowns of the cuspids in the young jaw impinge on the developing roots of the lateral incisors, driving the roots medially and causing the crowns to flare laterally. The roots of the centrals are also forced toward each other.

As the laterals erupt further, narrower portions of their roots are in proximity to the developing canines. Margolis has called the alveolar process "the servant of the tooth."[8] At this stage the maxilla is bulging in the canine region as the alveolar process develops around the forming canine. With the further migration of the canine occlusally, with its servant the alveolar process, the point of influence of the canine on the laterals shifts incisally, so that eventually the lateral crowns are driven medially, also effecting closure of the space between the centrals. With eruption of the crowns of the canines, more room is left in the bone, apically, for the roots of the laterals to move laterally.

The difficulty, again, is in determining whether the initial situation is within normal limits or whether faulty growth and development will not permit subsequent resolution of the problem. Periodic observation would seem to be a wiser course than immediate frenectomy to correct a circumstance that may be self-correcting.

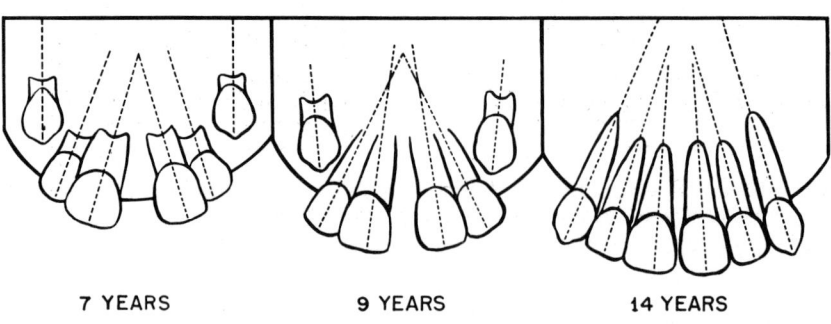

7 YEARS   **9 YEARS**   **14 YEARS**
Figure 14–21 "Ugly duckling" stage. (After Broadbent: Angle Orthodont., 7, 1937.)

＊　　＊　　＊　　＊　　＊

This chapter has been a brief condensation of information obtained as a result of much individual and group research and observation. Specific details and methods used have not been elaborated on. Rather, a broad and generalized approach has been used with the idea of giving the reader a background for better evaluation of changing conditions in the mouths of growing and developing individuals.

REFERENCES

1. Baume, L.: Physiological tooth migration and its significance for the development of occlusion. J. D. Res., *29*:123–132, 331–337, 338–348, 440–447, 1950.
2. Björk, A.: Facial growth in man, studied with the aid of metallic implants. Acta Odont. Scandinavica, *13*:9–34, 1955.
3. Broadbent, B. H.: The face of the normal child. Angle Orthodont., 7:183–208, 1937.
4. Broadbent, B. H.: Ontogenic development of occlusion. Angle Orthodont., *11*:223–241, 1941.
5. Brodie, A.: Growth pattern of human head from three months to eight years. Am. J. Anat., *68*:209–262, 1941.
6. Craven, A. H.: Growth in width of the head of the *Macaca rhesus* monkey as revealed by vital staining. Am. J. Orthodont., *42*:341–361, 1956.
7. Gans, B. J., and Sarnat, B. G.: Sutural facial growth of the *Macaca rhesus* monkey. Am. J. Orthodont., *37*:827–841, 1951.
8. Margolis, H. I.: Personal communication.
9. Moore, A. W.: Head growth of the macaque monkey. Am. J. Orthodont., *35*:654–671, 1949.
10. Watt, D., and Williams, C.: Growth and development of mandible and maxilla of the rat. Am. J. Orthodont., *37*:895–927, 1951.
11. Weinmann, J. P., and Sicher, H.: Bone and Bones. St. Louis, C. V. Mosby Co., 1947.
12. Weinmann, J. P., Sicher, H., Brodie, A. G.: The Temporomandibular Joint. Springfield, Ill., Charles C Thomas, 1951, pp. 47, 50.
13. Wheeler, R. C.: Textbook of Dental Anatomy and Physiology. 2nd ed. Philadelphia, W. B. Saunders Co., 1950.
14. Wilkinson, L.: Factors contributing to facial growth and development. Am. J. Orthodont., *26*:1019–1035, 1940.

15

PRELIMINARY STEPS IN PREVENTIVE ORTHODONTICS

by H. PERRY HITCHCOCK

Because the dentist wants to be of real service to his patients, he wants a "practical" course in preventive orthodontics. From this standpoint the most practical judgments he can make are whether a patient needs orthodontic care and whether he is the one to give that care. The steps leading up to these decisions involve examination, history, etiology and classification, which will usually lead to the correct diagnosis from which a treatment plan or referral can be made.

THE EXAMINATION

Examination will usually show whether any particular line of questioning should be used in obtaining the case history. The patient should be examined with the mouth closed, with the mouth wide open, and during the closing act. The three stages will give an idea of the presence or absence of a malocclusion, midline symmetry, or lower jaw shifts.

If the path of closure is not a smooth one, a note should be made of this fact to modify the eventual classification. Take a tongue blade and line it up with the midline between the eyebrows and the philtrum of the upper lip. Part the lips to see where the edge of the tongue blade comes in relation to the midline between the upper and lower incisors. Then have the patient once more open wide and close slowly. In this way any midline discrepancy can be observed. Furthermore, a lower midline discrepancy may prove to be the result of tooth shifting only, or of a lower jaw shift in the process of opening and closing. Make sure the closing act is in the patient's usual manner. Having him place the tongue far back in the roof of the mouth is sometimes a help in keeping him from biting too far forward.

332

A full mouth set of roentgenograms will disclose the number of permanent teeth present or absent, any supernumerary teeth, and the stage of eruption in the various quadrants.

HISTORY

A history may be more useful from the standpoint of what is left out of it, rather than what is in it. Whether chickenpox, mumps or whooping cough occurred at a particular age does not usually make much difference. On the other hand, if the mother had measles during the fifth to eighth weeks while pregnant with this child, it might be important.

A history of allergy associated with mouth breathing may be indicative of a nasal obstruction, which should be controlled if certain of the preventive orthodontic measures are to be successful. Calluses on the hands or a conspicuously clean thumbnail will often confirm a history of thumb or finger sucking. Primary tooth loss and secondary tooth eruption are normal within wide chronological limits, as indicated elsewhere. Therefore sequence of eruption would seem to be more important than exact time of eruption, as far as the development of a normal occlusion is concerned.

ETIOLOGY

If the etiology of a malocclusion is obvious from the history and the initial examination, it can be made part of the diagnosis then. Whole books have been written on etiology but some conditions are so obscure that to connect them with malposition of the teeth is to see a cause that may not be there.

Etiological factors within the control of the pedodontist are restorations of improper size and contact along with failure to maintain space when teeth have been lost prematurely. At the present time tongue habits are generally associated with protruding teeth and open bite.

Attributing a malocclusion without an obvious cause to heredity is justified, provided the judgment is based on a sound knowledge of genetics. Heredity is not to be used as a disguise for ignorance.

CLASSIFICATION

In recent years there has been a great deal of adverse but unjustified criticism in the literature of Angle's classification. Because of Angle's classification, the ranks of orthodontists have grown from a handful to nearly five thousand American Association members in this country alone. Planning treatment for a malocclusion without giving classification a prominent role in the diagnosis is like planning a trip without a map.

The average dentist referring a patient to an orthodontist cannot classify the patient's malocclusion. If he does not know the classification, he certainly *should* refer the patient to the orthodontist. If more dentists are to treat incipient orthodontic problems with any degree of success, it is important that they be able to classify malocclusion.

From the standpoint of preventive orthodontics, some class I cases, but not all,

UNIVERSITY OF ALABAMA SCHOOL OF DENTISTRY

Orthodontic Examination and Case History

Name _____ Age _____ Sex _____ Race _____ Date _____

Address _____ Phone _____ Case # _____

Musical instrument _____

HEALTH OF PATIENT

Present health _____

Has patient ever been very sick?

　　　　　　　　　　　　yes ☐ no ☐

With what? _____ age ___

Has patient ever been in hosp.?

　　　　　　　　　　　　yes ☐ no ☐

With what? _____

Is patient under special care of physician now? _____ yes ☐ no ☐

For what? _____

Is patient taking any special drug?

　　　　　　　　　　　　yes ☐ no ☐

What is it for? _____

Oral hygiene:　　good ☐ fair ☐ poor ☐

Instructions given _____

MOUTH, NOSE & THROAT

Caries rate:　　Mild ☐ Med. ☐ Exten. ☐

Breathe through both nostrils?

　　　　　　　　　　　　yes ☐ no ☐

If "no" why? _____

Any allergy _____

Many attacks of colds?　　yes ☐ no ☐

Tonsils or adenoids out?　　yes ☐ no ☐

UPPER LIP:		LOWER LIP:	
Normal	☐	Normal	☐
Short	☐	Short	☐
Functional	☐	Functional	☐
Nonfunctional	☐	Nonfunctional	☐

Mentalis:

　Normal　　☐　　Hyperactive　☐

Swallowing:

　Normal　　☐　　Abnormal　　☐

Mouth breathing:

　All time　☐　　Night only　☐

Other musculature _____

PRESENT DIET

Adequate　　　☐　　Inadequate　☐

Between meals:　yes ☐　　　　　no ☐

Sweets:　　　　yes ☐　　　　　no ☐

Soft drinks:　　yes ☐　　　　　no ☐

How often _____

ETIOLOGY

Habits

Thumb	_____	Mouth breathing	_____
Finger	_____	Foreign body	_____
Tongue	_____	Imitations	_____
Swallowing	_____	Other	_____

Missing teeth _____

Supernumerary _____

Malformed _____

Frenum space _____

Premature loss of dec. _____

Tardy erupt. of perman. _____

Poor dental restorations _____

Prolonged ret. of dec. teeth _____

Poor dental restorations _____

Loss of perman. teeth _____

Musical instrument _____

Relative with similar condition _____

Other factors _____

UPPER

Median line open:

　　　　　　　　right ☐ left ☐ center ☐

LOWER

Median line open:

　　　　　　　　right ☐ left ☐ center ☐

Median line closed:

　　　　　　　　right ☐ left ☐ center ☐

CLASSIFICATION _____

Dates:　　*before, progress, after, ret.*

Models	___	___	___	___
Photos.	___	___	___	___
Intra-orals	___	___	___	___
Cephalo-metrics	___	___	___	___

Figure 15–1　Example of a form that has proved useful for recording findings of the orthodontic examination and the case history.

can be treated without referral. All class II and class III malocclusions should be referred to the orthodontist. In cases of class II or III malocclusions, the orthodontist who will take over the case eventually, may advise the dentist to hold open spaces or take other interceptive measures. This procedure is acceptable provided the parents understand that further definitive orthodontic measures must be taken by the orthodontist.

Above all, the welfare of the patient must be considered. In setting the limits for testing one's abilities and experience, professional ethics and personal morality are the ultimate guides.

A classification can usually be made at the time of the examination. If there is some question about the classification, study models are a big help. There is no point, however, in making elaborate measurements and calculations for unerupted teeth if the case falls into a category which the dentist will send to the specialist anyway.

It would be rather short-sighted to use Angle's classification just as he used it sixty years ago. There are many modern diagnostic adjuncts now which were not available to Angle. Some of his premises were false, such as that of the stability of the maxillary first permanent molars. So Angle's original concept of his classification must be considered in the light of historical significance. Brought up to date, these concepts still may serve us well.

CLASS I

In a class I malocclusion, when the molars are in their correct relationship in the individual arches and the dental arches close in a smooth arc to occlusal position, the mesiobuccal cusp of the maxillary first permanent molar will be in correct mesiodistal relation to the buccal or mesiobuccal groove of the mandibular first permanent molar. (The correct position will depend to some extent on the occlusion of the deciduous molars, if they are still present. See Chapter 14, Face Development and Tooth Eruption.)

CLASS II

In a class II malocclusion, when the molars are in their correct position in the individual arches, and the dental arches close in a smooth arc to centric position, the mesiobuccal cusp of the maxillary first permanent molar will be in relation to the embrasure between the mandibular second premolar and the mandibular first molar. In other words the lower arch occludes distal to the upper arch, as exemplified by the occlusion of the molars. Angle recognized two divisions of class II according to the inclination of the maxillary incisors. He also recognized the existence of a class II relationship on one side and a class I relationship on the other side, which he called a subdivision. In general, orthodontists feel a subdivision case is more difficult to correct.

CLASS III

In a class III malocclusion, when the molars are in their correct position in the individual arches and the dental arches close in a smooth arc to centric position, the mesiobuccal cusp of the maxillary first permanent molar will be in relation to the distobuccal groove of the mandibular first permanent molar, or to the buccal embrasure between the mandibular first and second molars, or even further distal. In other words, the lower jaw occludes mesial to the upper jaw, as exemplified by the occlusion of the molars. Angle also recognized a one-sided condition in this class, which he referred to as a class III subdivision when the molars on one side follow the class III pattern and the molars on the other side meet normally in the mesiodistal relation.

RECOGNITION AND MANAGEMENT OF CLASS I MALOCCLUSIONS

Examining the definition for class I malocclusion will disclose some important criteria for a correct classification. First of all, "the molars are in correct relationship in the individual arches." If a maxillary second primary molar, or even a first molar, has been lost early, with subsequent drifting of the maxillary first permanent molar, the case is not necessarily a class II malocclusion (Fig. 15–6B). If the permanent molar drifts, it will usually drift more on the buccal than on the lingual. Therefore, mentally repositioning the molar will call for backward and turning movements of the tooth before a correct classification can be made. If there is any question, study models will allow the dentist to see the occlusion from the lingual. In normal occlusion the mesiolingual cusp of the maxillary first permanent molar should be in the central fossa of the mandibular first permanent molar.

The next criterion is: "the dental arches close in a smooth arc to occlusal position." This implies that there is no cuspal or joint interference with the closing motion. This closing act is a very important criterion in examination for malocclusion. As was mentioned earlier, any shift of the mandible in closing should be noted and taken into consideration in the eventual classification.

The occlusal position may exhibit lower incisors anterior to upper incisors. The path they take in arriving there may mean the difference between a class III and a class I type 3 malocclusion. Class I type 3 will usually show an interruption in the smooth arc of closing when the incisors meet edge to edge. From the edge to edge position the jaw has to shift forward in order to get the molars into occlusion. The class III malocclusion will usually show closure in a smooth arc from the wide open to the occlusal position, with the lower incisors anterior to the upper incisors. A patient with a posterior crossbite, or class I type 4, should be watched from the front during closure for a jaw shift prior to the arrival of the mandible at the occlusal position. If there is no jaw shift and the midlines are symmetrical, a single posterior tooth in crossbite might be expected to respond to simple treatment.

If there is a lateral jaw shift in closing, the patient with a posterior crossbite should be instructed to open wide, place the tongue as far back in the roof of the mouth as possible and close slowly until the teeth barely touch. At this point close examination of the mouth may reveal that the buccal cusps of both upper first molars are touching the tips of the buccal cusps of both lower first molars. When the patient is told to close all the way he slides laterally into his acquired crossbite. Such a situation would call for bilateral expansion of the maxillary dental arch, and the dentist has to make up his mind whether to tackle this or to refer the case to the orthodontist. Judicious spot grinding of interfering primary canines will often simplify the management of such a problem.

While the patient with a crossbite is in the initial contact position it is well to check again the mesiodistal relation of the molars for classification purposes. In a lateral mandibular shift, one condyle rotates, while the other condyle moves forward, thereby shifting teeth mesially on that side. Thus models of teeth in the full closed position do not represent the true mesiodistal relationship of the dental arches as they will be exhibited when the tooth contact interference is corrected.

The third criterion is: "The mesiobuccal cusp of the maxillary first permanent molar will be in correct mesiodistal relation to the buccal or mesiobuccal groove of the mandibular first permanent molar." Many dentists use this as the sole criterion in classifying. Without the two previous qualifying phrases, however, a judgment based on this criterion will be false in many cases. It is made without taking into account the knowledge gained since Angle originally thought of the molars as being fixed and correct in the individual arches. Notice that the Angle classification refers only to the mesiodistal relationship of the molars. It does not involve buccolingual relationships.

This brings us to the types of class I malocclusion. (The Dewey-Anderson modification of Angle's classification should be well known.) This discussion of the various types of class I malocclusion will indicate in broad terms the types that might be amenable to preventive orthodontic treatment.

Class I Type 1

Class I type 1 is a malocclusion that may have crowded and rotated incisors with no room for permanent canines or premolars in their proper position (Fig. 15–2). Quite often severe class I type 1 cases are complicated by many rotations and severe axial inclinations of teeth. The local cause for this condition appears to be too much tooth material for the size of the jawbones; the initiating cause is usually considered to be heredity.

The orthodontist treats this type of case in one of three ways or a combination of these ways: (1) He may expand the dental arch laterally or (2) he may expand it anteroposteriorly, in an effort to make the bony support equal to the quantity of

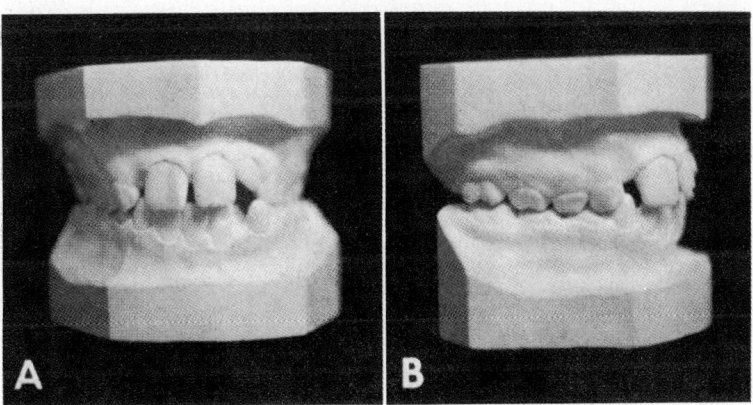

Figure 15–2 *A,* Class I type 1 case at age 7 years. There is not enough room for the maxillary right lateral incisor or the mandibular left lateral incisor. Midlines are off in opposite directions. *B,* Uprightness of deciduous canines helps confirm that there has been negligible mesial drifting of posterior segments. The condition is not subject to prevention. This is already a full-fledged orthodontic problem.

tooth substance, or (3) he may elect to remove some teeth in order to make the quantity of tooth substance equal to the bony supports.

Most class I type 1 cases should be referred to the orthodontist. The exceptions in the class I type 1 category which may be corrected, or at least improved, by preventive measures include some cases in the mixed dentition.

1. Mild anterior crowding can be relieved by slicing the mesial side of the primary canines.
2. A slight lack of room for the first premolar can be remedied by slicing the mesial of the second primary molar.
3. Finally, the use of separating wires on either side of a second premolar with almost enough room to erupt sometimes allows the tooth to erupt into its correct position.

Many "serial extraction" cases are class I type 1 cases. Almost all of them need some mechanical therapy before they are finished, and their treatment should ordinarily be left to the orthodontist.

Class I Type 2

Class I type 2 displays a correct jaw relationship as shown by the molar occlusion, if all previously mentioned criteria can be made to apply. The maxillary incisors are procumbent and spaced. Previous or current thumb sucking is often the initiating cause. The incisors are in an unsightly position and liable to fracture. This type of class I case can be treated by the general practitioner and the pedodontist (Fig. 15–3).

Class I Type 3

Class I type 3 involves one or more maxillary incisors lingually locked in crossbite. The lower jaw is shoved forward by the patient after initial contact of the incisors in order to get full closure. This situation can usually be corrected with inclines of one type or another. Regimented tongue blade exercise is the simplest method, if full cooperation can be expected. There must be room for the maxillary teeth to move labially, or for both upper and lower teeth to move reciprocally (Fig. 15–4).

Class I Type 4

Class I type 4 exhibits a posterior crossbite. Within limitations previously described, many crossbites involving one or two posterior teeth in each arch can be successfully treated without referral to the orthodontist, provided there is room for the tooth or teeth to move (Fig.15–5).

Class I Type 5

Class I type 5 often looks quite a bit like class I type 1. The essential difference is in the local etiology. In class I type 5, it is assumed that once upon a time there was room for all of the teeth. Drifting of teeth has deprived other teeth of the room

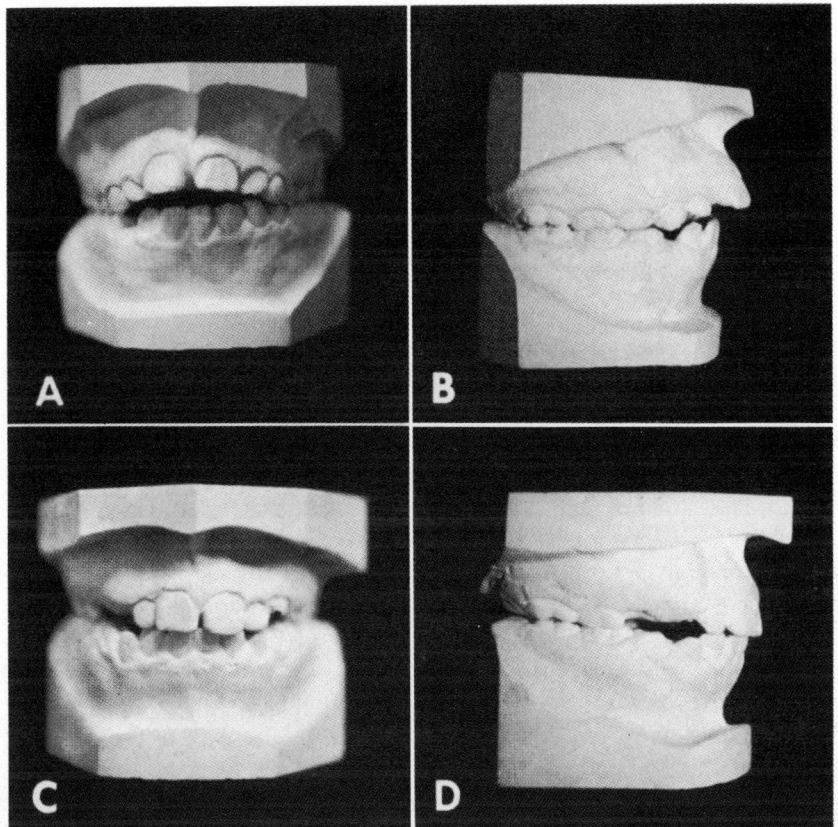

Figure 15–3   *A,* A class I type 2 case, amenable to simple therapy without bands or wires. Flared and spaced incisors due to thumb sucking. *B,* Ridge-groove relationship, plus axial inclinations of posterior teeth, confirm the case as a class I. *C,* Same case after five months. The only appliance ever used was an oral screen at night. *D,* Note that the mandibular permanent canine now has room (see Chap. 14, pp. 326 and 330).

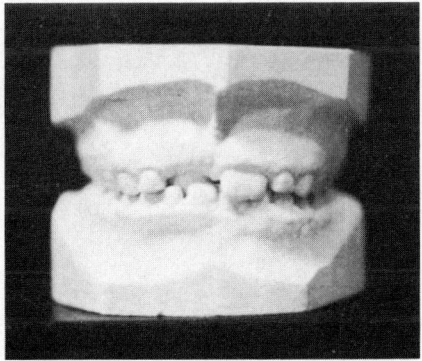

Figure 15–4   A class I type 3 case (sometimes called a pseudoclass III). There is plenty of room for the maxillary right central incisor to be moved over by simple means.

they need. Sometimes the crowding occurs more posteriorly (Fig. 15–6). One late stage may show the second premolars erupted toward the lingual.

In contradistinction to class I type 1, more cases of class I type 5 are amenable to preventive treatment. Take, for example, the case of a child who has lost a lower second primary molar early. A space maintainer was recommended, but the mother did not have the prescription filled. At the next regularly scheduled visit, the dentist pointed out the loss of space. The lower first molar was tipping forward and the second premolar was not in sight. The molar relationship may look like class III on that side. This is an instance where previous study models were definitely a help in convincing the mother that the dentist was right in having recommended a space maintainer earlier.

An x-ray taken at this time might show the first permanent molar tilted mesially, and the first premolar drifted distally or not. The position of the unerupted second premolar is, of course, important. Usually if there is room it can erupt into position. The position of the unerupted second permanent molar is of considerable importance. If the first permanent molar is to be positioned backward, either by an active fixed maintainer, an active removable maintainer or by separating wires, there must be room between the first molar and the second molar. Otherwise, backward tipping of the first molar may cause embarrassing impaction of the second molar. Within the above limitations, many potentially severe malocclusions can be prevented, even at such a late stage in the development.

A knowledge of classification enables the dentist to pick those cases for treatment with which he has the most reasonable chances for success. The range of operation is quite broad. There are more class I malocclusions than any other kind, and many if not most of these can be prevented from becoming full-fledged orthodontic problems.

Once it has been determined that a case falls into the class I category, the various analyses available for arch space-tooth size ratios can be applied. These analyses will be a help in determining if enough space can be saved by simple space maintenance, by active space maintenance, by slicing of deciduous cuspids or deciduous molars, or a combination of these methods.

In conclusion, let it be emphasized that often these conditions do not

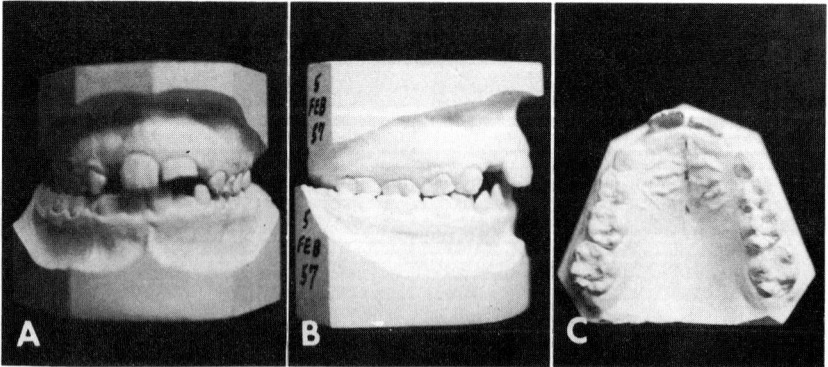

Figure 15–5   *A,* Class I type 4 case. Broken incisor needs repair. *B,* Mandibular shift to the right gives the impression of a distal relationship of the mandibular teeth. When the patient closes to initial contact, with the tongue far back in the roof of the mouth, the mesiodistal relation of the teeth is class I. *C,* Bilateral symmetry of maxillary arch indicates bilateral expansion is necessary to correct the crossbite.

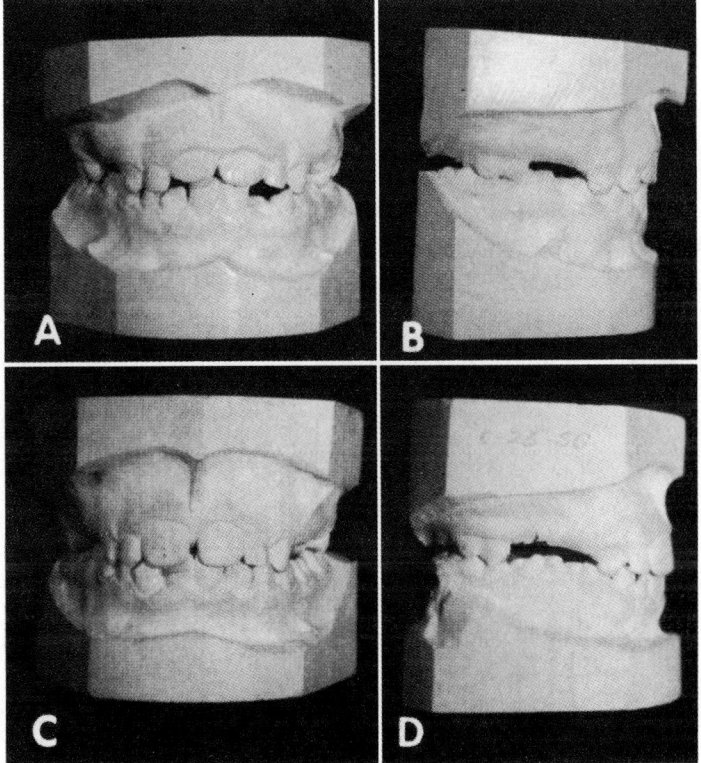

Figure 15–6 *A,* Class I type 5. *B,* Mesial drift of maxillary first permanent molar, after early loss of deciduous molars. Cuspid relationship confirms a class I situation. *C,* Same case five months later. *D,* Permanent molars now in correct relationship. Space between deciduous maxillary canine and maxillary first permanent molar has increased by 4½ mm. An active removable wire and plastic appliance was used to regain the lost space. (Courtesy of Dr. Wilson C. Bellenger.)

occur singly. The operator should not let one glaring situation dominate his treatment plan to the exclusion of other obvious conditions which need correction. For instance, in the example of the posterior crossbite (Fig. 15–5) the patient would also need disking of the mesial of the lower deciduous canines and protection for the fractured maxillary left central incisor. This patient is not only a class I type 4, but also a class I type 1, and needs treatment accordingly.

REFERENCE

Anderson, George M.: Practical Orthodontics. St. Louis, C. V. Mosby Co., 1960, p. 144.

16

PREVENTIVE ORTHODONTICS

by H. PERRY HITCHCOCK

By tradition and repetition the term "preventive orthodontics" is, to many, limited to procedures implied by the term "space maintenance." Preventive orthodontics certainly encompasses space maintenance, but speculatively it involves much more. The speculation comes in deciding whether certain measures belong within the scope of the general practitioner or whether they are full-fledged orthodontic procedures to be handled by the specialist.

This chapter will not deal with all of the orthodontic procedures which may legally or ethically be used by the general practitioner. It will indicate some simple procedures which will involve a minimum of instruments, time, and materials. These procedures will be indicated in cases where intervention may prevent or make less severe certain conditions which, if left unattended, would reasonably be expected to develop into full-fledged orthodontic problems.

SPACE MAINTAINERS

TYPES OF SPACE MAINTAINERS

Space maintainers may be classified in various ways:
1. Removable or fixed or semi-fixed.
2. With bands or without bands.
3. Functional or nonfunctional. (Can the patient chew on part of it?)
4. Active or passive. (Is the maintainer supposed to move teeth?)
5. Certain combinations of the above.

INDICATIONS FOR SPACE MAINTAINERS

If lack of a space maintainer would lead to a malocclusion, or to the encouragement of detrimental habits, or to psychic trauma, then a space maintainer is indicated. Placing maintainers routinely will do less harm than routinely not placing them.

1. When a second primary molar is lost before the second premolar is ready to take its place, use a space maintainer.

A space maintainer need not be used if the second premolar is already erupting or gives every indication by roentgenography that it soon will erupt.

The amount of space between the first molar and the first premolar may be greater than the roentgenographic width of the second premolar. This would allow a greater than usual late mesial shift of the first permanent molar and would still provide room for the second premolar to erupt. In this event, the space should be measured by means of dividers. Then, preferably monthly, the space should be measured and compared with the original measurement. If it is closing at a more rapid rate than the second premolar is erupting, insert a space maintainer.

2. The preceding method, with measuring and waiting, may be enough to take care of early loss of the first primary molar. Statistics indicate that space closure following premature loss of the first primary molar is less in degree and frequency than that following premature loss of the second primary molar.[6] Nevertheless, statistics applied to the total population, however comforting, should not lead to the neglect of a situation which can give trouble in an individual case.

3. In the case of congenitally missing second premolars it is probably better to let the permanent molar drift forward naturally and fill the space. It is better to make this decision later than early, since sometimes the second premolars are not bilaterally symmetric in the time of their development. Some do not show on the roentgenogram until 6 or 7 years of age.

4. Maxillary lateral incisors are very often congenitally missing. Almost always a mesially drifted cuspid can be dressed down to make a better looking lateral replacement than a fixed bridge in a space held open. Let the space close up.

5. Early loss of anterior primary teeth should be remedied by the placing of a space maintainer. Many sources indicate that the location of the developing permanent teeth prevents closure in the anterior part of the arch. *This is not true in all cases.* Not only may space close, with loss of arch continuity, but other factors enter the picture. The tongue will seek out spaces and thus habits may be encouraged. Defects in speech may be accentuated and prolonged. The absence of teeth in the front of the mouth before their loss in other children of the same age makes that child different and handicapped psychologically, if his temperament is vulnerable.

6. Many individuals are still in childhood when they lose one or more of their first permanent molars. This situation is deplored but in many sections of the country it is an actuality. If the loss should occur several years before the due eruption of the second permanent molar, the latter may move forward and erupt into normal occlusion, taking the place of the first permanent molar. If the second permanent molar is already erupted or partially erupted than there are two choices. Move the second molar forward orthodontically (in this case, probably by an orthodontist), or hold the space open for a permanent bridge later on.

7. If the second primary molar is lost only a little while before the eruption of

the first permanent molar, a bulge on the crest of the alveolar ridge will indicate the site of eruption of the first permanent molar (Fig. 16–1*A*). Roentgenograms will help to determine the distance from the distal surface of the first primary molar to the mesial surface of the unerupted first permanent molar. A removable inactive functional space maintainer constructed to impinge on the gingival tissue just anterior to the mesial surface of the unerupted first permanent molar is particularly useful in a bilateral case of this kind, or even when the first primary molar is lost on the other side (Fig. 16–1*B*). Reinforcing the anchorage of the labial bow with self-curing acrylic resin helps to keep the free-saddle distal end in contact with the alveolar ridge.

8. Most of the above situations in which space maintenance is indicated would make use of passive maintainers. There are situations in which an active maintainer can be used to advantage by the general practitioner. When a patient comes to the practitioner for the first time and it is found by manual examination and by roentgenography that there is not enough room for the lower second premolar but that there is a space between the first premolar and the cuspid, the first premolar is slanting distally and is in end to end relationship with the maxillary first premolar—an active space maintainer is useful here. It will open a space for the second premolar and restore the first premolar to normal occlusion.

An active space maintainer may be used to push distally or upright a first permanent molar that has moved or tipped mesially, preventing the eruption of the second premolar.

SELECTION OF SPACE MAINTAINERS

Generally speaking, most space maintenance can be accomplished by inserting removable, passive space maintainers made of wire and acrylic resin. The use of self-curing acrylic makes this an easy, fast office procedure. Bands are involved in the use of some space maintainers. The general practitioner usually shuns the making of bands, but band making is certainly not as complicated as some other procedures accomplished by the dentist. A well fitting tailor-made band, con-

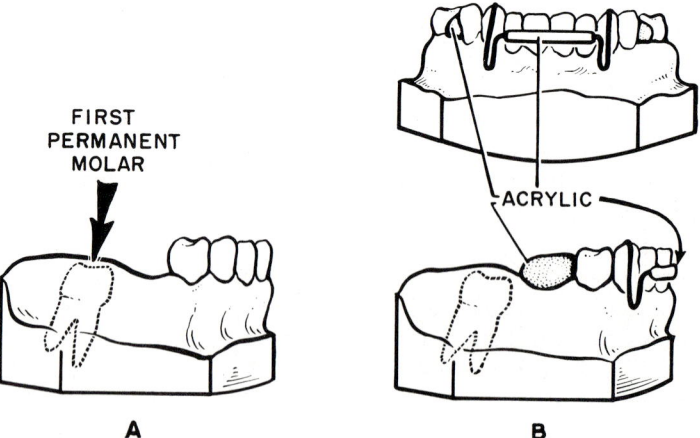

FIRST
PERMANENT
MOLAR

ACRYLIC

A

B

Figure 16–1   Loss of second primary molar just prior to eruption of first permanent molar.

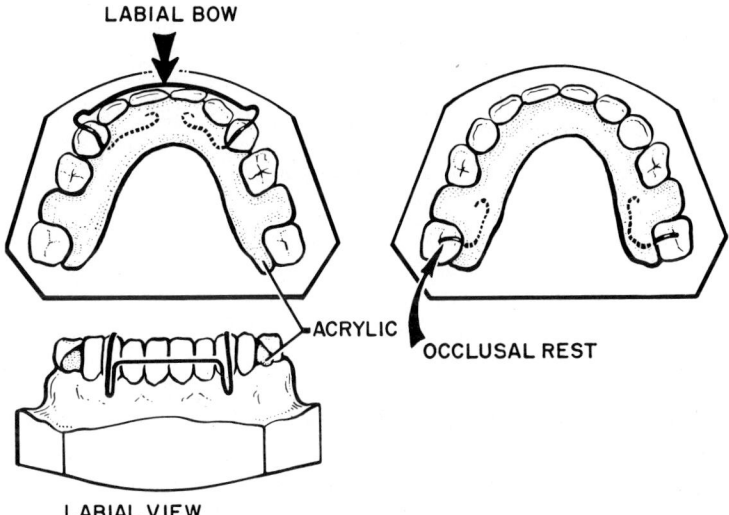

LABIAL BOW

ACRYLIC

OCCLUSAL REST

LABIAL VIEW

Figure 16–2 Simple retention for space maintainers.

structed in the patient's mouth, is usually more satisfactory than one made on a stone model by a commercial laboratory. Even preformed bands available in different sizes can be used advantageously by the dentist.

The loss of a second primary molar can usually be remedied by inserting a removable acrylic and wire space maintainer. This may replace loss on one or both sides. This might be made with or without a labial bow (Fig. 16–2), but occlusal rests on the molars (if present) are recommended, particularly in the lower arch of a unilateral case. The rest will prevent the maintainer from slipping down into the floor of the mouth.

The advantages of a removable type of space maintainer are as follows:

1. It is easy to clean.
2. It permits the teeth to be cleaned.
3. It maintains or restores vertical dimension.
4. It can be used in combination with other preventive procedures.
5. It can be worn part time, allowing circulation of the blood to the soft tissues.
6. It can be made esthetically desirable.
7. It facilitates chewing and speaking.
8. It helps keep the tongue in bounds.
9. It stimulates eruption of permanent teeth.
10. Band construction is not necessary.
11. Dental check-ups for caries are easily made.
12. Room can be made for eruption of teeth without making a new appliance.

The disadvantages of a removable space maintainer are:

1. It may be lost.
2. The patient may not wear it.
3. It can be broken.
4. It may restrict lateral growth of the jaw, if clasps are incorporated.
5. It may irritate the soft tissue.

Disadvantages 1, 2, and 3 point up the necessity of impressing upon the parent and the child the importance of the maintainer and the cost of replacement.

Usually if the space is filled with a reasonable facsimile of a tooth, the space maintainer becomes esthetically desirable and the maintainer and child are parted with difficulty.

If a crossbite seems to be developing (disadvantage 4), then it may be feasible to dispense with molar clasps and shift to anterior retention or interproximal spurs. Or, a new maintainer may be necessary to meet changing oral configuration.

Irritation to the soft tissue (disadvantage 5) may necessitate the substitution of a fixed or semi-fixed maintainer, although usually this situation can be fully or partially eliminated by making the removable space maintainer partly tooth-borne.

CONSTRUCTION OF SPACE MAINTAINERS WITHOUT BANDS

Construction of removable, functional, passive space maintainers should be kept as simple as possible. It is time saving to the dentist and the lower cost makes the benefits of the service available to more people.

The Labial Bow

Often a simple labial bow (Fig. 16–4A) is the only wire bending involved. This aids in keeping the appliance in the mouth, and in the upper jaw keeps the anterior teeth from moving forward.

Other things being equal, in a case with normal jaw relation and a deep or medium overbite, a labial bow is not necessary in a lower space maintainer. Forward migration of the lower anterior teeth will be inhibited by the lingual surfaces of the maxillary anteriors.

Because the labial bow is used for retention, it should be far enough toward the gingiva to accomplish this, but should not impinge on the interdental papillae. The passage of the wire from labial to lingual may pose some problem. Usually it can go in the occlusal embrasure between the lateral incisor and the cuspid, or distal to the cuspid. Ordinarily, if the labial bow includes the incisors, sufficient retention is obtainable. Cases arise, however, in which there will be occlusal interference by the wire. Examination of models, or natural teeth in occlusion, may indicate that it would be better to bend the wire directly over the cusp of the canine (Fig. 16–3) and follow closely the lingual ridge on the upper model, or the labial ridge on the lower. This is possible where the lingual ridge on the upper canine is opposite a labial embrasure in the lower arch or the labial ridge of a lower canine is opposite a lingual embrasure in the upper arch, when the teeth are in occlusion. The problem of fitting the wire is also a function of the size of the wire used.

Ordinarily 0.032 or 0.028 chrome nickel wire will be used. If occlusal interference is a problem, 0.026 stainless steel wire may be used. It is harder to bend than the Nichrome, so it will not distort as easily and a smaller size may be used.

Occlusal Rests

The next item of complexity would be the addition of occlusal rests on the molars (Fig. 16–2). These may be advisable in the lower jaw even though a labial bow is not used.

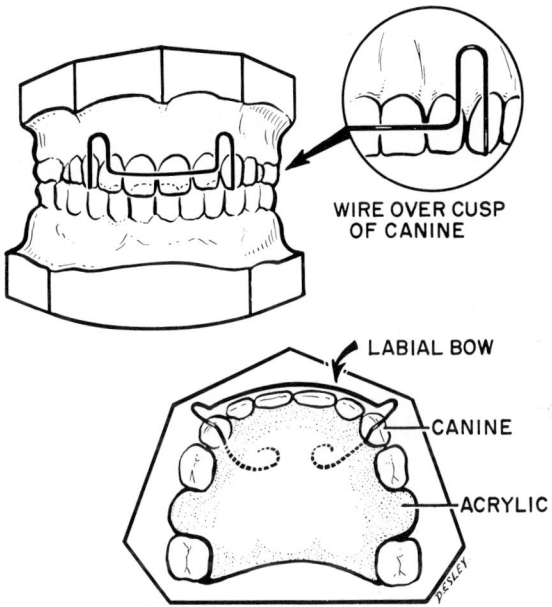

WIRE OVER CUSP
OF CANINE

LABIAL BOW

CANINE

ACRYLIC

Figure 16–3   Labial bow bent to avoid occlusal interference in the opposite arch.

Interproximal Spurs

After occlusal rests would come interproximal spurs for additional retention (Fig. 16–4*B*). In the lower, retention is not usually a problem, but owing to the child's constant playing with his tongue or inability to keep the maintainer in while eating, a labial bow and interproximal spurs may be necessary, as well as occlusal rests.

Clasps

Progressively complex are clasps. Clasps may be simple or of the modified Crozat type. Where space maintenance only is involved, the more complicated, super-retentive, modified Crozat is not usually necessary. Simple clasps may be interproximal clasps or wrap-around clasps. Interproximal clasps cross over the occlusal embrasure from the lingual acrylic and terminate by means of a loop in the buccal embrasure (Fig. 16–4*C*). Because of tooth contour, the wrap-around clasp should usually terminate with its free end to the mesial surface (Fig. 16–4*D*). Axial inclination and other possible factors may influence one to let the free end be distal.

Exclusive of retention, there is another reason for using or not using clasps. This involves the buccal-lingual relationship of opposing teeth. The presence of acrylic on only the lingual aspect of a tooth will often make this tooth move buccally.

For example, Figure 16–5*A* illustrates a case in which there is a problem of space maintenance in the upper jaw *plus* an end to end cusp relation, buccolingually, of the opposing molars. It would be advantageous, if possible, to dispense with clasps in the upper jaw in order to permit the maxillary molar to

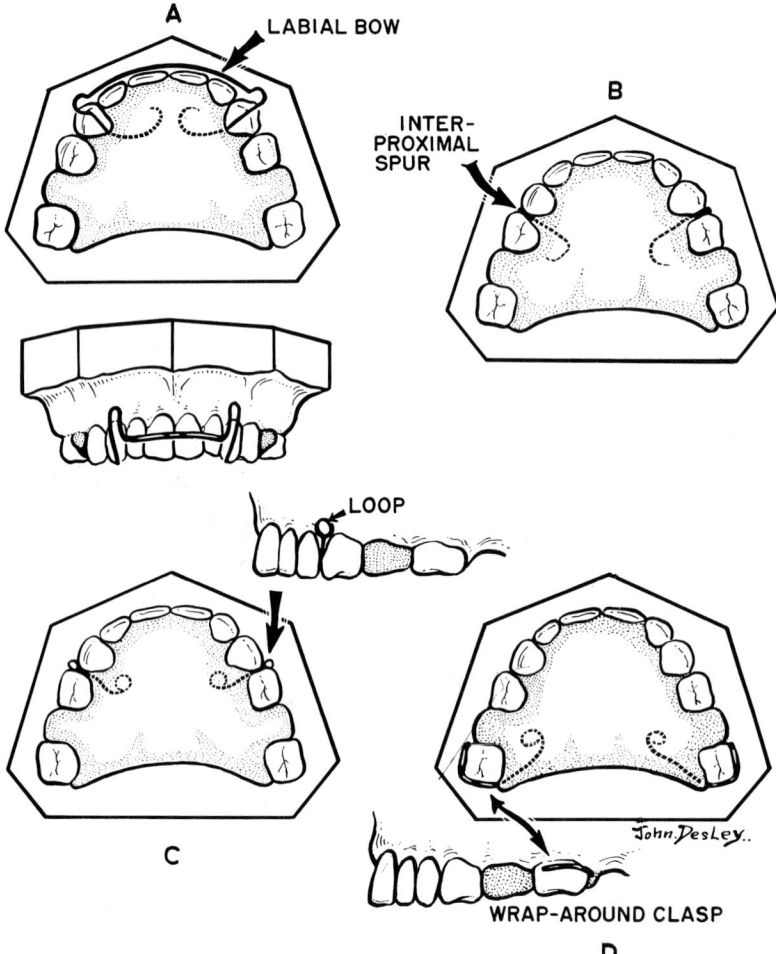

Figure 16–4 *A* through *D* show progressively complex means of retention.

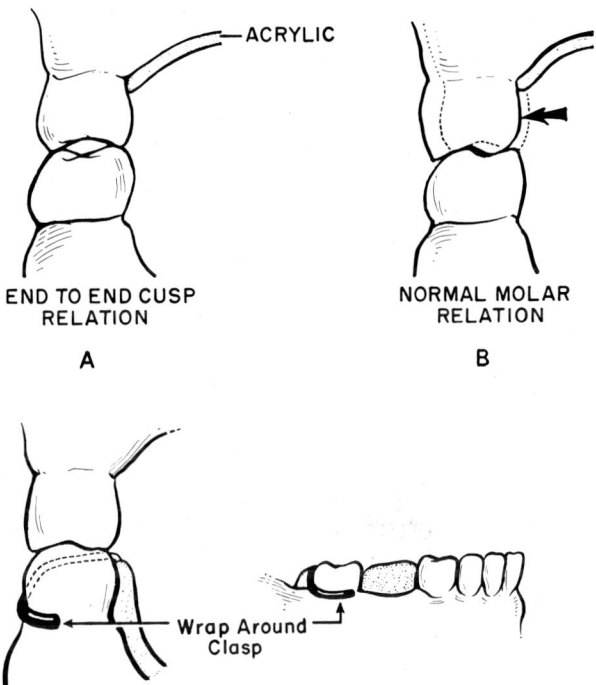

Figure 16–5 Rationale for clasping or non-clasping when a cusp to cusp molar relation exists buccolingually.

move buccally, either as a natural growth phenomenon or because of the influence of the lingual acrylic.

If, however, the space problem is confined to the lower jaw but the same molar relation exists as previously cited, a clasp on the lower molar would inhibit lateral movement of the lower molar. This would prevent a crossbite and even allow the maxillary molar to achieve normal buccolingual molar relation by natural physiologic expansion, if potentially present (Fig. 16–5B).

Sometimes the maxillary molars are almost in complete buccal version to the mandibular molars. This condition borders on what may be referred to as a "reverse crossbite." In such an instance, if space maintenance is a problem in the upper arch, clasps on the molars may inhibit further lateral movement. This, in combination with natural physiologic expansion in the lower jaw (if potentially present), may achieve normal buccolingual molar relation.

SPACE MAINTAINERS WITH BANDS

Considering the advantages of acrylic removable space maintainers, there have to be excellent reasons for using bands.

One such reason is lack of cooperation by the patient from the standpoint of loss, breakage, or failure to wear the maintainer. In such a case, bands are used as part of the appliance.

Another use for bands is in unilateral loss of primary molars. Here, both teeth on either side of the space may be banded and a bar may be soldered between them

(Fig. 16–6*A*) or a loop and band combination may be used (Fig. 16–6*B*). Sometimes a single band will suffice in a unilateral case. This is particularly true in early loss of a second primary molar before the first permanent molar erupts. If possible, the band on the first primary molar should be made, and an impression of the quadrant taken, with the band in place, before extraction of the second primary molar. Then, on the poured-up model, a wire can be soldered to the distal side of the band and bent down into the distal aspect of the socket of the second primary molar (cut out from the model) (Fig. 16–7).

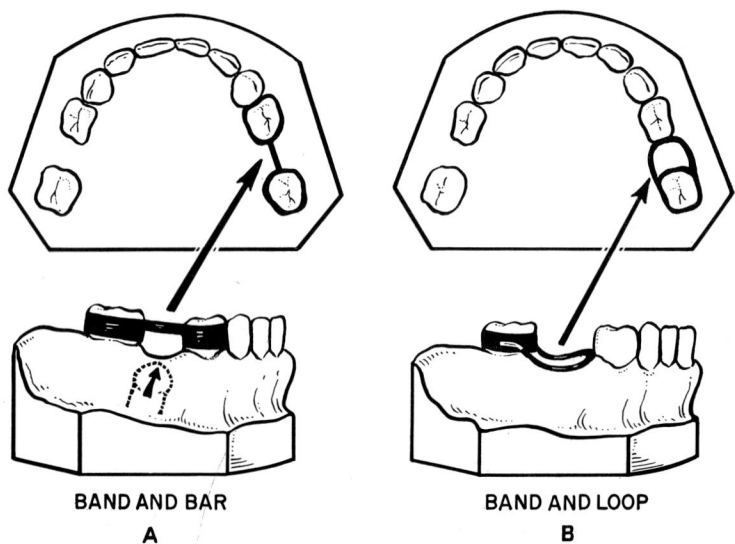

BAND AND BAR   BAND AND LOOP
A   B

Figure 16–6   Two types of space maintainers utilizing bands.

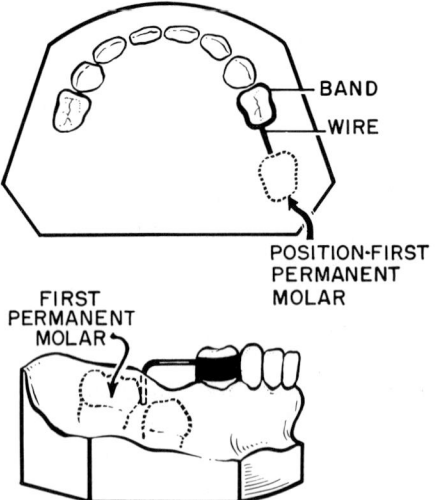

Figure 16–7   Space maintainer for guiding eruption of first permanent molar.

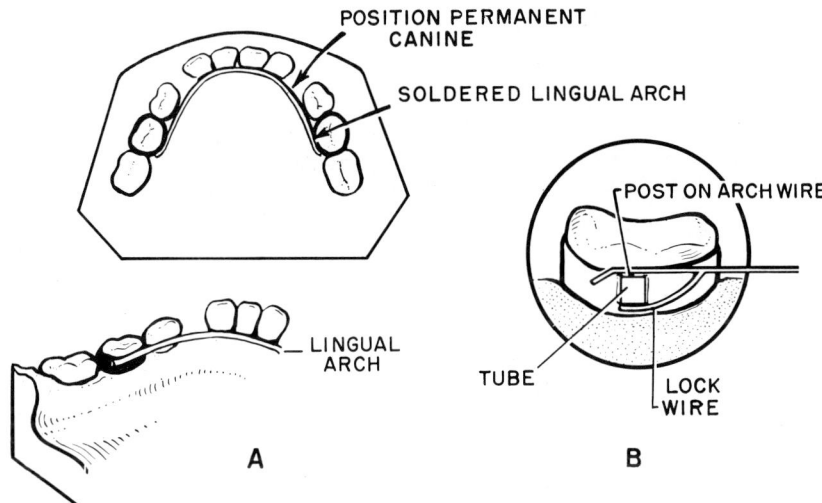

Figure 16–8   Fixed or semi-fixed space maintainers utilizing a lingual arch wire.

The removal of the second primary molar is accomplished with the space maintainer ready to be cemented on the first primary molar. With the socket sponged for visibility, the wire can be adjusted to touch the mesial surface of the usually visible first permanent molar.

If the dentist sees the patient only after the second primary molar is out, the proper length and bend of the wire can be estimated by examining the roentgenogram. The band is placed in the mouth and the position of the wire in the punctured tissue is checked roentgenographically.

Early loss of primary cuspids is sometimes accomplished artificially, in order to let the central and lateral incisors rotate and move forward into their proper position. If this is done early, there is danger that the posterior segments will move mesially, blocking out the room for the permanent canines and premolars. A fixed, banded, nonfunctional passive maintainer is indicated here (Fig. 16–8A). The use of molar bands on the second primary molars and a soldered lingual arch, adapted to the junction of the cingulum and gingiva of the incisors, will hold the space open. Use of vertical lingual tubes and posts soldered to the lingual arch would make this a semi-fixed maintainer (Fig. 16–8B). This usually is not necessary, if space maintenance is the only object to be accomplished. Tongue pressure plus natural development will usually allow the central and lateral incisors to straighten themselves out before the permanent canines and premolars erupt.

It is almost axiomatic that if a banded space maintainer of the above-mentioned type is to be used, then the second primary molars may be banded instead of the first permanent molars. Bands are easily made on second primary molars. Their position, more anterior than first permanent molars, and the fact that they erupt earlier than first permanent molars, give better access to the operator. The natural bell shape of the second primary molar lends itself to construction of a tight fitting, well contoured band.

Very often the amount of space needed to accommodate lower incisors is very slight. In such a case, the additional space is obtained by disking the mesial surfaces of the primary cuspids, rather than extracting them (Fig. 16–9). This procedure,

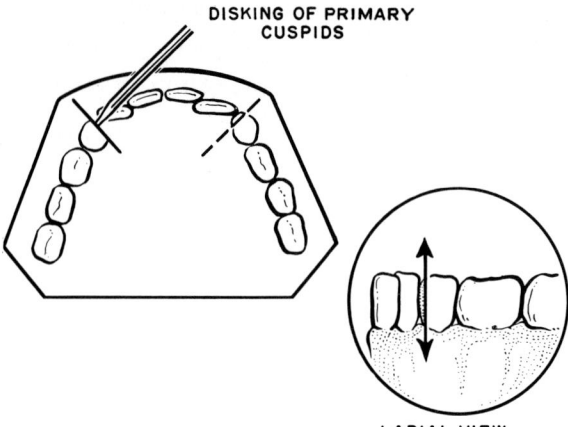

Figure 16-9 Disking mesial surface of primary cuspids to alleviate crowding of permanent incisors.

when applicable, eliminates the necessity for a space maintainer. Disking of primary teeth is beneficial in other situations, for example, when a maxillary first premolar is partially erupted and the maxillary permanent cuspid is also trying to erupt (Fig. 16-10). Disking the mesial surface of the maxillary second primary molar will allow the maxillary first premolar to move distally, under the influence of the erupting permanent canine. Care must be taken not to reduce the mesiodistal dimension of the second primary molar beyond the width of the unerupted second premolar.

Sometimes there is necessity for construction of a banded space maintainer in the anterior part of the mouth. Such an instance is represented by early loss of the maxillary primary central incisors. This maintainer should not be of a rigid type, as that would prevent any physiologic expansion of the maxillary arch in this region.

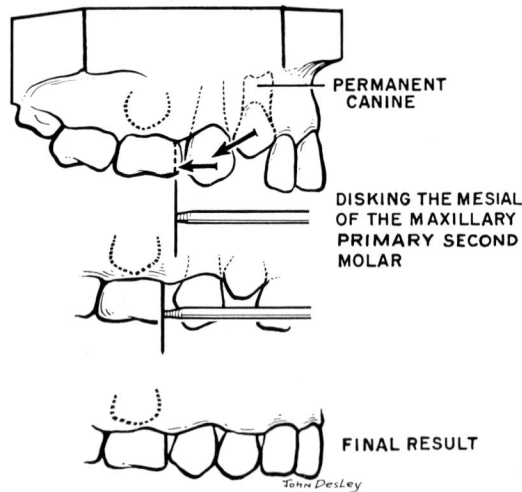

Figure 16-10 Disking mesial surface of primary second molar to allow room for permanent canine to erupt.

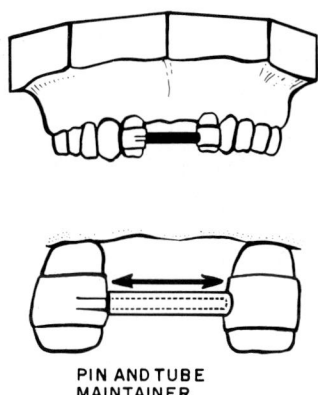

PIN AND TUBE
MAINTAINER

Figure 16–11   Anterior space maintainer that allows lateral growth.

The soldered pin and tube maintainer (Fig. 16–11) is possibly the best type here; the pin is allowed to slide partially out of the tube in response to lateral growth of the arch.

Retarded eruption of a permanent central incisor may call for a space maintainer. A pin and tube may be used here, and an acrylic tooth may be processed to the tube for esthetic purposes. Ordinarily, however, the removable, passive, acrylic maintainer with an artificial tooth suffices. It has the advantage of allowing natural, individual adjustment of the adjacent teeth, and the stimulation of the gingiva over the unerupted tooth may hasten eruption.

ACTUAL MOVEMENT OF TEETH

Preventive orthodontics involving actual movement of the teeth is the next consideration. Active space maintainers will be considered first. There are fixed and removable types in this category, also.

ACTIVE FIXED MAINTAINER

Consider a case (Fig. 16–12*A*) in which there is not enough room for a lower second premolar, but there is a space between the distally slanting first premolar and the cuspid, and the first molar is slanting slightly mesially.

A band is made on the first permanent molar. A spot welder, if available, is a helpful adjunct in construction of a band. The spot welder is also used to fix buccal and lingual tubes to the band. These tubes, about ¼ inch long, come equipped with flanges for spot welding, or precious-metal tubes may be soldered on the band. The band itself may be soldered, of course, if a spot welder is not available. The tubes should be parallel to one another in all planes, and their lumina should be aimed at the junction of the crown and gingiva on the first premolar.

An impression of the band and tubes is taken with the band seated on the tooth, and the band is then removed. The holes in the tubes are plugged with carding wax, to prevent stone from getting in them. The bands are seated in the impres-

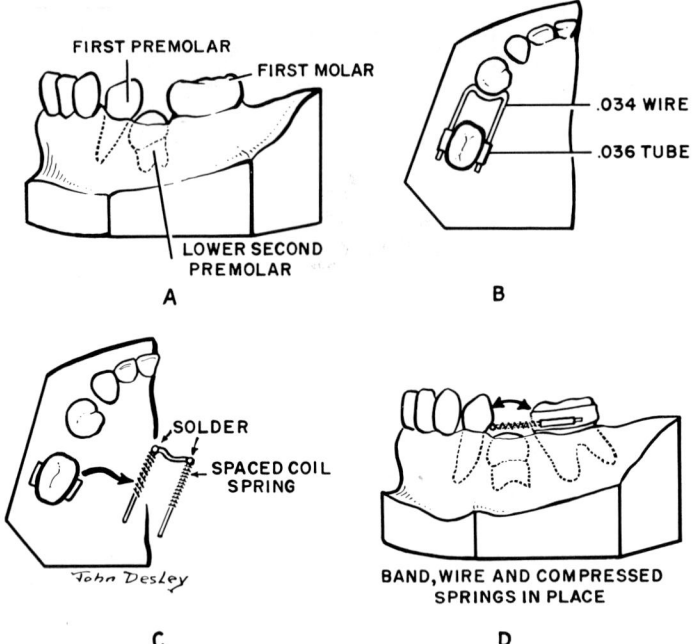

Figure 16–12   Regaining space for unerupted second premolar.

sion, and a model is poured up in green or buff stone. (Green stone is easier on the eyes.) A wire is bent to a U shape which will fit passively in both the buccal and the lingual tubes. The anterior curved part of the U should have a reverse bend where it contacts the distal outline of the first premolar (Fig. 16–12*B*). If the tubes have been aimed correctly, the wire will contact the distal surface of the first premolar below its greatest convexity. The size of the wire should be slightly smaller than the size of the tube; for instance, a 0.036 tube might be used with a 0.034 wire. A rectangular tube, if used, will readily accommodate a 0.0215 by 0.025 rectangular wire. These sizes are mentioned because they are easily obtained from the dental supply houses. A rectangular wire, however, is harder to bend.

At the junction of the straight part and the curved part of the wire, both buccally and lingually, flow enough solder to make a stop. Then cut enough spaced coil spring to extend from the stop to a point about 3/32 inch distal to the anterior limit of the tube on the molar (Fig. 16–12*C*). A 0.010 wire wrapped on a 0.036 spindle may be used. The band is removed from the model by heating the stone tooth inside the band, plunging the model into water, and carefully cutting away the resulting softened residue. The coil spring is slipped on the wire. The wire is put in the tubes and the band with the wire and compressed springs is cemented on the molar (Fig. 16–12*D*). The compressed springs try to become passive, and exert reciprocal pressure mesially to the premolar and distally to the molar.

A word about cementing a band: The tooth should be clean and dry. A thin coating of collodion, or sandarac or copalite varnish, will protect the tooth against initial decalcification from the free phosphoric acid in the cement before the cement hardens. Cement is mixed to the consistency for inlays, not the consistency for cement bases. The inside of the band is coated evenly with the cement and the thumb or finger is placed over the occlusal part of the band as the band is pushed into place. This forces the cement down around the tooth and squeezes it out gingivally.

Many special instruments can be obtained for final seating of the band, but a Mershon adaptor is usually adequate. A lower posterior band should be finally seated only from the buccal aspect (because of the lingual slant of the lower posterior teeth).

The band adaptor's serrated end is placed on the buccal occlusal edge of the band. A tongue blade is put on top of the band adaptor and the patient is asked to close (Fig. 16–13). The upper teeth close on the tongue blade, which transmits the pressure to the band adaptor and thence to the band, and the band moves down to its predetermined position.

On an upper band the seating pressure is applied both buccally and lingually, but on a lower band it is applied only from the buccal aspect.

After the cement has hardened, the excess, both occlusal and gingival, is chipped off with a hefty scaler.

ACTIVE REMOVABLE MAINTAINER

A removable wire and plastic space maintainer is sometimes used for the active backward repositioning movement of a molar to allow a second premolar to erupt.

A labial bow is constructed for the anterior teeth on the model.

On the affected side a U-shaped wire is bent to conform to the alveolar ridge between the first premolar and the molar. The mesial end of the U-shaped wire should have a small loop to be embedded in the lingual acrylic. The distal end is free and rests against the mesial surface of the molar (Fig. 16–14A). The curved part of the wire is adapted approximately to the buccal part of the alveolar ridge. Active distal pressure is obtained in the final product by flattening the wire. With an appliance of this type, additional retention is needed to keep the retainer in place.

On the opposite molar, a modified Crozat type clasp is constructed (Fig. 16–14B). It is modified to the extent that the 0.028 Nichrome wire clasp is not continuously adapted to the tooth on the lingual side but has two free ends, looped and embedded in the acrylic (Fig. 16–14C). Buccally, the gingival part of the stone model is

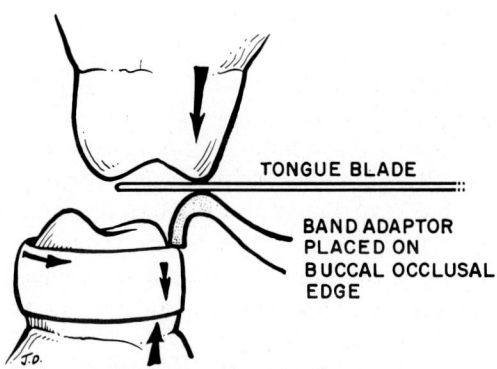

TONGUE BLADE

BAND ADAPTOR PLACED ON BUCCAL OCCLUSAL EDGE

Figure 16–13 Seating of a lower band.

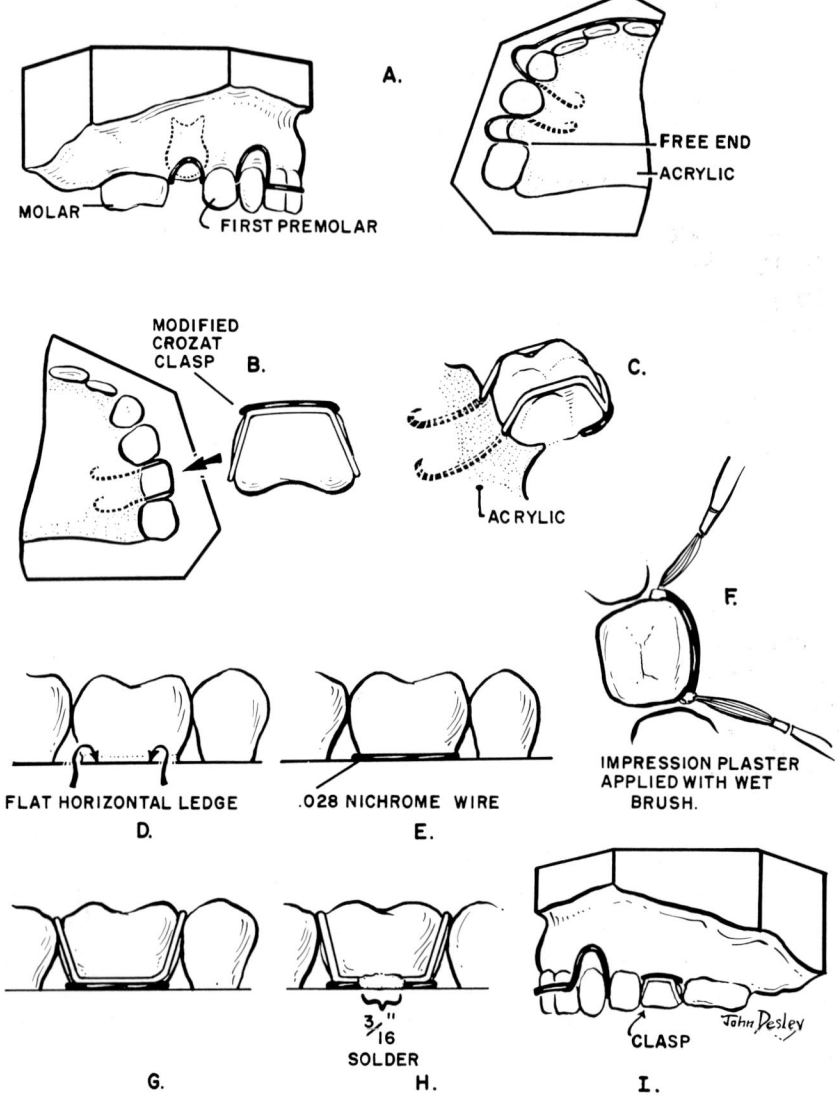

Figure 16–14   *A*, Active spring against mesially drifted molar. *B*, Construction of modified Crozat clasp.

trimmed down interproximally, mesial and distal to the molar, so a flat horizontal ledge extends around the molar from the mesial to the distal aspect (Fig. 16–14*D*). A piece of 0.028 Nichrome wire is adapted to fit against the buccal surface of the tooth. It lies flat on the ledge and extends part way interproximally (Fig. 16–14*E*). This crescent-shaped crib is sealed mesially and distally with a small amount of impression plaster, applied with a small wet brush (Fig. 16–14*F*). The main part of the clasp wire is adapted to pass from lingual to buccal at the mesial and distal occlusal embrasures. Then it is adapted to the buccal surface of the tooth so that the horizontal part just touches the crescent (Fig. 16–14*G*).

Before going further, it is well to coat the lingual or palatal surface of the model with separating medium. The labial surfaces of the anterior teeth are also coated. A thin layer of self-curing acrylic is applied by sprinkling lightly with powder and wetting it with monomer. Premature evaporation of monomer leaves a porous, granular finish, but recently improved material eliminates much of it.

Once this first layer of acrylic is set, the wire portions of the appliance are placed in their positions on the model. They are sealed buccally and occlusally with quick-setting impression plaster, applied by a small wet brush. The main part of the modified Crozat clasp should be sealed occlusally and part way buccally, even beyond where it joins the crescent or crib. A space only ³⁄₁₆ inch wide should be showing where the two wires are parallel and touching.

The main part of the clasp and the crib are then soldered at this ³⁄₁₆ inch space. A low-fusing solder is used with a fluoride and borax flux (the type which can be diluted with water). Some operators may prefer to use 450-fine gold solder, which takes a little longer (Fig. 16–14*H*).

The remainder of the appliance is sprinkled with self-curing acrylic powder and wet with monomer. Sometimes it may be preferable to do this in stages in order to get a more even thickness. Between stages, the model should be covered by a bowl to prevent evaporation of the monomer.

Sometimes, even more retention is desirable. This can be obtained if the anterior teeth are fully erupted and fairly regular in arrangement. Tooth-colored, self-curing acrylic is sprinkled over the horizontal part of the labial bow. The labial surfaces of the stone anteriors have previously been coated with separating medium. The powder is wet by the monomer. Additional layers are added until the grayness of the wire no longer shows through the tooth-colored acrylic.

Originally it was thought that an additional smaller-sized wire should be soldered to the labial bow, parallel to the horizontal wire and gingival to it, in order to keep the acrylic on the wire. This is not necessary in most instances. The labial bow has a curvature following the anterior part of the dental arch. This makes the acrylic occupy three planes of space, and it will not slip around the round wire.

When the appliance is completely built up to the desired thickness, it may be well to set it in warm water and then raise the temperature. A compound heater is ideal. This tends to complete the setting action and helps reduce unpleasant taste and smell.

After complete processing, the appliance is evened by an acrylic stone or bur, and polished with medium grit pumice, followed by powdered chalk or whiting, if desired. The rough finishing may be done while the appliance is on the model. Then the appliance is gently pried off the model after the sealing plaster has been removed. Care should be taken not to distort the labial bow assemblage.

Spicules of acrylic around clasps, labial bow, and molar spring should be removed by a *stiff wheel-shaped bristle brush,* which will remove the acrylic *without* nicking the wires. The acrylic on the labial bow is trimmed down occlusally and gingivally, parallel to the labial bow wire, and keeping about 1 mm. away from it. Sharp edges are rounded. The two vertical legs of each end of the labial bow should be separated by the bristle brush, if during the processing they were stuck together by the acrylic.

The appliance just described will have excellent retention (Fig. 16–14*I*). Adjustment in the spring should not be very great and the spring should not be activated more often than at three week intervals. An adjustment should not be any greater than to allow the patient to snap the appliance into place without manually

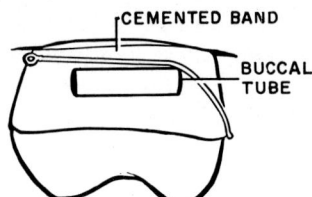

Figure 16–15 Band and tube to increase retention of clasp on removable appliance.

compressing the spring forward. The free end of the spring can be raised or lowered, depending on whether a definite tipping movement of the molar is desired, or a more nearly bodily movement. The free ends of the crib on the modified Crozat clasp can be bent in or out to adjust retention.

Of course, a cemented band with a buccal tube can be used instead of the modified Crozat clasp. Then a simple clasp on the appliance can be used to slip gingival to the buccal tube and thus hold the appliance in place (Fig. 16–15).

The advantages of using the modified Crozat clasp are that the patient can brush that tooth and the dentist can easily examine the tooth. Also, the construction may seem easier to some dentists than that of a band.

Sometimes a second premolar is partially erupted, correctly positioned buccolingually, and needs only a very slight amount of wedging action to make room for itself. This situation can be met by using brass separating wire, mesial and distal to the erupting tooth. A curved piece of 0.020 brass wire is carefully rolled between the second premolar and the first molar, gingival to the contact. The two free ends are twisted tightly at the bucco-occlusal line angle (Fig. 16–16A). The twisted ends are cut off to within ⅛ inch, and the stub is pressed down between either tooth and the free gingival margin (Fig. 16–16B).

The same thing is done between the second premolar and the first premolar. The ends must be twisted tightly enough so that the wire will not slip or roll when the stub is pressed down. In a week's time these wires will be loose. Probably they will break if one tries to tighten them further. Replace them with new wires. It may

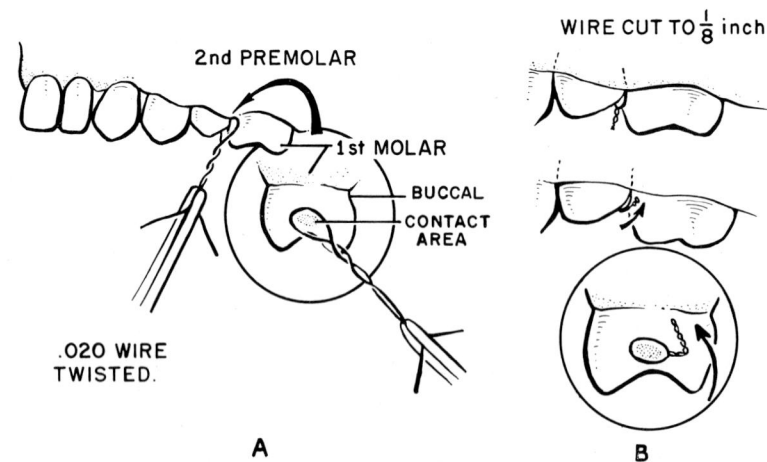

Figure 16–16 Use of separating wires to gain slight amount of space needed for tooth to erupt.

even be necessary to go to 0.022 thickness wire. This method is quite simple and, where applicable, is a real service to the patient. Once the tooth is free to erupt, the separating wires should be removed.

CROSSBITES

Both posterior crossbites and anterior crossbites of single teeth should be treated by the general practitioner.

Kutin and Hawes[9] have given ample evidence of the benefits of early correction of posterior crossbite.

If the results of their large sample can be carried over into the total population, then there is ample work to keep crossbite correctors in business. One out of thirteen children, or 7.7 per cent, have a posterior crossbite in the primary and mixed dentition.

Hanson, Barnard and Case[6] make an even better case for giving particular attention to this problem. In a sample of 193 four year olds, 24 subjects, or 12 per cent, had buccal crossbite, and 23 subjects or 11.8 per cent had lingual crossbites.

In almost all cases studied by Kutin and Hawes, crossbite of the permanent dentition followed uncorrected crossbite of the deciduous or mixed dentition, and added a crossbite of the first permanent molar.

In cases where crossbite is corrected in the deciduous and mixed dentition, premolars and molars erupt into normal relationships.

Kutin and Hawes[9] make another very shrewd observation in class I type 3 cases. If there are both an anterior and a posterior crossbite, the anterior crossbite should be corrected first. This will point up the extent of the posterior crossbite, and keep from overexpanding the buccal segments.

I would also point out that correcting a posterior crossbite first might lead to a situation in which there is not enough overbite anteriorly to retain the anterior correction.

Posterior Crossbites

A single molar in crossbite is most simply corrected by placing bands on the upper and lower molars. To these bands have been soldered hooks of 0.030 gold wire. On the upper band, the hook is on the palatal side of the band and the free end is directed upward but not impinging on the soft tissues. On the lower band, the hook is soldered on the buccal side and directed downward, but not impinging on the mucobuccal fold (Fig. 16–17). The ends of the hooks can be balled by holding over a hot flame till the ends just start to melt.

After cementation of the bands, the patient is instructed in the use of a medium, or small, heavy crossbite elastic. It goes from the palatal hook on the upper band to the buccal hook on the lower band. During the day, the patient may bite through one or more of these elastics, so he should be instructed to carry some spares with him. After a time, the upper tooth will roll buccally with some lingual movement of the lower molar. Then the bands are removed, and function will upright and settle the molars. Sometimes a lingual arch soldered to bands may be used to keep one of the molars from moving, usually the lower, if it already is in correct alignment in the arch.

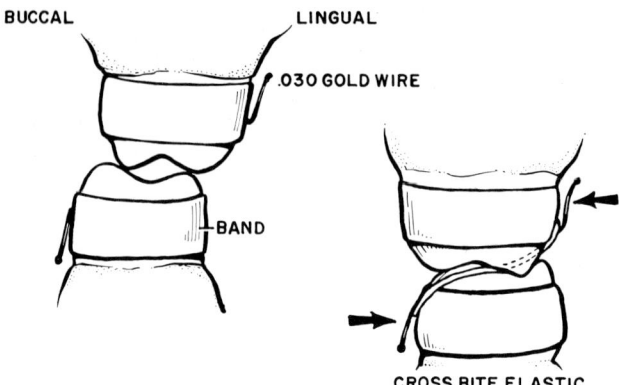

Figure 16–17   Correction of simple posterior crossbite.

Anterior Crossbites

The diagnosing of anterior crossbite is sometimes a problem. Frequently, one is led to believe the case is a simple class I type 3, when in reality it may be a true class III malocclusion. The patient is instructed to open his mouth with his mandible in the most posterior position. It is sometimes helpful to have the patient curl the tongue up and back to touch the posterior part of the palate. Then the patient is instructed to close slowly. If the mandible moves up in a smooth arc until the incisors meet edge to edge, and then the mandible has to slip forward to get complete closure, the case is most likely class I type 3 – in other words, an anterior crossbite. If, however, the mandible closes in a smooth arc to the closed position without having to slip bodily forward, then one is quite possibly dealing with a true class III condition. The patient should be referred to an orthodontist.

Anterior crossbites should respond readily to treatment. The hard way to separate a class I type 3 case from a class III case is to start treating it. If treatment is successful in three weeks (often sooner), then one is safe in assuming that one has dealt with a class I type 3 case. If treatment seems to be prolonged without much change, then an orthodontist should be consulted to see if it is a true class III case.

The Tongue Blade as a Lever.   There are various ways of correcting an anterior crossbite. An incipient case, in which the maxillary incisor is still erupting and is just caught lingual to the lower incisors, may be dealt with by using a tongue blade as a lever. The patient and parent should be instructed to press down with the hand on the tongue blade, and the other end is inserted between the upper and lower incisors. This should be repeated twenty times before each meal, the patient counting to five each time. Any exercises of this type must be done a certain number of times and at certain periods of the day. Otherwise the patient forgets, loses interest, and has no definite discipline to follow. If this method is not successful within a week or two, other procedures should be instituted.

The Bite Plane.   One of the most popular methods is to construct an acrylic bite plane on the lower front teeth, including the canines if present. The plane should be steep enough to give a definite forward thrust to the upper tooth or teeth (Fig. 16–18). This means that the mouth will be propped open quite a lot, in most cases, during the active treatment. Once the acrylic is set on the model, it is

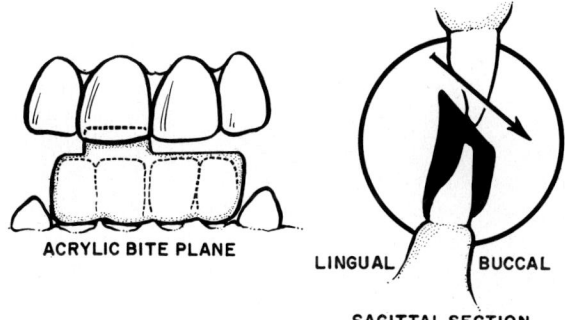

Figure 16–18 One type of inclined plane to correct anterior crossbite.

trimmed down so as not to impinge on the gingival papillae. It is tried in the mouth and the inclined plane is cut down and polished to the proper angulation and height. Then it is cemented in the mouth. If this method is to be successful, the maxillary incisor will usually move far enough labially in a week or two to remove the acrylic inclined plane.

Putting the incline on the lingually locked upper incisor or incisors is sometimes successful when the previous method is not. Here a band may be made for the tooth, and a strip of band material soldered or spot welded to the lingual portion of the band so that the free end sticks out of the patient's mouth. The patient is instructed to close slowly and gently until he strikes the protruding band material (Fig. 16–19*A*). About $1/16$ inch behond this point, the band material is bent until it contacts the labial part of the band. Excess is cut off and the labial connection made by spot weld or solder. Then solder is flowed into the sharp angle and along the inner surface of the lingual portion of the extension to reinforce the bite plane against bending during function. Then the band with its bite plane is cemented in the mouth (Fig. 16–19*A*). Pictures are shown of such a case (Fig. 16–20).

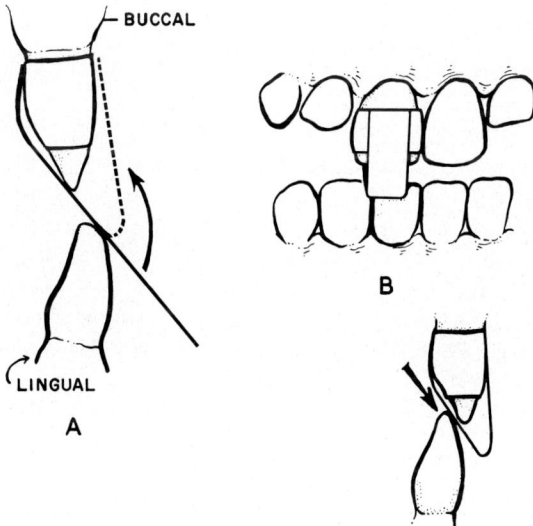

Figure 16–19 Banded incline to correct anterior crossbite.

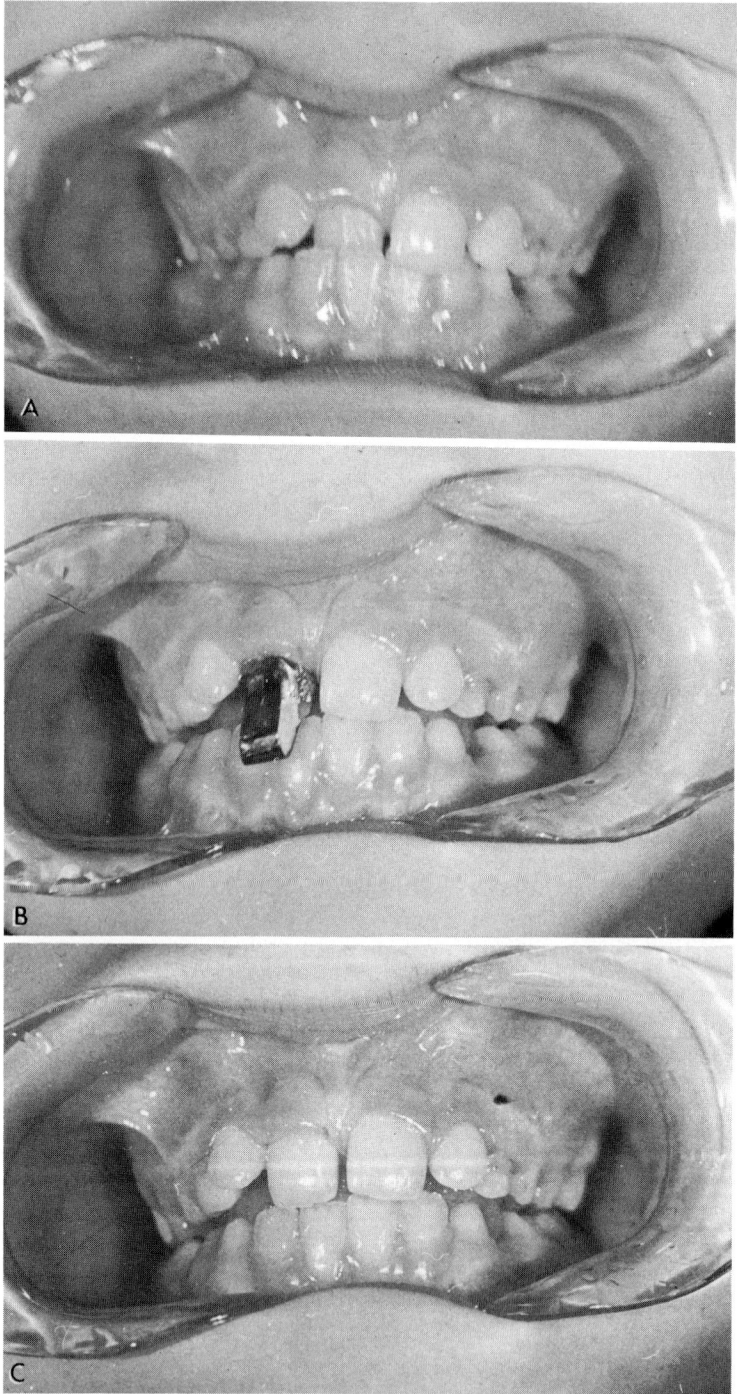

Figure 16–20   *A,* Single tooth in anterior crossbite with enough room to move. *B,* The banded incline cemented to the incisor. The bite is open posteriorly. *C,* The central incisor over after three weeks; it now acts as its own incline and the bite will close. (From Hitchcock: Dent. Clin. N. Amer., July 1968.)

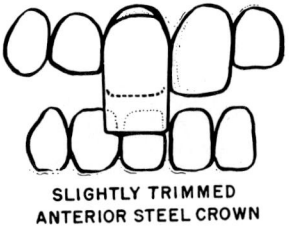

**SLIGHTLY TRIMMED
ANTERIOR STEEL CROWN**

Figure 16–21 Use of stock crown to correct anterior crossbite.

The Steel Crown.   Nowadays, the use of an untrimmed or slightly trimmed anterior steel crown eliminates the time necessary for making a band and soldering a bite plane extension. These steel crowns, ordinarily available for the protection of fractured natural crowns, are extremely simple to use and are a boon to the dentist (Fig. 16–21).

The Hawley-type Appliance.   Still another method is the construction of an acrylic Hawley-type appliance in the upper dentition with springs pressing against the incisors from the lingual aspect (Fig. 16–22).

Of course, regular labiolingual orthodontic technique may be used (Fig. 16–23). This method is most effective when used with the horizontal mesial incisal guide plane as advocated by Dr. Oren Oliver.[13] Such an appliance, however, gets a bit beyond the realm of preventive orthodontics and the general practitioner.

PROTRUDING MAXILLARY INCISORS

The Hawley-type Appliance.   Another situation in which the general practitioner may use his influence is that of protruding upper incisors. *Provided these are spaced* they can gradually be retracted by adjusting the labial bow on a maxillary Hawley-type acrylic appliance. On such an appliance, modified Crozat-type clasps are advisable for retention. The acrylic, lingual to the incisors, *must* be cut back to allow movement of the teeth in a lingual direction.

If a deep bite is present with the lower incisors touching the palate or cingula of the upper incisors, an acrylic bite plane may be built up on the applicance (Fig. 16–24). This will allow the molars to erupt further, or depress the lower incisors, or a combination of both of these movements may take place.

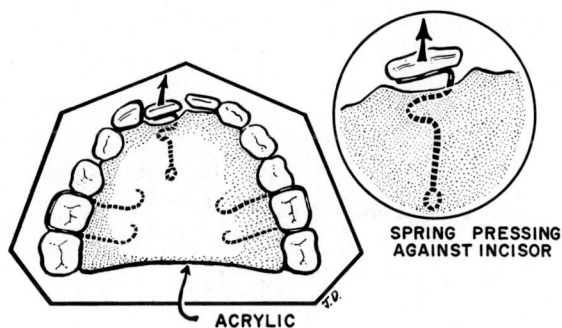

**SPRING PRESSING
AGAINST INCISOR**

ACRYLIC

Figure 16–22 Use of a finger spring to correct an anterior crossbite.

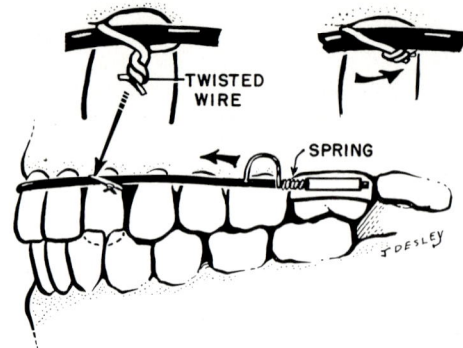

Figure 16–23 Labial orthodontic appliance to correct anterior crossbite.

Extreme care should be used in moving upper incisors lingually by the above method. A check on the roentgenograms should be made to be sure the permanent cuspids will not be interfered with or space for them encroached upon. Also, lingual adjustments to the labial bow should be very gradual so as not to injure the developing root ends or the pulp.

The Oral Screen. For the sake of safety, the use of an oral screen may be preferable. An oral screen is made from Plexiglas 1/16 or 3/32 inch thick. It fits the vestibule of the mouth and transfers muscular pressure from the lips through the screen to the teeth. The screen is constructed on articulated models, which are held together by pouring plaster from the lingual aspect at the rear of the models while they are in occlusion. After the plaster sets up, a line is drawn on the gingiva toward the mucobuccal fold, avoiding any muscle attachments (Fig. 16–25A). A translucent paper pattern is made from this (Fig. 16–25B), and the pattern is scratched on the Plexiglas. Heating the Plexiglas allows it to be readily cut to shape with scissors. Further heating is used to adapt it to the models. A wet towel is wrapped around the models and twisted like a tourniquet to adapt the screen closely to the anterior teeth. The finished appliance should touch only the maxillary anterior teeth, and should stand away about 1/16 inch from the buccal gingiva, upper and lower.

The patient wears this screen at night. One important requirement is that the patient have no nasal obstruction which would prevent normal breathing. Even some mouth breathers benefit from this appliance, because many of them *can* breathe through the nose but find it more convenient to have the mouth open most of the time. The patient should be seen about once every three weeks or once a

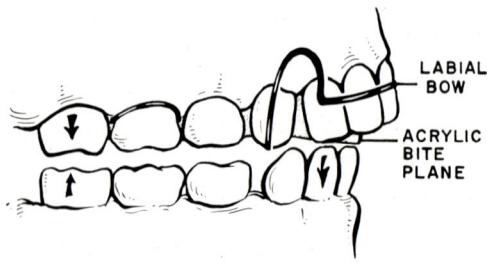

Figure 16–24 Bite opening and retraction of protruding maxillary incisors.

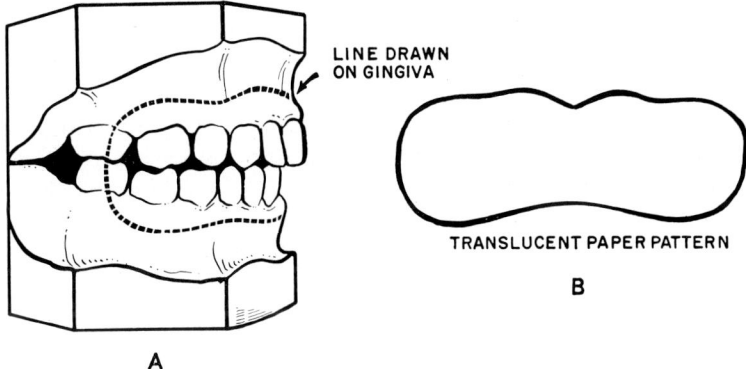

Figure 16–25 Construction of an oral screen.

month. At subsequent visits, the models are adjusted by scraping a little stone from the labial surfaces of the upper anterior teeth. The oral screen is then readapted to the new position with heating and toweling. One can get very enthusiastic about this device, for it is so simply made and cannot harm the patient. Tooth movement takes place slowly, because the patient wears it only one-third of the time. *This movement is of a truly physiologic nature,* as it makes use of the patients' own muscles. If the upper lip is short, both lips can be taped together with cellophane tape at night when the applicance is worn.

Better lip posture habits and better breathing habits are encouraged by use of the oral screen. In some cases it even influences the maxillary posterior teeth to move distally, helping to lessen the severity of an incipient distoclusion.

Protruding upper teeth without spacing should generally be supervised by an orthodontist.

EXCESS SPACING IN MAXILLARY INCISORS

The presence of excess space between nonprotruding upper incisors poses a problem. Some authorities feel that the frenum is at fault here and recommend its excision. (See Chapter 14, Face Development and Tooth Eruption.)

Oftentimes, if the incisors are brought together and held there, excess frenum tissue will atrophy. After the permanent cuspids have erupted, the centrals may move together as a result of changing root angulation due to a shift in the point of application of the cuspid crown pressure. If the centrals are still apart at this stage or if they separate again after being artificially moved together, a frenectomy may be advisable.

It should be borne in mind that forces other than the frenum may be operating to keep central incisors apart:

1. Spacing may be a component of a deep overbite when properly aligned lower incisors are firmly enough fixed to influence the maxillary centrals.

2. It is held by some authorities that the teeth which develop in the premaxilla are a distinct genetic entity, not subject to the same variable laws which govern the proportionate size of the lower teeth, for example. Thus, when maxillary anteriors are forcibly brought together they will occupy an arc of a smaller circle. The result

may be a slight to moderate crowding of a previously properly arranged lower anterior segment. Or, the result may be that after retention, the teeth will separate again owing to their being small in a bony arch which is more than large enough to accommodate them.

Several methods may be used to bring maxillary central incisors together, if such a move is indicated. Wrapping an elastic around the incisors is *not* one of them. The patient cannot be counted on to keep the elastic away from the gingiva. Sometimes this method wreaks havoc on the periodontium.

A band with a hook on each incisor may be used to carry such an elastic (Fig.16–26*A*), but this method sometimes permits a unilateral excess tipping of one incisor or the other. A better method is to have some kind of bracket attachment on each band into which a wire is tied (Fig. 16–26*B*). The elastic is placed over the free ends of the wire, which thus provides a track to control the direction of the tooth movement. Sometimes only a wire with an adjustable loop in the center need be activated and tied in; in trying to become passive, this wire moves the teeth together.

The acrylic removable appliance can be equipped with adjustable finger springs to move centrals together. These springs may be stainless steel (0.022 diameter) imbedded in the acrylic, protruding in a labial direction, and engaging the distal surfaces of the central incisors (Fig. 16–27*A*).

The acrylic on the palatal side of the active end of the spring is removed with a wheel-shaped bristle brush. The wires are activated just enough so that the patient can snap in the appliance. If the spring is activated too much, it will bind on the in-

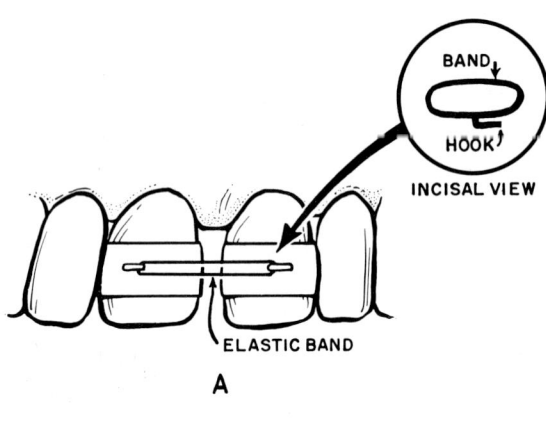

A

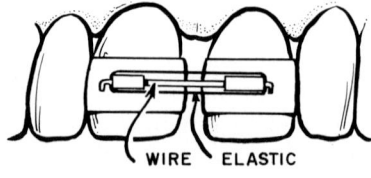

B

Figure 16–26 Closing space between maxillary incisors.

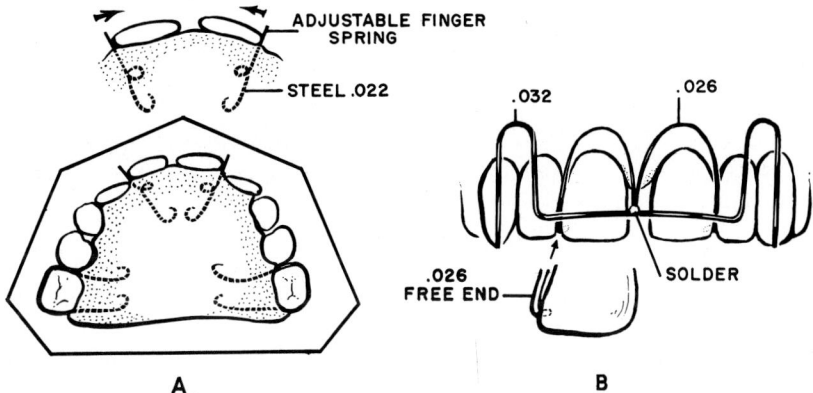

Figure 16–27 Closing space between maxillary incisors.

cisal edge of the central instead of slipping down distal to it. This is a good safe-guard against applying too much pressure.

The springs may also be of the loop variety soldered to the labial bow (Fig. 16–27B). Owing to the length and free action of these, however, a 0.026 diameter wire should be used.

Remember that when tipping crowns together, the roots have to go someplace. The roentgenograms should always be checked carefully to make sure the roots will not be impinging on unerupted crowns.

ORAL HABITS

This author had a page of comments on "oral habits" in the first and second editions of this book. It was omitted from the 3rd edition.

Some relatively recent work makes it worthwhile to introduce a changed point of view about thumb or finger sucking habits, and their control.

Gale and Ayer[2] suggest that so-called "punitive" measures can be successful in eliminating the habit without much danger of serious trauma to the psyche. Haryett, Hansen, and Davidson[7] seem to present the experimental proof of Gale and Ayer's contention. They indicate that palatal cribs, with or without spurs, are effective in stopping thumb sucking. It makes no significant difference to have psychological treatment along with the mechanical restraint. They suggest that if there is a tendency toward tongue thrusting, the crib without spurs may be less effective than the crib with spurs. The use of socially unacceptable mannerisms was not increased in those children with palatal cribs. To be most effective, the patients needed to wear the palatal cribs from six to ten months.

If the child wants to stop a habit, then the appliance can be called a "reminder." There is now no factual evidence to deter the dentist from helping patients to break the digit sucking habit. *The important proviso is the meticulous fabrication of a well-fitting appliance.* This will make the period of adjustment for the patient as smooth as possible.

When it comes to treating the tongue thrust habit, no such optimistic green light can be given. We are only a little further ahead in diagnosing the etiology of this distressing complication than we were ten years ago. Most of the progress is negative. That is, some supposed factors of etiology have been eliminated. Hanson, Barnard and Case[6] could find only two items out of 22 which were associated with tongue thrusting. These were lingual crossbite and enlarged tonsils. In their sample of 193 cases of preschool children, 45 cases had open bite, whereas 70 were judged to be tongue thrusters. The future results in their five year study should prove interesting, though possibly iconoclastic.

I still hold to the idea (which is probably naive) that an open bite associated with tongue thrust has a better chance of being successfully closed by simple measures, if the patient gives a previous history of having had a thumb or finger sucking habit.

Figure 16–28A shows a patient with open bite and spaced incisors. The patient had been a thumb sucker and now was a tongue thruster. I felt that the tongue was simply an opportunist, taking advantage of the space created by the previous thumb sucking. A lingual arch with pronged "reminders" was placed. The patient also wore an oral screen at night. The results are shown in Figure 16–28B after three months of wearing the screen. At that time the oral shield was broken, as shown in Figure 16–28C, and therapy was discontinued with removal of the tongue trap.

As was stated at the beginning of this chapter, not all methods or situations have been enumerated, but the dentist who wholeheartedly participates in a program of preventive orthodontics, at the level presented, will enliven his practice.

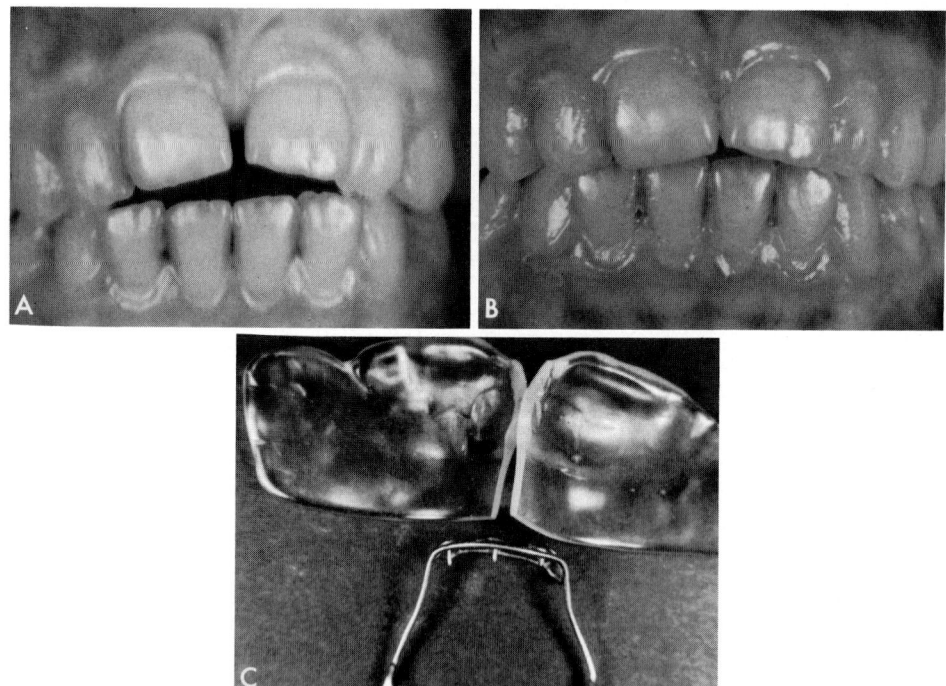

Figure 16–28 A, Former thumb sucker still has protruded spaced incisors with open bite. The tongue does go into the space. B, Results after three months of wearing a lingual arch with pronged "reminders," plus an oral screen at night. C, Broken oral screen and the lingual arch with "reminders."

He will prevent many children from becoming dental cripples. If further orthodontic work is necessary, he makes the task easier for the orthodontist. He earns the good will of his patients and their parents. He earns for himself the satisfaction that comes from doing something which benefits his fellow man.

Except in rare instances, it is very difficult in an undertaking of this nature to give credit to original sources of the ideas in this chapter. Preventive orthodontics is an accumulation of lore rather than an enunciated credo. A great debt of gratitude is hereby acknowledged to all those, past or present, whose aggregated contributions make up the warp and weft of what has come to be known by the term "preventive orthodontics."

REFERENCES

1. Brown, W. E.: The diagnosis, supervision and treatment of minor malocclusions and arch irregularities. Dent. Clin. N. Amer., pp. 723–738, November, 1961.
2. Gale, E. N., and Ayer, W. A.: Thumb-sucking revisited. Am. J. Orthodont. 55:167, 1969.
3. Gore, S. D.: Treatment of class II malocclusion in mixed dentition with the use of removable appliances. Am. J. Orthodont. *40*:359, 1954.
4. Graber, T. M.: Orthodontics: Principles and Practice. Philadelphia, W. B. Saunders Co., 1961, pp. 516–581.
5. Graber, T. M. (ed.): Symposium on Interceptive Orthodontics. Dent. Clin. N. Amer. pp. 279–447, July, 1959.
6. Hanson, M. L., Barnard, L. W., and Case, J. L.: Tongue-thrust in preschool children. Part II. Dental occlusal patterns. Am. J. Orthodont. 57:15, 1970.
7. Haryett, R. D., Hansen, F. C. and Davidson, P. O.: Chronic thumb-sucking. Am. J. Orthodont. 57:164, 1970.
8. Kohn, S. I.: Space maintenance. Dent. Clin. N. Amer. pp. 703–721, November, 1961.
9. Kutin, G., and Hawes, R.: Posterior crossbites in the deciduous and mixed dentitions. Am. J. Orthodont. 56:491, 1969.
10. Lundstrom, A.: The significance of early loss of deciduous teeth in the etiology of malocclusion. Am. J. Orthodont. *41*:819, 1955.
11. MacGregor, S. A.: Interception of malocclusion. J. Canad. D. A. *11*:301, 1945.
12. Massler, M.: The oral screen. J. Dent. Child., *19*:100, 3rd quart., 1952.
13. Oliver, O. A., Irish, R. E., and Wood, C. R.: Labio-lingual Technic. St. Louis, C. V. Mosby Co., 1940, pp. 128–133.
14. Ibid. pp. 318–327.

17

ORAL HABITS
IN CHILDREN

*by JOSEPH M. SIM
and SIDNEY B. FINN*

Oral habits in children have concerned dentists for many years. Dentists see in these habits the possibility of harmful unbalanced pressures which may be brought to bear upon the immature, highly malleable alveolar ridges, the potential changes in position of teeth, and occlusions which may become decidedly abnormal if habits are continued for long periods of time.

Also interested in these problems are the pediatrician, the psychiatrist, the psychologist, the speech pathologist, as well as the parents of the children. In general, it might be said that the dentist and the speech pathologist are interested more in *oral structural changes* resulting from prolonged habit patterns. The pediatrician, psychiatrist, and psychologist may place more importance on the deeper seated *behavioral problems* of the child, of which the oral habit may be only a symptom. The parents appear to be more concerned that a child with an oral habit is exhibiting *an act which is socially unacceptable.*

While it is of great importance for the dentist to be able to diagnose the changes in oral structures which appear to result from oral habits, it is of equal importance that he understand the voices of other professional people as they look at the same problems. In this chapter an attempt is made to orient the dentist to some of the prevailing opinions in these areas.

The dentist rarely sees these children until after the oral habits are well established. In some cases he sees the child then only to act as an arbitrator in a family dispute over whether or not the particular habit is harmful to the child patient. Because of this it is instructive to review how the infant relates to his external environment through his oral activities.

Freud and his followers emphasized this by delineating certain phases of childhood as oral and anal periods. Others have spoken of the "essential orality of the child."

370

THE SUCKING REFLEX

Engel emphasizes that direct observation of infants in the first year has revealed that their organization is predominantly an oral and a clinging one. At birth the child has developed a reflex pattern of neuromuscular functions called the sucking reflex. Even before birth, oral contractions as well as other reflex responses have been observed fluoroscopically.

This early neural organization of the infant allows it to nurse and to cling to the mother, as evidenced by the sucking and grasp reflexes and the Moro reflex, all of which are present at birth. Certainly the infant's sucking pattern has the quality of a need. Not so well understood is the need to cling. However, although both these reflexes influence the child in his early learning situations and contribute to his psychic development, the warmth of milk brought into his body and the relief from hunger which follows the sucking make this reflex clearly the dominant one.

As his hearing and vision develop, the baby tries to reach and transport to its mouth what it has seen and heard at a distance. Despite poor limb and digital coordination, the baby tends to persist until all possible objects are carried into his mouth to be licked, tasted, and, in effect, examined by oral sensations. If the object feels good he may attempt to eat it. If it feels bad, he spits it out and signifies his disgust by making a wry face and turning his head away from the object. The attempt to take into his mouth a "good" object is termed *introjection*. The rejection of a "bad" object is termed *projection*. In this behavior we see an elaboration and an accentuation of the oral behavior originally associated with the feeding and sucking experiences of the neonatal child. This oral "testing" apparently not only serves to relieve the hunger tension inside the child, but also is a means of testing by the senses available to him what is good and bad. Things placed in his mouth, particularly if they are warm and soft, have all the past associations of food and comfort. Using these past satisfying experiences, he is able to provide himself with some secondary gratification to relieve the frustration of hunger or other discomfort by putting his finger or thumb into his mouth. The thumb held in the mouth becomes the substitute for the mother who is not available with the warm food. It satisfies both the need for something in his mouth and the need to cling, and it is considered by some to be one of the earliest signs of developing separateness or independence from the mother.

Interesting findings have been elicited from studies done by pediatricians to determine what the incidence of thumb and finger sucking actually is in a cross section of patients seen in a pediatric practice. In one such study, Traisman and Traisman observed some 2650 infants and children, from birth through age 16 years, and noted that 46 per cent of them sucked their thumbs at some time during this period. Of these, 25 per cent began during the remainder of the first year. On an average, most had stopped by age four years. There were some, however, who continued the habit as late as 12 to 15 years.

In a serial study conducted by Rakosi, of 693 children who were considered thumb suckers, 60 per cent had dropped the habit after less than two years. The majority of this group had normal occlusion. Of the 413 children in this same group who were classified as having some type of malocclusion, it was found that they had continued a finger or thumb sucking habit for more than four years. This led the researcher to conclude that thumb sucking could be a causative factor in the development of a malocclusion, particularly that of class II. However, in many of these cases it was noted that when the habit was discontinued, the permanent dentition gradually became normalized and the continued effects of early abnormal pressures on the teeth and jaws brought about by the habit appeared to be of slight significance.

NONCOMPULSIVE ORAL ACTS

Children appear to undergo continuing behavior modification which permits them to release certain undesirable habit patterns and form new and more socially acceptable ones. Early success may reinforce the new patterns, or the changes may be accomplished by the parents using cajolery, flattery, or in some cases threats of punishment. The subtle and unsubtle molding of a child's personality continues into adulthood, as he is subjected to the external pressures brought about by parents, his playmate peers, and school associates. Habits which are easily added or dropped from the child's behavior patterns as he matures are termed *noncompulsive*. No abnormal responses usually result from these situations in which the child is being retrained to change from a formerly accepted personal habit to a new pattern of behavior more consistent with his increased level of maturity and responsibility.

COMPULSIVE ORAL HABITS

It is generally agreed that an oral habit is *compulsive* when it has acquired a fixation in the child to the extent that he retreats to the practice of this habit whenever his security is threatened by events which occur in his world. He tends to suffer increased anxiety when attempts are made to correct the habit. That these compulsive habits express a deep seated emotional need must be made clear. The habit act serves as his bulwark against the society about him. This is his safety valve when emotional pressures become too much to cope with. He literally turns inward upon himself, and from a body extremity placed in his mouth he may achieve the satisfaction he craves.

While specific etiologies of compulsive oral habits are difficult to isolate, some writers feel that early feeding patterns might have been too rapid, or that the child was fed too little at a time. Too much tension at feeding time also may have occurred, and indeed, even bottle feeding itself has been indicted. Moreover, it is generally accepted that insecurity in the child, brought about by lack of love and tenderness displayed by the mother, plays a large role in many cases.

PSYCHOLOGIC METHODS USED FOR RETRAINING

While these personality problems are clearly within the working area of those who deal with the psychologic aspects of health, the dentist many times is asked by the parents to intervene in cases in which it is found that alveolar bone and tooth positions are being distorted by an abnormal oral habit pattern. Some orthodontists have said that the duration, frequency, osteogenic development, genetic endowment, and the state of health of the child must be carefully examined before any intervention is attempted. It is a clinical rule of thumb that the thwarting of a habit such as that of thumb sucking can be consciously accomplished by the child himself, guided by the dentist and the parents, *only* if the child is ready psychologically and wants to break the habit.

Children often combine *primary oral habits,* such as thumb and finger sucking, with *secondary habits,* such as hair pulling or nose probing. Frequently, the primary oral habit can be broken by making the secondary habit impossible to perform. This is illustrated by the case of the ten year old schoolgirl patient who sucked her thumb and at the same time pulled out the hair on one side of her head. This had continued until she had almost denuded that side of her head. After the child's head was shaved she lost the desire to suck her thumb, and the habit was discontinued.

Other less dramatic methods are occasionally just as effective, however. One author proposed that children call him on the telephone at the dental office (after arranging this with the parents). By simply suggesting, after some conversation, that the caller sounded so "grown-up" that of course, he couldn't possibly be the one who had "formerly" sucked his or her thumb, a positive start toward retraining was made. A reinforcement office visit was also arranged for the child, if he desired. This was to make sure that no thumb was being sucked, so this information could be placed in "the special record in our office." After one short friendly visit at the office it was found that many of these children had been encouraged to break the oral habit. Obviously, this whole procedure implies that the parents are willing to cooperate and follow the dentist's suggestions in the home:

1. Set a short-term goal for dropping the habit (one to two weeks).
2. Do not criticize the child if the habit continues.
3. Offer a small reward for the child if the habit is extinguished.

Without such understanding cooperation little progress toward habit retraining will be noted.

EXTRA-ORAL METHODS FOR RETRAINING

Some simple methods which have brought success to other dentists and which do not include placing appliances in the child's mouth are: painting the child's thumb or finger with an unpleasant-tasting substance commercially available for this purpose; arranging for the offending digit to be taped or a glove to be taped at the wrist to hold it in place. All of these devices have one thing in common, though. They depend on the child's acceptance that the habit will be broken. The parents should be told that there is always the possibility that another more deleterious habit will spring up in its place if the present one is suppressed.

The attitude of the parents during such a procedure is of unquestionable importance. If they demand a perfection in the child with which he cannot comply, the process is doomed to failure. Indeed, such a parental attitude may have been partly responsible for the tenacity of the oral habit in the first place. However, if the parents in some way reward the child for "growing out of the habit" during the procedure, both by their actions and by some small token prize, it makes a deep impression on the child and orients him toward a definite goal. In this matter the dentist can certainly help the parents decide on the choice of methods or alternatives.

USE OF INTRA-ORAL APPLIANCES FOR HABIT RETRAINING

Most intra-oral appliances fabricated by the dentist and placed in the child's mouth with or without his overt permission are viewed by the child as punishment devices. They can produce emotional disturbances more difficult and costly to cure than any displacement of teeth brought about by the habit. In most children these appliances serve to fix a "guilt" complex to the original habit which can result in the apparent suppression of the habit, only to have the child change overnight from a seemingly happy youngster to a "nervous child." In these cases it is not worth the cost.

FIVE QUESTIONS TO ASK

Five questions that the dentist should ask himself before attempting to place a habit retraining appliance in a child's mouth are as follows.

1. Child's understanding: Does the child clearly understand the need for the appliance and does he express a desire to be helped?

2. Parents' cooperation: Do *both* parents understand what you are attempting to do and have you been promised full cooperation by them?

3. Friendly rapport: Have you set up a friendly rapport with the child so that a "reward" situation and not a feeling of "punishment" exists in the child's mind?

4. Goal orientation: Have you and the parents chosen a definite "goal," both in *time* and in form of a material *prize,* toward which the child can work?

5. Maturity: Has this child acquired the *maturity* to deal with a retraining period which may well produce an increased short-term anxiety?

The discerning dentist who asks himself these questions and one by one ascertains that the answer to each is in the affirmative can usually feel free to place a necessary habit-retraining appliance. Most men who report successes with these appliances agree that lack of care in preparing the child and the parents for the procedure almost certainly dooms the habit retraining episode to failure.

DENTAL EFFECTS OF LONG-TERM THUMB AND FINGER SUCKING

There remains a broad range of opinion as to the deleterious effects of long-term thumb and finger sucking. It is generally agreed that if the habit is discontinued before the permanent anterior teeth erupt, no residual damage to the alignment or the occlusion of the teeth is likely to result. If, however, the habit persists during the mixed dentition period (age 6 to 12) some disfiguring consequences can occur. The severity of the displacement of the teeth usually will be dependent upon the force, frequency of indulgence, and duration of each sucking period.

It must be emphasized that the displacement of the teeth or the inhibition of their normal eruption can come from two sources: (1) from the *position* in the mouth of the thumb or finger, and (2) from the *leverage* effect the child gains against the other teeth and the alveolus by the force he generates if he presses against the teeth as well as sucks (see Fig. 17–1).

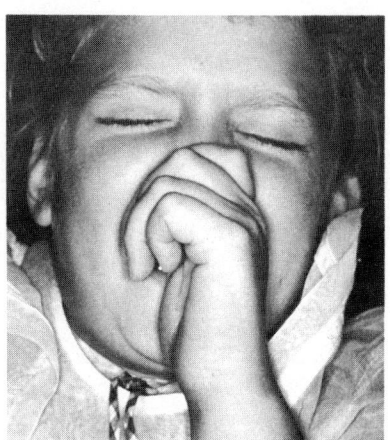

Figure 17–1   The thumb sucker often uses the index finger and middle finger as a fulcrum to exert considerable pressure against the teeth and the palatal surface of the alveolar ridge. Note the index finger clasping the nose.

One can almost tell from the contour of the open bite present on which hand the offending digit belongs. This can usually be confirmed by casually lifting the child's hands and checking for the cleanest finger or thumb or the hand with the tell-tale callus on the back of the finger or thumb.

The malalignment of the teeth usually produces a pronounced labial flare of the upper anteriors. This increases the overjet and opens the bite; and, depending upon the leverage produced, a lingual inclination and a flattening out of the curve of Spee of the mandibular anterior teeth can result. Some observers feel the maxillary posterior segments may be forced lingually, by buccal musculature held under tension, which can narrow the arch and produce a bilateral posterior crossbite.

Depending on the habit involved, there may be a tendency to produce an overeruption of the posterior teeth, thereby increasing the open bite. Whether thumb sucking produces a narrowing in the palatal region is open to some question. The resulting prominence of the labially posed upper permanent incisors does make them particularly vulnerable to accidental fractures. The open bite can lead to tongue thrusting problems and speech difficulties.

There can be a marked mentalis muscle contraction which compresses the lower lip inward on swallowing. The lower lip can slip up and make a seal (during the swallow) lingual to the upper anteriors, not labial as is usual. This increases the overjet and can make for a vicious circle perpetuating the open bite and upper labial protrusion. This is because the mentalis contracts on swallowing, flattening the lower lip strongly against the labial surfaces of the lower anterior teeth. At the same time the lower lip may contact the lingual surfaces of the upper anteriors with some force during the last of the swallowing spasm. This unequal force generated against the teeth by the *perioral musculature* may serve to perpetuate a malocclusion long after the original sucking habit has disappeared.

However, a certain perspective must be maintained where tooth and arch relationships are concerned in the child who exhibits oral habits. The fact that a child has developed a class II division 1 malocclusion, and just happens to be a thumb sucker as well, does not justify the conclusion that the thumb sucking per se produced the class II, malocclusion. Hereditary components must be considered carefully. Close observations of the parents' occlusions may disclose some valuable clues in this direction.

APPLIANCE CONSTRUCTION

There are many different types of oral habit-breaking appliances which can be constructed by the dentist. They are perhaps best separated into removable appliances and fixed appliances.

If the child expresses a desire to be helped the dentist should choose the most appropriate type of appliance after considering the child's age, dentition, and oral habit pattern. In children below age 6, where only the primary teeth are present, a removable appliance may not be as well accepted because of the child's immaturity. During the age of mixed dentition, clasping of incompletely erupted permanent teeth may also militate against a removable appliance. Speech maturation also occurs in this group, between 8 and 9 years of age.

However, a fixed appliance may cause a child to feel he is being "punished," whereas a removable one may allow him the freedom of wearing the appliance only during critical periods, such as at night. Certainly, for the dentist, most removable oral habit-breaking appliances are easier to fabricate and adjust than are the fixed types. The chief disadvantage of the removable appliance is that it is only worn at the option of the child.

CRIBS

A crib is a habit-retraining appliance which utilizes a blunt wire "reminder" which may prevent the child from indulging in his habit. The crib may consist of a wire embedded in a removable acrylic appliance similar to a Hawley retainer, or it may be a "fence" added to an upper lingual arch and used as a fixed appliance. (See Fig. 17–2*A*, *B*, and *C* and Fig. 17–3.)

Cribs can serve (1) to break the suction and force on the anterior segment, (2) to distribute the pressure to the posterior teeth as well, (3) to remind the patient that he is indulging in the habit, and (4) to make the habit nonpleasurable for him. The detailed construction of both types of these appliances is discussed in Chapter 16, Preventive Orthodontics.

RAKES

A rake may be a fixed or removable appliance, just as the crib. As implied by the term, however, this appliance more nearly punishes than reminds the child. It is constructed as is the crib, but has blunt tines or spurs projecting from the crossbars or acrylic retainer into the palatal vault. The tines discourage not only thumb sucking but tongue thrusting and improper swallowing habits as well.

OTHER ORAL HABITS

In sucking habits, not only are the thumb and other fingers employed in either conventional or nonconventional positions (Fig. 17–5), but other tissues, such as the cheeks, tongue or lips, are frequently used to take the place of the fingers.

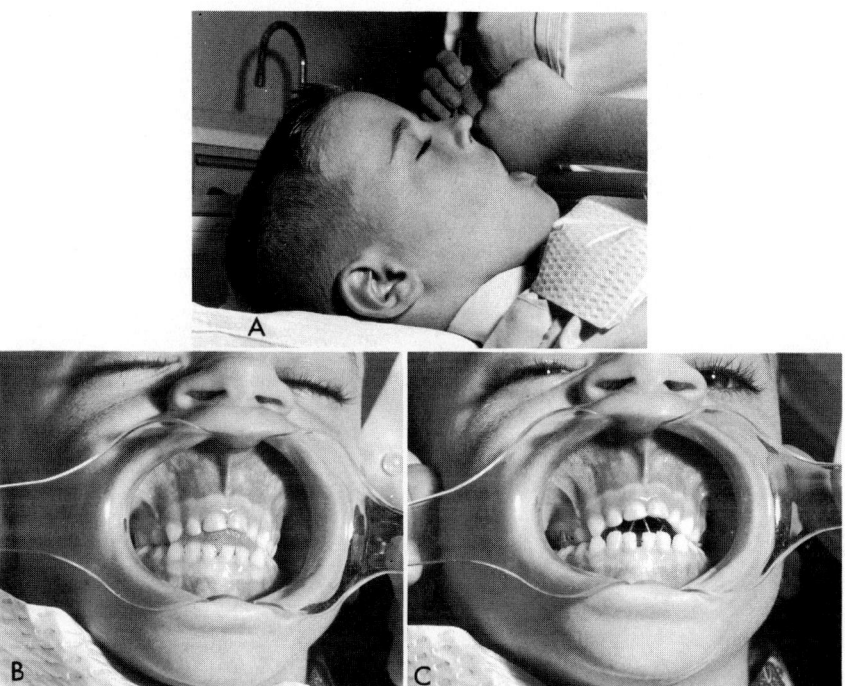

Figure 17–2 *A,* A 5 year old boy who indicated a desire to stop his thumb sucking habit. Here he is demonstrating the most "comfortable" position for his thumb. *B,* Same boy showing the anterior open bite which resulted from his habit. Note tongue position on swallowing. *C,* A fixed crib was constructed with molar bands and cemented in place. Despite care and frequent visits to the dentist, the crib was not successful in retraining him away from thumb sucking. The appliance was removed after six weeks.

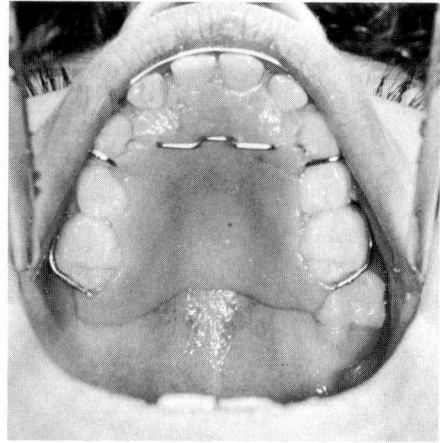

Figure 17–3 A "reminder" type of removable appliance to discourage thumb and finger sucking.

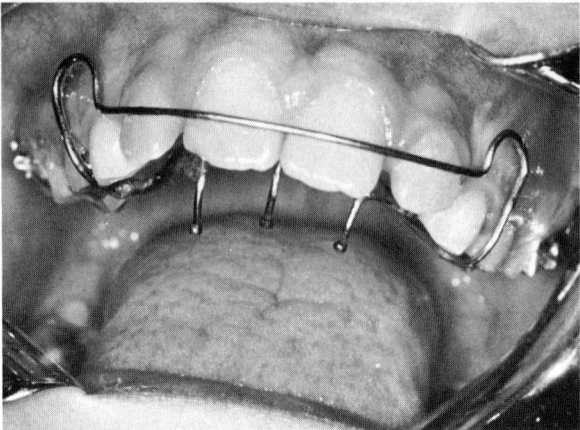

Figure 17–4   A removable rake fabricated to intercept a tongue thrusting habit.

Lip Sucking

Lip sucking or biting may lead to the same anterior displacement as finger sucking, although the habit usually occurs during the school age where an appeal to the child's own good judgment and cooperation can lead to its discontinuance. The dentist can assist by suggesting lip exercises such as extending the upper lip over the upper incisors and placing the lower lip forcibly over the upper. The playing of brass instruments assists in strengthening the lip muscles and in exerting pressure in the right direction on the upper anterior teeth.

Tongue Thrusting

Tongue thrusting is often observed in children with open bite and protruding upper incisors. However, it has not been conclusively proved whether the thrusting produces the open bite or whether the open bite permits the child to thrust his tongue forward into the space between the upper and lower incisors. Since the

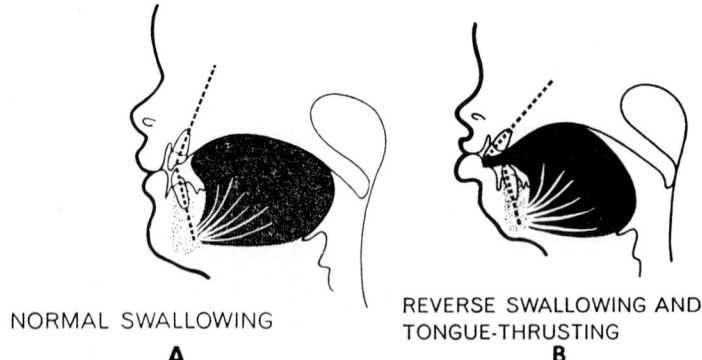

NORMAL SWALLOWING

A

REVERSE SWALLOWING AND TONGUE-THRUSTING

B

Figure 17–5   A, The tongue position in normal swallowing fills the palate behind the maxillary incisors. B, With reverse swallowing and tongue-thrusting where an open bite occurs, the tongue extends into the space between the maxillary and mandibular teeth resting on the lingual surfaces of the maxillary anterior teeth. (Courtesy of Rocky Mountain Dental Products Company.)

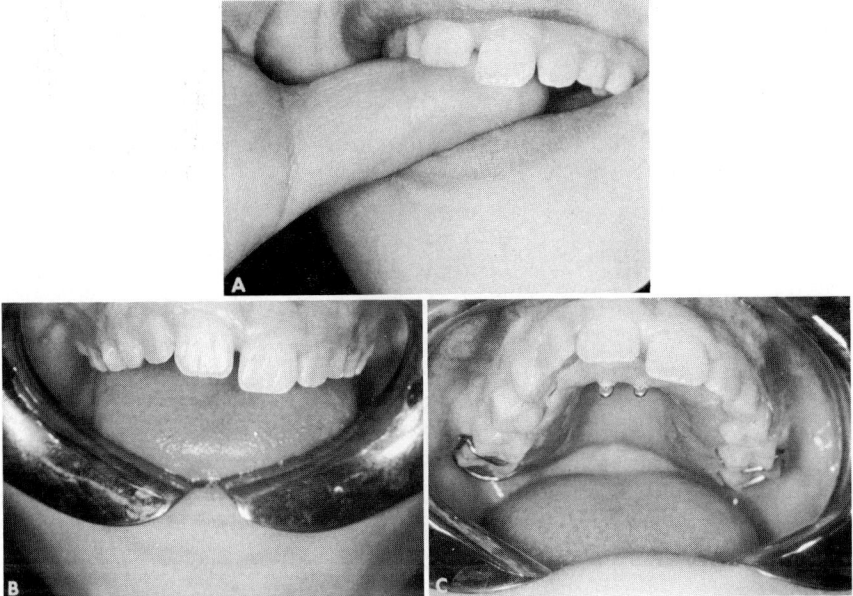

Figure 17–6 *A,* Lateral thumb sucking. *B,* The resultant malocclusion, with a marked unilateral anterior open bite. *C,* A removable appliance constructed to break the habit.

thrust involves only the tongue muscles, the tonus of the lower lip and mentalis muscle are not affected and, in fact, may be strengthened. As with thumb sucking, tongue thrusting produces a protrusion and a labial tipping of the maxillary incisors, although in the latter habit there may be depression of the lower incisors with marked open bite and lisping. In diagnosing an anterior open bite the dentist frequently is overly concerned with the thumb sucking habit and fails to notice a tongue thrusting habit or an enlarged tongue, which may be just as important in the formation of the open bite and protruding anterior teeth.

The treatment of tongue thrusting is training the child to hold the tongue in proper position during the swallowing motion. This will be difficult to accomplish until the child is old enough to cooperate. Myofunctional exercises like those employed in limiting the effects of thumb sucking can be used to bring the incisors into proper alignment. An older child who is concerned about his appearance and lisping speech may be taught to place his tongue tip on the incisive papilla on the roof of his mouth and swallow with his tongue in this position. A vertical crib may be constructed. It is made similar to that suggested for preventing thumb sucking, except that the palatal bars are soldered in a horizontal position extending down from the palate to prevent the forward thrusting of the tongue.

Frenum Thrusting

A habit rarely seen is that of frenum thrusting. If the upper permanent incisors are spaced slightly apart, the child may lock his labial frenum between these teeth and permit it to remain in this position for several hours. This habit probably starts as idle play but may develop into a tooth-displacing habit by keeping the central incisors apart, the effect being similar to that produced in certain instances by an abnormal frenum. One patient proudly boasted that he could lock his frenum between his teeth and keep it there for two hours after he had had a good rest.

Nail Biting

A normal habit that develops after the sucking age is that of nail biting. Frequently a child will go directly from the thumb sucking stage into the nail biting stage. It has been estimated by studies in the armed services that about 80 per cent of all individuals have been or are nail biters. This is not a pernicious habit and does not assist in the production of malocclusion, since the forces or stresses applied in nail biting are similar to those in the chewing process. However, in certain cases of nail biting where grit remains under the nails, a marked attrition of the lower anterior teeth has been observed. Nail biting is a normal tension release and although parents may not find it quite socially acceptable, one should remember that neither was cigarette smoking for women a few years ago. A habit, like behavior in general, should not be considered bad unless it does actual harm either physically or morally to the child himself or to others about him. Nail biting generally does neither. As the child grows older and enters adulthood, other objects are substituted for the fingers. Chewing gum, cigarettes, cigars, snuff, pencils, erasers, even the person's own cheeks or tongue may be utilized as substitutes for the fingers, for every age has its own pacifiers.

Postural Habits

Postural habits leading to malocclusion are rare and must be diagnosed or treated orthodontically on an individual basis. Certain orthopedic postural aids fall into this category. The Milwaukee brace as used for children with scoliosis is an example.

Masochistic Habits

On occasion, one finds a child with habits of masochistic nature. One child observed by one of the authors used the fingernail to strip away the gingival tissue from the labial surface of a lower cuspid. The habit had completely denuded the tooth of marginal and unattached gingival tissue, exposing the alveolar bone. The treatment consisted of psychiatric assistance and taping the finger.

Bobby-pin Opening

Another deleterious habit which once was prevalent among teen-age girls was the practice of opening bobby-pins with the anterior incisors to place them in the hair. Notched incisors and teeth partially denuded of labial enamel have been observed in girls with this habit. At this age, calling attention to the harmful results is generally all that is necessary to stop the habit.

Mouth Breathing

Continual mouth breathing is rather uncommon in children. These mouth breathers can arbitrarily be classified into three categories: (1) obstructive, (2) habitual, and (3) anatomical. Obstructive mouth breathers are children who have an increased resistance to, or a complete obstruction of, the normal flow of air through the nasal passages. Because of the difficulty of inspiring and expiring air through the nasal passages, the child is forced by sheer necessity to breathe through his mouth. The habitual mouth breather is a child who continually breathes through his mouth by force of habit, although the abnormal obstruction has since been removed. The anatomical mouth breather is one whose short upper lip does not permit complete closure without undue effort. One must distinguish between these types of mouth breathers. One must also distinguish the second type from the child who breathes through his nose but because of a short upper lip, continually keeps his lips apart. Obstructive mouth breathing is frequently observed in ectomorphic children who possess long, narrow faces and nasopharyngeal spaces. Because of this genetic type of tapering face and nasopharynx, these children are more prone to have nasal obstruction than those with wide nasopharyngeal spaces, such as are found in the brachycephalic individuals. Resistance to breathing through the nose may be caused by (1) hypertrophy of the turbinates caused by allergies, chronic infections of the mucous membrane lining the nasal passages, atrophic rhinitis, hot and dry climatic conditions, or polluted air; (2) deviated nasal septum with blocking of the nasal passage; (3) enlarged adenoids. Since adenoidal or pharyngeal tonsillar tissue is physiologically hyperplastic during childhood, mouth breathing from this cause in young children is not unusual. However, the mouth breathing may be self-correcting as the child grows older and as the natural physiologic process causes the adenoidal tissue to shrink.

The Oral Screen. Although correction of the nasopharyngeal obstruction may take place through surgical intervention or physiologic shrinkage, the child may continue to breathe through his mouth from mere force of habit. This may be especially evident when the child sleeps or is in a recumbent position. When this situation prevails the dentist may decide to intervene with an effective appliance which will cause the child to breathe through his nose. This may be done by the construction of an oral screen (oral shield) which will block the passage of air through the mouth and force the inspiration and expiration of air through the nares (Fig. 17–7).

Before one attempts to force a child to breathe through the nose by use of an oral screen, one must ascertain if the nasopharyngeal passage is sufficiently patent to allow for the exchange of air even with forced breathing resulting from extreme emotion or physical exercise. Massler and Zwemer suggest the use of a wisp of cotton or tissue paper held in front of the child's mouth and nostrils to test this. The child should close his eyes before the cotton is held to his nostrils and mouth, so that breathing will be entirely natural and not forced as when the child is deliberately instructed to breathe through his nose. If the child cannot breathe through his nose or does so only with great difficulty when instructed to do so, he should be referred to a rhinologist for diagnosis and correction. If the child has no difficulty breathing through his nose when requested to do so, even after violent exercise, the chances are that the mouth breathing is habitual and should be corrected by means of an oral screen.

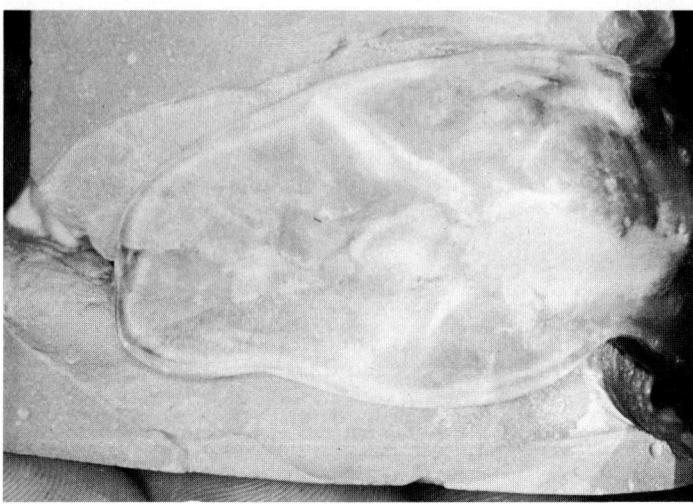

Figure 17-7   An oral screen on the working model is made from Plexiglas, $^5/_{64}$ inch thick, 4 inches long and 1$^1/_2$ inches wide.

Mouth breathers have a typical appearance, sometimes referred to or described as an "adenoid facies," although it has not been shown satisfactorily that mouth breathing causes the facies. The face is narrow, the upper anterior teeth protrude labially, and the lips are open with the lower lip extending behind the upper incisors. Because of the lack of normal muscular stimulation from the tongue and owing to the increased pressure on the cuspid and primary molar areas by the strained orbicularis oris and buccinator muscles, the buccal segments of the maxilla collapse, giving a V-shaped maxilla and a high palatal vault.

It has not been shown definitely that mouth breathing causes malocclusion, although a tendency toward malocclusion is seen quite frequently in children who are mouth breathers. The same genetic factors contributing to the production of class II malocclusion may also contribute to the production of mouth breathing.

In correcting habitual mouth breathing, the passive oral screen is recommended. The oral screen is a solid shield inserted in the mouth (Fig. 17–8). It rests against the labial folds and is employed to prevent mouth breathing and encourage breathing through the nose. It is generally inserted at night before going to bed and worn throughout the night, so that the child is forced to breathe through the nose while asleep.

The oral screen, when worn at night, prevents lip biters from placing the lower lip lingual to the upper incisors, tongue thrusters from forcing the tongue between the upper and lower anterior teeth, mouth breathers from breathing through the mouth, and thumb suckers from placing their fingers in the mouth. The oral screen, therefore, can serve a multiplicity of purposes, and should be used more extensively than is done today. The screen can be made out of any material compatible with the oral tissues, The simplest to utilize and the most commonly employed are the synthetic resins. The construction of an active screen is presented in Chapter 16, Preventive Orthodontics.

Bruxism

Another habit observed in children is bruxism, or the grinding of teeth. This is generally a nocturnal habit, occurring during sleep, although it may be observed during the waking hours as well. The grinding may be so forceful that the grating sounds can be heard for some distance. The child may produce considerable attrition of the teeth and may even complain of some soreness in the temporomandibular area upon arising in the morning.

The exact causes of bruxism are somewhat obscure. Perhaps it has an emotional basis, for it generally occurs in children who are high strung and irritable and who may evidence other habit patterns such as thumb sucking and nail biting. These children are generally fitful sleepers and seem to suffer from anxieties.

Bruxism has also been observed in such organic diseases as chorea, epilepsy, and meningitis, as well as in gastrointestinal disturbances.

The treatment belongs in the realms of the family physician, the psychiatrist, and the children's dentist. The dentist can assist in breaking the habit by constructing a soft rubber splint to be worn over the teeth at night. The soft rubber does not form a resistant and hard surface for grinding; thus the habit loses its satisfying effectiveness. The construction of a soft rubber splint is the same as that of the mouth protector and is described in Chapter 16.

Precautions Concerning "Too Early and Too Much" Treatment

After having developed a rather skillful technical approach to the problem of treating oral habits in children, the dentist commonly finds himself oriented to treating "too early and too much." Klein offers a more cautious approach with his suggestion that the "meaningful" sucking habit be differentiated from the "empty" sucking habit. He defines the meaningful habit as one which functions as an im-

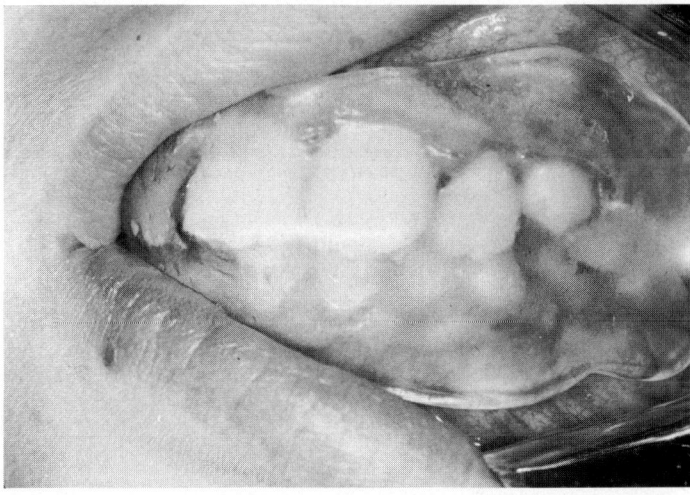

Figure 17–8 The oral screen in the mouth with cheeks retracted to show the area involved.

portant psychological prop for the child. The treatment to correct such a habit should be psychologically oriented. On the other hand, the empty sucking habit is one that is pursued even though it has been determined that the child has no deep need for the support the habit seems to provide. Correction in these cases is best accomplished through a dental approach, that is, by the fitting of a reminder appliance. Klein emphasizes that the child should evince a sincere desire to correct the habit in question before the appliance is fitted by the dentist.

SUMMARY

In this chapter concerning oral habits in children a deliberate attempt has been made to move somewhat outside the realm of routine dental treatment. The reasons are fairly obvious. The pediatrician and the psychiatrist deal in a different terminology when they discuss the compulsive oral acts of children. Instead of attempting to make the dentist an expert outside of his chosen field, it was decided rather to incorporate some of the terminology the dentist might be exposed to when he talked to the pediatric or psychiatric specialists preparatory to referring his patients to their offices for possible therapy.

Some of the background of the oral life of a child as he passes from neonate to the age of speech maturation at age 8 or 9 years has been touched on. The influence of early affection or rejection on children and the parents' attitudes have been emphasized. A number of questions have been posed which should be answered in the affirmative by the treating dentist before he attempts to place a habit-retraining device in a child's mouth.

REFERENCES

1. Baalack, I., and Frisk, A.: Finger-sucking in children: A study in incidence and occlusal conditions. Acta Odont. Scand., *29*:499–512, 1971.
2. Cimring, H.: Management of finger-sucking habits. J.A.D.A., *50*:191, 1955.
3. Davidson, P. A., Haryett, R. D., Scandilands, M. A., and Hansen, F. C.: Thumbsucking: Habit or Symptom. J. Dent. Child., *34*:252–259, 1967.
4. Emslie, R. D., Massler, M., and Zwemer, J. D.: Mouth breathing. I. Etiology and effects (a review). J.A.D.A., *44*:506, 1952.
5. Engel, G. L.: Psychological Development in Health and Disease. Philadelphia, W. B. Saunders Co., 1962.
6. Graber, T. M.: Orthodontics: Principles and Practice. 2nd ed. Philadelphia, W. B. Saunders Co., 1966.
7. Graber, T. M.: The finger sucking habit and associated problems. J. Dent. Child., *25*:145, 1958.
8. Henry, R. G.: The effect of thumb-sucking on the dentition. D. Practitioner & D. Record, *8*:300, 1958.
9. Klein, E. T.: The thumb-sucking habit: Meaningful or empty? Am. J. Ortho., *59*:283–289, 1971.
10. Korner, A. F., and Reider, N.: Psychologic aspects of disruption of thumb-sucking by means of a dental appliance. J. Dent. Child., *24*:119–127, 2nd quart., 1957.
11. Larson, E.: Dummy- and finger-sucking habits with special attention to their significance for facial growth and occlusion. Swed. Dent. J., *65*:1–5, 1972.
12. Lundstrom, A.: Tooth size and occlusion in twins. A–B. Stockholm, Fahlcranty Boktryckeri, 1948.
13. Massler, M., and Zwemer, J. D.: Mouth breathing. II. Diagnosis and treatment. J.A.D.A., *46*:658, 1953.
14. Massler, M., and Wood, A. W. S.: Thumbsucking. J. Dent. Child., *16*:1, 1949.
15. Moyers, R. E.: The role of musculature in orthodontic diagnosis and treatment planning. Vistas in Orthodontics, Ed. by Krauss, B. S., and Riedel, R. A. Philadelphia, Lea & Febiger, 1962.

16. Picard, P. J.: Bottle feeding as preventive orthodontics. Calfornia D. A. & Nevada D. Soc., *35*:90, 1959.

17. Rakosi, T.: Thumbsucking and malocclusion. D. Abst., *4*:1, 1959.

18. Ruttle, A. J., Quigley, W., Crouch, J. T., and Ewan, G. E.: A serial study of the effects of finger-sucking. J. D. Res., *32*:739, 1953.

19. Sillman, J. H.: Thumb-sucking and oral structures; serial study from birth to 14 years of age. J. Pediat., *39*:424, 1951.

20. Straub, W. J.: Malfunction of the tongue. I. The abnormal swallowing habit: Its cause, effects, and results in relation to orthodontic treatment and speech therapy. Am. J. Orthodont., *46*:404, 1960.

21. Traisman, A. S. and Traisman, H. S.: Thumb- and finger-sucking: a study of 2650 infants and children. J. Pediat., *52*:566, 1958.

18

ORAL SURGERY FOR CHILDREN*

by CHARLES A. McCALLUM, Jr.

The general principles of oral surgery remain the same whether applied to adults or to children. However, in the child we are dealing with a developing organism in both its physical and its psychological aspects. Techniques, therefore, must be modified to conform to the needs of this growing patient. Some factors to be considered in oral surgery for children as compared to adults are:

1. The oral cavity is small and there is greater difficulty in gaining access to the field of operation.

2. The jaws are in the process of growth and development and the dentition is in a continuous state of change, with the eruption and resorption of primary teeth and eruption of permanent teeth taking place simultaneously. Any interference with the growth centers in the jaw or premature extraction of primary teeth may lead to malformations of the jaw, the permanent teeth or both.

3. The bone structure of a child contains a higher percentage of organic material, which makes it more pliable than adult bone and not as likely to fracture.

LOCAL ANESTHESIA

It is unfortunate that many practitioners refer children to the oral surgeon for extractions under general anesthesia without first making an effort to perform the extraction themselves under local anesthesia. The general practitioner or pedodontist should refrain from instructing parents that general anesthesia is the method of choice, when with proper handling the work could be done under a local anesthetic with less difficulty.

We have found that many children can be handled under local anesthesia, provided that parents cooperate and there are no other contraindications. The

---

*Originally written for the first edition by Joseph P. Lazansky.

child should be told in simple words what is going to be done. He should never be told an untruth; a child can be disappointed only once and his confidence is lost forever. It is safer to tell the child he will experience some slight discomfort like a scratch or mosquito bite than to promise complete painlessness and not be able to abide by our promise.

If a child complains of pain during an injection or operation, believe him, reconsider the situation, reinject if necessary, but never submit him to pain by force.

A great percentage of even the more difficult and frightened children can be persuaded to take a local anesthetic. The remainder, often extremely young children, must be handled under general anesthesia.

When elective surgery is to be done, it is best to see the patient at least once prior to the operation. This gives the operator time to talk to the patient and presents an opportunity to establish rapport. This visit will permit discussion of the procedure with the child and parents. By taking time to explain what needs to be done, the dentist can keep apprehension and fear to a minimum.

PREPARATORY MEASURES

Most states have laws which make it mandatory to obtain permission from a parent or guardian of a child before any type of anesthesia, local or general, is to be used. The consent should be in written form and should include the type of anesthesia to be used and the operation to be performed. In an emergency, a telephone call will suffice, but it should be confirmed by a written statement as soon as possible. It is a safe precaution to note the number of the telephone and the name of the person giving the oral consent on the record of the patient, preferably in the presence of an assistant who can act as a witness.

Children seem to tolerate *local* anesthetics better after a moderate food intake, about two hours prior to the operation. If it is felt that the child might require a *general* anesthetic, the parents should be told not to give the child food or fluids for at least six hours prior to the procedure.

Appointments for surgery should be made whenever possible in the early morning when the child is well rested and does not have the opportunity to brood over the operation for hours. The office appointment should be scheduled so that the child does not have to wait because he tends to become restless.

The operating room should be set up with all instruments on the tray covered with a towel and out of sight of the patient. We have found it best to place the instruments on a tray behind the patient. A display of needles, knives, forceps and other instruments upsets not only a child but any patient. There is never a need to load syringes in front of patients; to do so only leads to further fear and apprehension.

Premedication has proven invaluable and an operator should not hesitate to use it as described in Chapter 7, The Problem of Pain and Sedation. Immediately before the operation, the child should be sent to empty the bladder and bowels whether local or general anesthesia is used.

Clothing should be loosened and protected with a gown or a protective apron. We prefer linen aprons, as rubber or plastic coverings make patients perspire more freely and this makes any patient, including a child, more uncomfortable. Relatives and friends should be sent out of the operating room unless it is felt that their presence may be of benefit in handling the child. The child's position should be adjusted for comfort and support and should be slightly reclining.

INJECTION TECHNIQUE

Some clinicians advise the use of topical anesthetics before injection. It is difficult to determine how effective they are. They certainly have a psychological value, but they do not substitute for a good injection technique. If they are used at all they should be used properly:[9]

1. The mucous membrane should be dried to avoid dilution of the topical anesthetic solution.

2. The topical anesthetic should be held in contact with the surface for at least 2 minutes, allowing at least another minute for it to act. One of the errors made in the use of topical anesthetics is the operator's failure to permit sufficient time for the topical agent to produce any effect before he injects. It is wise to wait at least four minutes after the topical anesthetic is applied before starting the injection.

3. A topical anesthetic should be selected which does not cause local necrosis at the site of application. No irritation has been found from the use of 5 per cent Xylocaine (lidocaine) ointment.

4. A sharp, fine needle with a relatively short bevel should be used, attached to a smoothly working syringe. We feel disposable needles should be used, for they assure both sharpness and sterility. Their use eliminates the possibility of transferring infection from one patient to another by means of a contaminated needle.

5. The tissues should be stretched if loose, as they are in the mucobuccal fold; they should be compressed if densely attached, as they are on the hard palate. The use of tension and pressure helps produce a certain degree of anesthesia and thus lessens the pain associated with the introduction of the needle. If the tissue is loose, we prefer to pull the tissue over the needle as we are advancing it.

6. When using an infiltration technique the anesthetic solution should be deposited slowly. Rapid injection tends to accentuate the pain. If more than one tooth in the maxilla has to be anesthetized, the operator can enter the initially anesthetized area and, by changing the direction of the needle to a more horizontal position, can gradually advance the needle and deposit the anesthetic solution. The palatal side may be anesthetized by injecting a few drops anterior to the greater palatine foramen, which can be found on a line connecting the last erupted upper molars. When anesthesia is necessary in the incisal region of the maxilla we have found it best to give the anesthetic on the labial first and then pass the needle from this anesthetized area through the interdental papilla between the centrals and gradually deposit the anesthetic solution as the needle is advanced. This technique seems to produce less pain than if the needle is inserted in or around the incisive papilla.

7. The vasoconstrictor should be kept at the lowest possible concentration, e.g., with 2 per cent Xylocaine, not more than 1:100,000 epinephrine should be used.

8. The symptoms of anesthesia should now be explained to the child. Numbness, tingling, a feeling of swelling may otherwise frighten a child who has not been forewarned.

9. Enough time (5 minutes) should be allowed to elapse before any operation is started. If tingling and numbness in the lower lip do not occur in 5 minutes following an inferior dental block, the injection should be considered a failure and repeated.

10. Aspirating syringes should be used to prevent intravascular injection of the anesthetic solution to keep toxic, allergic and hypersensitivity reactions at a minimum.

TYPES AND LOCATION OF INJECTION

Local anesthesia in children does not differ to a great extent from that in adults. The lesser density of bone hastens the diffusion of the local anesthetic through the compact layers of the bone. On the other hand, the smaller size of the jaws reduces the depth to which the needle has to penetrate in certain block anesthesias. One will find that, with the exception of the inferior dental block, no other blocks are necessary in children.

The bone density is such, especially in the region of the tuberosity, that anesthetic solutions easily pass through the cortex without the dentist having to resort to a deeper injection. Deep injections in this area may be followed by a hematoma due to injury of the adjacent pterygoid plexus, or, what is more likely, an injury of the superior posterior alveolar artery or of its external gingival branch, which runs downward and forward along the posterolateral wall of the maxilla close to the periosteum.[6] This is an unpleasant accident but it cannot always be avoided. A hematoma, once noticed, can be controlled by packing tightly compressed sponges behind and lateral to the tuberosity intra-orally while applying pressure from the outside against this pack with ice-cold compresses.

Mental and infraorbital blocks are usually unnecessary. They often lead to transient nerve injuries and hematomas which are painful. The block of the greater palatine foramen often causes a sensation of choking.

In terminal infiltration the puncture is made in the mucobuccal (labial) fold, slightly gingival to the deepest point, and the needle penetrates toward the bone in the direction of the apex of the particular tooth. One should consider the length of the root of each particular tooth as seen on the roentgenogram.

In the upper jaw, every tooth, even the permanent molars, can be anesthetized by terminal infiltration in the labial (buccal) fold. The palatal mucosa can be anesthetized by two different methods: a drop of anesthetic can be deposited slowly into the palatal mucosa about $1/2$ cm. above the gingival margin. This requires some pressure and is painful even in conjunction with a topical anesthetic. Another method uses the approach through the interdental papilla. Two to three minutes after the infiltration on the labial (buccal) surface, a fine needle is inserted into the labial (buccal) aspect of the papilla and slowly carried upward and palatally through the interdental spaces, releasing a few drops of the solution as the needle advances. This method is less painful and serves our purpose very well.

In the lower jaw, all of the six anterior teeth may be removed under terminal infiltration. Experience with 2 per cent Xylocaine has convinced us that even primary molars may be removed under infiltration, although a mandibular block is preferable. The lingual mucosa may be anesthetized as described above by passing the needle through the interdental papillae.

Permanent molars require a block injection; so do multiple extractions or larger operations involving the lower jaw. In making an inferior dental block injection, one has to bear in mind that the ascending ramus in the child is shorter and narrower anteroposteriorly than in the adult. The anteroposterior width may be estimated by palpation through the skin. The lesser height of the ramus has to be compensated for by inserting the needle a few millimeters nearer to the occlusal plane than in adults (Fig. 18–1).

The lingual nerve may be anesthetized during the retraction of the needle after the anesthetic has been deposited at the inferior dental nerve. The needle is withdrawn about 1/2 inch and the syringe is turned medially to account for the more anterior and medial course of the lingual nerve in relation to the inferior dental nerve.

As mentioned earlier, the child should be informed of the subjective signs such as tingling, numbness, and a feeling of swelling in the lip and tongue, either before or preferably after the anesthesia has been administered. Testing for anesthesia should be done carefully with slowly increasing pressure of an explorer or other instrument, keeping in mind that anesthesia in the superficial tissues does not necessarily mean anesthesia of the deeper tissues.

The long buccal nerve should not be anesthetized until definite signs of numbness in the respective side of the lip appear, as the child might give misleading information because he is confused by the tingling or numbness of the mucosa of the lip. The long buccal nerve should be anesthetized by terminal infiltration in the mucobuccal fold of the respective tooth.

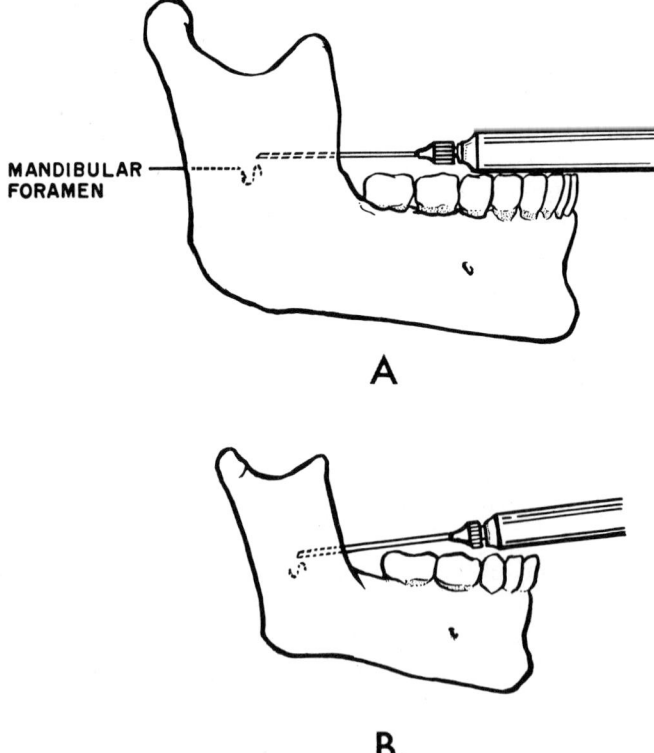

MANDIBULAR FORAMEN

A

B

Figure 18–1 Inferior dental block. Position of syringe in the adult (*A*) and in the child (*B*).

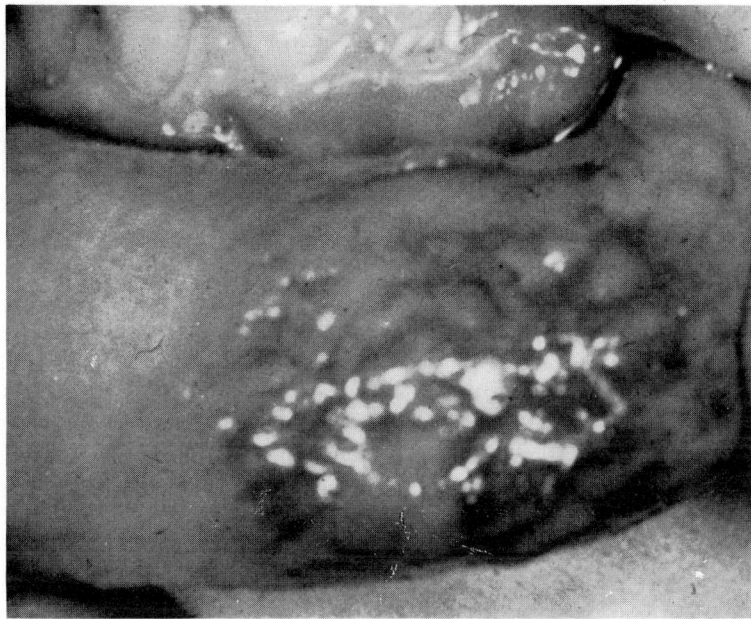

Figure 18–2 Ulcer caused by biting anesthetized lower lip.

COMPLICATIONS

Incidents and complications do not differ greatly from those occurring in adults. A relatively frequent sign of central stimulation may be retching and vomiting, which may be due to psychic or toxic reasons.[5]

Among the postanesthetic complications, the most frequently observed is formation of an ulcer in the lower lip due to biting on this anesthetized structure (Fig. 18–2). Also, herpetiform lesions sometimes appear on the lip, tongue or gingiva which can be explained by disturbance in the trophic innervation.

Parents should be warned to watch their child carefully after inferior dental block injections until sensation returns, to prevent him from biting his lips. They should also be told to be careful about giving the child any hot food until sensation returns lest the child burn himself severely.

EXTRACTIONS

INDICATIONS FOR EXTRACTION OF PRIMARY TEETH

In considering the advisability of extraction of primary teeth, one should always keep in mind that age per se is not an acceptable criterion in determining whether a primary tooth should be removed. A primary second molar, for example, should not be removed just because a child is 11 or 12 years of age, unless there is a special indication. For some patients the second premolars are ready to erupt at 8 or 9 years of age while in other cases these same teeth do not show sufficient root development at the age of 12. A primary tooth that is firm and intact in the arch should never be removed unless a complete clinical and radiographic evaluation has been made of the entire mouth and especially of the particular area (see Chapter 8, Operative Dentistry for Children).

Occlusion, arch development, size of teeth, amount of root, resorption of the primary tooth involved, the state of development of the underlying permanent successor and adjacent teeth, presence or absence of infection—all of these factors must be considered in determining when and how a primary tooth should be removed.

With the above considerations in mind, indications for extraction of primary teeth are as follows:

1. If the teeth are decayed beyond possible repair; if decay reaches down into the bifurcation or if a sound hard gingival margin cannot be established.

2. If infection of the periapical or interradicular area has occurred and cannot be eradicated by other means.

3. In cases of acute dentoalveolar abscess with cellulitis.

4. If the teeth are interfering with the normal eruption of the succeeding permanent teeth.

5. In cases of submerged teeth.

In considering conservative treatment of primary teeth with infected pulps or periapical tissues, the systemic condition of the patient is as important as local conditions. Since we cannot, with certainty, eradicate infection in or about the teeth, conservative procedures are unwise and dangerous for patients with rheumatic fever and its sequelae, such as rheumatic heart disease. Conservative procedures are contraindicated also in congenital heart disease, in kidney disorders and in cases of suspected focal infection. It is known that primary foci of infection and their manipulation cause transient bacteremias which may be followed by subacute bacterial endocarditis in patients with rheumatic and congenital heart disease and may cause a flare-up of diseases in other organs.

Extractions may be rendered relatively free from danger by the judicious use of antibiotics before and after the operation (see Chapter 19, Antimicrobial Agents).

CONTRAINDICATIONS TO EXTRACTION OF PRIMARY TEETH

Contraindications to extraction, except for the considerations mentioned above, are more or less the same as in adults. Many of these contraindications are relative and may be overcome with special precaution and premedication.

1. *Acute infectious stomatitis, acute Vincent's infection or herpetic stomatitis,* and similar lesions should be eliminated before an extraction is contemplated. Exceptions to this are conditions such as acute dentoalveolar abscesses with cellulitis, which demand immediate extraction.

2. *Blood dyscrasias* render the patient susceptible to postoperative infection and hemorrhage. Extractions should be performed only after adequate consultation with a hematologist and proper preparation of the patient.

3. *Acute or chronic rheumatic heart disease, congenital heart disease and kidney disease* require proper antibiotic coverage.

4. *Acute pericementitis, dentoalveolar abscesses and cellulitis* should be treated as will be explained later, when and if indicated, with preoperative and postoperative antibiotic medication.

5. *Acute systemic infections* of childhood contraindicate elective extractions for the child because of a lowered resistance of the body and the possibility of secondary infection.

6. *Malignancy,* if suspected, contraindicates dental extractions. The trauma of extraction tends to enhance the speed of the growth and spread of tumors. On the other hand, extractions are strongly indicated if the jaw or surrounding tissues are to receive radiation therapy for malignancy; this is done to avoid the risk of an infection in the bone which has been exposed to radiation.

7. *Teeth which have remained in irradiated bone* should be extracted only as a last resort and only after the consequences have been fully explained to the parents. If the teeth must be removed, consultation with the radiologist who gave the irradiation might be wise. Infection of the bone will follow extractions in most cases even after antibiotic therapy, owing to the avascularity which follows the radiation. The infection is followed by a slowly progressing osteomyelitis which is very painful and which cannot be controlled except by wide resection of the whole irradiated bone. It is, therefore, very dangerous to remove teeth after exposure to radiation.

8. *Diabetes mellitus* poses a relative contraindication. Consultation with the physician is a wise precaution to make certain that the child is under control. In controlled cases of diabetes, one does not observe more infections than in normal children and therefore antibiotics are not a prerequisite to extraction. It is important that the diabetic child retain his diet in the same qualitative and quantitative composition after an operation. Changes in these respects may change the sugar and fat metabolism of the child.

INDICATIONS FOR EXTRACTION OF PERMANENT FIRST MOLARS

When making a decision about the fate of permanent first molars, the following considerations should be kept in mind. If a permanent first molar is removed before the permanent second molar has erupted through the gingiva, the chances that this second molar will move mesially and occupy the space of the extracted first molar are very good. If, on the other hand, the permanent second molar has erupted through the gingiva at the time of the loss of the permanent first molar, the second molar will probably tilt forward into the space of the first molar, causing conditions favoring periodontal disease and orthodontic problems such as closing of the bite.

The procedure in practice, therefore, should follow the rule that when the second molar has not yet broken through and one or two first molars are diseased beyond repair, they should be removed. But if three first molars are diseased beyond repair, all four first molars should be removed with the expectation that a more symmetrical dentition will result.

In cases in which the second molars have broken through, every attempt should be made to save the first molars. If extraction is necessary, only the destroyed teeth should be removed and space maintainers should be inserted.

The routine extraction of first molars has been recommended in England under the phrase "extraction for prevention." It has been claimed that this procedure reduces the incidence of dental caries (see Chapter 24, Prophylactic and Operative Techniques in Dental Caries Prevention). It has also been claimed that extraction of first molars prevents impactions of third molars. No controlled studies have been undertaken to substantiate this latter claim, and we feel that only broken-down or badly infected first molars should be removed.

Transplantation of the unerupted third molar into the extraction site of the first molar has been tried with variable degrees of success.

EXTRACTION TECHNIQUE FOR PRIMARY TEETH

If sufficient resorption of the roots has occurred, extractions may be very simple. On the other hand, if a tooth, especially a molar, has to be removed prematurely, the roots may have undergone little or irregular resorption, and this situation can make these extractions difficult. It must be borne in mind that the crown of the succeeding tooth is situated in close relationship to the roots of the primary tooth. The widespread roots of the primary molars surround the crowns of the permanent teeth, and we may dislodge, if not extract, the forming tooth if great care is not exercised during the extraction. The permanent tooth will offer little opposition because of the lack of development of its roots. Not infrequently the resorption of a primary molar root occurs halfway between the apex and the cemento-enamel junction (Fig. 18–3). This weakens the root considerably and fractures of such roots are not uncommon. Good radiographs are of great importance and should be studied carefully before the extraction is planned. If such a root is broken, the question arises whether it should be removed immediately or whether an attitude of watchful waiting should be taken. The decision hinges upon the skill of the operator and the accessibility of the root tip. If the tip can be removed without trauma to the bud of the permanent tooth, it should be elevated with small spear-point elevators. Occasionally it is desirable to elevate a mucoperiosteal flap and remove buccal bone to approach such a tip. The commercial elevators are usually too heavy and large. We prefer an instrument which has been ground into a point from a straight root tip elevator (Fig. 18–4).

Many a broken root tip will be resorbed or, more often, brought to the surface and shed when the permanent tooth erupts. In some cases a root tip may act as a wedge and prevent the eruption of the permanent successor, necessitating surgical removal.

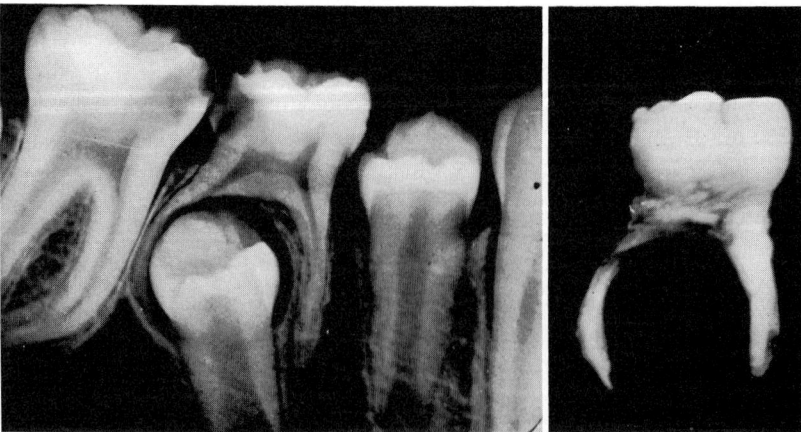

Figure 18–3 Irregularly resorbed distal root of primary second molar.

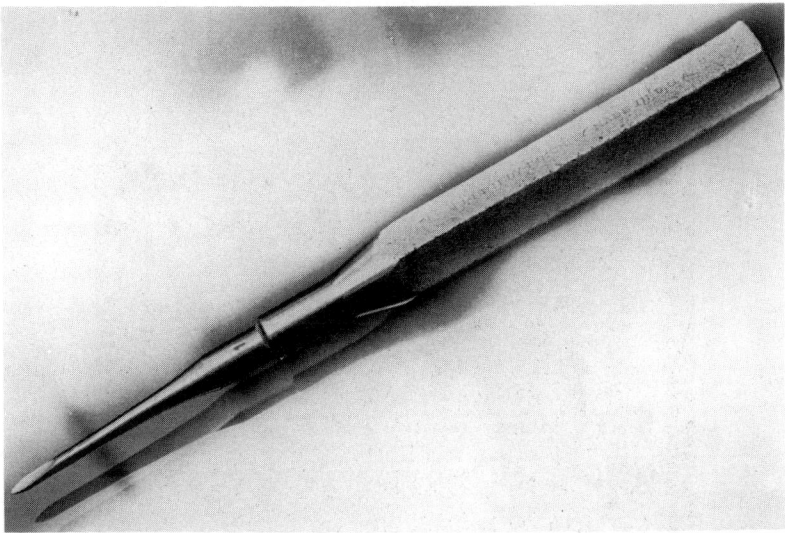

Figure 18–4   Root elevator.

If a permanent tooth bud is *moved* during an extraction, it should be carefully pushed into its original position and the socket closed with one or two sutures. Some operators cover the bud with Gelfoam. Should a permanent tooth bud be erroneously extracted, it should be reinserted immediately without disturbing the tooth follicle or dentinal papilla. Care should be taken to orient the tooth in the socket in the proper buccolingual position, and the socket should be closed by sutures. Pulp tests should be made of the tooth after eruption.

If an already erupted permanent tooth with an insufficiently formed root has been dislodged during the removal of a primary tooth, it should be reinserted and immediately splinted. After healing, pulp tests should be made, although the radiographic findings of further root development and of eventual narrowing of the root canal are proof that the vascular supply has been reestablished.

The forceps used in the extractions of primary teeth are the same as in adults. Some operators prefer special child forceps because they can be hidden in the palm. It is not felt that this is necessary, as an explanation should precede the extraction and the forceps with the larger handles can be controlled better.

The removal of anterior primary teeth and roots is simple, usually requiring a steady rotation in one direction which disengages the tooth from its attachment. This can be accomplished in the upper jaw with a No. 150 or bayonet forceps, and in the lower jaw with a No. 151 forceps.

For posterior teeth, the same instruments are used. In some cases, an English-type forceps with narrow beaks is advantageous for lower molars, because it allows better support of the lower jaw.

Upper and lower primary molars are removed with a buccolingual motion; the motion toward the lingual aspect quite often offers less resistance. Difficulties in the application of forceps may be encountered, especially on lower molars, because of a lingual inclination of the crown and the inability of a child to open his mouth sufficiently.

If a radiograph shows locking of the premolar within the roots of the primary

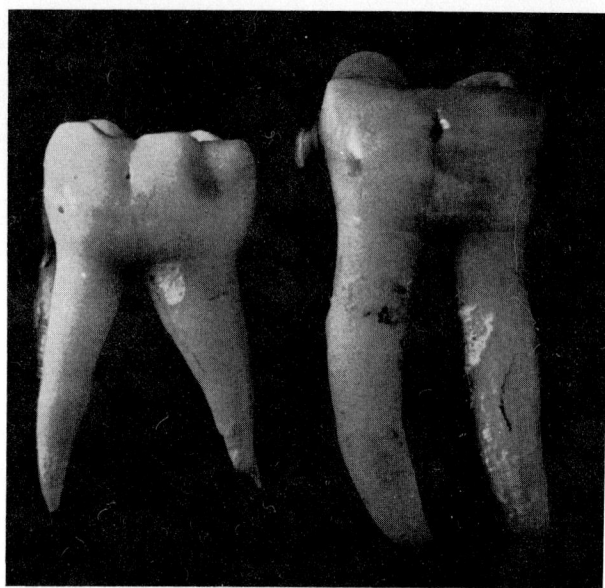

Figure 18–5   Location of bifurcation in primary and permanent molars.

molar, the tooth should be sectioned and each root removed carefully. It should be remembered that the bifurcation of a primary tooth is located much closer to the coronal portion than in permanent teeth so that only a very narrow bridge of tooth substance has to be divided (Fig. 18–5).

Chronic periapical lesions and sinus tracts should not be curetted, as they heal after removal of the infected tooth and curettage of the socket may damage the tooth follicle and may cause disturbances in the calcification of the enamel of the crown. Cysts, however, should be removed.

The technique for removal of permanent first molars does not differ from that in adults, except that space maintenance has to be considered if the second molar has already erupted through the gingiva.

It is the duty of the dentist who has removed primary teeth prematurely to take care that space is maintained for the successors.

POSTOPERATIVE EXTRACTION COMPLICATIONS

Postoperative extraction complications are the same as in adults and are treated accordingly. Fortunately, dry sockets are a rarity in children. If a child under ten years of age develops a dry socket the operator should immediately think of an unusual infection, e.g., actinomycosis or a complicating systemic disorder (anemia, nutritional disturbance, etc.).

Aspiration or swallowing of teeth or roots may occur, especially under general anesthesia with the mouth forced open. If possible most loose teeth should be removed before general anesthesia is started or the endotracheal tube is introduced orally. The same untoward incidents may occur during extraction under local anesthesia. In explosive, forceful extractions, a tooth may be suddenly released from the bone and, owing to its shape and the wedging action of the forceps, may be squeezed out of the beaks of the forceps and aspirated or swallowed. This accident can often be prevented by controlled pressure on the handles of the forceps and by using a 4 by 4 inch sponge as a curtain behind the tooth to be extracted. If a tooth or a part of it cannot be accounted for during or after an extraction, radiographic examination of the chest and abdomen should be requested immediately. Absence of cough is not proof that a tooth has not been aspirated. A tooth or part of it in the bronchial tree must be removed as soon as possible by bronchoscopy to prevent serious complications. If the tooth or other foreign body is in the alimentary canal, its elimination should be ascertained by having the stools examined for the tooth. Should the tooth not be recovered and abdominal symptoms develop, consultation with the physician should be obtained.

INFECTIONS

Infections in children are of special importance to the pedodontist, because he is often in a position to prevent or intercept them. He can shorten their course and prevent their spread.

The differences in the progress of infections of the jaws in the child and in the adult, especially as they concern the upper cuspid region and the molar region, have been described by Sicher.[7]

Infection in a young jaw: (1) may spread owing to the wide marrow spaces; (2) may involve the buds of permanent teeth, as in the brown discoloration of enamel produced in chronic infection (Turner's hypoplasia). Infection can also cause complete destruction of permanent tooth germs; (3) may reach the growth centers of the jaw, especially the condylar region in the mandible, resulting in disfigurement (sequestration of large pieces of bone in any part of the jaws may have the same effect); and (4) may produce cellulitis and abscess formation which will require incision and drainage.

PROGRESS OF INFECTION

Infection may spread by various pathways, the most frequent being by continuity. Here the infectious process proceeds from the periapical region of a tooth through the marrow spaces, breaks through the cortical plate and elevates the periosteum from the bone, forming a subperiosteal abscess. From the beginning of an acute pericementitis until it breaks through the periosteum, pus is confined to a limited space, causing pressure upon the surrounding tissues. This factor expresses itself clinically as an intense throbbing pain, with the tooth feeling elongated and very sensitive to pressure. Slight mobility can usually be found upon testing the tooth. During this stage, there is usually no marked edema present. In a subperiosteal abscess, a hard, circumscribed, painful swelling can be palpated on the bone, either in the mucobuccal folds or from the external surface. Lymph node enlargement may occur very early. Eventually the pus breaks through the confining barrier of the periosteum and, owing to collateral edema, a sudden swelling of soft tissues of the face appears. At this stage, the pressure has been relieved and pain usually decreases in intensity. Infection now spreads through more or less loose areolar tissue. Thenceforth, the extension of infection is determined by gravity and by anatomic pathways as dictated by the location of muscle attachments, fascia and fascial planes.

The next step in the progress of infection may be formation of an abscess accompanied by a cellulitis. The abscess may form in the mucobuccal fold, sublingual area, or palatal region, or progress toward the skin. The swelling first becomes pitting and later fluctuant. It is especially important to recognize pitting and fluctuation in abscesses progressing toward the skin because spontaneous breakthrough should be prevented by an incision at the proper time.

Spontaneous rupture of abscesses through the skin destroys the subcutaneous tissues and deprives the skin of its normal structure. Unsightly, irregular scars result. A sharp, well executed incision at the right time will leave a linear scar which usually becomes barely visible after a few months.

The second most frequent avenue of spread of infection is by the lymphatics. A tooth may or may not be sensitive to percussion, yet suddenly the lymph nodes under the mandible may become palpable and tender. It is important to stress the fact that clinically and even roentgenographically negative teeth may be infected and send their products of infection to the regional lymph nodes.

These lymph nodes are at first discrete and movable, but later on become more enlarged and matted. A diagnosis of whether an infection is an extension by continuity or via the lymphatics can be made only in the beginning when the nodes are still movable. In an infection by continuity, as in subperiosteal abscesses or cellulitis, the swelling will be attached to the bone. When considering the etiologic factors in lymph node enlargement the dentist usually thinks of only odontogenic infection. One must remember to consider other factors such as cat-scratch disease, lymphomas, infectious mononucleosis, etc.

During the course of extra-oral incisions, it can be determined whether the extension is by continuity or through the lymphatic system. In an involvement of nodes only, the hemostat, which is used to find deeply seated pus, will not encounter rough exposed bone. When the extension is by continuity, pus has to break through the cortical plate and periosteum which has been elevated and partially destroyed, exposing the rough, uneven bone surface.

Extension of infection occurs also by way of the blood stream in the direction of the heart. Invasion of the blood stream produces septicemia with or without metastatic abscesses in other parts of the body (pyemia).

Retrograde extension through veins may also occur. Veins in the face have no valves and will allow a back flow of blood or extension of thrombophlebitis toward the orbit and the cavernous sinus. This is especially true if the originating point is from the triangle formed by the upper lip and nose up to its root (Fig. 18–6). There are, however, other communications between the anterior and posterior facial veins, the pyterygoid plexus and again the cavernous sinus.

Propagation of septic thrombi through arteries has also been described. A thrombus forming in an artery running through infected tissue may become loose and lodge in the peripheral area supplied by this vessel. Local necrosis with infection will follow and manifest itself in a sudden swelling and pain in the peripheral part of the jaw. Observation has shown development of an independent and isolated sequestrum in the lower cuspid region following an acute osteomyelitis in the molar region. with healthy bone remaining between the two damaged parts.

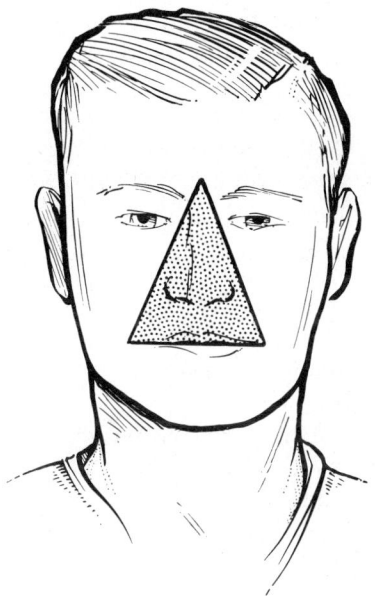

Figure 18–6 Danger triangle of the face.

MANIFESTATIONS OF INFECTION

A serious infection is always accompanied by certain systemic manifestations:

1. Fever, which especially in small children tends to reach higher levels than in adults, with rapid pulse and rapid but shallow respiration.

2. General malaise, nausea and vomiting, the latter two seen more frequently in children.

3. An increase in the white blood count, especially the neutrophils. In longer-lasting serious infections, such as osteomyelitis, anemia may follow.

4. Dehydration due to loss of water through perspiration and lack of fluid intake. Other signs and symptoms of systemic involvement through infection are anorexia, constipation or diarrhea, and pain in the abdominal region.

MANAGEMENT OF INFECTION

The management of infection consists of (1) local treatment and (2) systemic treatment.

Local Treatment

Local treatment depends on the local and systemic signs and symptoms, their severity, and the stage of the disease. Proper prevention of infections through operative dentistry and the removal of broken-down, irreparable teeth is all-important and will save the child and dentist much grief.

If an acute condition such as pericementitis occurs without pronounced systemic involvement, the first question which has to be answered is: Should we attempt to save the tooth? Retention of a permanent anterior tooth is of paramount importance and should be attempted even if the life span of that tooth, after treatment, may be relatively short. The importance of retaining the natural anterior teeth cannot be minimized.

If the tooth is painful to percussion and elongated and presents spontaneous throbbing pain, the pulp chamber should be opened. The use of high speed instruments permits this to be done with minimal pain. Whether or not antibiotics are used will depend upon the health of the individual, extent of infection, complicating systemic factors, etc.

Local anesthesia is not preferred for this purpose because it tends to produce ischemia above the apex, with diminished blood flow. If pus is present in the periapical tissue, it will be evacuated through the canal after a fine broach has removed the pulp debris. Usually one or more drops of pus will appear, followed by some hemorrhage. This hemorrhage contributes to the evacuation of the pus and brings about faster relief. Ischemia will inhibit this hemorrhage. If anesthesia must be used, it should be by inhalation; the analgesic state is usually sufficient, especially in a well premedicated child.

One will find that by using proper care and instruments and complete fixation of the tooth, the pulp chamber can be opened in the majority of children without any anesthesia.

If pus appears from the pulp chamber, the prognosis for early relief is very good. If only serous fluid appears, the outlook for such relief is not bright, for some of these teeth remain sensitive to pressure for a long time. After the pus has been evacuated, the parents should be instructed to insert a small pledget of cotton into the pulp chamber before eating and remove it immediately after eating.

The cotton prevents solid food particles from obstructing the drainage. The cotton, if left in the pulp chamber too long, will act as an obstruction as it quickly becomes clogged with coagulated pus. After the acute symptoms have receded, root canal treatment may be instituted, if necessary, followed by apicoectomy or periapical curettage (see Chapter 10, Pulpal Treatment of Primary Teeth).

In the presence of acute dentoalveolar abscess with cellulitis, when teeth are destroyed beyond repair or when a history of rheumatic and congenital heart disease, kidney disease and other diseases contraindicates conservative procedures, the teeth should be removed after the patient has received adequate antibiotic coverage. Antibiotics should continue for at least 24 hours after the patient has become afebrile.

The decision as to how to proceed becomes more difficult when the pericementitis has progressed through the bone beneath the periosteum. In cases in which, for reasons mentioned above, the tooth cannot be saved, extraction should be performed with proper antibiotic premedication and postoperative protection. Pus will usually escape through the socket and the patient will be relieved. General anesthesia is preferable.

If an abscess in the mucobuccal fold, palate or sublingual space has formed, it should be incised and the tooth should be opened for drainage or extracted if so indicated.

Intra-oral abscesses should be opened. If a general anesthetic is necessary, extreme care must be taken to prevent aspiration of pus. The use of a throat pack is advisable. Samples of the pus should be taken for smear, culture and sensitivity tests. If penicillin had been used prior to extraction, it should be stated so on the slip sent to the laboratory so that penicillinase can be used on the culture.

If the infection progresses toward the skin, extra-oral incisions may be necessary. Hospitalization is usually advisable and these cases are better referred to an oral surgeon.

A cyst or tumor must be considered when swellings which are painless and of long duration suddenly become acute.

Some controversy still exists on the use of cold or heat in dental infection. It seems that cold serves only one purpose, to reduce traumatic edema and to help prevent hemorrhage. It should be used, therefore, only after trauma, be it due to surgery or accident. Twenty-four hours after injury, cold should be discontinued and heat should be used to hasten the process of absorption of the exudate.

Cold should never be used in infection, as it counteracts nature's process of defense: vasodilatation and the mobilization of phagocytes.

The opinion that heat will draw pus toward the skin and that cold will prevent this occurrence is unfounded. Pus will progress along anatomic pathways and it is impossible to change the course.[7] Cold may delay this progress, heat may hasten it. Certainly, faster progress is preferable to a slow-down which does not cure but only postpones.

A similar consideration exists when the resolution of an abscess is effected through the use of antibiotics without surgical interference. In the beginning of the antibiotic era great expectations were laid upon the ability of penicillin to help resolve abscesses without incision, either by injection of the drug into the abscess or by its systemic use.

Injections of antibiotics into closed infected areas have proven to be hazardous and have been discontinued. Systemic use of antibiotics without proper surgical drainage has taught us that the infectious process may be arrested but the abscess continues to exist and is walled off. After discontinuation of the antibiotic, the abscess occasionally flares up and must be incised. Necrotic tissue, which often proves to be aseptic, is eliminated slowly through the incision or sinus tract.

Systemic Treatment

1. Antibiotics are administered as described in Chapter 19, Antimicrobial Agents. If fever persists and the other systemic signs and symptoms do not improve within 24 to 48 hours after drainage, the infective agents may be resistant to the antibiotic and consideration should be given to changing the drug. At this time the results of the sensitivity test will usually be known and one can choose the proper antibiotic. If, on the other hand, the response to the first antibiotic used was good, it should not be changed even if the sensitivity test shows the particular microorganisms to be resistant. The local tissues should be checked carefully for retention of pus.

It has been our experience that the best antibiotic for the treatment of most oral infections is penicillin. Should the patient be sensitive to penicillin, we like to use erythromycin.

Care should be taken to prevent dehydration, as in some cases even swallowing of fluids may be difficult. The child must be encouraged to drink water, fruit juices, etc. If this cannot be accomplished, intravenous fluids must be given. This will require hospitalization.

2. A diet rich in vitamins B and C and protein should be given; vitamin supplements can be administered orally or by injection.

SUPERNUMERARY TEETH

Supernumerary primary teeth are very rare. Supernumerary permanent teeth, on the other hand, are relatively frequent. They are found most frequently in the region of the upper anterior teeth, especially the central incisors. If in the midline, they are called mesiodens (Figs. 18–7 and 18–8). A third lower premolar is next in the order of frequency except for fourth molars, which are of no concern in this book.

Supernumerary teeth frequently cause a delay in eruption of permanent teeth or anomalies of position such as diastemas or rotations. Other complicating factors are the development of dentigerous cysts, or, if degeneration of the forming enamel organ occurs before laying down of any enamel, of primordial or follicular cysts. Primordial cysts are epithelium-lined cavities which do not show any signs of calcified tooth structure; they may present a diagnostic problem.

Pressure of supernumerary teeth on adjacent teeth may cause resorption of their roots with subsequent pulp damage. Infection in the tooth follicle may occur, but it is infrequent.

In some cases, the supernumerary teeth have the appearance of normal teeth; in some, they are rudimentary and peg-like. Some show dens in dente formation, others resemble abnormal root formations (Fig. 18–9).

In some cases, the crowns of these supernumerary teeth are erupted at least partially through the gingiva, but not infrequently they are found high up in the apical region of the upper central incisors, usually lingual to them.

In cleft palate patients, supernumerary teeth are found frequently either in the premaxilla or just distal to the cleft.

Before removal is attempted, good periapical, occlusal and cross-section radiographs should be taken to aid in the localization of these teeth. Clark's method[3] of radiographic localization is very useful. In the anterior region we like an occlusal view and a lateral view of the anterior maxilla. The latter can be taken by having the patient hold an occlusal film parallel to the cheek. This view tells us

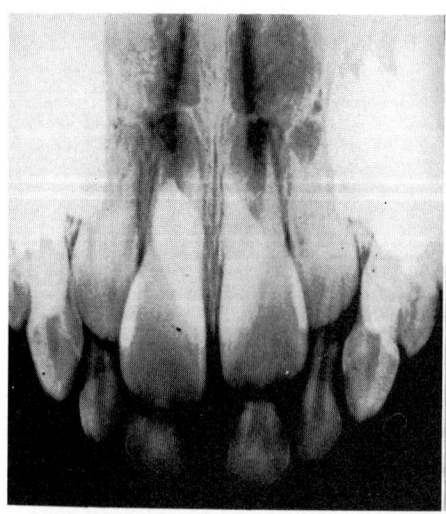
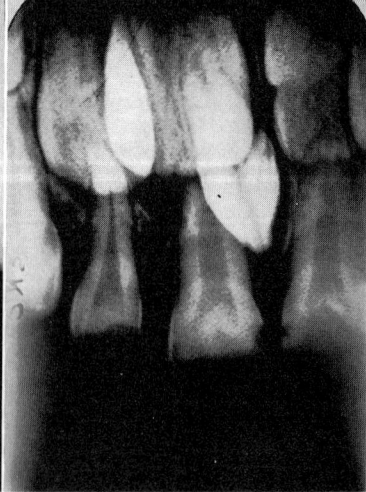

Figure 18–7 Inverted mesiodens.   **Figure 18–8** Mesiodens.

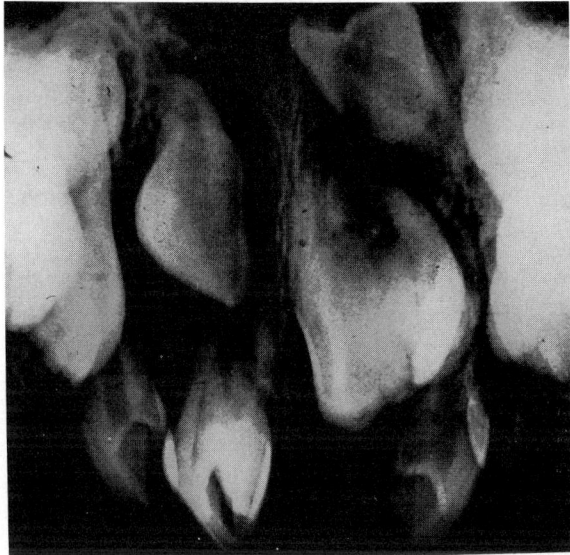

Figure 18–9 Supernumerary teeth with dens in dente formation.

whether the supernumerary teeth are palatal or labial to the permanent teeth, and the height of each. Another consideration before removing a supernumerary tooth is the condition of the apices of the permanent teeth adjacent to it. Are they fully formed or still incomplete? Removal of a supernumerary tooth lying near open apices should be postponed until closure of these canals occurs, unless the supernumerary tooth prevents the eruption of these teeth or is causing extreme rotation of a permanent tooth.

During removal of teeth from the neighborhood of apices of other teeth, damage to the vessels supplying the pulp may occur. Root canal therapy is difficult in teeth with open canals.

The radiographs must be studied very carefully to determine which tooth or teeth represent the supernumerary structure and should, therefore, be removed. Difficulties are sometimes encountered if the additional teeth are well formed and well developed. As a general rule, the supernumerary tooth lies lingual to the normal tooth.

Large flaps should be made to assure good access and visibility. Whether to operate from the labial or the lingual aspect depends upon the radiographic localization of the tooth and the position of the crown, which is the widest part of the tooth and must be exposed first. Wherever possible, avoid the removal of both lingual and labial plates, because bone regeneration is very slow in such instances. The tooth follicle should be removed in its entirety to prevent the development of a cyst or ameloblastoma.

If there are unerupted permanent teeth whose eruption has been delayed by the supernumerary teeth, removal of the bone overlying the crowns of these permanent teeth will frequently aid in their eruption. The space into which these teeth will erupt must be maintained. The progress of the eruption of the permanent teeth should be followed by radiographic examination. Should these teeth fail to show evidence of eruption, surgical exposure of the crowns and the use of wire and traction to move the teeth into position may be necessary.

IMPACTIONS

RELATIVE INCIDENCE OF IMPACTIONS

The most frequently encountered impactions in children are those of the upper permanent cuspids. Next in order of prevalence are impactions of lower second premolars and upper second premolars. Other impactions are rare except those of upper incisors due to supernumerary teeth. Many impacted or unerupted teeth are found in children who have cleidocranial dysostosis. Impaction of upper cuspids is 18 to 20 times more frequent than impaction of lower cuspids, and a greater percentage occurs in girls than in boys. The most frequent position is in the palate (Fig. 18–10); about 85 per cent of the remainder are located buccally and a few cases about halfway between the lingual and labial flare. Lower cuspid impactions are rare and usually they are located labially.

The frequency of occurrence of upper cuspid impactions may be explained according to Dewel[1] in the following manner:

1. The lingually displaced cuspid has to travel a long distance through the dense palatal bone. The root is usually more completely formed than in other permanent teeth that are ready to erupt. The roots of the primary cuspid very often show delayed resorption, which may lead to a deflection of the permanent successor. The delayed resorption may be caused by a faulty position of the permanent tooth bud, which does not cause resorption in an apical direction parallel to the bone and in the long axis of the primary cuspid.

2. The permanent cuspid erupts after the lateral incisors. With both premolars and first permanent molars already in occlusion, any deviation of the neighboring teeth will deprive the permanent cuspid of space formerly occupied by the primary cuspid, a tooth which is much smaller in its mesiodistal diameter. The second molar, which erupts at the same time as the permanent cuspid, exerts pressure in a mesial direction and can make this difficult situation worse.

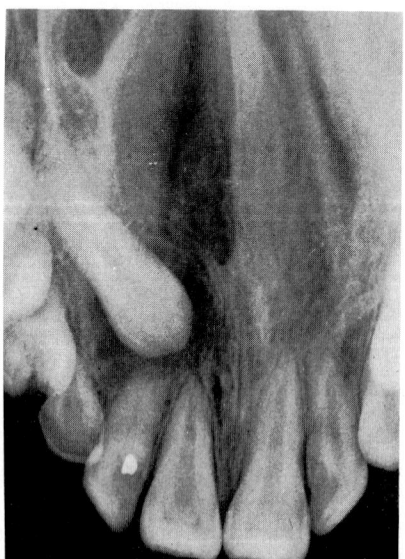

Figure 18–10   Palatal impaction of upper cuspid with resorption of the root of the lateral incisor.

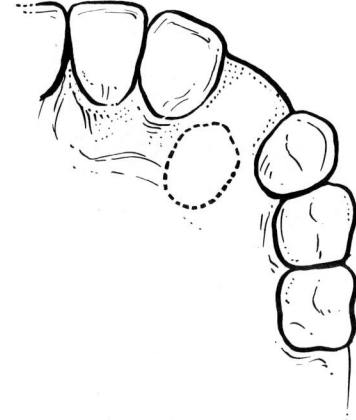

Figure 18–11 Excision of mucoperiosteum for exposure of impacted upper cuspid.

SURGICAL EXPOSURE OF IMPACTED MAXILLARY CUSPIDS

In impactions of upper cuspids in children the decision will have to be made whether they should be surgically exposed so that orthodontic treatment can be instituted or whether they must be removed.

This decision hinges upon the judgment of the operator and, very often, on orthodontic consultation. Electrosurgery for the exposure of impacted teeth is contraindicated because damage to the bone may occur, with prolonged healing time and much more discomfort. The roentgenogram will not always supply the complete information, and very often it is only after exposure of the crown of such teeth that a final conclusion can be drawn and the right decision made.

In the surgical exposure of upper cuspids located palatally, two methods may be followed:

1. If the crown of the permanent cuspid or the elevation caused by it can be definitely palpated, the overlying mucoperiosteum is excised and the bone over the crown removed carefully with burs so as not to damage the enamel of the permanent cuspid (Fig. 18–11). After the crown is exposed the pericoronal space down to the cemento-enamel junction is widened with periodontal scalers to make a space about 2 mm. wide around the crown. A celluloid or, preferably, an aluminum shell crown is adapted over the crown until it approaches the cemento-enamel junction and is cemented with zinc oxide-eugenol. The occlusal part of the shell should protrude through the excised portion of the bone and mucoperiosteum to maintain this opening.

Before this method was developed, either iodoform gauze dressings or surgical cements were used to keep the exposure open. Many changes of these dressings were necessary and caused a great deal of discomfort to the patient. The use of fine metal hooks cemented into the crown of the exposed tooth has been discouraged by Oppenheim, who demonstrated that this method is followed by pulp necrosis in an overwhelming number of cases. After slight eruption of the tooth has occurred, an impression of the crown may be taken with a copper band, a casting carrying one or two hooks can be made and cemented in place, and orthodontic treatment can be instituted.

2. When the position of the impacted cuspid cannot be ascertained by palpation, a large flap should be made as described later. After the shell has been

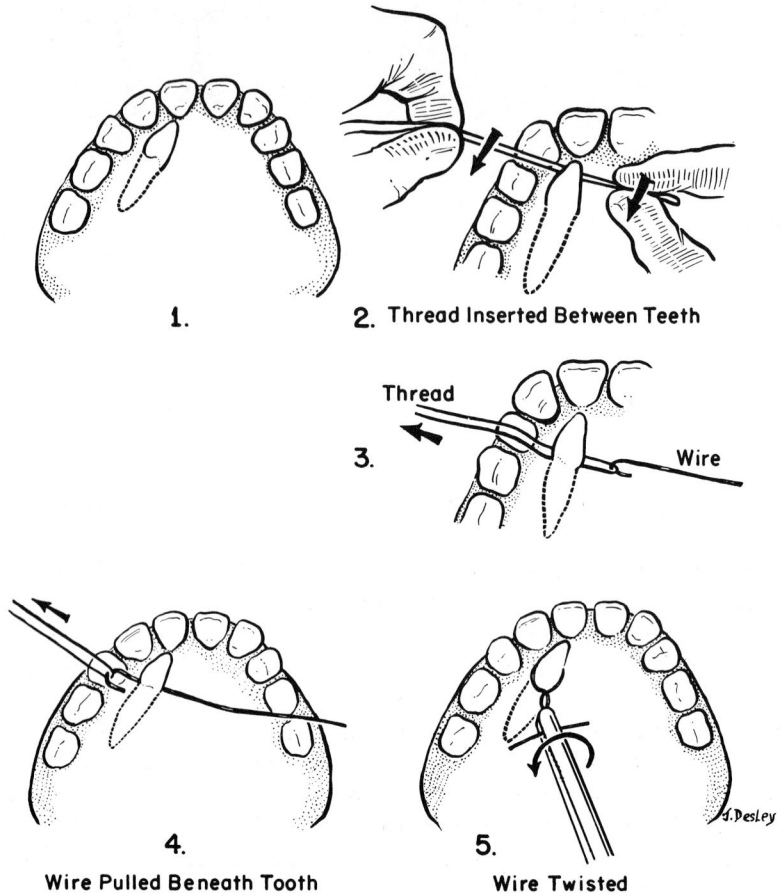

1.

2. Thread Inserted Between Teeth

Thread

3.

Wire

4.

Wire Pulled Beneath Tooth

5.

Wire Twisted

Figure 18–12 Exposure of upper cuspid and insertion of wire around cervical portion to be used for orthodontics.

adapted and cemented, the flap is repositioned and an opening is cut into it. Then the flap is sutured into position.

As there will always be some cases in which surgical exposure followed by orthodontic treatment will be found to be impossible after the crown has been exposed, the parent should be warned before the operation that removal of the impacted tooth may become necessary during the operation.

Pain and swelling following exposure are minimal.

If, upon exposure of the crown, the position is found to be so unfavorable that a shell cannot be slipped upon the crown (i.e., if the tip of the canine contacts a neighboring root), then a stainless steel wire must be applied and twisted around the neck of the exposed crown. The two ends extruding into the oral cavity are used for the orthodontic procedure.

It is not always simple to get the wire around the crown. A strong silk suture (about No. 00) may be pushed up between the cusp of the canine and the adjoining root. Enough motion in the cuspid can usually be obtained to let the silk suture slip through even if the contact is very close. The silk suture should be double so that the wire can be pulled into the space by bending the end sharply upon itself and pulling it into the area around the neck (Fig. 18–12).

REMOVAL OF IMPACTED MAXILLARY CUSPIDS

Although the technique for removal of impacted upper cuspids in children does not differ from that used in adults, it will be described in some detail because it is an operation that is frequently performed on children in the age group 12 to 16 years. As mentioned above, careful study of good radiographs is indispensable.

Anesthesia may be obtained by infiltration in the mucobuccal fold, starting above the central incisor and proceeding distally to the second premolar or even the first molar. An incisive canal block and an injection somewhat anterior to the greater palatine foramen are used to anesthetize the palatal tissues. If pain occurs during the operation it may originate from nerves entering the hard palate from the nasal cavity. A spray with 5 per cent Pontocaine into the appropriate nostril, followed by the insertion of two cotton applicators soaked in the same solution into the inferior meatus for about five minutes, will generally achieve the desired effect.

Palatal Impactions

An incision is carried along the gingival margin, starting palatally at the lateral incisor of the opposite side and continuing to the first permanent molar on the side of the impaction (Fig. 18–13*A*). In bilateral impactions the incision extends from the first permanent molar on the right side to the first permanent molar on the left side (Fig. 18–13*B*). The periosteum is carefully elevated from the hard palate and the incisive canal structures, nerves, arteries and veins are cut if necessary. Bleeding in this area is usually stopped by compression, or with a piece of bone wax. No permanent sensory disturbances due to the cutting of the nasopalatine nerves are experienced by the patient. The incision is extensive, but experience has shown that both the operation and the healing process are expedited by making a large instead of a small flap, which must be forcefully retracted and, therefore, damaged. The retraction of the flap is best done by a No. 00 suture taken through the palatal flap and held in place by tying to the opposite premolars or molars.

In our hands the bur has proven to be the best method of removing the bone; however, it may be removed with mallet and chisel. The crown is exposed beyond the cemento-enamel junction. If the cusp of the cuspid crown wedges against an adjoining tooth it should be sectioned at the cemento-enamel junction with a bur.

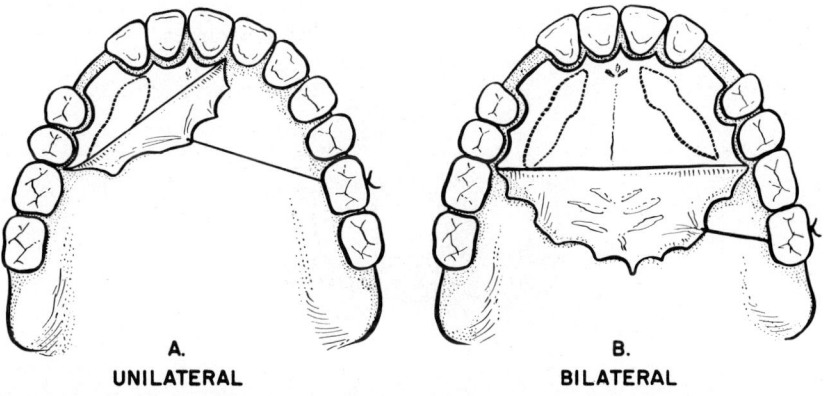

A.
UNILATERAL

B.
BILATERAL

Figure 18–13   Incision for removal of palatally impacted cuspids. *A,* Unilateral; *B,* bilateral.

At least 3 mm. should be removed between crown and root to allow the crown section to be pushed toward the root. This permits disengaging the cusp from the neighboring roots and preventing their injury. Before sectioning with a bur, the tooth should be moved slightly to make it easier to mobilize the root later on. Elevators should be used with discretion, as their injudicious use has caused luxation and permanent damage to central and lateral incisors.

After removal of the crown, the root is removed with fine-pointed elevators. If the root is not released easily a curvature at the apex may be present, requiring the removal of additional palatal bone.

After removal of the root follicle and débridement, the palatal flap is returned into its original position and sutured through the interdental spaces to the labial part of the gingiva. This procedure may be simplified by taking a suture through the palatal flap in the region of a papilla, passing the tied ends of the suture mesially and distally around the tooth and tying them. This tie is repeated around every other tooth. A preoperatively constructed acrylic palatal splint insures good adaptation of the soft tissue flap. This refinement in technique prevents blood from pooling between bone and periosteum. It is much more desirable than temporary compression with sponges. In addition, the splint will help protect the palatal flap from hot foods until the nerve supply to the area has completely returned.

Postoperative pain and swelling are usually of a minor degree. Sutures may be removed after five days.

Labial Impactions

Removal of buccally located impacted upper cuspids is simple, provided a distinct bulging of the buccal surface of the alveolar plate can be felt. A flap which will cover the socket after the removal of the cuspid should be raised (Fig. 18–14); then the usually thin bone is removed with fine, sharp chisels and the tooth is delivered by forceps. The flap should then be returned into its position and held with a few sutures.

Cuspids lying above the premolar roots are difficult to remove and should be handled only by the oral surgeon. Frequently the roots of these cuspids may partially encircle a bicuspid root, and unless care is exercised the premolar may be devitalized.

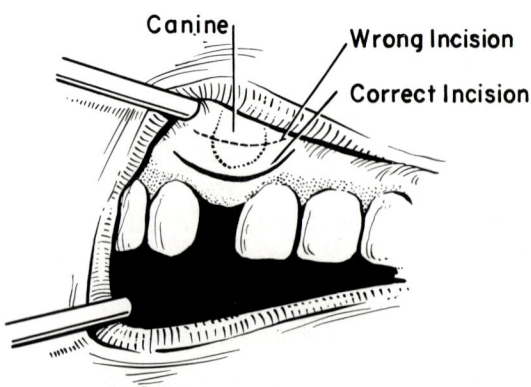

Figure 18–14   Incision for removal of a labially impacted upper cuspid.

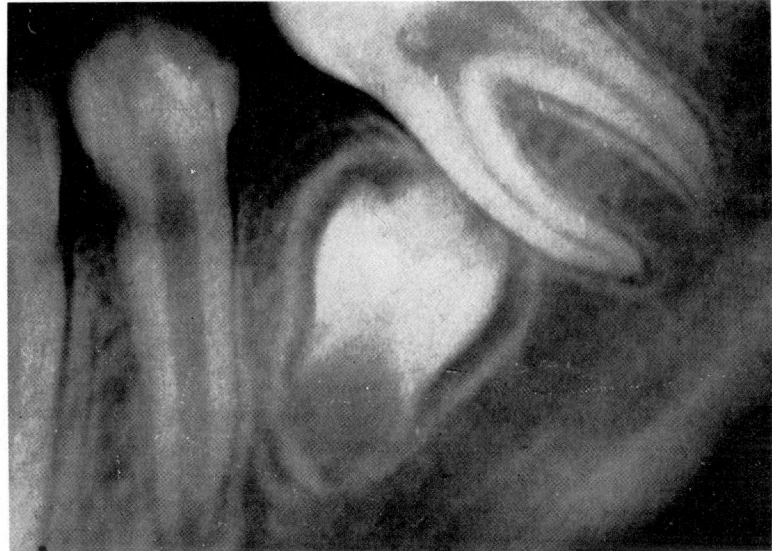

Figure 18–15 Impaction of lower second premolar with crown pointing lingually and distally.

REMOVAL OF IMPACTED OR MALERUPTED LOWER SECOND PREMOLARS

These teeth are usually situated between the first premolar and first permanent molar, with the crown pointing lingually (Fig. 18–15). Very often they are partially erupted, the crown being wedged between the two neighbors. In some cases an elevation caused by the erupting crown can be palpated on the lingual aspect. The tooth may, however, be lying beneath the roots of the two adjoining teeth, in which case removal is more difficult. Occlusal radiographs are very helpful in the location of these teeth (Fig. 18–16).

If the crown is slightly erupted the tooth can usually be removed with a narrow beak forceps. A bayonet forceps can be used with one beak lingually and the other in the triangular space formed by the crown of the three adjoining teeth (Fig. 18–17A). Sometimes a mesiodistal application can be used (Fig. 18–17B). A slight displacement lingually with the help of a small pointed elevator will create some space for the labial beak of the forceps. The adjoining first premolar must be supported by pushing it into the socket with a finger of the left hand. Sutures or dressings are unnecessary in these cases.

If the tooth is still covered with mucoperiosteum and a lingual bulging is evident, a small incision is made on the lingual gingival attachment from the first molar forward to the cuspid. One may then detach this tissue and retract the flap, taking care not to penetrate the sublingual tissues with the retractor.

The crown is exposed with burs and removed by forceps. If the crown is lingually placed but still deep in the bone, one should expose it, then make an incision on the buccal surface, locate and expose the root apex and, with a blunt instrument, carefully expel the apex with a mallet toward the lingual. The mental nerve should be avoided by making vertical incisions in the cuspid and first molar regions; this approach allows better exposure and protects the mental foramen (Fig. 18–18). The mucoperiosteal flap is then approximated with No. 000 silk. If it

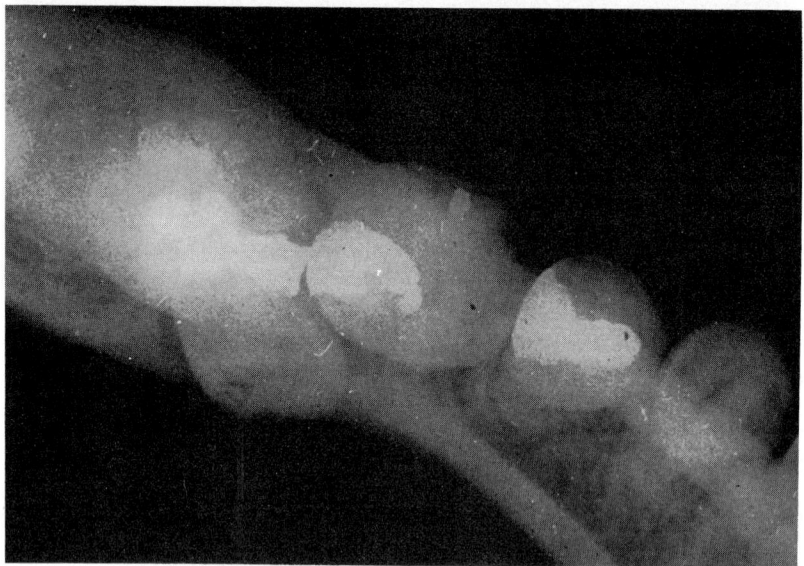

Figure 18–16 Occlusal radiograph of lingually impacted lower second premolar.

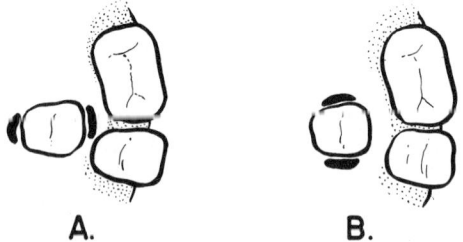

A. **B.**

Figure 18–17 Removal of lingually impacted lower bicuspid. *A*, Buccolingual application of forceps. *B*, Mesiodistal application of forceps.

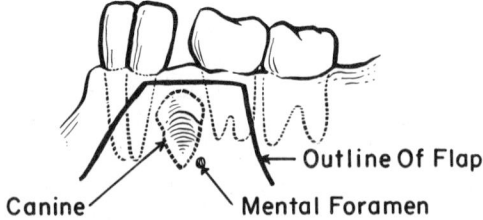

Figure 18–18 Incision for removal of lingually impacted lower premolar and cuspid, if tooth has to be expelled from the buccal aspect of the alveolar process.

has been necessary to do the procedure under general anesthesia because of lack of cooperation by the patient, absorbable sutures such as plain catgut are indicated.

CYSTS

CYSTS IN THE SOFT TISSUES OF THE ORAL CAVITY

Mucous Cysts

Mucous cysts occur in the lips and cheeks, usually at the line of occlusion. They also occur on the hard and soft palate, due to obstruction of the ducts from injury. These cysts are usually bluish in color and, on the surface, vesicular in appearance. They have an elastic consistency and collapse when drained but refill as soon as the incision heals (Fig. 18–19). A similar, somewhat larger cyst occurs on the lower aspect of the tongue, originating from the glands of Nuhn and Blandin.

The treatment of small mucous cysts consists of excision in toto. When enucleated they frequently recur.

Ranulas and Dermoid Cysts

A cyst in the floor of the mouth, called a ranula, may become quite large and may be located superficially, appearing as a thin-walled, blue-red, vesicular prominence in the anterior portion of the floor of the mouth (Fig. 18–20). If the cyst forms in the deeper planes, a submental swelling may be palpated; if it is growing posteriorly, it will be felt in the submaxillary region. Dermoid cysts occur in the same region and must be considered in the differential diagnosis.

Dermoid cysts, although congenital, usually are noticed later in life. Intra-orally they do not appear as a vesicle. The color is yellowish, and on palpation they are of rubber-like consistency. Ranulas contain viscous fluid, dermoid cysts a cheesy yellow material, sometimes with hair and teeth included.

Ranulas that are treated by enucleation may recur. Marsupialization, the preferred method, consists of removing the portion of the cyst sac seen as part of the floor of the mouth, including the overlying mucosa. Wharton's duct must not be cut or involved in suturing. A lacrimal probe in Wharton's duct identifies the course of this structure. The probe should remain in position throughout the operation. Sutures are employed to connect the remaining cyst sac and the cut edge of oral mucosa, transforming the cyst into an accessory cavity of the oral cavity. During healing the surgically created opening must be maintained by a stent or narrow gauze packing. It must be remembered that more than one cyst may be present in a ranula.

Complete removal of the cyst, with excision of the involved gland, may be indicated in deep-seated cysts, especially if they are made up of more than one cavity. This operation requires considerable surgical experience.

Cysts of the large salivary glands are rare in children.

Fig. 18–19

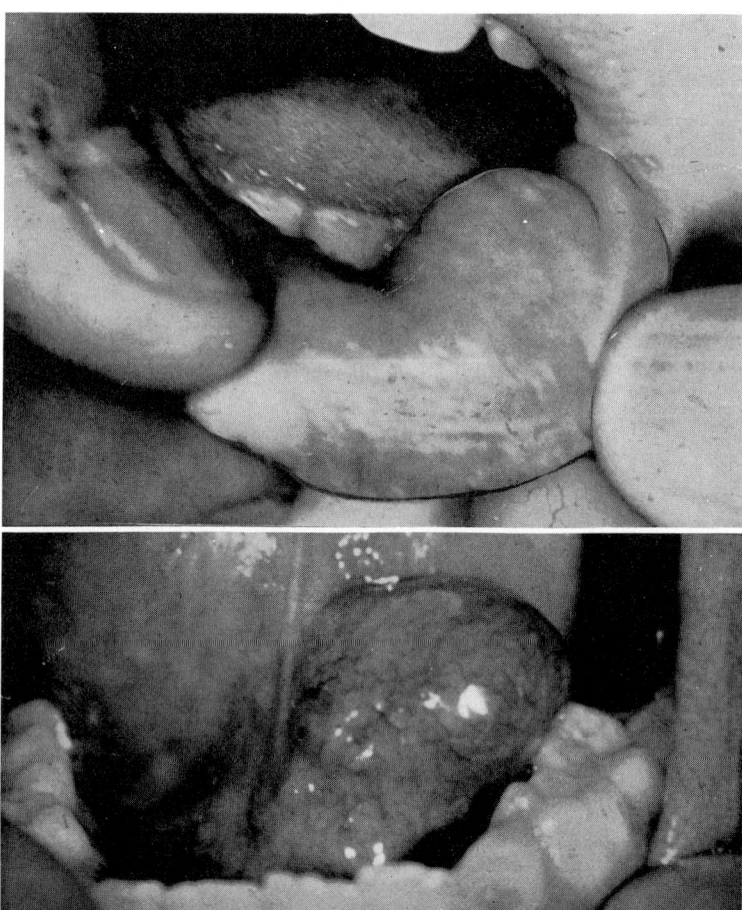

Fig. 18–20
Figure 18–19 Mucous cyst of lower lip.
Figure 18–20 Ranula.

Cysts of Bone

Cysts in the jaws occur quite frequently in children. These cysts may be of odontogenic or nonodontogenic origin or they may be cyst-like cavities in the bone, not lined by epithelium (traumatic, hemorrhagic, extravasation cyst) (Figs. 18–21 and 18–22).[4, 8]

In any cyst-like radiolucencies of bone, such as those produced by an ameloblastoma, a central fibroma, a central giant cell tumor, hyperthyroidism, monostotic fibrous dysplasia, Hand-Schüller-Christian disease, and eosinophilic granuloma, a differential diagnosis must be made by careful radiographic, clinical and histopathologic examination. In many instances certain laboratory tests, such as determination of calcium, phosphorus, and alkaline phosphatase, are indicated.

The problem of damaging or destroying neighboring teeth in contact with the pathologic area is of prime importance in choosing the proper surgical technique. Esthetics and function have to be considered because irreparable harm can be done by radical procedures. Enucleation is the method of choice with most oral surgeons and should be used in cysts which do not involve the roots of adjoining vital teeth. The Partsch operation or marsupialization is, in our opinion, preferable to total enucleation of large cysts in close proximity to teeth because it helps to preserve the vitality of these teeth. Some authorities feel that an ameloblastoma or a cystic recurrence can develop from cyst membrane left behind in the Partsch operation, and this possibility should be kept in mind. The solution of the problem may be to compromise by using the two-stage procedure of Waldron, who recommends, first, drainage of the cyst by the Partsch method, and later, when enough bone has formed around the roots of the surrounding teeth, the enucleation of the remaining cyst sac.

Whichever operation is performed, it is mandatory that parts of the cyst sac be removed for histopathologic examination. In large cysts portions of the cyst from various locations should be preserved, identified, and inserted into labeled bottles.

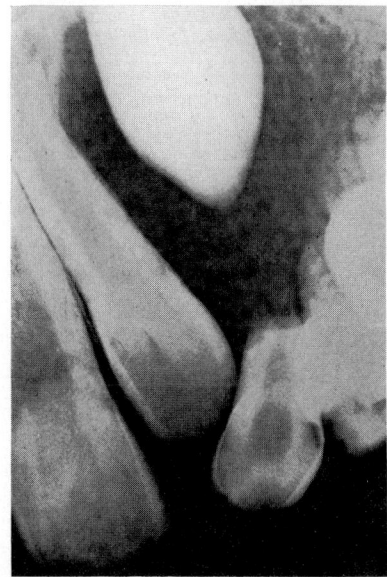

Figure 18–21 Dentigerous cyst originating from the upper cuspid.

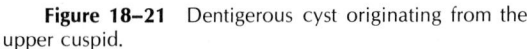

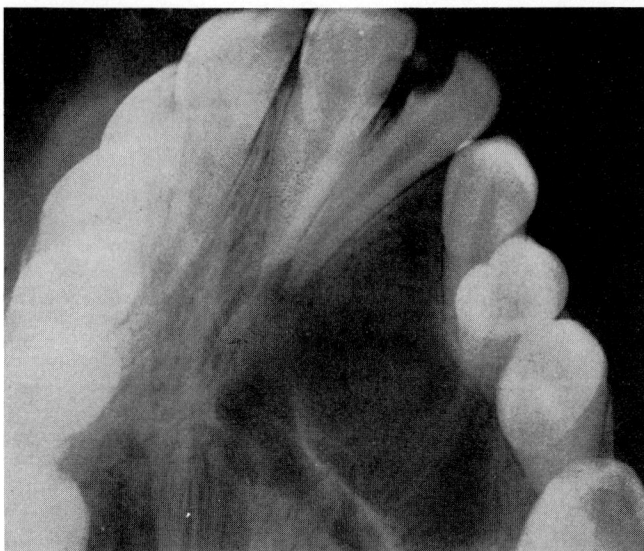

Figure 18–22   Globulo-maxillary cyst.

A diagram showing the location of each of the specimens should be submitted to the pathologist and a copy kept in the office. We have seen a few cases in which one portion of the cyst sac showed characteristics of a cyst, while another portion showed those of an ameloblastoma.

In dentigerous cysts, immediate removal of the tooth contained in the cavity is not always the procedure of choice. A survey of the time involved in the healing of dentigerous cysts has shown that healing and flattening out of the cyst's cavity occur three times faster when the tooth is left in position. Besides this fact, it is worth mentioning that many teeth contained in the cyst's cavity can be brought to normal eruption provided there is space for them in the dental arch.

TRAUMATIC CYSTS

Traumatic or hemorrhagic cysts are not true cysts because the cavity is not lined by epithelium (Fig. 18–23). Traumatic cysts occur most frequently in young people, and usually an antecedent history of trauma to the area can be elicited. One explanation for their occurrence is that hemorrhage occurs into the wide spaces of the cancellous bone and the subsequent breakdown of the clot leaves a cavity within the bone. Usually there are no symptoms and the traumatic cyst may be first detected by routine radiographic examination.

On surgical exploration of a traumatic cyst, the usual finding is a large hollow space containing no lining, but there may be a few cobweb-like fibers and dark reddish fluid at the bottom of the cavity. If an operator could predict that he would be dealing with a traumatic cyst, there would be no need for surgical exploration because these cysts usually resolve gradually and are filled in with bone. However, when one observes a large radiolucent area, it is necessary to explore it in order to rule out a pathologic process such as tumor, odontogenic cyst, etc.

VITALITY TESTS

Vitality tests should be performed on teeth adjacent to a cyst before an operation is contemplated. The vitality tests should be repeated about one week after the operation, and then at three month intervals. Immediately after the operation, some teeth close to the cyst may not respond but will in a few months. If a tooth gives a nonvital response but appears normal on inspection and transillumination, it should be left. Do not confuse a nonvital pulp with a pulp that is not reacting because of an interruption of nerve impulses due to the surgical procedure. This response is often transient. The best method to test the vitality of teeth, short of using a bur and drilling into the tooth, is to use heat and cold. The electrical pulp test is the least reliable method.

It is also important to realize that in large cysts the cyst membrane often carries the vessels and nerves to the pulps. The loss of sensation after an operation is due to the anatomic fact that, especially in the upper jaw, the nerves reach the apices of the teeth through the labial or buccal plate and are, therefore, cut during the operation. Vessels, on the other hand, because of the existence of many anastomoses and collateral pathways, remain intact unless there is interference with the tissues, bone or cyst membrane close to the apex.

In some cases the affected teeth may be saved by endodontic treatment, with or without apicoectomy, as indicated by the circumstances

FRENAL ABNORMALITIES

ABNORMAL LINGUAL FRENUM

Occasionally one observes in a child an abnormally short lingual frenum which binds the tongue down to the floor of the mouth so that it cannot be projected

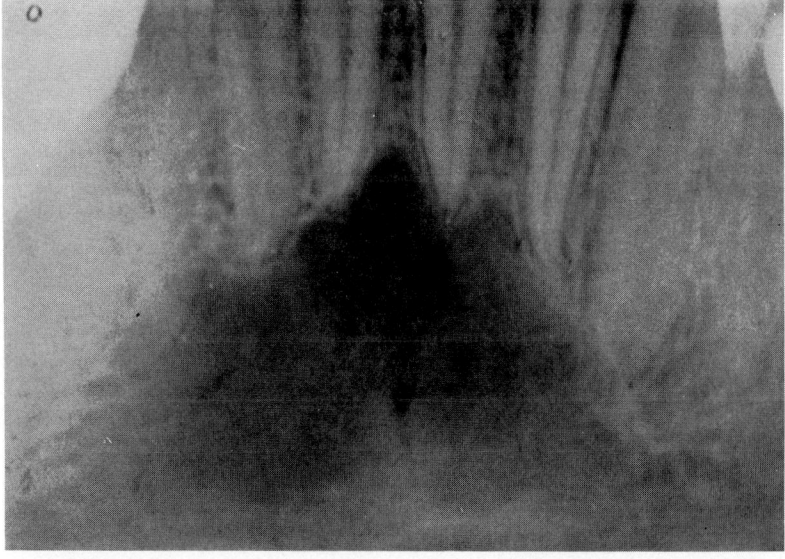

Figure 18–23 Traumatic cyst; all incisors and cuspids vital on pulp testing.

forward from the oral cavity or moved upward to make contact with the hard palate. Speech and deglutition may be impeded and, in addition, the frenum may be injured by contact with the lower incisors and an ulcer may develop. The fact remains, however, that too many frenums are cut unnecessarily and an operator should always be hesitant in promising improvement in a child's speech following frenectomy.

Treatment

Under infiltration anesthesia, a horizontal incision through the frenum is made, the tongue being held upward so that the frenum is stretched. The wound margins are gently undermined with curved scissors and the wound is transformed into a vertical one by suturing it from left to right, as shown in Figure 18–24.

Another, more simple, method consists in applying a small straight-pointed hemostat over the frenum just at the under surface of the tongue, and another, but curved, hemostat near the attachment to the floor of the mouth, taking care that the salivary ducts and caruncle are not pinched by the hemostat. The triangular piece between the two hemostats is excised with scissors, the margins are undermined, and the incision is closed with interrupted sutures (Fig. 18–25).

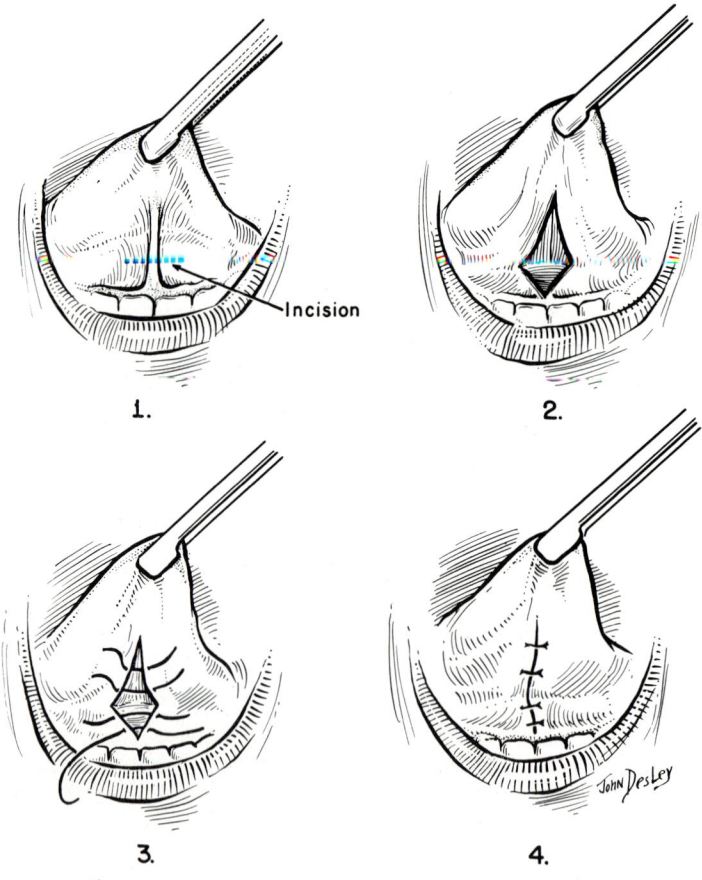

1.   Incision   **2.**

3.   **4.**

Figure 18–24   Operation to lengthen short lingual frenum.

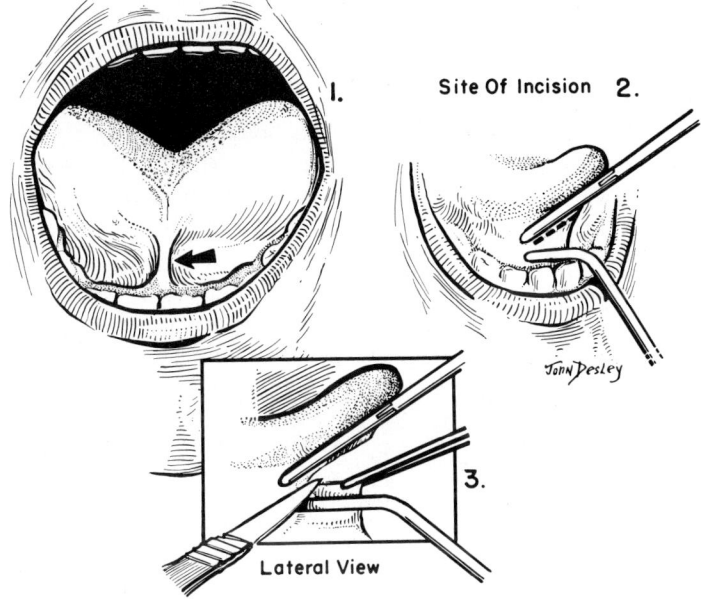

Figure 18–25 Modified operation for short lingual frenum.

LABIAL FRENUM OF THE UPPER LIP

An abnormally large frenum of the upper lip will be seen frequently in children, associated with a diastema between the primary central incisor or the erupting or erupted permanent centrals. A space between the upper primary centrals is common and normal, owing to growth of the anterior segment of the upper jaw, and should cause no concern. In addition, the separation of erupting or erupted permanent centrals may be absolutely normal at the time before the upper lateral incisors and cuspids have erupted.

In the newborn the frenum attaches at the crest of the alveolar ridge and as the alveolar process grows downward and the primary teeth erupt, the attachment of the frenum moves upward but may remain stationary in some cases, so that what appears to be an abnormal frenum at the age of 4 may be normal at the age of 8. Pressure from the erupting permanent laterals and cuspids usually results in closure of the space without any orthodontic or surgical interference (see Chapter 16, Preventive Orthodontics).

Treatment

If the labial frenum is removed, closure of the space should be attempted at the earliest possible time to prevent scar tissue formation between the two incisors, which would make the closure of the space more difficult. Frenectomy should be fixed upon only after a thorough discussion with a pedodontist or orthodontist.

Frenectomy can usually be accomplished under local anesthesia by infiltrating the frenum on the labial surface of the alveolar process, then sliding the needle through the interdental papilla toward the incisive papilla. After two or three minutes have elapsed, a few drops of anesthetic should be deposited in the incisive foramen. A triangular incision should be made, with the base anterior to the incisive papilla and the apex in the interproximal space between two central incisors. Care should be taken not to cut into the gingival attachment on the mesial surface of the centrals. The incision should be carried down to the bone, and elevation of the tissue by means of a periosteal elevator should be started anterior to the incisive papilla and carried forward into the interdental space between the two centrals, as far anteriorly as to the labial surface of the crest of the alveolar ridge. Now the lip is drawn forward and upward to tense the frenum and the incision is continued on either side of the frenum toward the lip up into the mucolabial fold (Fig. 18–26). The tissue which had been elevated is held with a hemostat and the whole mass is dissected free up into the fold. The periosteum on the labial side of the alveolar process should not be injured. A hemostat is now applied to the remaining frenum on the inner surface of the lip, and the part held by the hemostat is cut off with a

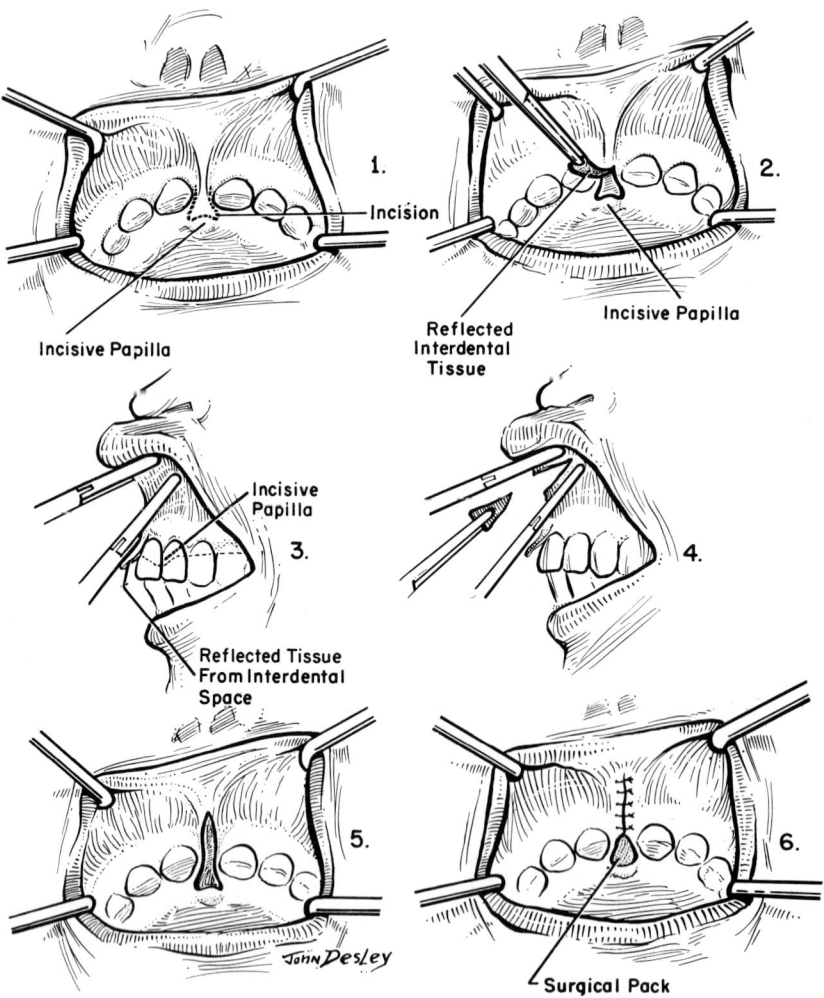

Figure 18–26   Labial frenum operation.

sharp scalpel. Only a few 3-0 silk or plain catgut sutures are necessary, especially in the lip. The exposed parts on the hard palate and the interdental space can be covered with a surgical pack. Some men prefer to perform the cutting part of the operation with the electrosurgical knife. This method requires more experience, and in the hands of the inexperienced may cause damage to the bone and surrounding teeth. It is difficult to see any advantage in it.

DIAGNOSIS OF TUMORS

Even in childhood the oral cavity and surrounding areas are subject to both benign and malignant neoplasms, and in many instances even a careful clinical examination does not conclusively identify the oral lesion as inflammatory, degenerative, or neoplastic. Biopsy followed by histopathologic examination is the only certain method of diagnosing questionable lesions of the oral cavity. The principles of biopsy technique are relatively simple and usually well within the limits of the pedodontist. The question whether a biopsy may hasten the growth or dissemination of a tumor is still moot, except in the case of malignant melanoma. If there is a suspicion of malignant melanoma, any manipulation of the tumor should be avoided and the patient should be immediately referred to a surgeon qualified to remove the tumor radically without previous biopsy, as dissemination of melanomas after biopsy is a frequent occurrence. In other lesions the dentist should make every effort to obtain the report of the biopsy at the earliest possible time, and if malignancy has been found, he must refer the patient, without delay, for treatment of the lesion.

TYPES OF BIOPSY

1. Excision Biopsy

When the lesion is small, it should be totally excised (Figs. 18–27 and 18–28). The excision should be wide enough and deep enough to include a border of healthy tissue along the entire cut surface, so that no further surgery is required if the pathologist's report is that of a benign tumor. If, on the other hand, a malignancy has been found, immediate referral to a competent surgeon is necessary, as recurrence is likely.

2. Incision Biopsy

When the size of the lesion is such that complete excision is not possible or feasible, a specimen which is representative of the lesion should be obtained (Figs. 18–29 and 18–30).

a. That portion of the lesion which demonstrates all of the pathologic changes noted clinically should be selected. If this is not possible with one tissue section, several areas must be selected.

b. Thin, deep sections should be removed rather than broad, shallow sections,

Fig. 18–27

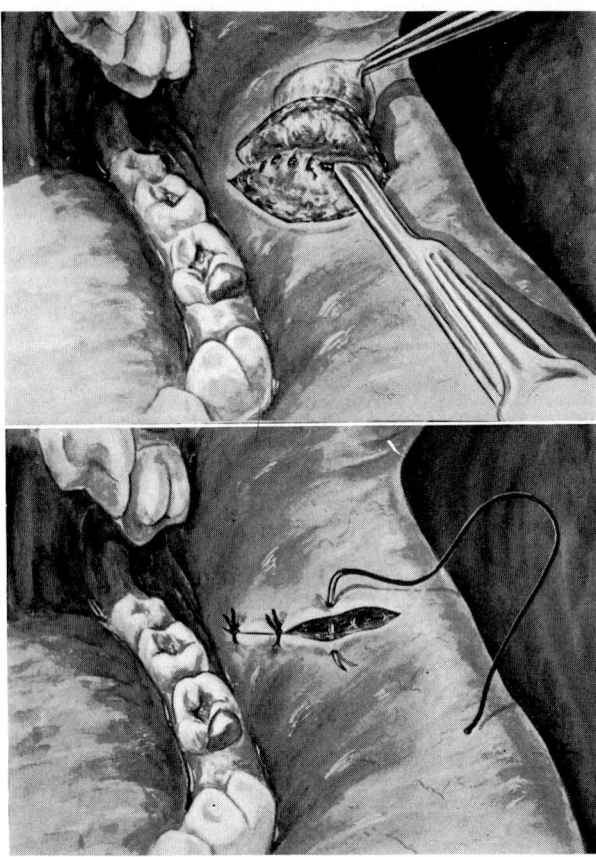

Fig. 18–28

Figure 18–27   Excision biopsy.
Figure 18–28   Excision biopsy, sutured.

because a small superficial tab of tissue may show nothing more than degenerative, inflammatory or necrotic changes. Never perform a biopsy just in the center of a lesion, because the tissue may show only necrosis and not provide the pathologist with enough cellular detail to establish a diagnosis.

c. The section should include tissue at and beyond the lateral margins and the base of the lesion. In this way the transition from healthy tissue to tissue showing pathologic changes can be followed (e.g., expansion or infiltration of tumors).

3. Aspiration Biopsy

If the lesion is deep seated, as in salivary gland tumors, aspiration biopsy may be used. This method is not too effective and has been modified by Silverman, who uses a special needle which enables the operator to remove a larger portion of intact tissue. This method should not be used by pedodontists, but should be reserved for an operator who is trained in the method.

4. Biopsy by Exploration

If the lesion is deep seated, especially in the bone, a flap is raised and a portion of the lesion is removed (Figs. 18–31 and 18–32). Often curettage is necessary in order to obtain material from bony cavities and sinus tracts. In addition, a part of the compact plate and surrounding cancellous bone from the tumor area should be removed and submitted for biopsy. The use of trephines is valuable in obtaining a biopsy of a central lesion in bone.

5. Punch Biopsy

Punch biopsy is of limited value in the oral cavity. It is more applicable in the removal of small tissue specimens in inaccessible areas, such as the maxillary sinus and the lateral or posterior pharyngeal walls. The punch forceps tends to crush tissue, and so make the diagnosis more difficult. On the other hand, it helps in the control of hemorrhage.

If the biopsy is done in a hospital, a frozen section may be obtained which may

Fig. 18–29

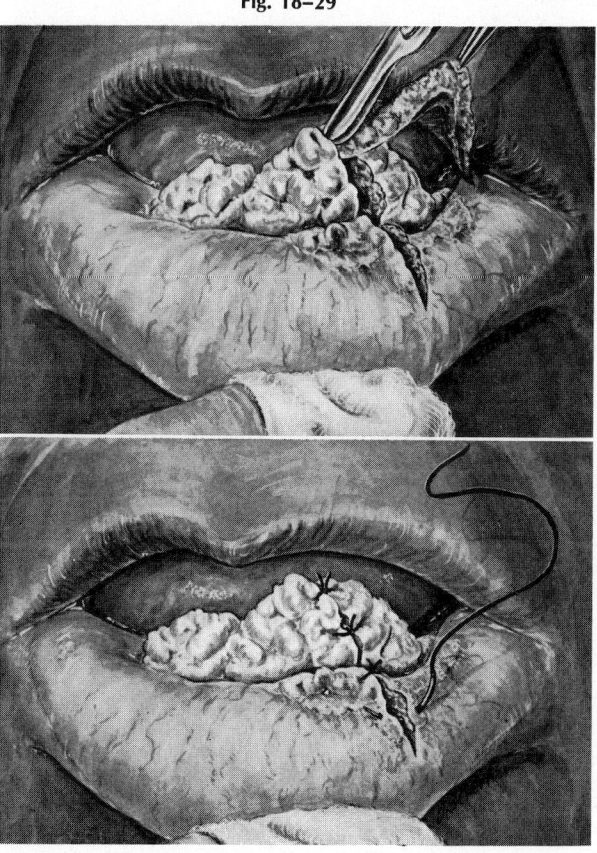

Fig. 18–30
Figure 18–29 Incision biopsy.
Figure 18–30 Incision biopsy, sutured.

Fig. 18–31

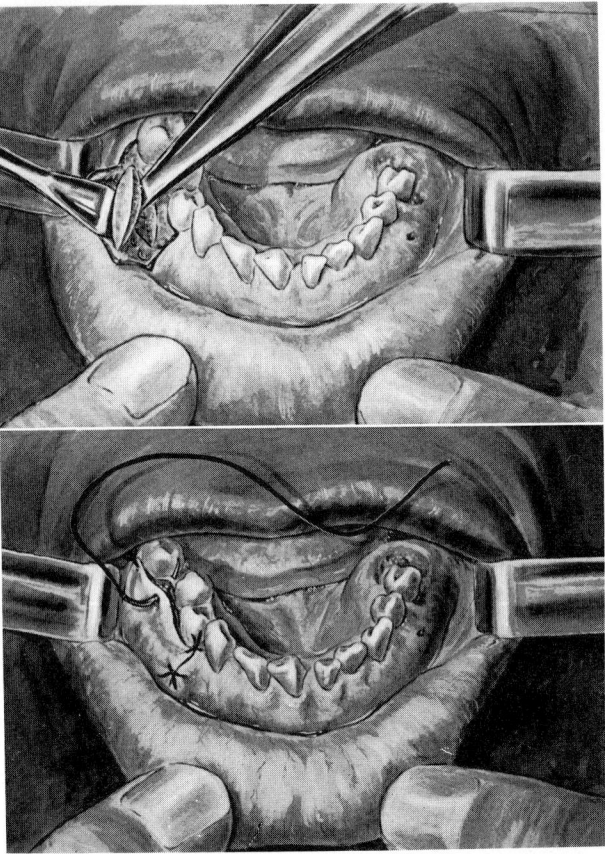

Fig. 18–32
Figure 18–31   Biopsy by exploration; removal of bone.
Figure 18–32   Suturing of incision after biopsy by exploration.

enable the operator, provided he is qualified, to continue with the complete removal of the lesion at the same operation if necessary. Very often the frozen section will not show all of the details necessary for accurate diagnosis, and the final operation will have to be postposed until a pathologist has had a chance to examine the routine sections.

TECHNIQUE OF BIOPSY

1. Anesthesia

Most biopsies can be performed under local anesthesia. In the preparation of the field, no strong antiseptics should be used because they tend to cause changes in the tissues and so influence their staining qualities. The anesthetic should not be injected into the tumor, because infiltration with the anesthetic tends to balloon the tissues and distort their structure, and if the lesion is malignant may cause its dissemination.

2. The Incision

If only a small piece of tissue need be removed, the scalpel is preferable to the high frequency cutting current, because the latter tends to coagulate the specimen and destroy its characteristics. On the other hand, if a section is large enough, the high frequency cutting current may be used to advantage, especially in highly vascular tumors. If malignancy is suspected, it may be a good procedure when using the scalpel to coagulate the cut surface afterward with the high frequency coagulating current, to seal off severed blood and lymph vessels and tissue spaces and so prevent possible dissemination of tumor cells. Electrocoagulation also helps in the control of hemorrhage.

3. Removal of the Specimen

During removal of the specimen, extreme care should be taken not to crush or to mutilate the tissue. This can be avoided by not using hemostats, tissue forceps, or similar instruments to hold the tissue, unless the piece removed is large, so that only a small part is damaged. Fine hooks or explorers are much more advantageous for this purpose.

4. Suturing

The wound should be closed with sutures wherever possible. In friable tumors some difficulty will be encountered in applying the sutures, and they may have to be taken through the surrounding normal tissue.

HANDLING OF THE TISSUE SPECIMEN

1. The specimen should be placed in the fixing solution as soon as it is obtained. Delay may result in loss of cellular detail and prevent the pathologist from rendering a diagnosis. Ten per cent formalin is the fixative used most frequently. The volume of fixative should be approximately 20 times the volume of the tissue specimen. If the pathologist to whom the biopsy specimens are submitted prefers another fixative, it would be wise to keep on hand several small bottles containing this fixative. Care should be taken that the solutions are always fresh, as all of them tend to deteriorate.

If the specimen is too thick, only the peripheral portions of the tissue will be completely infiltrated and fixed, while the central areas will undergo degenerative changes. Therefore, the large specimen should be cut in several sections before being immersed.

2. The specimen bottle should be properly labeled to indicate whether the tissue specimen is soft tissue only or whether it contains bone. It is good practice to keep soft tissue and bone specimens in separate marked bottles whenever possible.

If a large tumor or large cyst has been removed, the specimen should be cut in portions, the individual pieces inserted in numbered bottles, and a diagram made of the lesion and labeled accordingly, as some cysts or tumors may show various characteristics in different parts.

3. A brief history should accompany the specimen. This should include the name, age, and sex of the patient, the location and gross description of the lesion, its duration, rate of growth or change in growth rate, and the method used in obtaining the specimen.

Reports on soft tissue will usually be available in from two to four days. Bone specimens require from one to three weeks, depending upon the degree of calcification.

HOSPITAL PROCEDURE FOR THE DENTAL PATIENT

Not infrequently a dentist is called upon to perform either operative or oral surgical work in the hospital. Up until a few years ago, very little instruction was given in dental schools concerning the relationship of the dentist to the hospital and his prerogatives and duties within the hospital. The following paragraphs deal with matters which may be of interest to the dentist when admitting his own patients to the hospital or when called as a consultant.

ADMISSION PROCEDURES

Responsibility for Admission

1. If the dentist is a member of the staff of the hospital and desires to hospitalize a patient, he must call the admitting office and obtain a bed. Otherwise, he should contact the patient's family physician, who will arrange for the admission.

2. If the dentist is called for consultation the physician will be responsible for the admission.

Admission Orders

Routine admission orders to be given in writing for a simple procedure include:
1. Complete blood count (CBC), which usually includes the following:
   a. Hemoglobin.
   b. Hematocrit.
   c. WBC (white blood count) with differential.
2. Urinalysis.
3. Antibiotics (if needed).
   Example: Procaine penicillin 300,000 units daily intramuscularly (i.m.).
4. Analgesics.*
   Example: Codeine and aspirin capsules, one every 4 hours if necessary for pain.
5. Sedatives.*
   Example: Secobarbital 30 to 100 mg. at night (h.s.).
6. Regular diet.

Hemoglobin Level

Most hospitals have a rule that the hemoglobin must be 70 per cent before general anesthesia is permitted. Transfusion may be necessary. This is solely the responsibility of the admitting physician or dentist to determine prior to surgery. When in doubt consult an internist, hematologist or anesthetist.

---

*For dosage, see Chapter 7.

Admission Note

Chief Complaints **(CC).**   The main presenting symptoms of the present illness together with the duration of each should be enumerated in the order of their development. The complaint should be listed briefly and in the patient's own words.

> Example: 1. Toothache—2 weeks.
> 2. Swollen jaw—1 week.

Present Illness **(PI).**   Use opening sentence to summarize the following: previous admissions, age, sex, occupation, duration and severity of illness.

> Example: This is the first admission to the University Hospital for this 12-year-old white male child who has been in excellent health until he experienced a toothache two weeks prior to admission.

Continue the present illness to complete the story of the patient's present trouble, including events in the past that are definitely or probably related to the present illness.

Past Medical History **(PMH).**   A complete history should include a sentence giving the parent's estimate of the child's general health before the present illness, plus history of infection or infectious diseases, immunizations, drug idiosyncrasies, previous hospital admission and injuries. If PMH is of no significance, one may use, for example: "Non-contributory except for blow against mandible three years ago."

Physical Examination (PE).   This should include intra-oral and extra-oral examination.

> Example: The patient is a well developed, well nourished 12-year-old white male with gross swelling of the right lower face. The warm, tender and fluctuant swelling extends *superiorly* to the zygomatic arch, *inferiorly* to include the right submandibular area and across the midline to involve the left submandibular area, *posteriorly* to the angle of the mandible and *anteriorly* to the corner of mouth, etc.
>
> *Intra-oral examination* revealed poor oral hygiene and an extremely carious lower right second molar which was mobile and extremely sensitive to percussion.
>
> *X-ray examination* reveals radiolucent areas approximately 2 mm. in size associated with apices of lower right second molar.

Impression.   List the disease or diseases which are most likely present:

> Example: Cellulitis of face secondary to dentoalveolar abscess of lower right second molar.

MEDICAL CHECK-UP

It is a hospital rule to have a physician examine the patient prior to a general anesthetic.

PREOPERATIVE ORDERS

1. The quantities vary with the size, age and health of the patient, but routine preoperative orders for healthy children prior to surgery at 7:00 A.M. are:
   a. Nothing per os (NPO) after midnight.
   b. Phenobarbital 30 to 100 mg. at bedtime (h.s.) according to age.
   c. Demerol, Atropine, Scopolamine. A sedative is usually given the night

TABLE 18-1 PREMEDICATION FOR CHILDREN*

	Sedative	Atropine	Scopolamine
Newborn	None	None	None
5 months	None	grain 1/600 0.1 mg.	grain 1/600 0.1 mg.
6 months	None	grain 1/400 0.15 mg.	grain 1/600 0.1 mg.
1–2 years 21–26 pounds	Luminal grain i (64 mg.) hypo.	grain 1/300 0.2 mg.	grain 1/400 0.15 mg.
3–4 years 32–40 pounds	Luminal grains ii (130 mg.) hypo.	grain 1/250 0.24 mg.	grain 1/400 0.15 mg.
4–5 years	Demerol 25 mg. (½ cc.) or Morphine S grain 1/24 (2.5 mg.)	grain 1/200 0.3 mg.	grain 1/300 0.2 mg.
6–7 years 42–48 pounds	Demerol 37 mg. (¾ cc.) or Morphine S grain 1/16 (4 mg.)	grain 1/200 0.3 mg.	grain 1/300 0.2 mg.
8–10 years 50–60 pounds	Demerol 50 mg. (1 cc.) or Morphine S grain 1/12 (5 mg.)	grain 1/150 0.4 mg.	grain 1/200 0.3 mg.
11–12 years	Demerol 62 mg. (1-¼ cc.) or Morphine S grain ⅛ (8 mg.)	grain 1/150 0.4 mg.	grain 1/200 0.3 mg.

*To be given one hour before scheduled time of surgery. When an "on call" order must be left, Demerol is the best agent to use. If in the age group for Luminal, two hypos may be necessary; Luminal must not be given on call. Since Luminal is long acting, some estimate can be made of the time of surgery and the Luminal given in advance, even if the time elapsed is considerable; the atropine or scopolamine must then be given on call; otherwise, give only one hypodermic.
Courtesy University of Alabama Medical Center, Alice McNeal, M.D., Department of Anesthesiology.

before and nothing taken by mouth for approximately six hours prior to the operation. If the time of operation is not definite, leave preoperative medication orders as follows: "On Call to Surgery."

OPERATING ROOM

1. Patient should be seen prior to surgery to determine if everything is in order and that no complications have developed.

Scrub Technique

2. After changing into scrub suit, cap and mask, the hands and arms, up to the elbows, are thoroughly washed and scrubbed for 10 minutes, preferably with Septisol. Each surface of the finger should be scrubbed individually and rinsed, then the water is allowed to run off the elbows. When the operating room is entered the scrub nurse will give you a towel to dry the hands. One hand should be dried first and then the arm up to the elbow.

Gowns and Gloves

3. Hospitals differ in operating room procedures, but for dental extractions the operating gown is often omitted. Gloves should be worn in the operating room. The hands should always be held above the level of the operating table, as anything which drops below this level is considered as being in a contaminated area.

Drapes

4. Many methods are advocated. A simple technique is to place four towels around the mouth, each towel held with a towel clip. The rest of the patient and table are covered with drape sheets.

Procedure

5. The main difference in extracting teeth under general anesthesia is the fact that the reflexes are lost and a foreign body can easily drop into the oral pharynx and be aspirated. Thus, an oropharyngeal pack is mandatory. If the patient is intubated (the placement of a tube into the trachea through the mouth or nose by the anesthesiologist), a throat pack can be used. This can be placed with thumb forceps or index finger. The pack is placed first on one side and then on the opposite and packed well into the tonsillar fossa anterior to the pharyngopalatine arch at the base of the tongue. If the patient is not intubated, two large sponges may be tied together and placed between the tongue and the soft palate. The tongue should be pulled forward to prevent obstruction to the airway. The surgeon must cooperate with the anesthesiologist, and prevent any obstruction to the vital airway. In the presence of massive swelling around the airway, general anesthesia for incision and drainage of abscesses is contraindicated unless the patient is intubated or a tracheotomy is performed. Rupture of the abscess intra-orally often occurs and aspiration may result.

TABLE 18–2   NORMAL VALUES OF CLINICAL AND LABORATORY FINDINGS*

Pulse Rate		Blood Pressure (mm. Hg.)		
Age	Pulse Rate Per Minute	Age	Systolic	Diastolic
6–12 months	115–105	4– 5 years	58–104	40–74
2– 6 years	105– 90	6– 8 years	74–110	42–74
7–10 years	90– 80	9–11 years	75–120	44–76
11–11 years	80– 75	12–14 years	82–126	48–86

Hemoglobin

Age	Hemoglobin (Gm. %)	Hematocrit (Vol. of Packed RBC/100 cc.)
1– 3 years	12.2–13.1	39–39
4– 7 years	13.1–13.3	40
8–12 years	13.6–14.1	41–42

Complete Blood Count

Age in Years	Reticulo- cytes per 100 RBC	WBC	Granu- locytes	Lym- pho- cytes	Mono- cytes	Platelets per cu. mm.
1– 3	0.5–1.0	8,500–10,000	40–55	50	5–8	200,000–300,000
4– 7	0.5–1.0	8,000	60	40	5–8	200,000–300,000
8–12	0.5–1.0	8,000	62–65	30	5–8	200,000–300,000

Bleeding time	1–3 minutes
Coagulation time	
capillary tube	2–6 minutes
Lee and White	5–10 minutes
Clot retraction time	1 hour
Prothrombin time	12–15 seconds

Value for Blood Constituents of Value in the Diagnosis of Diseases of Bone

	Adults	Children
Serum alkaline phosphatase	Bodansky units, 1.5–5.0 per 100 cc. King-Armstrong units, 5.0–17.5 per 100 cc.	Bodansky units, 5.0–15.0 per 100 cc. (depending on rate of growth)
Serum inorganic phosphorus	2.5–4.0 mg. per 100 cc.	4.0–6.0 mg. per 100 cc. higher in infants
Total serum calcium	10.0–11.5 mg. per 100 cc.	11.0–12.5 mg. per 100 cc.

*Compiled from various sources, especially Holt and McIntosh, Pediatrics, Appleton-Century-Crofts, 1962.

POSTOPERATIVE ORDERS

In most hospitals, when the patient returns from surgery a complete new set of orders is necessary. Thus, we must repeat preoperative orders if we wish them continued, as well as the routine postoperative orders. For example:

1. Take and record blood pressure (BP), pulse (P), respiration (R), every (q) 15 min. for an hour, then every 30 min. until the patient has reacted and is stable.
2. Suction to bedside. Suction when necessary (prn).
3. Semi-Fowler position.
4. Antibiotics (if necessary).
5. Analgesic* (if necessary).
6. Sedative* (if necessary).
7. Diet (liquids after nausea has passed).

POSTOPERATIVE CARE

Usually after short procedures on a healthy patient, he may be discharged the next day. If the procedure was long, it is very important to turn the patient every hour after the operation to make him cough up secretions. This may be written on the order sheet as one of the postoperative orders. If in doubt, the cooperation of the Department of Anesthesiology should be sought.

After the patient has been returned to his room, the operator should visit him to make certain that all of his orders are being observed and that the patient is in good condition.

NORMAL VALUES

Frequently the dentist finds it necessary to evaluate case histories of patients. He should, therefore, acquaint himself with the normal values of the most important clinical and laboratory findings. Table 18–2 presents normal averages of these findings in children of various ages. For evaluation of abnormal values the reader is referred to textbooks on oral and dental diagnosis, hematology, pediatrics and pathology.

REFERENCES

1. Dewel, B. F.: Clinical diagnosis and treatment of palatally impacted cuspids. D. Digest, *51*:492, 1945.
2. Holt, L. E., Jr., McIntosh, R., and Barnett, H. L.: Pediatrics. 13th ed. New York, Appleton-Century-Crofts, Inc., 1962, pp. 592–593.
3. Ivy, R. H.: Interpretation of Dental and Maxillary Roentgenograms. St. Louis, C. V. Mosby Company, 1918, p. 146.
4. Robinson, H. B. G.: Classification of cysts of the jaws. Am. J. Orthodont. & Oral Surg., *31*:1370, 1945.
5. Sadove, M. S., et al.: Classification and management of reaction to local anesthetic agents. J.A.M.A., *148*:17, 1952.
6. Sicher, H.: Oral Anatomy. 3rd ed. St. Louis, C. V. Mosby Company, 1960, p. 419.
7. Ibid., pp. 462–463.
8. Thoma, K.: Oral Surgery. 3rd ed. St. Louis, C. V. Mosby Company, 1958, p. 1020.
9. Zur, J. E.: Topical anesthesia for children. J. Dent. Child., *17*:13, 3rd quart., 1950.

*See Chapter 7.

19

ANTIMICROBIAL AGENTS

by CHARLES A. McCALLUM, Jr.

INTRODUCTION

Antimicrobial agents are an important adjunct in the management of infection in the oral cavity and the prevention of complications following surgical operations involving the oral cavity. However, their indiscriminate use can result in serious complications. With the myriad agents available today, it is important that the modern practitioner of dentistry use a scientific approach and sound rationale in selecting and prescribing antimicrobial agents.

It seems appropriate to spend a short time discussing the philosophy of antimicrobial agents and their place in the practice of dentistry. The use of these drugs is not without inherent dangers, and it behooves the practitioner to become thoroughly familiar with their action and use. In no instance should an antimicrobial agent be substituted for sound surgical judgment in the management of odontogenic infections but it should be used to complement the operator's scientific knowledge, judgment, and skill.

Some of the dangers associated with the use of antimicrobial agents are the development of (1) sensitivity by the patient to the agent, (2) hypersensitivity and anaphylactic reactions, (3) toxic reactions, (4) resistant strains of microorganisms, and (5) superinfections.

Sensitivity of the Patient

Whenever an antimicrobial agent is prescribed, the patient may become sensitized to it, which will preclude its future use. Any time a drug is given, it has the ability to evoke an antibody response; and if subsequently prescribed for a sensitized patient, it can produce a severe allergic reaction. Fortunately, most patients can have repeated exposure to a specific antimicrobial without ever manifesting evidence of sensitivity. There have been some cases in which people have been sensitized to an antibiotic without knowingly having previously received it. This can

430

result when a drug with a chemical configuration similar to that of the antibiotic has been given to the patient; thus the sensitivity. Another possible explanation is that the patient may have received the antibiotic as a contaminant in food or some other substance. The important point to remember is that one should not prescribe an antimicrobial agent indiscriminately. Any dose could be the one to sensitize the patient to the drug and preclude its future use. For example, if penicillin were given for treatment of a mild gingivitis and the patient developed a severe rash due to the agent, its subsequent use would probably be contraindicated. If, at a later date, the same patient needed penicillin for the treatment of pneumococcal meningitis, could you then still defend your original decision in prescribing the agent for a relatively minor infection which might have been managed satisfactorily without using the penicillin?

Hypersensitivity and Anaphylactic Reactions

Once a patient has been sensitized to a drug, its subsequent use could evoke either a hypersensitivity or an anaphylactoid reaction. One can help to avoid these allergic reactions by taking the time to review the patient's previous drug therapy in detail with him. However, just because a patient has had a particular antibiotic previously and did not experience a reaction does not mean he could not have a reaction the next time the drug is prescribed. Therefore, a negative history to a specific drug does not give one absolute assurance that the patient will not have a reaction to that drug. The importance of taking a detailed history regarding drug therapy is that it permits you to identify those patients who have positive sensitivities as manifested by previous skin reactions, drug fever, or other allergic phenomena. In such patients, the drug which caused the positive reaction must be avoided. Similarly, one should exercise discretion when prescribing an antimicrobial to any patient who gives a history of multiple allergies or severe asthma.

If a patient is hypersensitive to a drug, even a minute amount of it can evoke a severe allergic reaction. Therefore, in sensitive patients, one is not justified in giving even minute amounts of the drug as the reaction is not dependent upon the quantity of the drug prescribed. There have been fatal reactions in patients who have been given minute amounts of the drug during skin testing.

The most severe type of reaction that a patient may have following the administration of an antibiotic is the anaphylactic reaction, which may cause severe morbidity or death. This reaction is characterized by the development of immediate profound shock which may be accompanied by impalpable pulse and loss of consciousness. Facial or laryngeal edema and a generalized urticaria may or may not accompany it. Therefore, it is imperative that the dentist or physician take time to make certain that the patient is not sensitive to a drug before prescribing it. Information concerning drug sensitivity is best obtained by taking a detailed history and asking specific questions about previous drugs which the patient may have taken or any reactions which he may have experienced.

Toxic Reactions

Almost every antimicrobial agent has the ability to produce a toxic response in the host. A toxic reaction is due to an overdose of the drug. Therefore, in prescribing antibiotics, it is important to use the minimal amount of the agent that will give the desired therapeutic response and thus reduce the possibility of reactions from an overdose. An example of a toxic manifestation of an antimicrobial agent is the bone marrow depression that has been noted with chloramphenicol and the sulfonamides. Toxic reactions may also result when certain antimicrobial agents are used in what might be considered normal dosages in patients who have serious systemic involvement of organ systems which may prevent the detoxification and elimination of the drug. An example of this is the effect of tetracyclines in severe renal insufficiency.

Development of Resistant Strains

Every antimicrobial agent has certain organisms against which it is effective. This is frequently spoken of as antimicrobial spectrum. For example, penicillin is considered to be particularly effective against the gram-positive bacteria, but less effective against the gram-negative bacteria.

It is not uncommon, however, for organisms to become resistant to antimicrobial agents. There are two main theories concerning the development of drug resistance by the microorganisms, namely, mutation and adaptation.

Most large bacterial colonies give rise to a few mutant strains which are more resistant to a particular antibiotic than the rest of the bacteria in the colony. These mutant strains arise independently of exposure to antimicrobial agents and are thought to be due to normal genetic variations during the reproduction of the bacteria. Such mutant strains may not be affected by the antimicrobial agents, and in turn, the organisms which they produce also exhibit this drug resistance. The important thing is that the second and third generations of these resistant mutants can become extremely resistant to and totally unaffected by the highest possible concentration of the antibiotic.

The second theory concerning drug resistance concerns the ability of the organism to develop alternate metabolic pathways which are completely unaffected by the mechanism of action of the antimicrobial agent. Although this theory of adaptation has been postulated, it still lacks definite proof and most authorities feel that the development of mutant strains is the most common cause of drug-resistant organisms. An example of a drug-resistant organism is the penicillin-resistant staphylococcus which is commonly encountered in hospital-acquired infections.

One can prevent the development of highly resistant strains of bacteria by utilizing an adequate concentration of the antimicrobial agent to provide a therapeutic level that not only inhibits or kills the sensitive bacteria in a certain colony but which may also be effective against first generation mutant strains. Intermittent therapy with ineffective concentrations of the drug aids in the development of resistant strains and should be avoided.

Superinfections

When prescribing an antimicrobial agent for treatment of a specific infectious process, all bacteria within the body that are sensitive to that antibiotic will either be killed or their growth will be inhibited. As a result of this suppression of the sensitive bacteria by the antibiotic, there may be an overgrowth of other nonsusceptible microorganisms which could produce an infection of greater consequence than the one for which the antibiotic was prescribed. The development of concomitant yeast infections (for example, those caused by *Candida albicans*) which may result when certain antibiotics are used for a long period of time has been well documented. In particular, the possibility of superinfection should be remembered when treating infections in the oral cavity in patients who might concomitantly have a chronic disease of the respiratory, urinary, or gastrointestinal tract. Suppression of sensitive organisms in the normal flora by the prolonged use of antimicrobial agents may permit a multiplication of other pathogens and cause a severe superimposed infection.

Therefore, before prescribing an antimicrobial agent, one has to weigh the possible risks of sensitizing the patient; the development of toxic, hypersensitive, or anaphylactic reactions; the emergence of resistant strains of microorganisms; and the development of superinfections against the benefit to be obtained by prescribing the agent. If more individuals would take the time to weigh the consequences versus the benefits, there would be a more rational approach to the use of antimicrobial agents.

DEFINITION

There is considerable confusion about the use of such terms as chemotherapeutic agents, anti-infective agents, and antibiotics. For the purpose of clarity, it might be helpful to briefly review what is meant by these terms.

Chemotherapy is the treatment of a disease process by the use of a chemical agent. For example, the use of aspirin in the treatment of arthritis is chemotherapy. On the other hand, the use of the sulfonamides in the treatment of infection also represents chemotherapy, but here we are using an agent specifically for the treatment of infection.

Antibiosis is the inhibition of growth of one organism by another, and the term antibiotic as presently accepted was proposed by Waksman in 1941 and is thought of as a chemical substance produced by a microorganism which has the capacity to inhibit the growth of or destroy other microorganisms in dilute solutions. In its broad usage, an antibiotic is a chemotherapeutic agent, but the term in its specific usage is reserved for a chemical agent produced by a microorganism that is effective in controlling the growth of other microorganisms. Recent identification of the chemical structure of certain antibiotics has made it possible for some to be produced synthetically; thus the term synthetic antibiotics.

In this chapter we will be discussing chemotherapy as related to anti-infective agents, which will include chemical substances produced artificially, e.g., sulfonamides, semi-synthetic penicillins, and the antibiotics produced by microorganisms. Put another way, the chemotherapeutic agents which are presently available for the treatment of infectious diseases can be divided into two main groups on the basis of their origin, (1) the synthetic substances and (2) the substances produced by various microorganisms, some of which might also be synthetically produced subsequent to their identification. Therefore, this chapter is termed Antimicrobial Agents, which includes not only the antibiotics but also the various chemotherapeutic agents that are used as anti-infectives.

HISTORY

Chemotherapy in the treatment of infection is not new. In South America, the Inca Indians actually practiced chemotherapy by treating malaria with cinchona bark. Another example of the early use of a chemotherapeutic agent is ipecac, which was introduced in the seventeenth century for the treatment of amebiasis. Chemotherapy formally became a science when Paul Ehrlich (1854–1915), referred to as the father of scientific chemotherapy, defined the fundamental principles upon which our present day anti-infective therapy is based. The fundamental principle in chemotherapy is selective toxicity, which dictates that, for an agent to be useful in the systemic treatment of an infectious disease, it must be harmful to the parasite or microorganism but relatively innocuous to the host cell. Ehrlich spent his life searching for chemical agents which would destroy pathogenic organisms and not harm the tissues of the human host. He discovered that the organic arsenicals showed much promise and prepared one arsenical compound after another and tested it for its effectiveness against syphilis. On compound number 606 or salvarsan he was successful, and thus provided the healing arts with what was then and for some time thereafter the most effective agent for the treatment of syphilis. In 1935 Domagk introduced the sulfonamides, following which numerous organic chemical agents have been identified, introduced, and employed successfully in the management of infectious processes.

Another presently held misconception is that antimicrobial therapy was not used prior to 1941. However, it is known that over 2500 years ago the Chinese used the moldy curd of soybean in the treatment of boils, furuncles, and similar infections. They noted that this mold was extremely effective against these infections. Thus, unknowingly, they were utilizing antimicrobials. A review of the medical literature shows that other ancient civilizations used soil and various plants for the treatment of infected wounds. The English bacteriologist Alexander Fleming discovered penicillin in 1929; however, not until 1941 was it mass produced and made available for clinical trial. This formally ushered in the *antibiotics*, which have since come to be the most widely used anti-infective agents.

MECHANISM OF ACTION

Generally speaking, antimicrobial agents are frequently referred to as being either bacteriostatic or bactericidal when used in usual nontoxic therapeutic dosages. A bacteriostatic agent is one which has the ability to inhibit bacterial reproduction. Even though a drug is bacteriostatic, once it is removed from the immediate environment, reproduction by the organism may resume. On the other hand, bactericidal denotes the ability to kill the microorganism. This action is irreversible and is not dependent upon the continued contact of the drug with the microorganism. Some time might be spent reviewing more specifically the various mechanisms of action of the more commonly used antimicrobial agents.

The mechanism of action of all antimicrobial agents is based on their ability to interfere with a vital process in the microorganism without interfering with the cells of the host. Most effective antimicrobial agents act by interfering with or inhibiting the synthesis, function, or organization of the macromolecular components of the microbial cells. The known mechanisms of action of the antimicrobial agents would include: (1) a change in cell permeability, (2) interference with cell wall synthesis, (3) interference with nutritional requirements or essential metabolites, (4) interference with nucleic acid synthesis, and (5) interference with protein synthesis.

Changes in cell permeability are brought about by agents which alter or disrupt the cell membrane of certain bacteria or fungi and allow their intracellular substances to escape. These agents are relatively selective because of the differences in the cytoplasmic membrane of some gram-negative bacteria, most fungi, and all animal cells. Examples of antimicrobial agents having this mechanism of action are the polymyxins, which affect certain gram-negative bacteria, and nystatin and amphotericin B, which are particularly effective against certain fungi.

Other antimicrobial agents act by *interfering with cell wall synthesis.* These would include all the penicillins, cephalosporins, vancomycin, bacitracin, and ristocetin. Removal of the bacterial cell wall or inhibition of its formation will lead to lysis of the cell. Since animal cells do not have this rigid outer layer which is composed of a complex mucopolypeptide, they are not affected by the antimicrobial agents. Gram-negative bacteria do not depend solely on the integrity of the mucopeptide in the cell wall to maintain their tensile strength, thus explaining the resistance of these organisms to the penicillins, cephalothin, and other antimicrobial agents which primarily affect the integrity of the cell wall. The mode of action of penicillin explains why it is only effective against actively multiplying microorganisms and will have virtually no effect on already existent bacterial cell walls.

Examples of agents which *interfere with nutritional requirements or essential metabolites* would include the sulfa drugs, sulfones, and nitrofurans. Since sulfonamides are structurally similar to para-aminobenzoic acid (PABA) they can compete for the enzymes which are necessary for the conversion of PABA into folic acid, an important and necessary coenzyme to the bacteria. As a result, nonfunctioning analogs of folic acid are formed, preventing the further growth of the microbial cell. Animal cells are not affected by the sulfonamides since they do not synthesize folic acid but depend on extracellular sources. Similarly, some bacteria are also dependent on exogenous sources of folic acid and are not affected by sulfonamides.

Interference with nucleic acid synthesis occurs with antimicrobial agents such as actinomycin, mitomycin, idoxuridine (IDU), and griseofulvin. These drugs act on DNA synthesis (IDU) or on the structure of DNA already present (actinomycin, mitomycin). They also inhibit animal cells and therefore are not selective enough to be employed systemically in the treatment of infection. Idoxuridine (IDU) is employed only topically in DNA-virus infections such as herpetic keratitis of the eye. Griseofulvin is particularly effective against certain cutaneous fungal infections (dermatophytes).

The *interference with protein synthesis* explains the mode of action of one variety of antimicrobial agent. Tetracyclines, chloramphenicol, streptomycin, isoniazide, erythromycin, kanamycin, neomycin, and lincomycin are included in this group. It has been postulated that some of these drugs, e.g., chloramphenicol, are more selective for bacterial cell proteins since animal cell proteins have a more stable attachment of messenger RNA to the ribosomes, and it is felt that chloramphenicol interferes with the incorporation of amino acids into this newly formed protein on the ribosomes. Streptomycin also acts on the ribosomal surface, interfering with mRNA function but not with its attachment as does chloramphenicol. The entire field of protein synthesis is in a state of rapid change, and specific details concerning the mechanism of action of some of these drugs are not known.

In summary, these represent a few of the known mechanisms of action which illustrate the selective toxicity of antimicrobial drugs. In many instances the precise mechanism of action or site of action awaits further clarification.

INDICATIONS

The two indications for the use of antimicrobial agents in dentistry are the control and eradication of infections of the oral cavity and prophylaxis to prevent complications following surgical operation.

By complementing surgical judgment with proper antimicrobial therapy, most infections of the oral cavity can be controlled or eradicated. This forward step in the elimination of severe morbidity and mortality due to dental infection takes on added significance when one realizes that the development of cavernous sinus thrombosis secondary to dental infection is fortunately a rarity in present-day practice. Today, it is uncommon for anyone to die from odontogenic infection. This is due to the scientific approach of the practitioner of dentistry in the prevention, diagnosis, and treatment of odontogenic infection. The antimicrobials have played a major role in helping the dental profession to control the ravages of infections of the oral cavity and contiguous structures.

It is rather difficult to provide definite guidelines concerning the specific indications for placing a patient on anti-infective therapy, how long it should be continued, the type of drug to be used, and the ideal dose to be administered. This entire spectrum of questions depends on the judgment of the clinician treating the patient. When evaluating a patient with an infectious process, he must weigh not only the clinical evidence regarding the infectious disease but also the state of health of the patient. Once that is done, then decisions concerning the type, dose, route of administration, and length of treatment with chemotherapy can be made.

In evaluating the clinical evidence of an infectious process, the clinician takes into consideration both local and systemic factors. When judging local factors, he must consider such salient features as the extent, type, and location of swelling, the presence or absence of fluctuation, the presence or absence of regional phlebitis or lymphadenitis, and whether or not there is a loss of function of the involved part, e.g., trismus or dysphagia. If a patient had extensive cellulitis in the submaxillary triangle and involvement of the parapharyngeal space, the utilization of antimicrobials would be more justified than it would in the patient who had a chronic draining sinus tract opposite a deciduous molar. Septic thrombotic involvement of the angular or ophthalmic vein secondary to an infection of a maxillary incisor would dictate aggressive anti-infective therapy.

In attempting to judge the systemic effect of the infectious process, the clinician may use as guidelines the temperature, pulse rate, respiratory rate, and other signs of systemic toxicity which might include nausea, vomiting, anorexia, dehydration, lethargy, and so on. Intermittent shaking chills with spikes of high fever certainly make one suspicious of septicemia, a condition which demands intensive antimicrobial therapy.

Laboratory tests, including white blood count, differential white count, sedimentation rate, blood cultures, hemoglobin, etc., can also be extremely valuable adjuncts in evaluating an infectious process. An elevated white cell count, e.g., 18,000 with a differential that shows a shift to the left with a preponderance of neutrophils and immature polymorphonuclear leukocytes, should indicate to the clinician that the infection is no longer localized but has evoked a rather severe systemic response. In bacterial infections, the total white count is usually elevated above normal ranges and the differential count shows a preponderance of polymorphonuclear leukocytes. On the other hand, infections produced by viruses may actually show a normal or slightly depressed total white cell count and differential examination of the white cells reveals an increase in the number of lymphocytes and monocytes.

We have primarily mentioned the evaluation of those factors concerning the infectious process, both local and systemic; however, as mentioned previously, consideration must always be given to the general health of the patient. Although the infectious process might by all standards be considered rather insignificant in the healthy patient, the same infection in a patient with hypogammaglobulinemia or severe malnutrition would have a different connotation and perhaps warrant the use of anti-infective therapy.

One point should be emphasized. Once the decision has been made to use an anti-infective agent, then the dose of the drug should be high enough to provide a serum and tissue level of the agent that will be sufficiently therapeutic to assist the body in bringing the infection under control. One-day therapy with an anti-infective agent has no place in the modern practice of dentistry or medicine. If the patient gets well from one day of therapy with an antibiotic, in all probability he would have improved without the antibiotic and its use was unjustified.

When all factors regarding the infectious process, both local and systemic, have been judged individually and then collectively, one should then be in a position to make a fairly rational judgment concerning antimicrobial therapy.

Some infectious processes of the oral cavity that frequently warrant systemic antimicrobial therapy are severe cellulitis, osteomyelitis, bacterial infections of the salivary glands, compound fractures, infected cysts, infected oro-antral fistulas, and fulminating bacterial stomatitis or pericoronitis with an associated severe systemic response.

The prophylactic use of antimicrobial agents has its place in dentistry; however, the indications for the prophylactic use of these agents are limited to a rather small number of systemic disease states. Antibiotics should not be used prophylactically for the prevention of a local infection which "might result" if a tooth were extracted. You prevent local infections by asepsis and other surgical principles and not by the employment of antimicrobial agents. The use of a potent antibiotic for the sole purpose of preventing alveolar osteitis (dry socket) or osteomyelitis is unsound and without scientific validity. Similarly, using an anti-infective so that the operator may transgress sound surgical principles or "take chances" has no place in dentistry. Employment of such a practice has all the inherent risks involved in using antimicrobials and very few of the benefits. Unfortunately, the individual who suffers from such practices is the unsuspecting patient.

The main indication for the prophylactic use of antibiotics is to protect patients who have certain systemic diseases when the development of bacteremia could result in severe morbidity or mortality. It is a well established fact that the extraction of a tooth may produce a bacteremia in 85 per cent of the cases. In reality, the incidence of bacteremia following dental extraction probably approaches 100 per cent. In the healthy individual, the transient bacteremias produced by such operations as gingival curettage, gingivectomy, or exodontia cause no detectable harm to the patient. However, in patients with certain systemic disease processes, these bacteremias can produce severe consequences. In particular, the person with rheumatic heart disease, congenital heart disease, or valvular heart disease must be protected against possible bacteremias following surgical operations within the oral cavity. Bacteremia in these patients could lead to an acute or subacute bacterial endocarditis. For similar reasons, patients who have had cardiac surgery to correct congenital malformations or acquired defects, or patients who have had replacement of major vessels with prosthetic grafts, should be protected by antimicrobial therapy prior to any operative procedure of the oral cavity which might produce a bacteremia.

The uncontrolled diabetic should also be covered with prophylactic antimicrobial therapy. However, the well controlled diabetic should be treated as a normal patient.

People receiving cortisone therapy or who have adrenal insufficiency frequently show decreased resistance to infection. It is usually advantageous to cover these individuals with antimicrobial agents prior to surgical operations. Similarly, people with agranulocytosis, regardless of its cause, should be covered with anti-infective agents prior to intraoral surgery. Individuals with malglobulin states, e.g., multiple myeloma or hypogammaglobulinemia, should also be covered with prophylactic antibiotics prior to any procedure that might produce a bacteremia.

SELECTION OF THE AGENT

Scientific judgment and not conjecture should guide the clinician when selecting an appropriate antimicrobial agent for treating infection of the oral cavity. When one reviews the organisms that are primarily responsible, it becomes apparent that the great majority of infections of the oral cavity are due to the streptococcus and staphylococcus. It is then logical to assume that the appropriate antimicrobial agent would be the one that is most effective against these gram-positive cocci. It has·been proved that penicillin is the most efficacious agent in controlling these organisms; it is, therefore, the drug of choice. If the patient is allergic to penicillin, then a drug with an antimicrobial spectrum similar to that of penicillin should be chosen.

Academically speaking, it would be helpful if every infection could be studied from a microbiological standpoint. This could provide information concerning what specific antimicrobial agent would be most appropriate in the treatment of a particular infection. However, several reasons make this approach somewhat impractical. It is difficult to obtain a representative specimen of the organism causing an infectious process within the oral cavity. A sample taken from the oral cavity usually reveals a wide variety of organisms, and it becomes a guess as to which one is the primary infective agent. In some infections, the pus becomes localized and, by either incision and drainage or aspiration, it is possible to obtain a representative specimen. Such cases permit the laboratory to perform smear, culture, and sensitivity studies that are more valid. The gram stain will reveal whether or not the organism is gram-positive or gram-negative. This simple test can be an extremely valuable guide in selecting an agent with the desired antimicrobial spectrum. A specimen of the purulent material should be cultured both aerobically and anaerobically. Most infections involving the oral cavity are aerobic; however, identification of actinomycosis, a not infrequent cause of oral infection, requires anaerobic conditions for its growth. The appearance of bacterial colonies on various media frequently are characteristic enough to permit the identification of the organism. Subsequent use of discs impregnated with various antimicrobials is helpful in indicating the inhibition of the organisms by the various agents. As stated previously, it is frequently impossible and impractical to obtain a smear culture, and sensitivity study on an infection of the oral cavity. However, when treating a severe infection, particularly if the patient warrants hospitalization, it is always important to utilize these tests. This is a welcome adjunct when the infectious process fails to respond to the anti-infective agent originally prescribed. In vitro studies are helpful, but they can be misleading. One should not randomly accept the dictates of laboratory results and substitute them for clinical judgment. If a patient is improving clinically on an antimicrobial agent, then do not change the agent being used just because the laboratory may indicate that the organism identified is not sensitive to that agent. It is possible that they have identified the secondary rather than the primary infective agent. There is no substitute for clinical judgment, and information provided by the laboratory should only be interpreted as an adjunct in arriving at a decision.

In the treatment of infections in or about the oral cavity, it is usually appropriate that initially the patient be placed on only one antibiotic. Starting a patient on two or three antibiotics for the treatment of odontogenic infection is usually not justified. It is better to select one, give it an adequate therapeutic trial, and observe the clinical result. If the patient fails to improve, then the addition of a second antibiotic after the first 36 hours could be considered. Only in the critically ill would the employment of so-called shotgun therapy be defendable.

ROUTES OF ADMINISTRATION

Antibiotics may be administered either locally or systemically. When used locally, or topically, they have only a superficial action, and because of their inability to penetrate the tissues, their effectiveness is limited to the superficial microorganisms. No protection is provided against bacteremia. The topical application of any drug may cause severe local reactions which frequently make it difficult for the clinician to properly evaluate the infectious process. Additionally, repeated use of small amounts of antimicrobial agents is an excellent means of producing a sensitivity in the patient. Because of these reasons, it is the feeling of the author that the topical application of antimicrobial agents has a rather limited place in the treatment of dental infections.

If topical antibiotics are used, it is suggested that they be reserved as a means of reinforcing the systemic administration of the same drug. Occasionally, in an attempt to get a high concentration of the antimicrobial agent in certain areas of the body, topical administration along with systemic therapy could have certain beneficial effects.

If a clinician feels it appropriate to use a topical antibiotic by itself in the management of dental infection, a plea is entered that use be limited to those antibiotics which cannot be given systemically. Bacitracin, polymyxin, and neomycin would be drugs that fall in this category. When antimicrobials are used, their limitations should be remembered and a miraculous improvement should not be expected.

Systemic administration is the most effective means of gaining the maximum benefit from antimicrobial agents. The various routes employed are oral, intramuscular, and intravenous. For the most part, the intravenous administration of antimicrobials in dentistry is reserved for the treatment of severe infectious processes which frequently are accompanied by septicemia. The most commonly used routes of systemic therapy in dentistry are either oral or intramuscular. Fortunately, because of the advances made in the synthesis of the various antimicrobial agents, the oral route is usually satisfactory except in the most severe infections.

SULFONAMIDES

The sulfonamides represent a large group of chemotherapeutic drugs which have had the longest history of success in the management of bacterial infection. Although sulfanilamide, the parent drug, was first synthesized in 1908 from azo dyes, it was not until 1932 that the sulfonamides were used clinically to treat infection. Since that time, almost a hundred sulfonamide derivatives have been prepared and used in the treatment of infectious disease.

The sulfonamides have a wide antimicrobial spectrum, being effective against some gram-positive and gram-negative pathogens and certain fungi such as actinomyces and nocardia, all of which cause a significant number of infections in the oral region. The sulfonamides are bacteriostatic rather than bactericidal; therefore, one must consider the host resistance and defense mechanisms before selecting this group of drugs in the treatment of odontogenic infection. The mechanism of the bacteriostatic action of the sulfas is not completely understood. As stated previously, it is felt that they interfere competitively with the utilization of para-aminobenzoic acid (PABA) by some microorganisms, thereby preventing the formation of folic acid, a necessary metabolite for these organisms. Bacterial resistance to this group of drugs may develop.

Adverse effects of the sulfonamides are many and variable. The kidneys are probably the organs most commonly affected. This may be due to a plasma concentration-solubility relationship of the specific sulfonamide with resultant crystalluria or to toxic nephrosis and hypersensitivity reactions. The former may be prevented or reduced by (1) increased oral or intravenous fluid intake, (2) alkalinization of the urine, and (3) use of the sulfonamides in combination (Triple Sulfa, U.S.P.). Toxic nephrosis and hypersensitivity reactions are not preventable and require early recognition of signs and symptoms and discontinuance of the drug. Another organ system which also is affected by the sulfonamides is the hematopoietic system. Acute hemolytic anemia, aplastic anemia, agranulocytosis, and thrombocytopenia have all been reported during and following the administration of the various sulfa drugs. Therefore, the clinician who elects to use any of the sulfonamides in the treatment of infection must assume the responsibility of adequately monitoring the organ systems which are commonly adversely affected by these drugs. The urine should be examined for evidence of crystalluria or hematuria. Any decrease in urinary output may also indicate renal complications. The peripheral blood should be monitored for evidence of anemia, agranulocytosis, thrombocytopenia, and leukopenia.

Because of the subsequent introduction of the antibiotics, many of which have proved superior in the management of infection of the oral cavity, the sulfonamides are only rarely used by the dentist. If in the treatment of a resistant infection of the oral cavity, bacteriologic survey shows that a particular sulfonamide is the drug of choice, then its use is certainly justified. Cervicofacial actinomycosis, particularly if it involves the maxilla and mandible, seems to respond best to a combined therapy of penicillin and sulfadiazine. Sulfa therapy is usually the treatment of choice in nocardiosis.

Since there are many available sulfonamides, a detailed description of the individual drugs with their appropriate dosages is felt to be beyond the scope of this chapter. This information is readily available in *Accepted Dental Remedies, Physicians' Desk Reference* and most textbooks of pharmacology. Before prescribing the sulfonamides for children, it is always best to check the dosage, using a reliable source.

PENICILLINS

Penicillin, the first of the antibiotics to be identified, is still considered today by many authorities as the most effective agent available for the control of infection. In view of its bactericidal action and its effectiveness against gram-positive cocci, it is the drug of choice when treating dental infections. There are a variety of penicillins available, and for the purpose of discussion and clarity, these will be broken down into the naturally occurring penicillins and the semi-synthetic penicillins.

NATURALLY OCCURRING PENICILLINS

The naturally occurring penicillins are produced by the mold *Penicillium chrysogenum* In the early stages of the production of penicillin, it was found that four different types of penicillin were formed; namely F, X, K, and G. Of these, penicillin G or benzyl penicillin was found to have the most desired properties.

Penicillin G (Benzyl Penicillin)

As formed, penicillin G is an unstable acid, and in production is converted to a salt, usually potassium, which is more stable. This potassium salt of penicillin G is frequently referred to as crystalline or soluble penicillin G. When given intramuscularly (I.M.), it is rapidly absorbed, which results in a high concentration of the drug in the blood within 10 minutes. However, because of its rapid excretion by the kidney, the high blood level only lasts for one or two hours. In order to prolong its action, penicillin G has been combined with procaine which when given intramuscularly delays its absorption and prolongs its action. As a result, procaine penicillin G does not give peak concentrations in the blood for about two hours, but once obtained, the concentration will persist for about 24 hours. If one desires an immediate peak concentration of penicillin G in the blood by the intramuscular route, then crystalline penicillin G should be selected. To obtain concentrations within the blood that have a more prolonged action, the use of procaine penicillin G is indicated.

There is a combined preparation of procaine penicillin G and crystalline penicillin G. This injectable preparation has the advantage of giving a rapid peak in the blood due to the action of the crystalline penicillin G and a prolonged therapeutic level in the blood due to the action of the procaine penicillin G.

Benzathine penicillin is another type of depot penicillin which is very slowly absorbed. An adult dose of 1.2 million units of this preparation given intramuscularly will provide adequate blood levels for about 14 days. However, the levels are usually not sufficient to permit treatment of an acute infectious process, and benzathine penicillin is usually reserved for long-term prophylactic therapy. It has little or no place in the management and treatment of infections of the oral cavity.

The usual adult dose for the treatment of most infections is 600,000 units of procaine penicillin every 24 hours. In view of the low toxicity of penicillin, this dose is well tolerated by children. It should be emphasized that the amount of penicillin prescribed is dependent on the patient and the characteristics of the infectious process being treated. Guidelines concerning this have been discussed in detail previously under "Indications."

Penicillin V (Phenoxymethyl Penicillin)

By adding phenoxyacetic acid to the fermentation medium, penicillin V or phenoxymethyl penicillin was produced. The great advantage of penicillin V over penicillin G is that it is acid stable, therefore not destroyed in the stomach, which permits its use orally. Although it is not 100 per cent absorbed when given orally, it does give an adequate therapeutic blood level which will persist for four to six hours. Of the different forms of penicillin V, the potassium salt is the best absorbed and hence the most commonly used. When given for the management of infection, absorption is enhanced if it is given on an empty stomach. Therefore, when using this drug it should be given either one hour before or at least two hours after meals.

Penicillin V has approximately the same antibacterial activity as penicillin G. Because it is more slowly destroyed by penicillinase, it is more active against the resistant strains of staphylococci. On the other hand, it seems to be less effective than penicillin G against the streptococci.

Because penicillin V is incompletely absorbed, the dosages given orally must be greater than those usually given intramuscularly. As a rule of thumb, the oral dosage is usually four times as great as the intramuscular dosage. The usual adult oral dose is 250 mg. (400,000 units) every six hours. This same dose can be given to children for the treatment of infectious processes.

The oral preparations come in either drops, suspensions, or tablets. Many of the suspensions have a high concentration of carbohydrates and following their administration, the parents should make sure that good oral hygiene is observed to prevent any deleterious effect from the carbohydrates.

SEMI-SYNTHETIC PENICILLINS

As mentioned previously, crude filtrates of the mold *Penicillium chrysogenum* contain a variety of penicillins. They all have a common nucleus, 6-aminopenicillanic acid, but their other properties are dependent upon different side chains. It has been found that, by adding certain agents or precursors to the ferment, various side chains can be produced which have slightly different antibacterial properties. By using these techniques, it has been possible to produce the so-called semi-synthetic penicillins.

Although many semi-synthetic penicillins have been prepared, none are superior to penicillin G in their antibacterial activity against the usual penicillin-sensitive gram-positive cocci.

Phenethicillin and Propicillin

Two of the semi-synthetic penicillins, namely, phenethicillin and propicillin, should be mentioned. Both are acid resistant, which permits their oral administration. The antibacterial spectrum of phenethicillin and propicillin is similar to that of penicillin G. The main advantage that these two semi-synthetic penicillins have over penicillin G and penicillin V is that they are better absorbed when administered orally. Even though they are more completely absorbed from the gastrointestinal tract, they are not superior to penicillin G or penicillin V in terms of antibacterial activity. Therefore, when considering oral administration of penicillin, neither phenethicillin nor propicillin has any great advantage over penicillin V.

Methicillin

Methicillin is a semi-synthetic penicillin which is highly resistant to staphylococcal penicillinase. It is bactericidal in its action and is effective against both the penicillinase-producing strains of *Staphylococcus aureus* and the penicillin-sensitive strains of this organism. Although a few strains of *Staphylococcus aureus* have shown the ability to become resistant to methicillin, it is one of the drugs of choice when treating penicillin-resistant staphylococcal infections. Methicillin is not acid resistant; and therefore, it cannot be given orally but must be administered intramuscularly or intravenously. The usual adult dose is 100 mg. I.M. every 4 to 6 hours. The dose for children is 100 mg./kg. of body weight per day given in four divided doses every six hours (to change the dose per kilogram to the dose per pound, divide by 2). In no circumstance should the child's dose exceed the adult's.

Oxacillin (Isoxazolyl Penicillin)

Oxacillin is also resistant to staphylococcal penicillinase and should be reserved for treating infections caused by the penicillinase-producing staphylococcal organisms. Oxacillin is bacteriostatic in its action. It is resistant to acid and can be given orally. The usual adult dose is 500 mg. every six hours. The children's dose is 50 mg./kg. of body weight per day in equally divided doses given at six-hour intervals. When given orally, it is best absorbed during the fasting state; thus, the patient should be instructed to take it one hour prior to meals. The child's dose should not exceed the adult's.

Both methicillin and oxacillin are extremely valuable drugs for the treatment of penicillin-resistant staphylococcal infections. They should be reserved for this purpose and not used for the treatment of other infections. Since there is cross sensitivity between both methicillin and oxacillin, they should not be given to any patient who is sensitive to the naturally occurring penicillins, e.g., penicillin G.

Ampicillin

By the addition of certain side chains to the basic penicillin nucleus (6-aminopenicillanic acid) it has been possible to produce certain forms of semi-synthetic penicillins which show considerable activity against gram-negative bacilli. Ampicillin is a representative of this type of drug. Ampicillin is slightly less active against gram-positive organisms than penicillin G but considerably more effective against gram-negative bacilli. Like penicillin G, it is bactericidal. Because it is acid resistant, it can be given orally, and the usual recommended adult dose is 250 to 500 mg. every six hours. For children, the recommended dose is 100 mg./kg. of body weight per day in four divided doses. The child's dose should not exceed the adult's dose. This drug should not be used routinely but should be reserved for infections that have been shown by bacteriologic studies to be resistant to the other penicillins and sensitive only to this agent. As with the other semi-synthetic penicillins there is a cross sensitivity between ampicillin and penicillin G; and therefore, it should not be used in patients who are hypersensitive to the latter.

In summary, when selecting and using the penicillins, it is best to initially consider using the naturally occurring penicillins; namely, penicillin G and penicillin V. Penicillin G would be the drug of choice when it is desirable to administer the drug intramuscularly. If it is desired to use an oral preparation, then phenoxymethyl penicillin or penicillin V seems to be the drug of choice.

The main advantage that the acid-resistant semi-synthetic penicillins, phenethicillin and propicillin, have over penicillin V is that they are better absorbed from the gastrointestinal tract. However, this is counterbalanced by the fact that they are less active than penicillin V in terms of antibacterial activity.

Methicillin and oxacillin should be reserved for the treatment of proved penicillin-resistant staphylococcal organisms, and ampicillin should only be used when the infectious process has failed to improve on the other penicillins and bacteriologic studies have indicated it to be the drug of choice. Ampicillin would have certain advantages in treating mixed infections in which both gram-positive and gram-negative organisms are the causative agents.

It should be remembered that there is cross sensitivity between the naturally occurring and semi-synthetic penicillins; and if a patient is allergic to one preparation of penicillin, then the likelihood of having a reaction to another penicillin, whether it be natural or semi-synthetic, cannot be excluded.

COMPLICATIONS

The two main complications which can arise from the use of penicillin are toxic and hypersensitivity reactions. Toxic reactions from penicillin are extremely rare and usually do not occur unless there is severe renal insufficiency which would interfere with the excretion of the drug. This complication in persons with extensive renal disease can be avoided by decreasing the dose of the drug prescribed.

The most common complication associated with penicillin therapy is the hypersensitivity or allergic reaction. It is imperative, before administering penicillin, to obtain a detailed history to exclude the possibility of sensitivity in the patient to the drug. Although some tests have been developed which hold promise for detecting drug sensitivity in the patient, at the present time these sensitivity tests are not available for routine use. If there is any doubt concerning the possibility of sensitivity to penicillin, then an alternate chemotherapeutic agent should be prescribed.

Allergic reactions following penicillin therapy may be classified as being either immediate or delayed. The immediate reaction, or so-called anaphylactic reaction, is the most severe and accounts for most fatalities due to reactions to penicillin. It is suggested that if penicillin is to be prescribed, it is best to give the patient his initial dose while in the office, clinic, or hospital so that he may be observed for any untoward reactions. By keeping the patient under observation for 15 or 20 minutes, proper therapeutic countermeasures may be instituted without undue delay. A common misconception is that people do not have allergic reactions from oral administration of penicillin. Although the incidence of allergic reactions following the oral administration of the drug is less than that associated with its parenteral administration, patients may have allergic reactions following topical, oral, or parenteral administration of the drug.

The immediate or anaphylactic reaction is characterized by the signs of profound shock secondary to vasomotor collapse, an impalpable pulse, and difficulty with respiration. Facial and laryngeal edema or a generalized rash may or may not accompany this reaction. The specific therapy for the treatment of this reaction is the intravenous, intramuscular, or subcutaneous administration of 0.2 to 0.5 cc. of 1:1000 aqueous adrenalin. Because of the urgency of the situation, the intravenous route is highly desirable. When administering the 1:1000 aqueous adrenalin, it is advisable to dilute the solution with normal saline and gradually titrate the drug until the symptoms are relieved. If one were to take 0.5 cc. of 1:1000 aqueous adrenalin and give it rapidly intravenously, serious sequelae could result. If shock persists, then vasopressors may be used to support the blood pressure.

Some of the delayed reactions are characterized by fever, skin rash, swollen joints, and edema. Although these situations dictate treatment, they are not as severe as the anaphylactic reaction and do not require emergency measures. They are frequently alleviated by the utilization of antihistamines, e.g., diphenhydramine (Benadryl).

ERYTHROMYCIN

The antibiotic erythromycin was obtained in 1952 from a strain of *Streptomyces erythreus*. Depending upon the concentration used and the nature of the organism being treated, erythromycin is either bacteriostatic or bactericidal. In presently used doses, the drug is bacteriostatic, and its antimicrobial spectrum is similar to that of penicillin; namely, gram-positive organisms. It is felt that erythromycin acts by interfering with the protein synthesis of the bacteria. It has a rather high activity against pneumococci and the hemolytic streptococci of group A, the latter of which are responsible for numerous dental infections. Because bacteria seem to quickly develop resistance to erythromycin, it should be reserved for the treatment of infections which will only require a period of five to seven days of therapy.

Although erythromycin base is readily absorbed from the upper portion of the intestinal tract, it is partially inactivated by the gastric content of the stomach. To overcome this difficulty, it may be given in either enteric-coated capsules, which are acid resistant, or as erythromycin stearate which is resistant to gastric acid but easily broken down in the intestine, liberating the base. The oral administration of erythromycin base or erythromycin stearate produces a peak plasma level in one to two hours. The usual adult dose is 250 mg. by mouth every six hours. The recommended dosage for children is 20 to 40 mg./kg. of body weight per day, which is divided into four doses and given at six-hour intervals. The oral preparations are available in capsules, drops, or suspensions. Again, the child's dose should not exceed the adult's dose.

Preparations of erythromycin may also be given either intramuscularly or intravenously and have the benefit of attaining a more immediate effect and higher blood levels. The intramuscular route is accompanied by considerable pain at the site of injection. In the management of dental infections, it is rare that either the intramuscular or intravenous route would have to be employed.

When given in normal dosages, erythromycin has a very low degree of toxicity. When used orally, occasional gastrointestinal disturbances such as nausea, vomiting, diarrhea, and epigastric distress may develop. This is usually a result of a disturbance of the intestinal flora. At the onset of any of these symptoms, the drug should be discontinued. There have been reports of mild skin eruptions and drug fever associated with the drug, all of which disappear shortly after therapy is stopped. No severe toxic effects have ever been recorded from the administration of the erythromycin base. However, some hepatic involvement has been reported when the lauryl sulfate salt of the propionic acid ester of erythromycin is used. It is recommended that patients with hepatic insufficiency or dysfunction should not receive the lauryl sulfate salt of erythromycin, erythromycin estolate.

In dentistry erythromycin is an excellent substitute in the treatment of dental infections in those patients who are allergic to penicillin. This is due to the fact that it has approximately the same antibacterial spectrum as penicillin and because of its low toxicity and limited side effects. It should be remembered that organisms develop a resistance to the drug in a short period of time, and after five or six days of therapy it will probably be ineffective.

TETRACYCLINES

The tetracyclines make up a group of antimicrobial agents which has been used extensively in the management of infections since 1948. Chlortetracycline (Aureomycin), produced by *Streptomyces aureofaciens*, a soil bacterium, was the first to become available. Since that time, oxytetracycline (Terramycin), 1950, tetracycline (Achromycin), 1953, and demethylchlortetracycline (Declomycin), 1959, have been added to this group of antibiotics. Each of the tetracyclines may claim some superior qualities depending on the clinical problem for which it is intended. In general, however, their chemical, pharmacological, antimicrobial, and therapeutic properties are very similar. Therefore, the clinician who chooses a tetracycline for his patient may select the one with the most advantages for the particular infection without sacrificing efficacy in antimicrobial activity.

In usual doses, the tetracyclines are bacteriostatic. Because of their wide range of activity against various microorganisms, these drugs are frequently referred to as "broad-spectrum" antibiotics. Besides being effective against many gram-positive and gram-negative species, they are also effective against many of the rickettsiae.

The only large group of pathogenic organisms fully resistant to these drugs includes most of the fungi.

The tetracyclines are readily absorbed from the gastrointestinal tract, and therefore, are effective orally. They may also be administered intravenously or intramuscularly, but the latter route is usually avoided because of severe local irritation and pain. They may be used topically, but have the usual disadvantages and limitations associated with the topical use of antibiotics. Regardless of the route of administration, the tetracyclines are mainly removed from the plasma by the liver and kidneys. They should be used with care, if at all, in patients who have advanced hepatic or renal insufficiency. Failure to observe this precaution can lead to a rapid plasma accumulation of the tetracyclines, thereby enhancing toxic effects.

Because of the wide antimicrobial spectrum of the tetracyclines and their effect on the gastrointestinal flora, gastrointestinal irritation is not uncommon with tetracycline therapy. This is commonly due to an overgrowth of certain fungi, e.g., *Candida albicans*, and resistant coliform bacteria. Occasionally, suppression of the gastrointestinal flora may permit superinfection by resistant strains of *Staphylococcus aureus*. At the first signs of gastrointestinal irritation, the antibiotic should be discontinued. There seems to be less gastrointestinal disturbance with tetracycline hydrochloride (Achromycin); and as a result, this seems to be prescribed more frequently than the other tetracyclines.

Allergic and hypersensitivity reactions including skin rashes and drug fever have been reported with tetracycline therapy. Reactions of the skin in individuals treated with Declomycin who become exposed to sunlight have been reported. This phenomenon is referred to as a phototoxic reaction. Long-term therapy with tetracyclines may produce certain changes in the peripheral blood including prolonged coagulation time and thrombocytopenic purpura. Severe liver injury has been reported in patients who have received high doses of the tetracyclines.

The tetracyclines cross the placental barrier, and administration of these drugs to pregnant patients may result in a discoloration of the teeth in their offspring. Children receiving long- or short-term therapy with tetracyclines during a time when the teeth are being calcified may subsequently develop brown discoloration of the teeth. Large doses of the tetracyclines have been reported to cause hypoplasia of the enamel. The determining factor in the discoloration of the teeth and the enamel hypoplasia appears to be related to the total quantity of the antibiotic administered rather than the total duration of therapy. The tetracycline stain on the teeth is esthetically undesirable, and because of this effect on the dentition, this fact should be given careful consideration before prescribing. These drugs may produce a brown or black coating of the tongue, a hypertrophic glossitis, or moniliasis in the oral cavity. The tetracyclines are excreted by the salivary glands and sometimes this is helpful when managing infections involving the salivary glands.

Chlortetracycline (Aureomycin), oxytetracycline (Terramycin), and tetracycline (Achromycin) have basically the same potency, and therefore the doses are similar. The usual adult dose is 250 mg. by mouth every six hours. For children the dose is 20 to 40 mg./kg. of body weight per day, which is divided into four equal doses and given every six hours. These drugs are available in tablets, syrups, or pediatric drops. Declomycin, because of its potency and lower rate of renal clearance, is given in smaller doses and at less frequent intervals. The usual adult dose is 150 mg. by mouth every six hours. The dose for children is 6 to 12 mg./kg. of body weight per day given in three or four equally divided doses. Since all the tetracyclines are poorly absorbed in the presence of foods having a high calcium content, such as milk and some dairy products, they should be administered at least one hour before or two hours after meals.

In summary, it might be said the tetracyclines are particularly effective when dealing with a mixed infection caused by sensitive gram-positive and gram-negative organisms. However, in view of the deleterious effect that these drugs have on the teeth of the child, it is probably best that they be avoided unless the infectious process dictates their use.

STREPTOMYCIN

Streptomycin was initially produced from a strain of *Streptomyces griseus*. It is a bactericidal agent and is effective against the mycobacterium, gram-negative bacilli, and some strains of staphylococcus. The streptococci and pneumococci are relatively resistant to streptomycin. *Mycobacterium tuberculosis* is one of the organisms which is most sensitive to streptomycin and this agent has had a dramatic effect upon the treatment of tuberculosis.

Streptomycin is not absorbed from the gastrointestinal tract and is ineffective when administered orally, being excreted unchanged in the feces. When given intramuscularly, it reaches a peak level in the serum within one hour. The usual adult dose is 1 gm. per day, divided into two 500 mg. doses given intramuscularly every 12 hours. In children, the recommended dosage is 40 mg./kg. per day divided into two doses given intramuscularly every 12 hours.

Like most antimicrobial agents, streptomycin has both toxic and hypersensitivity reactions. Streptomycin is toxic to the eighth cranial nerve and particularly to the vestibular branch, which may lead to disturbances in equilibrium. At the first sign of vertigo, the drug should be discontinued. Although it is less common, streptomycin may also damage the auditory branch of the eighth cranial nerve, causing deafness. The incidence of vestibular disturbance is related to the total dosage of the drug and also the age of the patient. Older patients are more susceptible to vestibular injury. Prolonged therapy with streptomycin is not a prerequisite for vestibular impairment. Vestibular damage has been reported in patients receiving the drug for 10 days or less. The toxic effects of the drug are enhanced if the patient has associated renal damage.

Streptomycin may also produce mild skin reactions which are frequently characterized by a maculopapular type of rash. Cases of agranulocytosis and bone marrow depression have also been reported.

Streptomycin has little or no place in the treatment of dental infections. It is primarily used when treating a tuberculous infection, which is indeed rare in the oral cavity. The other occasion on which streptomycin may be indicated is in the treatment of a gram-negative infection of the oral cavity. Occasionally, it may be the drug of choice if so indicated by appropriate sensitivity studies of the organisms. In treating any dental infection with streptomycin, it should be remembered that organisms frequently develop rapid resistance to the drug. As a result, little or no benefit is to be gained in the treatment of the usual infections by continuing the therapy for more than five or six days.

CHLORAMPHENICOL

Chloramphenicol (Chloromycetin) was the first broad-spectrum antibiotic to be discovered. It was originally obtained from *Streptomyces venezuelae*. Since its original discovery, its structural formula has been identified, and it has been produced synthetically. It is the only antibiotic totally produced by synthetic means.

Chloramphenicol has a wide spectrum of antimicrobial activity and is effective against numerous gram-positive and gram-negative bacteria including all species of the rickettsiae. It is bacteriostatic in its action. Organisms have been slow to develop resistance toward this antibiotic.

Chloramphenicol may be given orally, intramuscularly, or intravenously. The usual route of administration is oral, and therapeutic plasma levels are obtained within one hour. The usual adult dose is 250 mg. orally every six hours. In children, the usual dose is 50 mg./kg. per day. If the child is under one month of age, the dose should not exceed 25 mg./kg. per day. These are given in four equally divided doses. An oral suspension is available for administering the drug to children.

Some of the reactions associated with chloramphenicol are skin rashes, edema, and atrophic glossitis. Spontaneous hemorrhage into the skin and mucous membranes has been reported. Gastrointestinal disturbances including epigastric distress, nausea, vomiting, and diarrhea have also been reported. Prolonged use of the drug may permit the development of moniliasis. Occasionally, the patient on Chloromycetin may complain of a bitter taste which is due to the fact that some of the drug is excreted in the saliva.

The major toxic reaction to chloramphenicol is bone marrow depression. Pancytopenia may develop, and some of the changes seen in the peripheral blood are anemia, thrombocytopenia, and granulocytopenia. Any patient receiving chloramphenicol should have a WBC, differential white count, hemoglobin, and reticulocyte count at least every 48 hours. Evidence of depression of either the total white cell count, granulocytes, red cells, or reticulocyte count dictates that the drug be stopped immediately. Failure to recognize bone marrow depression could lead to aplastic anemia which is fatal.

It is the feeling of the author that chloramphenicol has no place in the treatment of dental infections on an outpatient basis. It should never be used for the treatment of minor infections, but should be reserved for the treatment of serious infections which are resistant to the other commonly used antibiotics. Should the drug be prescribed, careful monitoring for bone marrow depression is required.

LINCOMYCIN

Lincomycin is a relatively new antibiotic with an antibacterial spectrum resembling erythromycin. Thus, it is effective against odontogenic infections which are caused by most streptococci and staphylococci. It is both bacteriostatic and bactericidal; and to date, there has been little evidence, either in in vitro or in vivo studies, that resistant strains develop. Lincomycin is synthesized by *Streptomyces lincolnensis*. It has displayed neither bacterial cross resistance with other antibiotics nor cross antigenicity with the various penicillins. To date, only a few serious side reactions have been reported. Of these, diarrhea is the most common. Abdominal cramps, nausea, vomiting, jaundice, leukopenia, and an elevated serum transaminase have been reported following its use. There is no evidence that lincomycin affects tooth development, but since it crosses the placental barrier, its effect in children and the newborn should be carefully observed.

Lincomycin may be administered orally, intravenously, or intramuscularly. Peak blood levels are obtained in one or two hours via the oral or intramuscular routes. It may be given orally in the form of capsules, syrup, or drops. The adult dose is 500 mg. orally every six hours. The oral dose for children depends on the severity of the infection and ranges from 30 to 60 mg./kg. per day, which should be given in four equally divided doses.

Recently, a newer antibiotic very similar to lincomycin has come on the market. This drug, clindamycin (Cleocin), is chemically and pharmacologically related to lincomycin. Clindamycin can only be given orally, and it is felt that the incidence of diarrhea commonly associated with lincomycin is less with the use of this drug. The usual adult dose of clindamycin is 150 to 300 mg. every six hours.

NYSTATIN

Nystatin (Mycostatin) is derived from *Streptomyces noursei,* and is effective only against yeast and fungi. Therefore, the drug has no place in the treatment of *bacterial* infections of the oral cavity. It is reserved for the treatment of certain yeast and fungal infections.

Nystatin is both fungistatic and fungicidal. The development of fungi resistant to this antibiotic has been reported in some strains, but *Candida albicans,* which occasionally produces an infection in the oral cavity of children, has not shown resistance in in vitro studies. However, when moniliasis occurs as a superinfection secondary to prolonged broad-spectrum antibiotic therapy, this disease may be refractory to treatment with nystatin.

Nystatin is poorly absorbed in the gastrointestinal tract; when taken orally, the drug is primarily excreted in the feces. It is not absorbed by the skin and mucous membranes, which makes it effective for topical use. Intramuscular and intravenous injection of nystatin produce untoward systemic reactions and a distressing local inflammatory reaction at the site of administration. Use of the drug in pedodontics should be limited to topical administration. Occasionally, its use is indicated under space maintainer appliances (acrylic), palatal obturators, and other such appliances with which there may be an associated moniliasis infection. The drug is also used as a mouth wash when superinfection occurs during broad-spectrum antibiotic therapy. In these cases, elimination of the broad-spectrum drug is recommended wherever feasible.

The drug is virtually free from side effects except in extremely large doses which may lead to gastrointestinal distress and diarrhea.

Nystatin is available as a cream, ointment, or powder containing 100,000 units per gram. It is also available as a suspension for use as a mouth wash containing 100,000 units per cc. of solution. The topical preparation should be applied liberally two or three times daily to the affected area. Oral tablets are available in 500,000 units, but this preparation is usually reserved for the treatment of intestinal moniliasis.

PROPHYLAXIS AGAINST BACTERIAL ENDOCARDITIS

On patients with rheumatic or congenital heart disease, bacteremia produced by surgical manipulation within the oral cavity could permit bacteria to be lodged on the heart valves or other portions of the endocardium and produce bacterial endocarditis. This carries with it a relatively high degree of mortality and morbidity. These patients should be protected with appropriate antibiotics prior to any surgical procedures in the oral cavity. The American Heart Association, through its Committee on Prevention of the Council on Rheumatic Fever and Congenital Heart Disease, published its opinion regarding prophylaxis against bacterial endocarditis in 1960. This statement appeared in *Circulation*, Volume 21, 1960. Although the exact dosage and duration of therapy are empirical, there is some evidence that for effective prophylaxis, high concentrations of penicillin must be present at the time the surgical procedures are performed in the oral cavity. Some authorities feel that prophylaxis should be started several days prior to the operative procedure. On the other hand, other authorities have been concerned that pretreatment could lead to the emergence of antibiotic-resistant microorganisms. The emergence of such organisms would present a very difficult therapeutic problem if they became implanted on the valves. It has, therefore, been argued that prophylaxis should not be instituted until immediately before the operative procedure.

In view of the lack of definitive evidence to support either method categorically, it has been suggested that the physician evaluate the likelihood of infection and decide whether a period of preliminary treatment prior to the operative procedure is indicated. It has been emphasized that there is no disagreement regarding the advisability of using antimicrobial agents immediately before and subsequent to the operative procedure. The following treatment schedule is recommended.

Oral Plus Intramuscular Penicillin

For Two Days Before Dental Procedure (Optional)
    500,000 units of buffered penicillin G or phenoxymethyl penicillin (penicillin V), by mouth four times a day.
Day of Dental Procedure
    500,000 units of buffered penicillin G or phenoxymethyl penicillin (penicillin V), by mouth four times a day, supplemented by 600,000 units crystalline penicillin I.M. one hour before surgical procedure.
Two Days Following Dental Procedure
    500,000 units of buffered penicillin G or phenoxymethyl penicillin (penicillin V), by mouth four times a day.

Oral Penicillin

Because of practical considerations some physicians and dentists rely on oral penicillin alone when full cooperation of the patient is assured.
    Each oral dose: 500,000 units buffered penicillin G or penicillin V.
    Oral dosage four times a day for two days before dental procedure (optional), on day of dental procedure, and on two following days.

If patients are sensitive to penicillin, it is suggested that erythromycin be used. If erythromycin is employed, the dose for adults and older children is 250 mg. by mouth four times daily. For small children, a dose of 40 mg./kg. of body weight per day in four evenly spaced doses is used. The dose of the erythromycin should not exceed 1 gm. per day.

NEWER ANTIMICROBIAL AGENTS

During recent years a number of newer antimicrobial agents have been developed. These inclue cephalexin (Keflex), gentamicin (Garamycin), carbenicillin (Geopen), spectinomycin (Trobicin), and others. These agents either have a narrow spectrum of coverage or are only indicated for certain specific infections which have been proved by culture and sensitivity. They are, therefore, agents which would not be the drug of choice in treating primary odontogenic and oral infections. For this reason, detailed descriptions of these agents are not included within this chapter.

SUMMARY

In summary it can be said that prior to prescribing any antimicrobial agent, it is important to evaluate the risks involved in using the agent versus the benefits to be obtained. This should prevent the indiscriminate use of the antimicrobial agents. Considering that most of the organisms responsible for dental infections are sensitive to penicillin, this antimicrobial is the drug of choice. If the patient is sensitive to penicillin, then erythromycin, because of its similar antimicrobial spectrum, should be considered as the next drug of choice. Occasionally, when dealing with a mixed infection composed of gram-positive and gram-negative organisms, the tetracyclines may be used. However, because of their effects upon the dentition, it is best to avoid their use while teeth are being calcified. Other antimicrobial agents which have been reviewed in this chapter should be reserved for the treatment of those resistant infections which have proved to be susceptible to a specific drug after adequate bacteriologic survey. For the treatment of moniliasis, nystatin has proved effective.

An attempt has been made to spend a considerable time on the philosophy of the use of antimicrobial therapy. It should be remembered that the dose of the drug must be individualized for each patient; and prior to prescribing the drug, the dosage should always be checked in a reliable text.

REFERENCES

1. Barber, M., and Garrod, L. P.: Antibiotic and Chemotherapy. London, E. & S. Livingstone, Ltd., 1963.
2. Brumfitt, W., and Williams, J. D., eds.: Proceedings of the International Conference on Therapy with the New Penicillins. Post. M. J., *40*:Supp., December, 1964.
3. Drug Letter, Bull. Hopkins Hospital, *116*:69–72, January, 1965.
4. Dubos, R. J., and Hirsch, J. G.: Bacterial and Mycotic Infections of Man, 4th ed. Philadelphia, J. B. Lippincott Company, 1965.
5. Gillespie, W. A.: Antibiotics for prevention of bacterial endocarditis during dental treatment. Lancet, *1*:686–688, 1966.

6. Goodman, L. S., and Gilman, A.: The Pharmacological Basis of Therapeutics, 3rd ed. New York, The Macmillan Company, 1965.

7. Harrison, T. R., et al.: Principles of Internal Medicine, 5th ed. New York, McGraw-Hill Book Company, 1966.

8. Jawetz, E., Melnick, J. L., and Adelberg, E. A.: Review of Medical Microbiology, 7th ed. Los Altos, Calif., Lange Medical Publications, 1966.

9. Prevention of rheumatic fever and bacterial endocarditis through control of streptococcal infections. Circulation, 21:151, 1960.

10. Rose, H. M.: Antimicrobial agents and chemotherapy. Curr. Ther. Res., 7:41–45, 1964.

11. Shirkey, H. C., ed.: Pediatric Therapy, 2nd ed. St. Louis, C. V. Mosby Co., 1966–67.

12. Simon, H. J., ed.: Treatment of superinfections. Mod. Treatm., 3, 1966.

13. Jaffe, S. J., and Back, N.: Pediatric pharmacology. Postgrad. Med., 40:193–201, 1966.

20

THE EPIDEMIOLOGY
OF DENTAL CARIES

by JOSEPH F. VOLKER
and DAVID L. RUSSELL

In 1970 around $4,383,000,000 was spent for dental care with the major expenditure going for restoration of carious teeth. This sum is approximately one half of 1 per cent of the total national income. In terms of the nation's health bill it may be conservatively estimated that approximately ten cents out of every health dollar is spent for dental care. Although there are now over 100,000 dentists serving the civilian and military population, it is probable that within each year less than 50 per cent of the population see a dentist. Even more discouraging is the realization that it would be necessary to double the present number of dentists if the dental defects that occur each year were to be corrected.

Since such a marked expansion of dental training facilities is not likely, the solution to our present dilemma rests in the development of effective techniques for the prevention of dental disease and for its early treatment. These techniques must be based on a sound knowledge of the factors that predispose to susceptibility and resistance. Because dental caries is the most common of the oral diseases and because the average individual has his first experience with this disease in childhood, it is particularly important that we review the accumulated knowledge of tooth decay from the first through the twelfth year of life. In this crucial period, the primary teeth erupt, function, and are exfoliated, and the permanent teeth, exclusive of the third molars, are formed and erupt into a functional pattern.

As a first step in the realization of this objective it is pertinent to review the epidemiology of dental caries. Epidemiology has been defined by one authority as "the science dealing with the relationships of the various factors which determine the frequency and distribution of a disease." It has been more simply stated by another as being "the study of occurrence and distribution of disease." In utilizing the epidemiologic approach one observes the disease in moderate- to large-sized groups of people. Subsequently, particular attention is paid to the persons who are most or least affected by the disease with the hope that a common denominator will be found among those who are disease susceptible or disease resistant. The possibility that this common factor is of etiologic significance is then tested under controlled experimental conditions.

There are numerous instances in which this approach has given clues to the cause of a disease and in this manner has ultimately led to its prevention. Even in those cases in which the technique has not resulted in the prevention and control of the disease, it has resulted almost invariably in more intelligent diagnostic procedures because it tells the practitioner when and where to look for initial disease lesions. Similarly, it enables the dentist or physician to anticipate the rate at which the disease will usually progress. Finally, it permits the practitioner to discuss the disease intelligently with his patient, since the accumulated information assists him in advising his patients what factors are significant or unimportant in causing the disease.

One of the first to utilize epidemiologic techniques in the study of the etiology of dental caries was Emile Magitot. More than ninety years ago this investigator published data showing the distribution of dental caries in the various permanent teeth. Even more surprising, he reported data on the frequency of dental caries in the primary dentition. From his personal observations he prepared graphs showing the relative frequency of dental caries of each of the permanent teeth. Indicative of his genius was his study and interpretation of the dental caries in men eligible for French military service. Noting that these followed a geographic pattern, he attempted to relate these differences to environmental factors, concluding: "We might pass in review and successively refute the other influences which have been named: the altitudes, the geological basins, the climates, the common alimentation, the conditions of wealth or of poverty, etc., and we should arrive at this result, that no one of these circumstances, taken by itself, can supply the explanation we seek."

In recent years the U.S. Public Health Service and the public health departments of the various states and cities, as well as individual investigators both at home and abroad, have extended and refined these techniques. Presently, we are in possession of information that permits comparisons between countries and within various sections of this country. More important, we can make comparisons within a mouth between individual teeth and even individual surfaces.

GEOGRAPHIC INFLUENCES ON DENTAL CARIES

The accumulated data suggest that the dental caries susceptibility of children in the United States is fairly comparable to that of the children of western Europe and the various English-speaking countries of the British Commonwealth, i.e., Canada, Australia, New Zealand. Consequently, observations made in these countries may be accepted as being applicable generally to children residing in the United States.

In evaluating the results of surveys within this country it should be borne in mind that dental caries in the United States follows a geographic pattern. The first reliable data in support of this conclusion were accumulated during the Civil War when military conscriptees were given dental examinations. Subsequently, the pattern has been reaffirmed on numerous occasions, particularly in the mouth examinations of prospective and actual members of the armed services in World Wars I and II. As a general statement it may be said that persons born and raised in the

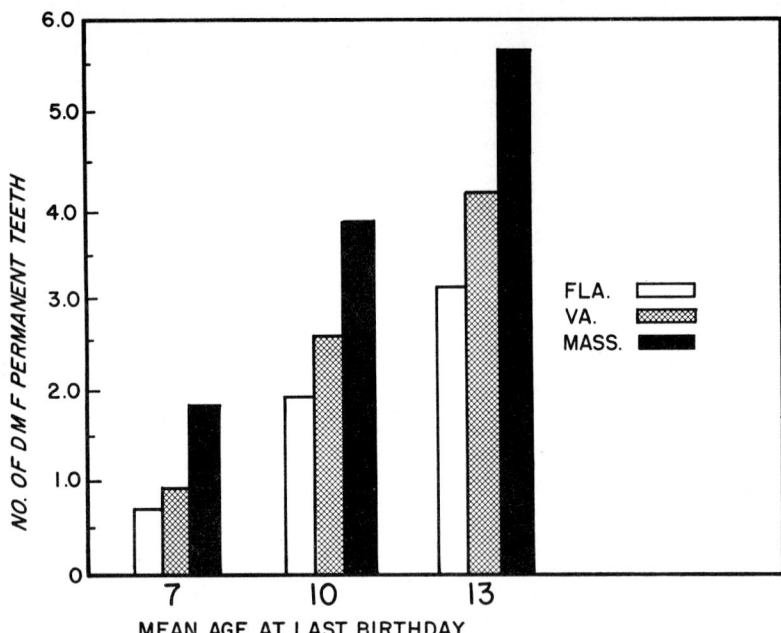

Figure 20–1   Mean DMF of the permanent dentition of boys residing in Florida, Virginia, and Massachusetts. (From East: Am. J. Pub. Health, *32*, 1942.)

New England, Middle Atlantic and North Pacific states have the greatest caries experience while those in the Rocky Mountain and Southwestern states have the least, and the Central and Southeastern states are intermediate.

The data relating geographic location to the variations in dental caries in children are rather meager. There is, however, evidence that such differences do exist, and they may be observed in the permanent dentition immediately after eruption. The data shown in Figure 20–1 summarize the mean DMF* rates of boys residing in Florida, Virginia, and Massachusetts cities of 100,000 or more at ages 7, 10 and 13.

Although the factors responsible for these differences are not fully understood, it is known that the presence of 1 part per million (ppm) of fluoride in the drinking water during the time when teeth are being formed reduces their liability to caries by as much as 60 per cent. Although fluoride is the only trace element for which unequivocal evidence exists supporting its importance in human dental caries, several other elements have been reported to effect a reduction or an increase in dental caries in both animals and humans. In addition, studies regarding the concentration of trace elements in soils and water supplies, temperature, soil pH, humidity, and contiguity to coastal areas have resulted in different epidemiological findings for caries rates in different geographical areas. For these reasons the sources of the data represented in the figures of this chapter are presented.

It should also be kept in mind in evaluating the figures that whereas averages give us an overall picture of the extent of a disease, they tend to minimize the well

─────────────

*For explanation of DMF, see paragraph headed Extent in Primary Dentition.

established fact that individuals with widely divergent disease patterns are included within the total. Unfortunately, many clinicians are prone to remember the patients who are exceptions rather than those who conform to the general rule.

CARIES IN THE PRIMARY DENTITION

ONSET IN THE PRIMARY DENTITION

One of the most important questions to be answered is the age at which the child should first be seen by the dentist. All too often the practitioner is willing for this to be delayed until the kindergarten stage of development. Such an attitude is inconsistent with the accumulated data concerning the onset of dental caries in the primary dentition. The findings of several investigators indicate that at 1 year of age approximately 5 per cent of the children exhibit dental caries. The percentage increases to approximately 10 per cent at 2 years of age. There is a further rise so that by the third and fourth years 40 and 55 per cent of the children, respectively, have tooth decay. The trend continues, and at age 5, three out of four preschool children have carious primary teeth. These data are shown in Figure 20–2. Many pedodontists, therefore, recommend that the child should first visit the dentist at 1½ to 2 years of age, before extensive cavities are established and while there is still a chance to practice preventive dentistry on the primary dentition.

EXTENT IN THE PRIMARY DENTITION

Two good indices of dental caries experience in the permanent dentition are the number of decayed, missing, and filled teeth and the number of decayed, missing, and filled tooth surfaces. For the sake of convenience these two indices have been designated with the abbreviations DMF and DMFS, respectively. When these

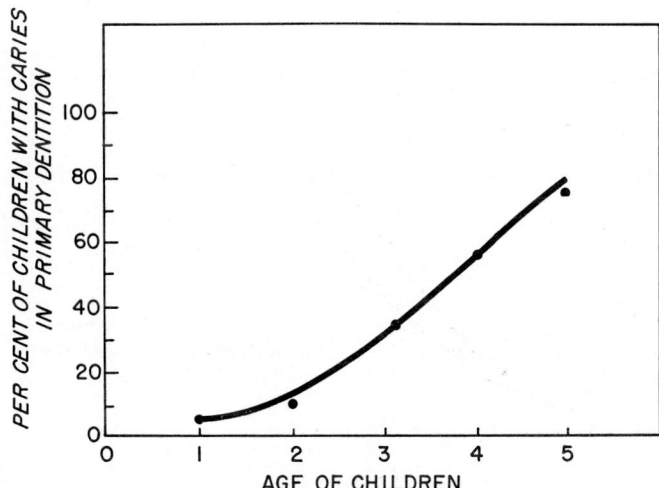

Figure 20–2 Caries in children; per cent of children with caries in primary dentition. (Toverud et al.: Survey of the Literature of Dental Caries, National Academy of Sciences-National Research Council.)

criteria are applied to the primary teeth, one recognizes immediately that beginning with age 5 an appreciable number of teeth may be missing, not because of caries but because of normal exfoliation. For this reason investigators often report the extent of dental caries in the primary teeth in terms of decayed and filled teeth (df teeth, which may be abbreviated dft) and decayed and filled surfaces (df tooth surfaces, which may be abbreviated dfs). The use of capital letters indicates the permanent dentition while lower case letters signify the primary dentition.

Available data indicate that the average 2 year old has 0.3 df teeth. The df teeth increase to approximately 1 at age 3, with acceleration to 2.5 and 4.6 at ages 4 and 5, respectively. The number of decayed, filled surfaces approximates the number of decayed, filled teeth until age 3. Beyond this point it increases significantly until at age 5 the dfs is about 8. These data are shown in Figure 20–3. Such figures are of importance from an epidemiological viewpoint; however, they should not be applied to the individual child. Recent studies have shown that while an average child may have a dft of 2 at age 3, the child who exhibits dental caries at that age may have four to five carious lesions.

LOCATION IN THE PRIMARY DENTITION

Since the early detection of dental caries is facilitated by a knowledge of the relative caries susceptibility of the various tooth surfaces, it is advantageous to be

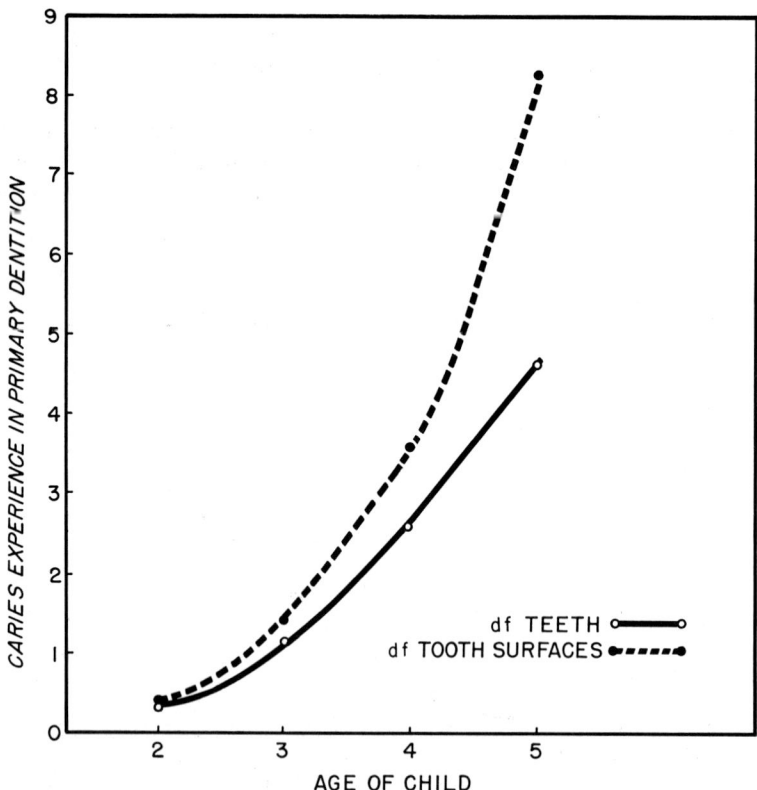

Figure 20–3 df teeth and df tooth surfaces in the primary dentition of 2 to 5 year old children. (Toverud et al.: Survey of the Literature of Dental Caries. National Academy of Sciences-National Research Council.)

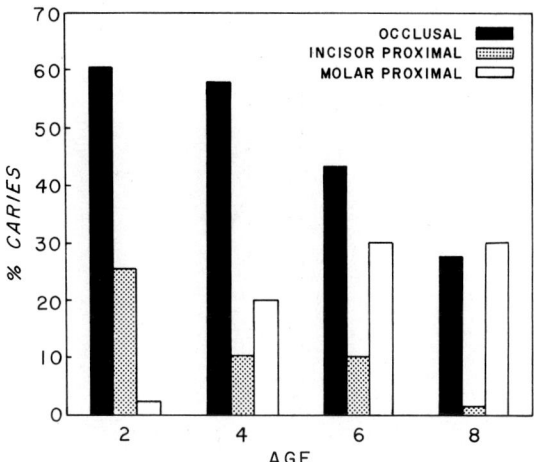

Figure 20–4 Distribution of caries in the primary dentition. (Adapted from Parfitt: Brit. D.J., 99:423, 1955.)

acquainted with our present knowledge of the phenomenon. It has been shown that at age 2 occlusal caries accounts for over 60 per cent of the carious lesions while proximal incisor caries accounts for 25 per cent of the primary tooth decay. The amount of proximal molar caries at this age is insignificant. The difference in susceptibility between occlusal and proximal surfaces may be associated with the normal spacing which exists between primary anterior teeth and the short period of exposure of primary second molars in most children of age two years. During the sixth year, however, proximal molar caries is as prevalent as occlusal molar caries. The distribution of occlusal and proximal caries in the primary dentition at various ages is shown in Figure 20–4.

Interrelation of Occlusal and Proximal Caries in Primary Molars

The data presented in Figure 20–4 give only a general picture of the location of caries in the primary dentition at various ages. Further analysis of the available data is necessary if we are to understand the relation or lack of relation between occlusal and proximal caries in molar teeth. Present evidence indicates that the factors that result in the development of both occlusal and proximal caries although they may be similar are quite independent of each other.

Over 400 six year olds have been subjected to intensive study and have been grouped according to the number of occlusal and proximal cavities present in their primary teeth. It has been observed that the group having as many as 14 occlusal cavities had on an average 3 proximal cavities. The latter figure is quite comparable with the number of proximal cavities found in 6 year olds having on an average 3, 7, and 9 occlusal cavities. From this we may conclude that the obvious presence of considerable occlusal caries in the primary teeth is not presumptive evidence of any unusual amount of molar proximal caries. These data are shown in Figure 20–5.*

---

*Multiple occlusal carious lesions on a single tooth were counted, thus allowing the possibility of more than eight occlusal lesions, which is the maximum number of primary molars at risk at age six years.

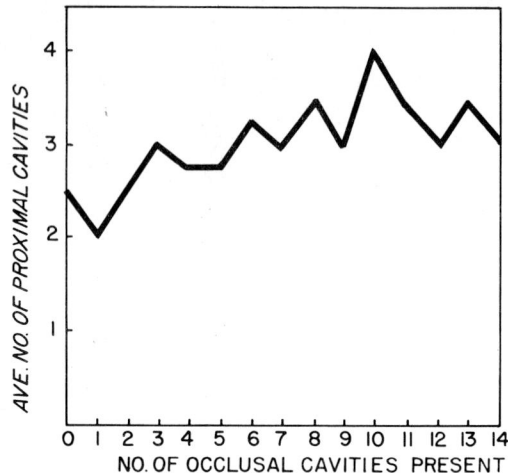

Figure 20–5   Proximal and occlusal caries in primary molars of 6 year olds. (From Parfitt: J. Dent. Child., 23:1956.)

Occlusal Caries in Primary Molars

The first primary molars, both maxillary and mandibular, are much less susceptible to occlusal caries than the second primary molars even though the former erupt at an earlier date (Fig. 20–6). Whereas at age 8 over 50 per cent of the second primary molars in one large study had occlusal caries, only about 20 per cent of the first primary molars had occlusal surfaces that were involved with decay. The difference in caries susceptibility is probably a result of the occlusal surfaces of the second molars being more fissured and pitted than those of the first molars.

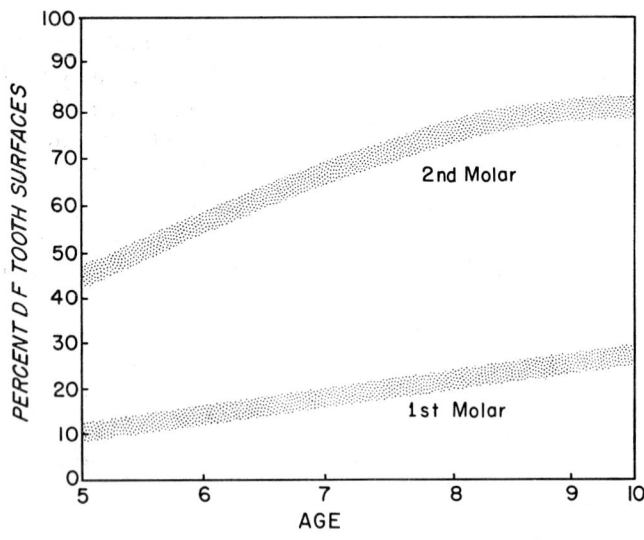

Figure 20–6   Occlusal caries in first and second primary molars. (From Walsh and Smart: New Zealand D.J., 44, 1948.)

Proximal Caries in the Primary Molars

When undertaking an examination for dental caries, the relative susceptibility of the distal surface of the first primary molar and the mesial surface of the adjacent second primary molar must be considered. The dentist may be faced with a situation wherein there is roentgenographic evidence of decay on the former and it is advantageous to know of the possibilities that the latter will suffer a similar fate. The present evidence suggests that the caries experience of the two surfaces is very similar. In most instances in which an unrestored carious lesion is present on the distal surface of the first primary molar, a lesion may be anticipated on the mesial surface of the second molar within the year. Although the first molar is usually erupted twelve or more months before the second molar, it seems probable that the factors determining caries susceptibility of their proximal surfaces affect them equally. This opinion is supported by the data presented in Figure 20–7.

Susceptibility of the Proximal Surfaces of the Second Primary Molar to Dental Caries

The distal surface of the second primary molar is unique in the primary dentition. From age 2, when it most often erupts, until age 6, when the first permanent molar erupts, it has no approximating tooth surface. Subsequently, it remains in position for approximately four years before being exfoliated. It is of interest, therefore, to know the relative caries susceptibility of the surface under the different conditions of presence and absence of an adjacent tooth. It has been shown that at age 6 there are ten times as many carious lesions on the mesial surfaces of second primary molars as there are on the distal surfaces of the same teeth. At age 9, however, there are almost half as many carious lesions on the distal surfaces as there are on the mesial surfaces. This is illustrated in Figure 20–8.

Proximal Caries in the Primary Cuspid and First Primary Molar

As seen in Figure 20–7, the caries susceptibility of the distal surface of the first primary molar is quite comparable to that of the mesial surface of the second primary molar. In contrast, the caries susceptibility of the mesial surface of the first primary molar is relatively moderate and resembles that of the distal surface

Figure 20–7 Caries on distal surface of first primary molar and mesial surface of second primary molar. (From Parfitt: J. Dent. Child., 23:31, 1956.)

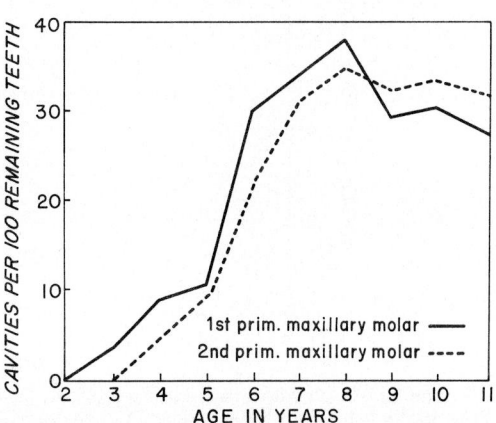

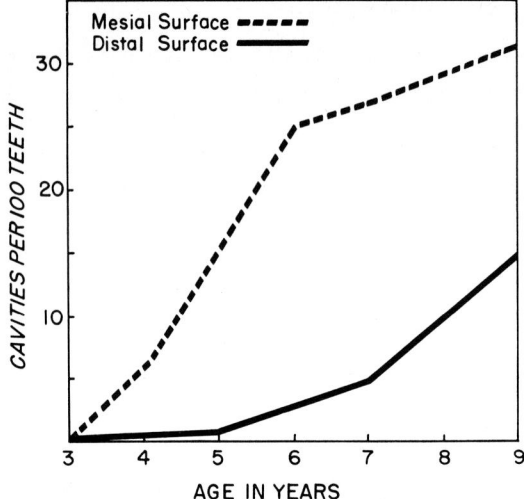

Figure 20–8 Caries on distal surface and mesial surface of the maxillary and mandibular second primary molars. (From Parfitt: J. Dent. Child., *23*, 1956.)

of the primary cuspid. It is likely that the broader area of contact between the first and second molars predisposes to conditions more favorable for the development of caries than exist between the primary cuspid and the first molar. In addition, spaces normally exist between the primary cuspids and first molars in many children, especially in the mandibular primary dentition. The general caries experience of the tooth surfaces of the two interproximal areas is illustrated in Figure 20–9.

A summary of the relative caries susceptibility of various surfaces of the primary teeth is illustrated in Figure 20–10. The summary is generally applicable to both maxillary and mandibular primary teeth.

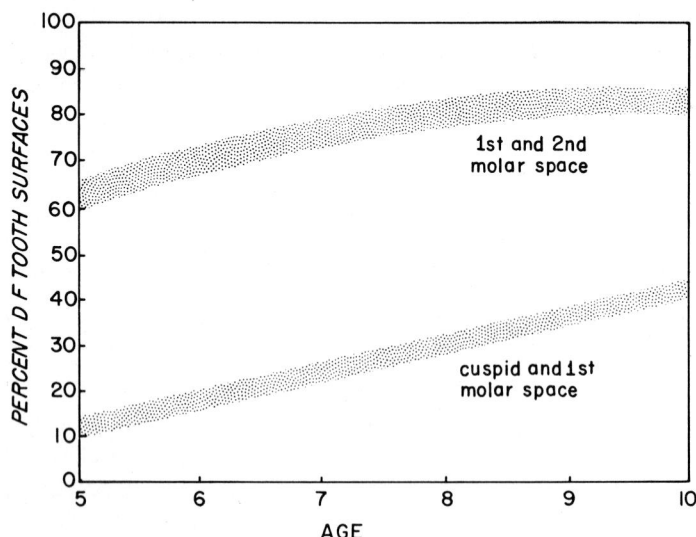

Figure 20–9 Proximal caries in the primary cuspid-first molar, and primary first molar-second molar. (From Walsh and Smart: New Zealand D.J., *44*, 1948.)

Figure 20–10 The relative susceptibility of various surfaces of the primary teeth. A < B, B = C, C < D, D = E, E > F (until G erupts), BC < DE, CD < EF.

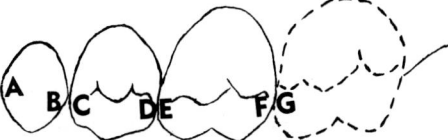

CARIES IN THE PERMANENT DENTITION

During the sixth year of life the permanent dentition starts to erupt and exfoliation of the primary dentition is begun. Both of these processes are usually completed, the third molars excepted, by age 12. Having considered the pertinent epidemiology of caries in the primary dentition, it is logical to attempt comparable observations for the permanent dentition, particularly in the 6 to 12 year age range.

ONSET IN THE PERMANENT DENTITION

A considerable number of surveys have been made of dental caries experience in the permanent dentition. These studies are in general agreement that 20 per cent of the children at age 6 have experienced tooth decay in their permanent teeth. A rapid increase follows so that 60 and 85 per cent of children at ages 8 and 10, respectively, have been affected by dental caries. At age 12, when most of the permanent dentition has erupted, over 90 per cent of school children have experienced tooth decay. These data are shown in Figure 20–11.

EXTENT IN THE PERMANENT DENTITION

The DMF rates of large groups of children indicate that at age 6 a DMF of 0.5 in the permanent dentition may be anticipated. The rate increases to 2.3 and 3.6 at ages 8 and 10, respectively. At age 12, when most of the permanent dentition has erupted, a DMF of 5.5 may be considered as being average. As a generalization, it may be said that for every year during the period when the permanent teeth are erupting we may anticipate a new carious permanent tooth. These data are shown in Figure 20–12.

The number of decayed, missing, and filled permanent surfaces approximates the number of decayed, missing, and filled teeth from ages 6 to 8. Beyond this point the DMFS increases at an accelerated rate until at age 12 a DMFS of 7.5 may be expected. These data may also be seen in Figure 20–12.

LOCATION IN THE PERMANENT DENTITION

The greatest portion of the dental caries in the permanent teeth of the 6 to 12 year old child is contributed by the 6 year molars. At age 7 approximately 25 per cent of the mandibular first permanent molars are carious. An increase to more than 50 per cent at age 9 and to 70 per cent at age 12 has been reported. At compa-

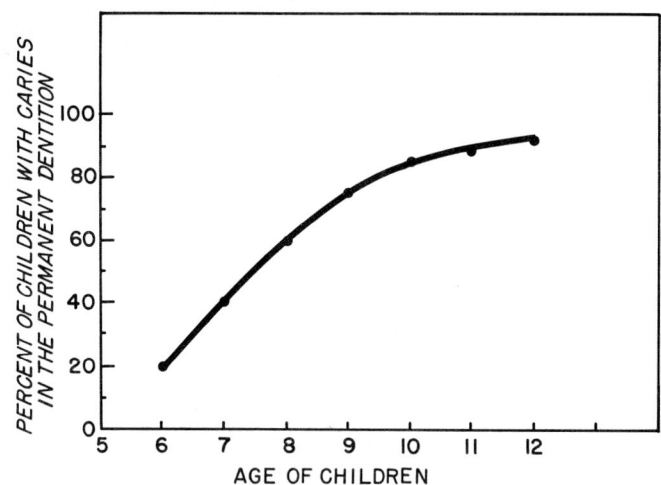

Figure 20–11 Caries in children (permanent dentition). (From Finn, in Toverud et al.: Survey of the Literature of Dental Caries, National Academy of Sciences-National Research Council.)

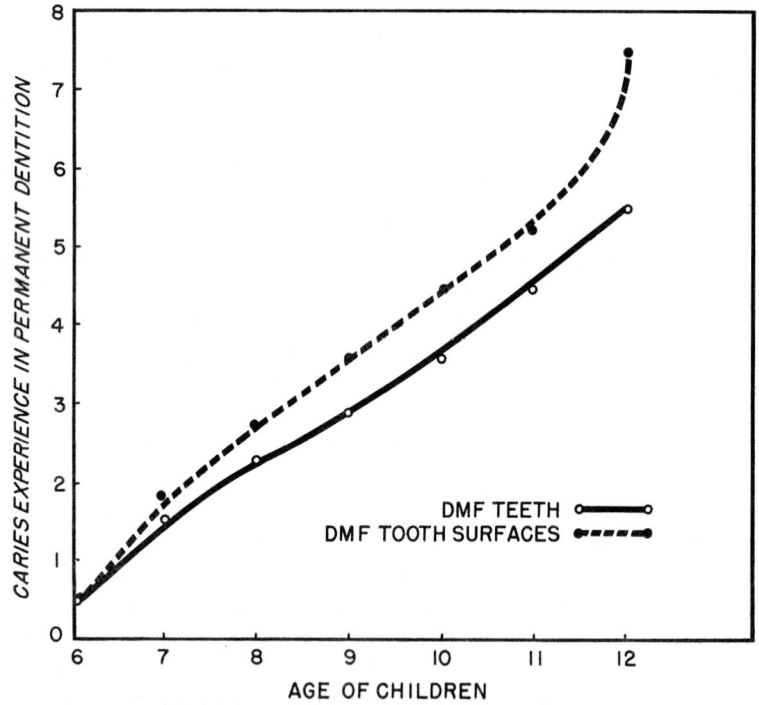

Figure 20–12 DMF teeth and DMF tooth surfaces in the permanent dentition of 6 to 12 year old children. (From Finn, in Toverud et al.: Survey of the Literature of Dental Caries, National Academy of Sciences-National Research Council.)

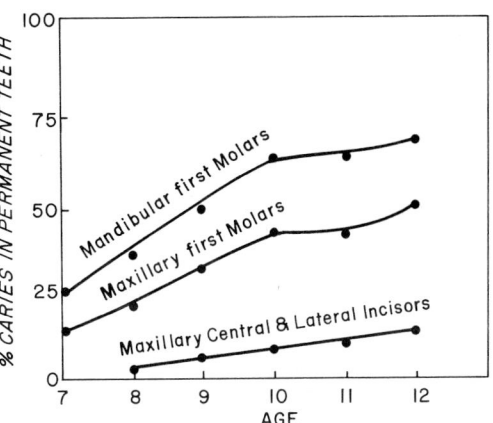

Figure 20–13 Dental caries in selected permanent teeth. (From Klein et al.: The Epidemiology of Dental Disease. U.S. Public Health Service, 1948.)

rable ages, 12, 35, and 52 per cent of the maxillary first permanent molars are carious. The maxillary permanent central and lateral incisors, although erupting at approximately the same age, are much less susceptible to caries. At age 8, an average of 1 per cent of these teeth will be found to be carious. An increase to approximately 10 and 15 per cent at ages 11 and 12, respectively, follows. Figure 20–13 shows the percentage of caries in selected permanent teeth at ages 7 through 12.

The caries experience of the permanent mandibular central and lateral incisors in young children is minimal. On an average, less than 2 per cent of these teeth are affected by age 12. Accordingly, the appearance of cavities on the mandibular permanent incisors in children may be an indication of rampant caries, necessitating prompt caries control measures.

During the 10 to 12 year age interval the eruption of the maxillary and mandibular permanent cuspids and first and second premolars may be anticipated. Although caries in the maxillary and mandibular permanent cuspids and mandibular first premolars is infrequent up to and including age 12, approximately 5 per cent of mandibular second premolars and maxillary first and second premolars may be expected to experience tooth decay at this age. In contrast, the second permanent molar, which usually erupts at 12 years, is quite caries susceptible. Approximately 20 per cent of the mandibular second permanent molars and 10 per cent of the maxillary second permanent molars have tooth decay within a year after they erupt.

Only a limited amount of information exists on the collective caries susceptibility of the various surfaces of the permanent teeth of children of ages 6 through 12. It is generally agreed that occlusal caries is the most prevalent form occurring in the permanent teeth of children. It may be anticipated on the molar surfaces shortly after their eruption. Proximal caries on the posterior teeth in most instances occurs subsequently. At age 12 about 50 per cent of the caries involving permanent tooth surfaces is occlusal, 30 per cent is proximal and 20 per cent is buccal and lingual. Less than 1 per cent is found on the labial, incisal, and cervical surfaces.

Since the first molar is by far the most caries susceptible of the permanent teeth, its pattern of tooth surface decay has been investigated in detail. In one careful study, it has been shown that 63 per cent, 75 per cent, and 93 per cent of 6, 7, and 8 year olds, respectively, showed occlusal fissure caries in their first permanent molars. Comparable data for the mesial surface of the same tooth show only 2

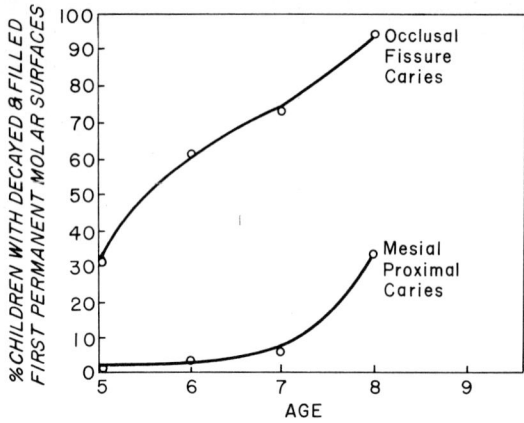

Figure 20–14 Relative caries susceptibility of the occlusal and proximal surfaces of first permanent molar. (Adapted from Walsh and Smart: New Zealand D.J., 44:17, 1948.)

per cent of 6 year olds, 5 per cent of 7 year olds, and 33 per cent of 8 year olds are affected. (See Fig. 20–14.)

SPEED OF DEVELOPMENT OF CARIOUS LESIONS

A knowledge of the length of time a cavity takes to develop is prerequisite for the intelligent practice of preventive and restorative dentistry. Instances have been observed wherein the crowns of primary and permanent teeth have decayed to the level of the gum tissues in less than a year after eruption. Similarly, caries has been observed on tooth surfaces within a month after the insertion of poorly constructed orthodontic or prosthetic appliances. In a study of over 100 institutionalized children whose DMF rate was approximately 0.75 teeth per year, it was observed that caries on the occlusal surface may take from less than three months to more than 48 months to progress from the state of incipient caries to a clinical cavity. Twenty-eight per cent of the incipient lesions progressed to a clinical cavity in less than six months, but as many as 53 per cent of occlusal cavities remained more than two years in the incipient stage. These observations support the need for establishing six months as the maximal interval between dental diagnostic visits with some individuals required to return at even shorter intervals of time. However, these data also suggest that many incipient lesions may never become clinical cavities. Consequently, they should be carefully observed before the decision is made to treat them as such, especially incipient proximal lesions in patients who drink fluoridated water or who routinely have adequate topical fluoride therapy.

SEX AND FAMILIAL RELATIONSHIPS IN DENTAL CARIES

SEX DIFFERENCES AND DENTAL CARIES EXPERIENCE

It has been a consistent finding that girls have a higher caries experience than boys of the same chronologic age. Such data are illustrated in Figure 20–15, which gives details relative to the permanent DMF teeth of several thousand school children. It has also been shown that the teeth of girls erupt at an earlier age than do those of boys. Thus, they are exposed to the risk of dental caries at an earlier average age. If one takes this factor into consideration, the caries susceptibility of boys and girls is probably comparable.

DENTAL CARIES IN SIBLINGS

The existence of a familial pattern of caries experience in child patients is sometimes questioned by parents. Fortunately, this has been studied in some detail by competent investigators. Over 4000 dental records of school children have been analyzed. From these, two groups were selected, one being relatively immune to dental caries and the other showing a relatively high susceptibility to dental caries. Next, the records of the brothers and sisters of the "immunes" and "susceptibles" were carefully examined for their caries experience. It was found that the brothers and sisters of the "susceptibles" had twice as much caries as the brothers and sisters of the "immunes." It should be stressed that this is an overall finding, and that caution must be used in interpreting it to parents.

DENTAL CARIES IN TWINS

Studies have been made of dental caries in monozygotic and dizygotic twins. Such an approach affords the investigator an opportunity to evaluate the influence of hereditary and environmental factors on dental caries. The rationale involved is that, if hereditary factors are predominant, identical twins should be more similar in their caries patterns than fraternal twins. Such "nature and nurture" studies indicate that there are genetic factors which influence the susceptibility of the child to dental caries.

Although it is generally considered that the actual amount of caries the teeth experience is largely under the control of environmental factors such as diet and oral hygiene, it is clear that genetically determined factors such as tooth morphology and, to some extent, tooth position must be of considerable importance in de-

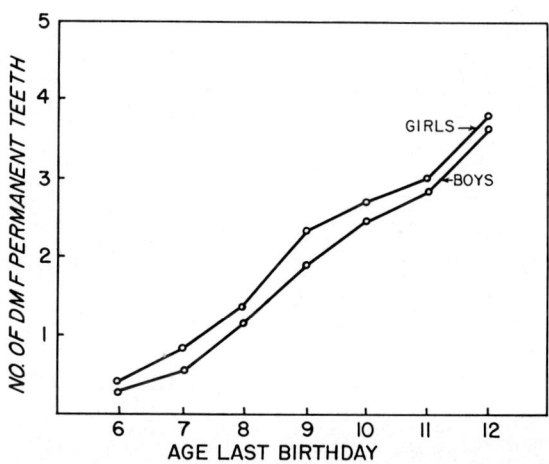

Figure 20–15 Dental caries experience of the permanent teeth of boys and girls. (From Klein et al.: The Epidemiology of Dental Disease. U.S. Public Health Service, 1948.)

termining dental caries susceptibility or resistance. (For further information on this subject, see Chapter 27, Hereditary Factors in Pedodontics.)

DENTAL CARIES IN PARENTS AND OFFSPRING

Often parents express interest in the possible relationship between their caries experience and that of their offspring. This possibility has been studied and certain generalizations are permissible, particularly where the mothers and fathers have had a similar caries experience. In one large study it was found that in the 10 and 14 year age groups, the sons and daughters of mothers and fathers of low caries experience had DMF's of 2.0 and 3.4, respectively. In contrast, sons and daughters of comparable age of parents with high caries experience had DMF's of 5.0 and 6.6, respectively. This is illustrated in Figure 20–16. From these data, it may be anticipated that children whose parents have a low caries experience will have only half as much caries as those whose parents have high caries experience. It should be mentioned that the total relationship in caries experience between parents and offspring does not necessarily indicate a hereditary factor. It has been said that "what is inherited is the cookbook," implying that the factor responsible is that members of the family eat the same foods and the children acquire eating habits similar to those of their parents. However, at least one investigation indicates that the parental-offspring caries experience probably does have a genetic factor not related to diet.

PARENT AGE AND DENTAL CARIES EXPERIENCE OF OFFSPRING

Another question that presents is whether children born of older parents tend to have a greater dental caries susceptibility than children born of younger parents.

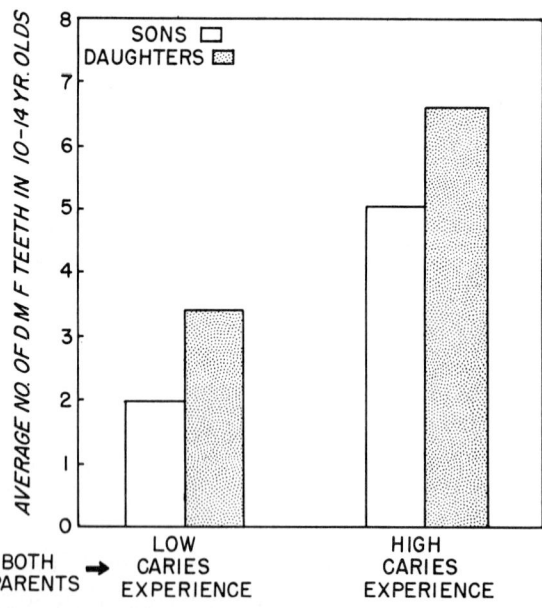

Figure 20–16 Relation of caries experience of adults and their offspring. (From Klein et al.: The Epidemiology of Dental Disease. U.S. Public Health Service, 1948.)

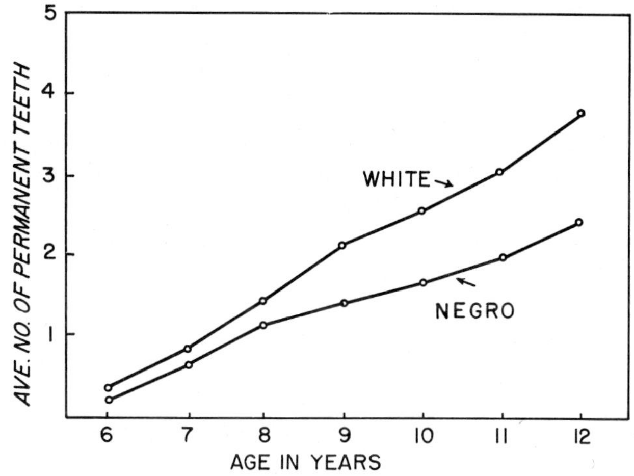

Figure 20–17 Dental caries experience of the permanent teeth of Negro and white children. (From Klein et al.: The Epidemiology of Dental Disease. U.S. Public Health Service, 1948.)

This possibility has been investigated in mothers aged 20 through 39 and fathers aged 20 through 49. It was found that the age of the father or mother at time of birth had no consistent relationship to the amount of dental decay experienced by their offspring.

SIZE OF FAMILY AND DENTAL CARIES EXPERIENCE IN THE OFFSPRING

Since there is some evidence that children from large families have greater numbers of physical defects than children of smaller families, the question of family size and dental caries experience in the offspring has received consideration. At least one investigation of this possibility has been reported. It was found that the offspring of families with one to three, four and five, and six or more children had comparable DMF rates from ages 10 through 18.

SOCIOECONOMIC FACTORS IN DENTAL CARIES

DENTAL CARIES IN NEGROES

Many people are of the opinion that Negroes have less dental caries than Caucasians, and it is well to be oriented in the matter. Most studies in this subject area support such a belief. Indicative of the findings is a report on two groups of almost 3000 each of white and Negro children with comparable age distribution from 3 through 17, wherein it was noted that the Negroes had approximately 25 per cent less caries. This is shown in Figure 20–17.

However, a recent report indicates that as the living standards of Negroes are raised this difference disappears.

COMMUNITY ECONOMIC STATUS AND DENTAL CARIES

Since the socioeconomic conditions in various communities differ widely, a knowledge of the possible relationship of these factors to dental caries in children is advisable. An intensive study of almost a quarter of a million children living in communities with very different economic levels within one state has been attempted. Comparisons between the 6 to 8, 9 to 11, and 12 to 14 year age groups were made in forty urban communities. Although considerable differences in the caries experience rates were apparent from community to community, they were not related to variations in the economic index. Children living in the communities with higher economic levels had better dental care and fewer lost teeth, but the total caries experience was unaffected by the level of dental care available. Many other studies have produced conflicting data; however, it now appears that socioeconomic conditions may affect the caries prevalence in the primary dentition more so than in the permanent dentition.

NATIONAL ORIGIN AND DENTAL CARIES

In many sections of the United States there are communities in which persons of one national origin predominate. Consequently, one should be informed on the relative caries susceptibility of offspring as related to the national origin of their parents. Since data accumulated as a result of dental examinations of Selective Service examinees from New England may be pertinent to this question, they are presented in Figure 20–18. Under these conditions it was noted that the average DMF of Chinese was between 6 and 7, of Russian Jews and Portuguese between 10 and 11, of Italians approximately 12, and of English and Irish between 16 and 17. In this study the socioeconomic factors were considered and were shown to be without effect on the findings. Although these data are from young male adults, it is believed that the differences in the caries pattern are detectable in children.

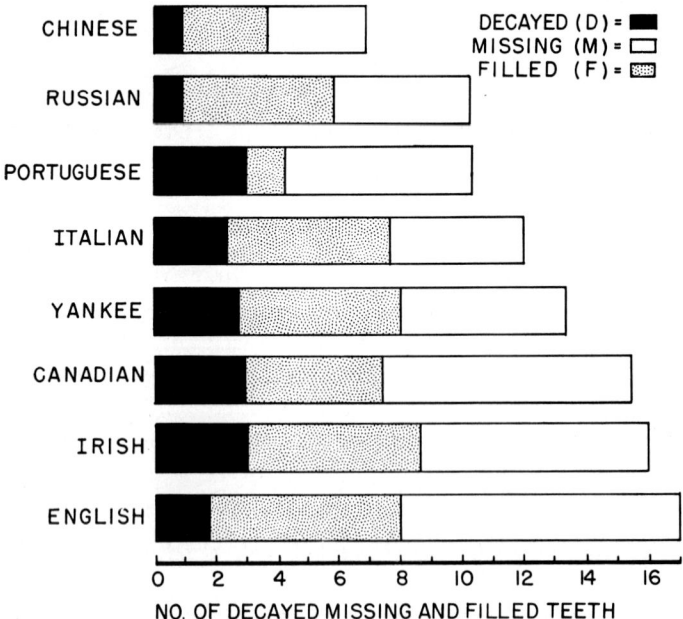

Figure 20–18 Dental caries and parents' nationality. (From Hyde: New England J. Med., *230*, 1944.)

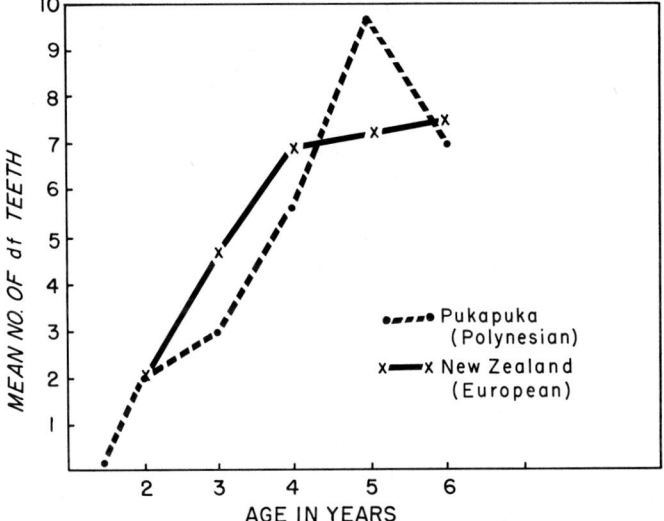

Figure 20-19 Dental caries experience in the primary teeth of children living on an isolated South Pacific island (Polynesian) and in New Zealand (European). (Davies, G. N.: International Association for Dental Research, Thirty-Fourth General Meeting, 1956.)

DENTAL CARIES IN ISOLATED AND PRIMITIVE PEOPLES

It is commonly believed that the caries attack rate in primitive and isolated peoples is almost negligible. Although many reports in the literature support this belief, there is a growing number of exceptions that should be noted, particularly as they relate to the primary dentition. Recently it has been shown that the number of decayed and filled primary teeth of isolated South Pacific Islanders, age 2 to 6 years, parallels that of the New Zealand children of European stock (Fig. 20-19). Similarly, it has been observed that the primary dentition of children in southern Thailand is comparable in caries susceptibility to that of children residing in New Jersey. Such observations suggest that generalizations should be avoided when commenting on the relationship of primitive cultures to caries susceptibility, particularly with reference to the primary dentition.

COMPARATIVE SUSCEPTIBILITY OF THE PRIMARY AND PERMANENT DENTITIONS

The question may be asked whether the extent of dental caries in the primary dentition is comparable to the caries experience that may be anticipated for the permanent dentition. In considering this problem one can utilize information that has been accumulated on the percentage of children with caries in the primary teeth at various age levels and compare it with similar data for permanent teeth. Referring to previous figures, it will be noted that at age 5 approximately 75 per cent of children have experienced caries in the primary dentition, whereas at age 10, 85 per cent of children have experienced decay in the permanent dentition.

If the point of reference is the number of decayed, missing, and filled teeth, it can be seen from previous figures that at age 5, 4.6 of the primary teeth are in-

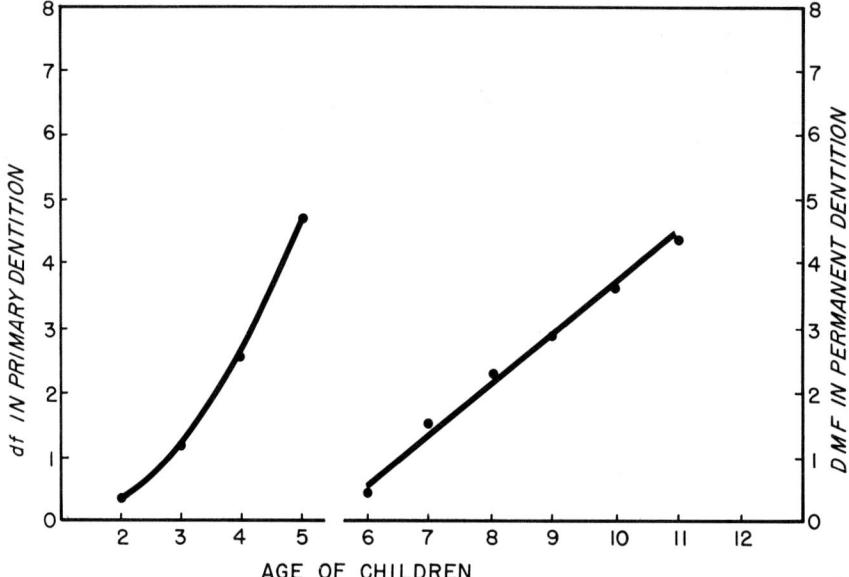

Figure 20–20   A comparison of caries in the primary and permanent dentition. (Toverud et al.: Survey of the Literature of Dental Caries, National Academy of Sciences-National Research Council.)

volved, whereas at age 10, 3.6 of the permanent teeth are involved. Recognizing the limitations of the comparison shown in Figure 20–20, there is support for the idea that in American children the caries susceptibility of the primary and permanent teeth has a general resemblance. The results of surveys in the Far East, however, show that although the dental caries experience of primary teeth of Asian children may be comparable to or may exceed that of American or European children, the caries experience of their permanent teeth is of a much smaller magnitude.

BILATERAL CARIES EXPERIENCE

The tendency for dental caries to occur bilaterally is a generally appreciated phenomenon. The extent to which this condition can be used in the location of incipient lesions is difficult to ascertain. The results of one careful study indicate that approximately 75 per cent of the permanent posterior teeth that were decayed, filled, or missing were bilaterally involved. Of these, 15 per cent were unilaterally carious on another surface. Only 25 per cent of posterior teeth were unilaterally affected with caries. We may, therefore, generalize that in three cases out of four in which dental caries occurs in a posterior tooth, the comparable tooth in the opposite arch will also be involved. We may extend this generalization to state that in four out of five of these cases it will be on the same surface.

SUMMARY

Since ten cents out of every health dollar is spent for dental care and since tooth decay, a major oral disease, begins at an early age, a knowledge of the epidemiology of dental caries in children is pertinent. Available evidence indicates that the dental caries attack rate in the United States is comparable to that of western Europe, Canada, Australia, and New Zealand. In the United States, dental caries generally follows a geographic pattern, being greatest in the New England states and least in the Southwest, with the remaining sections of the country in intermediate order. Although susceptibility to dental caries in the primary dentition does seem to be related to the socioeconomic level of the community, its role in the permanent dentition is unclear. Children whose parents are of English, Irish, and Canadian ancestry may be expected to have a high caries attack rate when compared with children whose parents' nationality is Russian-Jewish or Portuguese.

Dental caries in the primary dentition may occur as early as the first year. By age 5, 75 per cent of all children have had experience with the disease, with the average child having almost five primary teeth involved. Initially, most of the carious lesions in the primary dentition occur on the molar occlusal surfaces, but by age 6 the molar proximal surfaces are the most common site of attack.

Dental caries in the permanent dentition begins immediately after the eruption of the permanent teeth, and at age 6, 20 per cent of children have carious involvement of their permanent teeth. At 12, 90 per cent of children have had caries in their permanent dentition, with the average child having almost six teeth involved. The usual site of the initial carious lesion is the occlusal surface of the first permanent molar. Proximal caries tends to occur at a later date.

The caries pattern of a child is related to the caries patterns of his parents and his brothers and sisters. In general, children whose parents have low caries susceptibility have only half as much caries as children whose parents have extensive caries involvement. Similarly, the brothers and sisters of children who have low caries attack rates tend to have only half as much tooth decay as those whose brothers and sisters have high caries attack rates. The age of the father and mother at the time of birth of the offspring and the number of children in the family unit have no influence on dental caries susceptibility. Recent studies of dental caries in twins have shown genetic influences to be of considerably greater importance than had previously been suspected.

Since available evidence indicates that an appreciable number of cavities in children progress from the incipient lesion to the clinical cavity in six months or less, biannual clinical examinations are a minimum requirement. At any given age, girls show higher caries attack rates than boys. This difference is probably explained by the earlier eruption of their teeth. Dental caries tends to occur bilaterally in a similar tooth and tooth surface distribution, and it may be expected to occur in the opposite side of the arch in three out of every four carious teeth.

REFERENCES

1. Böök, J. A., and Grahnen, H.: Clinical and genetical studies of dental caries II. Parents and sibs of adult highly resistant (caries-free) propositi. Odont. Revy 4:1–53, 1953.
2. Bureau of Economic Research and Statistics: Expenditures and prices for dental and other health care, 1935 to 1970. J.A.D.A., 83:1334–1337, 1971.
3. Davies, G. N.: Dental disease among the Polynesians of Pukapuka. IV. Defective tooth structure and odontoclasia. International Association for Dental Research, Thirty-Fourth General Meeting, March 22–25, 1956, St. Louis, Missouri. Preprinted Abstracts, pp. 63–64.
4. East, B. R.: Some epidemiological aspects of tooth decay. Am. J. Pub. Health, 32:1242–1250, 1942.

5. Hennon, D. K., Stookey, G. K., and Muhler, J. C.: Prevalence and distribution of dental caries in preschool children. J.A.D.A., *79*:1405–1414, 1969.

6. Hyde, R. W.: Socioeconomic aspects of dental caries. New England J. Med., *230*:506–510, 1944.

7. Katz, S.: Socioeconomic factors and dental caries frequency. J. Indiana State Dental Assoc., *60*:57–60, 1967.

8. Klein, H., and others: The Epidemiology of Dental Disease. Collected Papers, 1937–47. Washington, D.C., Federal Security Agency, U.S. Public Health Service, 1948.

9. Jenkins, G. N.: Natural protective factors of foods, pp. 67–73. Symposia of the Swedish Nutrition Foundation III. Nutrition and Caries Prevention. Blix, G. N. (ed.). Uppsala, Almquist and Wiksells, 1965.

10. Magitot, E.: Treatise on Dental Caries. Boston, Houghton, Osgood and Company, 1878, pp. 59–82.

11. Parfitt, G. J.: Conditions influencing the incidence of occlusal and interstitial caries in children. J. Dent. Child., *23*:31–39, 1956.

12. Parfitt, G. J.: The speed of development of the carious cavity. Brit. D. J., *100*:204–207, 1956.

13. Parfitt, G. J.: The distribution of caries on different sites of the teeth in English children from the age of 2–15 years, Brit. D. J., *99*:423–427, 1955.

14. Toverud, G., Finn, S. B., Cox, G. J., Bodecker, C. F., and Shaw, J. H.: Survey of the Literature of Dental Caries. Publication 225. Washington, D.C., National Academy of Sciences–National Research Council, 1953.

15. Walsh, J. P., and Smart, R. S.: The relative susceptibility of tooth surfaces to dental caries and other comparative studies. New Zealand D. J., *44*:17–35, 1948.

21

THE ETIOLOGY OF DENTAL CARIES

by JOSEPH F. VOLKER
and DAVID L. RUSSELL

The primary lesion in dental caries begins at the tooth surface and, if not arrested or removed, progresses inward, ultimately involving the pulp. Initial carious lesions occur most frequently on those tooth surfaces that favor the accumulation of foodstuffs and oral microorganisms. It is now known that one of the earliest changes detectable at the research level is a loss of mineral from the subsurface enamel. In the majority of instances the first observable clinical change in enamel dental caries is a whitening of the surface at the point of attack. Although this whitening may escape notice when the tooth is moist, it is easily detectable when the tooth surface is dried carefully and examined. Subsequently, the chalky appearing area becomes further softened until it cavitates and is penetrable with a dental explorer.

There is general agreement that three major factors must be given consideration if we are to understand the carious process. These are fermentable carbohydrate foodstuffs, the oral microbial enzymes, and the physical and chemical composition of the tooth surface. The fermentable carbohydrates and the microbial enzymes may be considered as attack forces, the tooth surface as the resistance force The interplay of the various factors associated with the etiology of caries is illustrated in Figure 21–1 which shows that initiation of dental caries depends on the presence of a cariogenic oral microflora, a favorable substrate, and a susceptible tooth surface.

THE CARBOHYDRATE FACTOR

For centuries it has been noted that persons ingesting diets containing appreciable quantities of starches and sugars tend to have moderate to excessive tooth

475

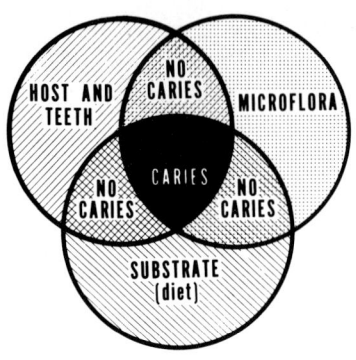

Figure 21–1 The interplay of factors in caries. (From Keyes: Inter. D. J., 1962.)

decay. It has also been noted that individuals subsisting on diets that are made up primarily of fats and proteins have little or no dental caries. These observations have pointed to the importance of certain carbohydrates as causative agents in dental caries but have left unsettled the question whether this action was a local or a systemic one. Whereas the majority opinion favored an essentially local etiologic concept, an articulate minority stressed that the carbohydrates were present in the diet at the expense of other foodstuffs which, if present, may have been responsible for caries immunity by contributing certain protective factors.

It was left to the beautifully conceived and executed research of the Harvard group to separate these two possibilities. These workers fed comparable carbohydrate-containing diets to laboratory rats. In one instance the animals were permitted to eat their ration normally; in the other instance it was fed to them by stomach tube. After a suitable period on the experimental regime the two groups were sacrificed and examined for evidences of tooth decay. Whereas the animals that ingested their food normally had a considerable number of carious lesions, those that were fed by stomach tube were free from tooth decay. These findings, shown in Table 21–1, indicate quite clearly that the action of fermentable carbohydrates in producing tooth decay is primarily a local one. Stated more simply, in order for fermentable carbohydrates to produce tooth decay they must be in contact with the tooth surface presumably for a reasonable period of time. This does not say that carbohydrates cannot modify dental caries via the systemic route. It does, however, seem to discount the notion that systemic carbohydrate can initiate the carious process.

TABLE 21–1   CARIES IN RATS FED A DECAY-PRODUCING DIET VIA NORMAL AND STOMACH TUBE ROUTES

Group	Method of Feeding	No. of Rats	Ave. No. of Carious Molars	Ave. No. of Carious Lesions
A	Normal	13	5.0	6.7
B	Stomach Tube	13	0	0

From Kite, Shaw and Sognnaes: J. Nutrition, 42, 1950.

ORAL CLEARANCE OF CARBOHYDRATES

The experiments with germ-free* and tube-fed animals bring into important focus the oral physiology of carbohydrates. The presence of such foodstuffs in and about the teeth is obviously dependent upon their being retained for varying periods of time following eating and drinking.

In a series of studies with human subjects it has been observed that several hours after eating, the quantity of carbohydrate (estimated as glucose) in the saliva is negligible. Subsequently, if a test carbohydrate glucose-containing substance is introduced into the mouth and repeated analyses are made, appreciable quantities of carbohydrates (calculated as glucose) persist for periods of a half hour or longer. Immediately after swallowing the bolus of carbohydrate foodstuff, values of several thousand milligrams per cent of glucose are not unusual. Typical experimental data may be seen in Figure 21–2. From observations like this we may conclude that there are numerous occasions when the amount of fermentable carbohydrate on the tooth surface is appreciable.

ACID PRODUCTION ON THE TOOTH SURFACE

It is most important to recognize that in the limited period carbohydrates are in contact with the tooth surface either they or their products can alter the nature of any adhering plaque. This has been adequately demonstrated. By employing an

*See Table 21–4.

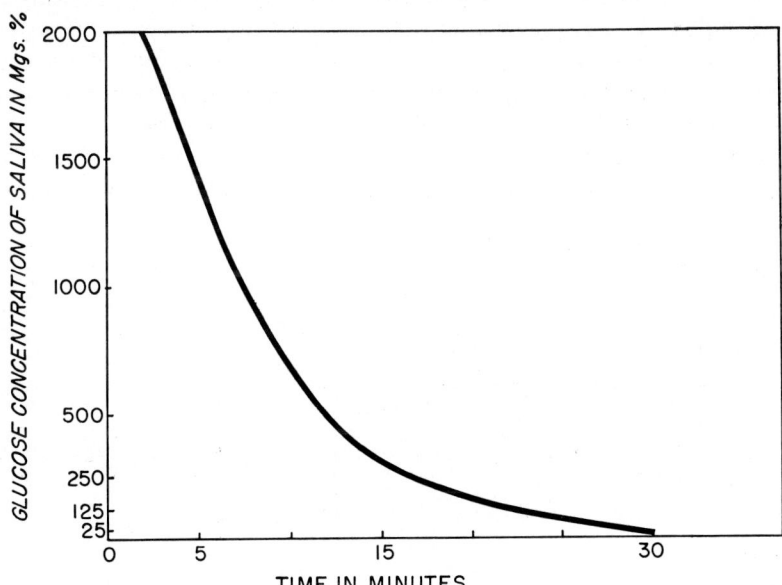

Figure 21–2 The clearance of glucose from the mouth following ingestion of a chewy candy. (From Volker: J.A.D.A., *51,* 1955.)

antimony electrode, it has been possible to measure the hydrogen ion concentration in dental plaque before, during, and after selected carbohydrate foodstuffs have been in contact with the tooth surface. Immediately following the bathing of the teeth with carbohydrate there is a drop in pH of the plaque. The return of the tooth plaque to its original base line pH is rather slow, being accomplished over a period of about an hour. Although this drop in pH, which is indicative of acid production, occurs to some degree in almost all dental plaque, it is much more pronounced in plaque from caries-susceptible individuals (Fig. 21–3). Similarly, the decreased pH is much more marked on the surfaces of maxillary anterior teeth than on the surfaces of mandibular anterior teeth.

It is also important to note the interrelatedness of the clearance of carbohydrates from the saliva and the presence of acids on the surfaces of teeth. Most investigators have concluded that bacterially produced acids are a major factor in the production of the incipient carious lesion. Others have expressed the opinion that the presence of acids on the tooth surface, although not directly responsible for caries, creates a favorable environment for some other enzymes that are etiologic or contributory to dental caries, i.e., phosphatases and proteases.

IDENTITY OF THE CARBOHYDRATES ASSOCIATED WITH DENTAL CARIES

Good evidence exists to indicate that carbohydrates associated with the formation of dental caries must (a) be present in the diet in meaningful quantities, (b) be cleared slowly and/or ingested frequently, and (c) be readily fermented by cariogenic bacteria. At least three carbohydrates meet these general qualifications: (1) polysaccharide starches; (2) the disaccharide sucrose; and (3) the monosaccharide glucose.

Starch is widely distributed in natural foods in the human diet. It is supplied chiefly from vegetable and cereal sources. The vegetable starches are usually purchased in the raw state and the only modification they undergo before ingestion is the cooking process. Although it is known that this procedure does make them more available for bacterial degradation, there are no substantial clinical observations that they contribute appreciably to dental caries incidence. The cereal starches are subjected to much more extensive alteration by manufacturing processes before they are available for food preparation. These alterations are both

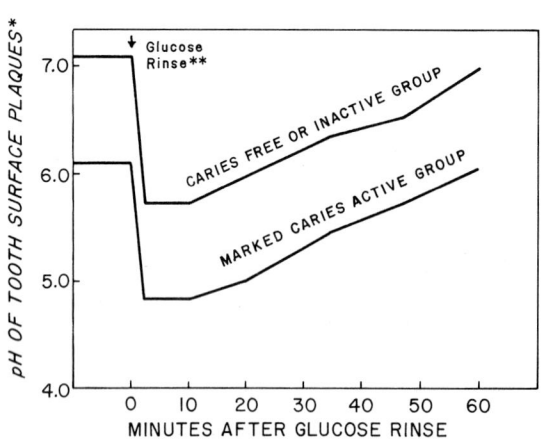

Figure 21–3 Intra-oral acid production. (From Stephan: J. D. Res., *23*, 1944.)

*Site Labial Surfaces Maxillary Incisors
**Test Solution - 2.5cc 10% Glucose

physical and chemical. This can easily be noticed if we compare white flour that is available for baking purposes with the whole wheat that arrives at the commercial mills for processing. It has been repeatedly demonstrated that these refined starch-containing foodstuffs are rapidly converted *in vivo* by oral microorganisms to organic acids. In the mouth at least the first step in this reaction is attributable to the salivary amylase. This enzyme has a pH optimum of 6.9, approximating that of saliva, and hydrolyzes starch ultimately to the disaccharide maltose. Subsequently, the enzyme maltase, produced by oral microorganisms, hydrolyzes the maltose to glucose.

The disaccharide sucrose is mostly available in the human diet as refined cane sugar and today constitutes nearly 90 per cent of the sugars consumed by Americans or an average of two pounds per week per individual. The British consume a similar amount. Sucrose may be used to sweeten prepared foods or may be cooked with them to effect the same result. It is quickly hydrolyzed by oral microorganisms, presumably by the action of an enzyme sucrase, to one molecule of glucose and one molecule of fructose.

Sucrose has been indicted as the "arch criminal" of dental caries because of its wide dietary usage in large amounts and its reported ability to support growth and proliferation of cariogenic bacteria more efficiently than any other known dietary ingredient. These reports have led some individuals to call for the substitution of sucrose in the diet by less cariogenic sugars. Such an approach would undoubtedly reduce the total amount of dental caries in the target population. However, other sugars such as glucose are cariogenic to some degree and other preventive measures would be necessary to reduce their destructive effect.

The monosaccharide glucose is available, but seldom utilized in the diet, in a crystalline form. It is more often used in the preparation of foods and confections as corn syrup or corn starch. These substances constitute around 10 per cent of the American sugar consumption and are somewhat less sweet than sucrose.

From the foregoing we may say the polysaccharides and disaccharides, some starches and cane sugar, are quickly converted to simple sugars, glucose and fructose. In addition, a meaningful quantity of glucose and a limited amount of fructose are introduced directly into the mouth. The conversion of these substances in turn to organic acids is accomplished at a remarkable rate, presumably by the usual anaerobic type of carbohydrate degradation.

FACTORS INFLUENCING CARBOHYDRATE RETENTION

The factors influencing the retention of carbohydrates in the oral cavity are many. One only has to remember that the cereal starches are used as a base in the preparation of adhesives to understand that such a property would greatly prolong the retention of these substances on and about the tooth surface. A rather extensive investigation has resulted in the measurement of adhesiveness of seventy-seven foods to tooth surfaces. The data are included in Appendix I at the end of this book. An examination of the relative adhesiveness of the various foodstuffs to the enamel surface is appreciable. Toffee and caramel adhere tenaciously to the tooth surface, while other carbohydrate foods such as whole wheat bread and oil-sprayed crackers are much less sticky. It is also apparent that although certain foodstuffs in themselves are not cariogenic, they may promote the oral retention of cariogenic carbohydrates when ingested along with them.

TABLE 21–2   GLUCOSE IN SALIVA (IN MILLIGRAMS PER CENT) AT INTERVALS
AFTER USING 500 MG. OF GLUCOSE

How Used	Time In Minutes				
	0	2	9	16	30
Eaten (Cake)	18	1425	68	20	14
Sucked (Wafer)	18	3304	1860	1125	229*
Rinsed (Solution)	21	832	105	25	17
Chewed (Gum Base)	23	725	204	144	27

*Three of the six subjects had not completely dissolved their wafer. The 30 minute average figure for dissolving the wafer was 91 mg. %
From Volker: J.A.D.A., *51*, 1955.

Other factors must be considered in the matter of food retention in the mouth. Among these are the physical form of the foodstuff, and limited attempts have been made to study this problem. In one instance young adult subjects were fed 500 mg. quantities of glucose in varying physical forms. These included a cake that was eaten, a wafer that was sucked, a solution that was rinsed, and a gum base that was chewed. Salivary samples were analyzed for glucose before and at stated intervals after the test substance was taken. Marked differences in carbohydrate clearance were observed, the extremes being represented by the solution, which was rapidly cleared, and the sucked wafer, which maintained elevated glucose levels for the duration of the experimental period. These findings, shown in Table 21–2, strongly suggest that the physical form of the carbohydrate is of greater importance in causing tooth decay than is its quantity.

This view is supported by studies in laboratory animals and humans. It has been shown in laboratory investigations that if two groups of hamsters are fed comparable quantities of milk, in one instance in the form of dry powdered whole milk and in the other as reconstituted milk (the dry powdered whole milk plus water), sharp differences in dental caries occur. Whereas animals in the former group developed moderate to severe tooth decay, the animals in the latter group were caries free. These results may be tentatively explained by assuming a prolonged retention of the milk sugar when fed in the powdered form and a rapid oral clearance of the milk sugar when ingested in a liquid form. The fluidity of the diet is of major significance in caries studies. It has been shown that, regardless of the diet ingested, animals maintained on a thin slurry of the diet have less than one-third as much caries as those receiving the diet in dry powder form.

The studies in human subjects by a group of Swedish investigators deserve special consideration. They determined the oral clearance of a variety of sugar-containing foodstuffs. Subsequently they arranged groups of institutionalized clinical subjects and added to their basic ration selected sugar-containing supplements. The extremes were represented by sugar given in solution form and sugar added in the form of a sticky candy. Whereas the sugar in solution caused only a minimal increase in tooth decay, most of the subjects receiving the sticky candy showed a marked increase in caries experience during the experimental period. Several other sugar supplements, shown to have oral clearance characteristics between the two extremes, were found to promote intermediate levels of caries increment. These studies are particularly noteworthy because they included observations covering a period of five years. Selected findings are shown in Table 21–3. It is important to note that sugar in sticky form caused six times as much caries as the same quantity of sugar in liquid form.

RELATIVE ABILITIES OF NATURAL AND REFINED CARBOHYDRATES TO CAUSE DENTAL CARIES

Because of the limited amount of tooth decay usually noted in people ingesting diets containing only natural foods, it is a common belief that unrefined carbohydrates do not contribute significantly to dental caries etiology. This in turn has led to the speculation that raw carbohydrates have antienzymatic substances which are removed in the refining process. Although there is evidence that such a presumption may explain in part the increased ability of refined as compared to natural starches to produce tooth decay, it is of little or no significance in modifying the ability of disaccharides and monosaccharides to cause dental caries.

It is easily demonstrated that mixtures of honey, which is a fairly pure mixture of the three sugars, sucrose, glucose, and fructose, when mixed with saliva will favor acid production. Similarly, maple syrup and raw cane syrup are easily fermented by oral microorganisms. In all probability the only reason they are not ordinarily associated with caries etiology is not that they resist enzymatic degradation but rather that they make up such a limited portion of the carbohydrate fraction of the diet. Similar logic should be applied to the notion that sugars and related substances found in natural fruits are not cariogenic. Whereas the digestible carbohydrate content of cakes, crackers, cane sugar, cornstarch, jellies, etc. ranges from 60 to 100 per cent, the value for most vegetables and fruits is 20 per cent or less.

OBSERVATIONS ON THE ROLE OF ORGANIC ACIDS IN TOOTH DECAY

Although acid production by the microorganisms of dental plaque is readily demonstrable, the exact metabolic pathway by which this is accomplished has not been established in the known strains of cariogenic bacteria. It seems highly improbable that with the variety of conditions found on different tooth surfaces the sequence of events and the end products in each instance are identical. As stated before, it is generally assumed that the pathways of acid formation which operate in the mouth are comparable to those observed in other biologic tissues and in particular are comparable to those of other bacterial strains in which the mechanisms of

TABLE 21–3   INFLUENCE OF ADDED DIETARY SUGAR OF DIFFERENT PHYSICAL FORM ON DENTAL CARIES

Groups	No. Of Subjects	Tooth Surfaces Becoming Carious Per Person Per Year
Control Diet	60	.30
Control Diet + Sugar In Solution*	57	.67
Control Diet + Sugar As Toffee (24 pieces/day)*	48	4.02

*Amount of added sugar consumed in the two experimental groups was comparable (over 100 lb. per year per person).

From Gustafsson et al.: Acta Odontol. Scandinavica, *11*, 1954.

acid formation are known. In the process of glycolysis there is an initial phosphory-lation of the monosaccharide and a subsequent stepwise degradation to pyruvic and lactic acid. Such views find considerable support in reports of investigators who have repeatedly identified lactic acid in plaque and saliva-glucose mixtures. A considerable number of other organic acids, however, have also been detected in such mixtures, including acetic, formic, propionic, malic and others, suggesting that various bacterial metabolic pathways are involved.

Accordingly, it seems reasonable to believe that dental caries is not specifically a lactic acid decalcification. Very possibly any one or several organic acids under specific circumstances might effect a dissolution of the enamel. In support of this concept it should be recalled that numerous experiments have demonstrated that enamel is dissolved by a variety of organic acids.

In the past, much emphasis has been placed on the fact that acids at low pH dissolve enamel. In the chemico-parasitic theory it is considered that this dissolution of the enamel is the first stage in dental caries. However, it has been known for many years that the inorganic fraction of enamel can be dissolved at widely varying pH's and indeed at a pH above neutrality. Recently a theory known as the proteolysis-chelation theory has been vigorously discussed in the literature. This theory explains the etiology of dental caries as two reactions: a microbial destruction of the organic matrix and a loss of the inorganic material due to the action of chelating agents which are released as breakdown products of the matrix.

At the present time there is no convincing evidence that the oral flora can destroy the organic matrix in enamel unless the enamel has been previously decalcified. Also, the chelating agents implicated in the proteolysis-chelation theory include acids which could dissolve the inorganic apatite through activity of their dissociated hydrogen ions. It seems feasible that at a higher pH certain acids and other agents released by the breakdown of the organic matrix could also act as chelating agents to dissolve the apatite. The available body of knowledge at present does not allow for an unequivocal statement on the role of organic acids in tooth decay. Acids are present on the tooth surface; acids dissolve enamel; acid is present in the carious lesion; but it remains for future research to establish the precise role of acid as well as proteolytic mechanisms in the causation of dental caries.

THE MICROBIAL FACTOR

It was not until the last century that people speculated on the relationship of microorganisms to the well-being of man. The researches of Pasteur and Koch focused attention on the possibility that bacteria were etiologic factors in many pathologic states, and it was only natural that their possible role in dental caries would be investigated. Shortly before the turn of the century, Miller accumulated presumptive evidence that certain oral bacteria were causative agents in dental caries. He showed that selected organisms recovered from the oral cavity thrived on carbohydrate media, and that included in the products of their metabolism were considerable quantities of organic acids. The latter substances in turn were capable of decalcifying enamel and dentin. As a result of these studies he formulated the chemico-parasitic theory of dental caries which in an abbreviated form states that fermentable carbohydrates are acted on by oral microorganisms to form organic acids. These organic acids progressively destroy the inorganic portions of the teeth. Subsequently, the same or other oral microorganisms utilizing other processes bring about the destruction of the organic portions of the tooth. Collectively these two destructive processes result in the carious lesion.

Despite strong circumstantial evidence, a limited number of people refused to concur in this reasoning, pointing out that the presence of bacteria on the tooth surface and in the lesion might be incidental rather than etiologic in tooth decay. Recent studies with germ-free animals have eliminated such a possibility. Research workers at Chicago cooperating with the Notre Dame group have reared rats under germ-free conditions and have fed them caries-producing diets. None of these animals developed dental caries. Control animals inoculated with selected oral organisms and maintained on the same cariogenic diet had excessive tooth decay (see Table 21–4). These findings indicate that the presence of microorganisms in the mouth is essential for the initiation of the carious lesion.

The use of the germ-free animal technique will be of great value in the future in testing the ability of single strains of microorganisms or known mixtures of microorganisms to produce dental caries and other oral lesions. The term "gnotobiotic" is now often used to describe a completely germ-free animal or a germ-free animal which has been inoculated with a known microbial flora.

IDENTITY OF THE MICROORGANISMS RESPONSIBLE FOR TOOTH DECAY

Although the experimental evidence indicates that bacteria are causative agents in the production of the carious lesions, we cannot make the assumption that all oral microorganisms are equally important in this connection. In fact, it has been shown that some acidogenic bacteria do not cause caries. Also we have only to recall that although everyone has microorganisms in the mouth, there are thousands of individuals who have never experienced dental caries. To understand this premise it is logical, therefore, to consider which oral microorganisms may be of primary importance in the etiology of tooth decay. In doing so it is relatively safe to say according to current evidence that oral microorganisms other than bacteria, such as fungi, yeasts, and protozoans, do not play an important role in the initiation of dental caries.

Until very recently there was no substantial scientific evidence that dental caries might be an infective process. However, in the past few years a most interesting series of experiments by Keyes and Fitzgerald has shown that dental caries in rats and hamsters is a transmissible disease. In so-called "caries-resistant" hamsters,

TABLE 21–4   DENTAL CARIES IN GERM-FREE RATS AND GERM-FREE RATS
INOCULATED WITH KNOWN BACTERIAL CELLS
(ENTEROCOCCI PREDOMINATING)

Group	Microbial State	No. of Rats	No. of Rats Developing Molar Caries
A	Germ Free	9	0
B	Inoculated With Enterococci Plus Others	13	13

From Orland et al.: J.A.D.A., *50*, 1955.

the supposed resistance could be overcome by introduction of a factor from the feces of "caries-susceptible" hamsters. Next it was shown that the same phenomenon could be achieved by inoculation with one or more streptococci isolated from carious lesions in a caries-susceptible animal. Such observations seem to indicate that a caries-resistant animal is one with an oral flora incapable of causing appreciable caries. When the appropriate flora is introduced into the mouth, caries will occur rapidly. Recently it has been demonstrated that bacteria can be transplanted from the human mouth into the mouths of rodents, resulting in the onset of dental caries. Thus, while cariogenic bacteria were first demonstrated in rodents, similar organisms have been found in man.

To establish the causative microorganism for a disease it is customary to insure that Koch's postulates are satisfied. This has now been achieved, according to Fitzgerald and Keyes, in the case of hamster caries. The causative microorganism is a previously undescribed streptococcus which does not have proteolytic activity but ferments glucose to lactic acid. Similar observations have also been made in studies of rat caries.

Of particular interest are the several observations by independent investigators that certain types of streptococci associated with dental plaque in the human mouth manufacture both intracellular and extracellular polysaccharides. These carbohydrate polymers have been identified as amylopectins, dextrans and levans. Sucrose appears to be the substrate of choice by cariogenic bacteria in the production of dextrans and levans. The extracellular polysaccharides are thought to form the sticky substance which binds the plaque together and keeps it attached to the tooth surface. The intracellular polysaccharides provide continuous nourishment to the plaque bacteria even when no substrate is being introduced into the mouth (between meals). The abilities of these organisms to produce acids and to form plaque are said to be necessary for the occurrence of rampant caries.

Many of the recent studies concerning the microbial factors in initiation and maintenance of dental caries have shown that several factors are important. These include host specificity and susceptibility; bacterial transmissibility; and the quality and quantity of available substrate (diet). Evidence indicates that one kind of bacteria may be more important in the initiation of the lesion while others are more important in maintenance. In addition, some strains of bacteria may be more likely to cause smooth surface caries than pit and fissure caries and vice versa. Of equal interest is the observation that some microorganisms seem to be more specific for initiation of enamel caries while others are more effective in producing caries of dentin and cementum.

All these reports seem to underline the obvious complexity of the caries process which involves an everchanging relationship between cariogenic bacteria, suitable substrate, and a susceptible tooth surface.

IN VITRO TOOTH DECAY

Our understanding of the caries process has been greatly expanded by experimental attempts to produce dental caries in extracted teeth. Even today there are persons who persist in the belief that dental caries is initiated only in vital teeth. To refute this one has only to recall the early observations of Magitot, who, in the era before prosthetic supplies were readily available, utilized extracted teeth for pivots, inserting them in roots and affixing others to denture bases. He recorded his observations very carefully and illustrated the tooth decay that occurred under such circumstances.

More recently, intensive investigations in this area have been carried on at the University of Alabama by using an "artificial mouth," so called because it simulates many of the conditions in the oral cavity. The extracted teeth are maintained in a moist environment and at body temperature. Carbohydrate-containing media are dripped over tooth surfaces previously inoculated with known strains of organisms. Special conditions permit the carbohydrate media to be periodically removed from the tooth surface in somewhat the same manner as occurs in the normal processes of digestion. Simulated conditions of mouth hygiene have been instituted with periodic brushing of the teeth. Under these circumstances it has been possible to produce lesions that by clinical and roentgenographic examination and in histologic sections resemble or are identical to in vivo caries. It seems pertinent that these structural alterations have been produced with a variety of oral microorganisms and that it has been possible to localize them on those surfaces of the teeth where one normally anticipates the appearance of carious lesions.

In an extension of these observations the action of the carbohydrates and oral microorganisms on the enamel, dentin, and cementum has been studied. It has been noted that, whereas certain of the organisms seem more effective in dissolving the enamel, others are more effective in altering the dentin. Furthermore, it appears that when one concentration of glucose is made available to the microorganisms it promotes decalcification almost exclusively, whereas a different and somewhat lower concentration may permit simultaneous decalcification of the inorganic material and proteolysis of the organic material.

SALIVA AND DENTAL CARIES

Although oral microorganisms and retained carbohydrates are etiologic factors in dental caries, it must be remembered that each of these exists in an environment which is constantly exposed to saliva. Accordingly, it is conceivable that the physical or chemical properties of saliva may influence susceptibility to dental caries. It is well known that in those instances in which normal salivary flow is greatly diminished—for example, as the result of radiation therapy for tumors—rampant tooth decay may ensue. The importance of this possibility is easily demonstrated in laboratory rodents. If these animals are divided into two comparable groups, the control with intact salivary glands and the experimental group with the major salivary glands rendered nonfunctional, the latter will develop much more tooth decay than the former when fed the same cariogenic diet. This is shown in Table 21–5.

TABLE 21–5   EFFECT OF DESALIVATION ON HAMSTER CARIES

Group	Number	Ave. No. of Carious Teeth	Ave. No. of Carious Lesions
A, Intact Salivary Glands	20	2.3	2.5
B, Desalivated	10	10.5	13.0

From Finn, in Sognnaes (ed.): Advances in Experimental Caries Research. American Association for the Advancement of Science, 1955.

RELATION OF RATE OF SALIVA FLOW TO DENTAL CARIES

It should also be noted that some workers have presented data indicating that the rate of salivary secretion is an important factor in caries etiology. Typical of their findings is the observation that persons with salivary secretion rates lower than average develop a greater number of carious lesions than persons with salivary secretion rates higher than average. It should be understood that these are only generalizations, and that conclusions in this area must be conservatively drawn.

Although it is generally agreed that increased salivary flow is of benefit in limiting tooth decay, very little information is available as to the factors associated with increased salivation. Investigations have been made of the effect of application to the tongue of optimal concentrations of acid (citric acid), salt (sodium chloride), sweet (sucrose), and bitter (quinine) stimuli on salivary flow for periods up to 130 minutes. Although all substances stimulated salivary flow, the greatest response resulted from citric acid and sodium chloride. It is conceivable that continuation of these experiments could result in the formulation of therapeutic agents that would be beneficial in the control of dental caries by accelerating oral food clearance. However, a clinical study of the effect of increasing salivary flow by sucking a tablet containing sorbitol and malic acid yielded disappointing results.

Considerable data have been accumulated on the relative contribution of the individual major salivary glands to the total amount of salivary secretion. It appears that the submaxillary, parotid, and sublingual glands contribute approximately 75 per cent, 20 per cent, and 5 per cent, respectively, to the "resting" salivary flow. In this connection it is interesting to note that in animal experiments in which selected salivary glands have been rendered nonfunctional the results indicate that removal of the submaxillary secretion results in the greatest increase in caries susceptibility, removal of the sublingual the least, and removal of the parotid intermediate. From data such as these it may be concluded that increased dental caries is related to diminished salivary flow whereas decreased dental caries is related to increased salivary flow.

In most textbooks of biochemistry the statement appears that the daily secretion of saliva in adults approximates 1500 cc. Regardless of the accuracy of this estimation it is well to know that the total amount of saliva secreted during sleep is negligible. If, as has been suggested, diminished salivary flow favors caries activity, the process of tooth decay should be accelerated during the nonwaking hours. During this period the mechanical clearance of carbohydrates and microorganisms would be minimal.

BIOLOGIC FACTORS IN SALIVA OF POSSIBLE IMPORTANCE IN TOOTH DECAY

It is also conceivable that saliva may contain certain substances which inhibit dental caries by modifying the oral flora. It is well known that human saliva contains substances which kill the organism *Micrococcus lysodeikticus* and have adverse effects on other species of oral flora. This action has been attributed to a substance called lysozyme. There is reason to believe that other substances of a similar nature are also present in the saliva. A bacteriolytic agent has been identified in the saliva of caries-immunes which is not found in the saliva of persons susceptible to dental caries. Further studies of the bacteriolytic properties of saliva may be of great importance in understanding the phenomenon of caries susceptibility.

Similarly, it has been shown that saliva increases capillary permeability and has the power of attracting leukocytes by a mechanism not yet understood. Furthermore, there are substances in the saliva, opsonins, that make bacteria more susceptible to phagocytosis by the leukocytes.

To date, several investigators have speculated on the possibility of immunizing persons to dental caries through the use of vaccine. The implications of a possible vaccine for the prevention of dental caries are underscored by the outstanding success demonstrated in recent years by both the poliomyelitis and smallpox vaccines. In most of the past efforts to develop a caries vaccine lactobacilli have been used. However, in one instance a streptococcus was studied. The presence of agglutinins in the saliva of persons receiving such a vaccine has been noted and some limited correlation has been established with caries experience. Also, studies on the salivary and serum antibody levels of individuals with a low caries experience have produced some optimism regarding the possibility of such a caries preventive measure.

Although they are intriguing, past studies involved with the actual production of antibodies to cariogenic bacteria have been limited to animals. Other factors, such as the multiple strains of bacteria which may cause dental caries and the low antigenicity of many of these bacterial strains, would seem to classify present attempts to produce a caries vaccine as being in the preliminary stages of investigation.

Considering collectively the lytic factors, leukocytes, and agglutinins we can only note the existence of these biologic entities and state that because of our limited knowledge we cannot currently attribute to them any significant role in the etiology of tooth decay.

CHEMICAL PROPERTIES OF SALIVA IN RELATION TO TOOTH DECAY

Having discussed the physical and biologic properties of saliva as they may be related to tooth decay, it seems logical to review the possibilities that certain chemical properties of saliva may influence tooth decay. Since the accumulated evidence indicates a probable etiologic role of acid in dental caries, it is pertinent to review the evidence that the buffering capacity of saliva may have an effect on the carious process. It has been reported in one study that the saliva of people immune to dental caries is capable of neutralizing considerable acid before the hydrogen ion concentration is altered to a point at which enamel is likely to be dissolved in appreciable amounts. Other reports are in general agreement with this statement. A recent investigation was undertaken to determine the relative importance of various buffer systems in human saliva. Included in the study were bicarbonate, phosphate, protein, mucin, and microorganisms. It was concluded that the buffering capacity of saliva is primarily due to the presence of bicarbonate. The only other buffer of any significance was phosphate. Contrary to the belief of some, salivary mucin was shown to have an insignificant role in the buffering mechanism. It should be noted that any buffering capacity of saliva would most probably have to take place within the dental plaque for it to be appreciably effective. It is here that cariogenic bacteria and sugars are present in sufficient quantity to produce concentrations of organic acids which would lower the pH to the degree necessary to result in dissolution of enamel. In general, the plaque assumes the qualities of a permeable membrane and will allow selective diffusion of various substances to and from the saliva. Reports indicate that approximately 90 per cent of the acids may be neutralized by buffers in the saliva and in the plaque. However, neutralization efficiency of saliva would depend upon the concentration of sugar, frequency of intake, and the thickness of the plaque.

It is also important to understand that saliva contains appreciable quantities of calcium and phosphorus. Under certain circumstances these and other inorganic ions in saliva may combine to form insoluble precipitates. This in all probability is the general explanation of the presence of calculus on those teeth that approximate the major salivary ducts. There is evidence to indicate an interrelationship between the presence of carbon dioxide in saliva and the precipitation of dental calculus, since it has been noted that on standing carbon dioxide is lost from the saliva and minerals are precipitated.

The ability of saliva to form, on a macroscopic scale, a calcified material bearing a distinct resemblance to tooth structure raises the question of whether or not such a process is continuously being accomplished on the tooth surface at a microscopic or submicroscopic level. With the advent of radioactive isotopes, researches on this problem have been attempted. There is now general agreement that the inorganic ions in saliva are constantly being exchanged with those of the tooth surface or are being adsorbed thereon. It seems safe to conclude that, unlike the underlying body of enamel, the surface is undergoing a continuous change in its chemical composition. Although we cannot say whether this phenomenon is definitely related to caries susceptibility, one investigator has presented evidence that the amounts of calcium and phosphate removed from the saliva of caries-free and caries-active persons by shaking with tricalcium phosphate follow distinctly different patterns.

From the foregoing we may conclude that two chemical properties of saliva may influence the carious process. They are its buffering capacity and the reactivity of certain inorganic ions, particularly calcium and phosphate, with the enamel surface. Theoretically at least, the salivas with good buffering capacity could neutralize some of the acids that play an etiologic role in tooth decay. Similarly, if the salivary calcium and phosphate are available, they should combine with the tooth surface in such a fashion as to help maintain its integrity.

THE TOOTH SURFACE FACTOR

Whereas retained carbohydrates and oral microorganisms may be considered as attack forces in caries etiology and salivary secretion may be considered an environmental force, capable of enhancing or detracting from the process, the enamel may be viewed as a resistance force. Many years ago the dental profession had a slogan, "A clean tooth does not decay." If by a clean tooth we mean one that is devoid of fermentable carbohydrates or oral microorganisms, or both, this statement as viewed in the light of the research with tube-fed and germ-free animals is essentially correct. We seem justified, however, in believing that susceptibility to dental caries is associated with certain physical and chemical changes in the enamel.

REFERENCES

1. Bowen, W. H.: A vaccine against dental caries. A pilot experiment in monkeys (Macaca irrus). Brit. Dent. J., *126*:159–160, 1969.
2. Caldwell, R. C.: Adhesion of foods to teeth. J. D. Res., *41*:821–832, 1962.
3. Chauncey, H. H., and Shannon, I. L.: Parotid gland secretion rate as method for measuring response to gustatory stimuli in humans. Proc. Soc. Exper. Biol. Med., *103*:459–463, 1960.
4. Day, C. D. M.: Nutritional deficiencies and dental caries in northern India. Brit. D. J. *76*:143–147, 1944.
5. Fitzgerald, R. J., and Jordan, H. V.: Polysaccharide-producing bacteria and caries. In Art and Science of Dental Caries Research. Harris, R. S. (ed.). New York, Academic Press, 1968, pp. 79–84.
6. Fitzgerald, R. J., Jordan, H. V., and Archard, H. O.: Dental caries in gnotobiotic rats infected with variety of lactobacillus acidophilus. Arch. Oral Biol., *11*:473–476, 1966.
7. Fitzgerald, R. J., and Keyes, P. H.: Demonstration of the etiologic role of streptococci in experimental caries in the hamster. J.A.D.A., *61*:9–19, 1960.
8. Gibbons, R. J., and Banghart, S. B.: Synthesis of extracellular dextran by cariogenic bacteria and its presence in human dental plaque. Arch. Oral Biol., *12*:11–23, 1967.
9. Green, G. E.: Bacteriolytic agent in salivary globulin of caries-immune human beings. J. D. Res., *38*:262–275, 1959.
10. Gustafsson, B., and others: The Vipeholm dental caries study. Acta Odontol. Scandinavica, *11*:195–388, 1954.
11. Jenkins, G. N.: The Physiology of the Mouth. Oxford, Blackwell Scientific Publications, 1954.
12. Keyes, P. H.: Infectious and transmissible nature of experimental dental caries. Arch. Oral Biol., *1*:304–320, 1960.
13. Keyes, P. H.: Bacteriological findings and biological implications. Inter. D. J., *12*:443–464, 1962.
14. Kite, O. W., Shaw, J. H., and Sognnaes, R. F.: The prevention of experimental tooth decay by tube-feeding. J. Nutrition, *42*:89–103, 1950.
15. Newbrun, E.: Sucrose, the arch criminal of dental caries. J. Dent. Child., *36*:239–248, 1969.
16. Nordsiek, F. W.: The sweet tooth. Amer. Sci., *60*:41–45, 1972.
17. Orland, F. J., Blayney, J. R., Harrison, R. W., Reyniers, J. A., Trexlar, P. C., Ervin, R. F., Gordon, H. A., and Wagner, M.: Experimental caries in germ-free rats inoculated with enterocci. J.A.D.A., *50*:259–272, 1955.
18. Pigman, W.: In vitro production of experimental caries. J.A.D.A., *51*:685–696, 1955.
19. Schatz, A., Karlson, K. E., Martin, J. J., Schatz, V., and Adelson, L. M.: Some philosophical considerations on the proteolysis-chelation theory of dental caries. Proc. Pennsylvania Acad. Sc., *32*:20–48, 1958.
20. Schneyer, L. H., and Levin, L. K.: The rate of secretion by individual salivary gland pairs of man under conditions of reduced exogenous stimulation. J. Appl. Physiol., 7:508–512, 1955.
21. Schour, I., and Massler, M.: The effect of dietary deficiencies upon the oral structures. Physiol. Rev., *25*:442–482, 1945.
22. Slack, G. L., Millivard, E., and Martin, W. J.: Effect on incidence of caries of tablets stimulating salivary flow. Brit. D. J., *116*:105–108, 1964.
23. Sognnaes, R. F. (ed.): Advances in Experimental Caries Research. Washington, D.C., American Association for the Advancement of Science, 1955.
24. Stephan, R. M.: Intra-oral hydrogen ion concentrations associated with dental caries activity. J. D. Res., *23*:257, 1944.
25. Volker, J. F.: Relation of oral biochemistry of sugars to the development of caries. J.A.D.A., *51*:285–292, 1955.
26. Zipkin, I.: Tooth chemistry. In Art and Science of Dental Caries Research. Harris, R. S. (ed.). New York. Academic Press, pp. 29–41, 1968.

22

THE PREVENTION OF DENTAL CARIES WITH FLUORIDE

by JOSEPH F. VOLKER
and DAVID L. RUSSELL

One effective approach to the control of a disease involves the identification of factors responsible for natural resistance or immunity and the subsequent utilization of such knowledge in preventive therapy. A classic example of this is the researches that have led to the utilization of fluoride in several forms in the prevention of tooth decay. Since a great portion of this work has involved clinical experimentation with children and since many of these techniques are directed toward the treatment of dental caries in the younger age groups, it is particularly pertinent that the subject be adequately presented in pedodontic textbooks. This chapter contains, in successive major sections, information on (1) historical background, (2) water fluoridation, (3) topical application of fluoride, (4) fluorides in dentifrices, (5) fluoride tablets and mouth washes, and (6) the action of fluoride in limiting tooth decay.

HISTORICAL BACKGROUND

Although the occurrence of fluoride in calcified tissues was already known at the beginning of the nineteenth century, one of the earliest references relating it to dental caries is that of Magitot. When this researcher was studying the action of various organic acids on extracted teeth he noted that a solution of 1:100 acetic acid was "without action upon the enamel, but vigorously attacks both the cement and the ivory." He offered the following tentative explanation of this finding: "The fact itself of the alteration undergone by the cement and ivory of teeth exposed to acetic acid is explained by the property this agent has of dissolving the earthy phosphates, a property singularly favored, according to Deherain, if they are found in the presence of carbonic acid or the carbonates, as is precisely the case with the ivory and bone. As to the integrity preserved by the enamel, it is owing perhaps to a smaller proportion of the phosphates, and doubtless also to the minute quantity of fluoride of calcium it contains, or perhaps to certain combinations of these substances of a nature calculated to resist all alteration."

Another early investigation that deserves particular consideration was the demonstration that fluoride had a marked affinity for calcified tissue. In this study bone was exposed to dilute fluoride solutions for a five month period and showed an increase in the fluoride content from 0.31 parts per 100 to 4.7 parts per 100. Two more late nineteenth-century papers are also worthy of special comment. In one of these, the incorporation of fluoride in the diet was suggested as a means of limiting dental caries. In the other, analytical results were reported showing that noncarious teeth contained greater fluoride concentrations than carious teeth.

Despite the meagerness of acceptable investigations substantiating a fluoride-tooth decay relationship, the idea was widespread at the advent of the twentieth century. A variety of fluoride-containing therapeutic agents was available for public consumption, including tooth powders, toothpastes, mouth washes and pastilles. Almost a half century was to elapse before adequate research would help clarify the role of fluoride in the prevention of dental caries and furnish a more sound basis for its therapeutic use.

In the intervening years, unfortunately, a series of events focused attention on the possible toxic effects of fluoride on the dentition. These began in 1901 when the occurrence of disfigured teeth was reported among people residing in the vicinity of Naples, Italy. The disfigurement was believed to be due to a substance in the water that altered the calcification process. Subsequently, reports indicated that the same or similar conditions prevailed in many other sections of the world. In the United States it was noted to be particularly common in those persons residing in certain sections of Colorado, Arizona, New Mexico and Texas. Although repeated attempts were made to associate the composition of the drinking water with the defect, it was not until 1931 that American and French investigators working independently showed that minimal quantities of fluoride were responsible for the abnormality.

The immediate reaction to these observations was to focus attention on the toxicity of fluorides. Often water supplies containing levels of fluoride that produced mottling were replaced with those that were fluoride free. In certain instances this was not economically feasible. Accordingly, researchers were directed toward the development of methods and techniques that would remove the excess fluoride from the water. As a consequence the possible benefits of fluoride in caries control were largely forgotten.

Although mottling of the enamel focused attention on the toxicity of fluorides, it played a major role in pinpointing the relationship of the element to caries prevention. Even before the etiologic role of fluoride in mottling was established, it had been observed by such eminent investigators as Black and McKay that teeth so affected had a limited susceptibility to dental caries. Subsequently, similar and more detailed observations were made in China, in England, in Japan, and in Argentina. Of even greater significance were the continuing observations of the U.S. Public Health Service in the continental United States. The extensive clinical examinations for dental caries of Dean and his associates and accompanying water analyses by Elvove not only clearly illustrated the epidemiology of dental fluorosis but carefully documented the reduction in dental caries liability that accompanied such a state.

Ultimately in 1939 Dean and co-workers studied the relationship of the fluoride content of the water and dental caries in 12 to 14 year old children in four Illinois cities. Two of the cities, Galesburg and Monmouth, had 1.8 and 1.7 ppm of fluoride in the water. The other two cities, Macomb and Quincy, had 0.2 ppm and 0.1 ppm in their water. The results are shown in Table 22–1.

Even more significant, they observed that of the 243 Galesburg children studied, 114 had mottled enamel while the remaining 129 were without mottled enamel. Since the group with mottling had a caries DMF rate of 200 per 100 children and those without mottling had a rate of 186, they concluded, "It would appear that the factor responsible for the low amount of caries in this city was operative irrespective of whether the child showed macroscopic evidence of mottled enamel." As a natural consequence of this finding, it became obvious that the level of fluoride in the domestic water effective in inhibiting tooth decay was below that which caused unsightly mottling of the enamel.

Beginning in the 1920's, attention was directed to the possibility of studying dental caries in rats under controlled laboratory conditions. Numerous investigations were conducted and many of the findings seemed to contradict one another until it became clear that the physical as well as the chemical nature of the carbohydrates in the experimental ration modified its ability to produce caries in the rat. Finally the problem was resolved and the use of coarse-particle diets became a standard caries-producing ration by the late 1930's. This in turn permitted the screening of potential caries inhibitors. One of the first investigations involved a study of the effect of fluoride and iodoacetic acid on coarse-cereal caries in rats. These substances were selected because it was believed they would inhibit the mechanism of carbohydrate breakdown by oral bacteria. This in turn would minimize the acid formation which was assumed to be responsible for the initial carious lesion. A reduced caries incidence was noted when fluorides were added to

TABLE 22–1 DENTAL CARIES IN CHILDREN AND THE FLUORIDE CONTENT OF THE DOMESTIC WATER

City	F ppm in Water	No. of Children	% With no dental Caries Experience	DMF Permanent Teeth per 100 Children
Galesburg	1.8	243	36.2	194
Monmouth	1.7	99	36.4	208
Macomb	0.2	63	14.3	368
Quincy	0.1	291	4.1	628

All Subjects Were 12-14 Years Old And Had A History Of Continuous Residence In Their Respective Communities.

From Dean et al.: in Moulton (ed.): Dental Caries and Fluorine. American Association for the Advancement of Science, 1946.

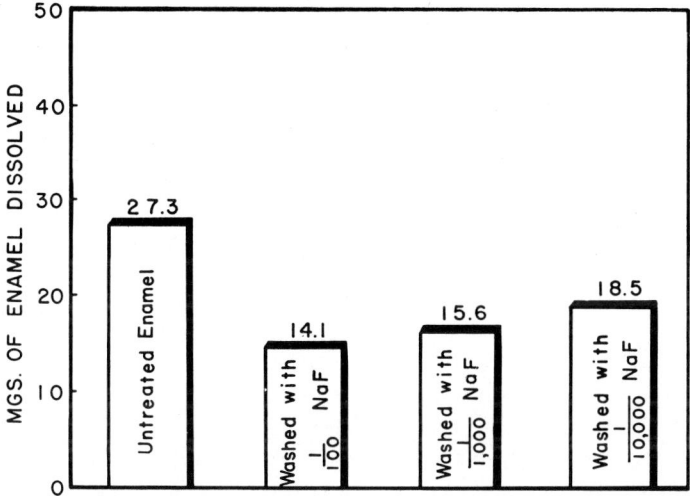

All enamel samples 50 mgs.

Acid used 20 cc. of 0.2 m. acetic acid sodium acetate buffer pH 4.0

Time of exposure 1 hr.

Figure 22–1   Acid solubility of fluoride-treated enamel. (From Volker: Proc. Soc. Exper. Biol. Med., 42, 1939.)

the ration and water. Shortly thereafter, other investigators reported that the oral administration of soluble fluoride by dropper greatly reduced the amount of experimental rat caries produced as a result of the administration of the coarse-particle diet.

These findings focused attention on the mechanism of fluoride action in limiting tooth decay. Clinical studies showing a relationship between mottling of the enamel and reduced tooth decay seemed explainable on the basis that the fluoride present at the time of calcification was incorporated in the tooth and in some way made it more resistant to caries. In the animal studies such a conclusion seemed untenable because the teeth were fully formed and erupted before the fluoride was administered. It seemed logical to assume that, in this instance at least, fluorides were acting posteruptively to inhibit dental caries.

At about the same time, Volker was investigating the problem of enamel acid solubility. Having rather carefully reviewed the literature, he was aware of the classic observations of the affinity of fluoride for calcium phosphate. He also knew that when fluoride was combined with calcium phosphate it reduced its solubility. Recognizing the similarity between these substances and tooth structure, he studied acid solubility of normal enamel and compared it with samples of enamel exposed to varying dilutions of sodium fluoride in distilled water. The findings are shown in Figure 22–1. He reported that "the natural surfaces of whole teeth treated with sodium fluoride were much less affected by acid than those of untreated teeth."

In explanation, Volker suggested: "These observations seem to establish that fluorine reacts with tooth substance to produce a less soluble product. This reaction is probably similar to that occurring between fluorine and bone or other calcium phosphates and may consist of change to a fluorapatite, an adsorption of fluorine or a combination of both." In summarizing his researches he stated: "It is believed that these preliminary findings point to the use of controlled applications of fluorine-containing compounds as a means of preventing dental caries."

WATER FLUORIDATION

Once the United States Public Health Service teams had accumulated the initial evidence that certain minimal levels of fluoride in the drinking water could inhibit dental caries in children without producing disfiguring mottling, they expanded their researches, studying new areas and re-evaluating information accumulated in their earlier investigations. By 1942 they had confirmed the hypothesis in studies involving 21 cities selected on the basis of varying concentrations of fluoride in their public water supplies. These data are summarized in Figure 22–2.

It will be noted that 12 to 14 year old children with a history of continuous residency in a city having less than 0.5 parts per million of fluoride in the domestic water had on an average more than 7 decayed, missing and filled permanent teeth. A similar group of children residing in cities where the fluoride concentration of the public water supply was between 1.0 and 1.4 ppm had on an average slightly less than 3 teeth so affected. The presence of concentrations of water fluoride greater than 1.4 ppm made for only a slight further reduction in caries susceptibility. There was, however, evidence pointing to considerable tooth decay inhibition when the communal water supply had between 0.5 and 0.9 ppm of fluoride. Since levels of fluoride in the drinking water of approximately 1 ppm caused a marked inhibition of dental caries without producing significant mottling of the enamel, these findings resulted in the initiation of clinical experiments wherein water supplies with less than 0.5 ppm were supplemented with fluoride. It should be added that paralleling research had shown (1) that the reductions in dental caries were not attributable to any other factors, i.e., solar radiation or water hardness, and (2) that this level of fluoride did not produce any other alterations in physical state.

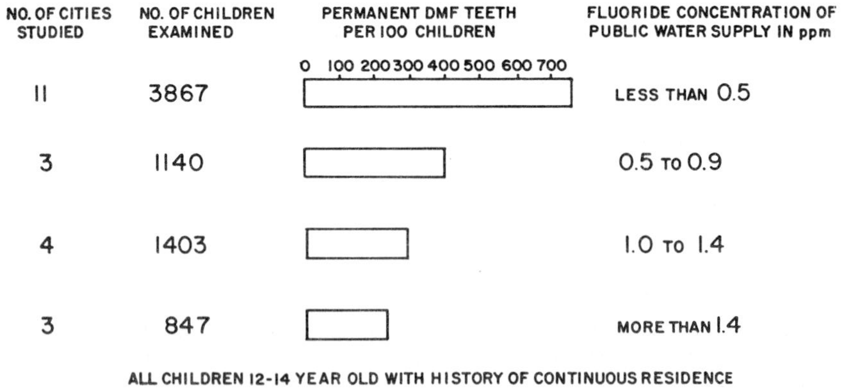

NO. OF CITIES STUDIED	NO. OF CHILDREN EXAMINED	PERMANENT DMF TEETH PER 100 CHILDREN	FLUORIDE CONCENTRATION OF PUBLIC WATER SUPPLY IN ppm
		0 100 200 300 400 500 600 700	
11	3867		LESS THAN 0.5
3	1140		0.5 TO 0.9
4	1403		1.0 TO 1.4
3	847		MORE THAN 1.4

ALL CHILDREN 12-14 YEAR OLD WITH HISTORY OF CONTINUOUS RESIDENCE

Figure 22–2 Dental caries in children and fluoride concentration in the public water supply. (Dean et al.: in Moulton [ed.]: Dental Caries and Fluorine. American Association for the Advancement of Science, 1946.)

TABLE 22–2   DENTAL CARIES IN CHILDREN DRINKING DOMESTIC WATER
WITH ADDITIONS OF 1.0 TO 1.2 PPM OF FLUORIDE

AGE	CITY	PPM OF F ADDED	DMF TEETH PER 100 CHILDREN WITH PERMANENT TEETH	% REDUCTION
6– 9[*]	NEWBURGH	1.0 TO 1.2	98.4	57.9
	KINGSTON	0	233.7	—
10–12	NEWBURGH	1.0 TO 1.2	328.1	53.0
	KINGSTON	0	698.6	—

[*]NEWBURGH CHILDREN IN THESE GROUPS EXPOSED TO FLUORIDATED WATER
SINCE BIRTH

From Ast et al.: J.A.D.A., 52, 1956.

CLINICAL TRIALS

Beginning in 1945, three clinical studies were undertaken. One of these was at Brantford, Ontario, another at Newburgh, New York, and the third at Grand Rapids, Michigan. In each instance the fluoride level of the water was supplemented to approximately 1.0 ppm. The Brantford study was under the direction of the Brantford Health Department and utilized the city of Sarnia as a control. The Newburgh study was under the direction of the New York State Health Department and the neighboring city of Kingston was selected as a control. The Grand Rapids study was under the joint sponsorship of the U.S. Public Health Service, the University of Michigan, and the Michigan State Department of Health, with the city of Muskegon being utilitized as a control. In each of the control cities repeated water analyses had indicated that fluorides were either absent or present in negligible amounts. Immediately thereafter these studies were supplemented by an increasing number of investigations undertaken by state and local agencies.

The 10 year findings from the Brantford, Newburgh and Grand Rapids studies are in general agreement, and no attempt will be made to present each of them in detail. Rather, selected data indicative of the general conclusions will be presented. Since the pioneer efforts of the U.S. Public Health Service in earlier investigations have been duly acknowledged, the illustrations have been limited to the Ontario and New York studies.

In viewing these data it should be remembered that when fluorides are added to the communal water supply they presumably must be available during the developmental stages of tooth calcification and eruption as well as post-eruptively to be maximally effective in limiting dental caries. Since formation of the primary and permanent teeth covers a span of more than ten years, a "complete" fluoride effect on tooth decay can be anticipated only after 12 to 13 years of water fluoridation. In the intervening time there should be a gradual, but progressive, reduction in the dental caries experience of the children drinking the fluoride-containing water.

Table 22–2 summarizes the 10 year findings relative to dental caries in Newburgh children. Those in the 6 to 9 year age group represent persons who have been exposed to fluoridated water since birth. Consequently, all of the permanent teeth present in their mouths were formed at a time when they were drinking public water with added fluoride. The children in the 10 to 12 year age group could

TABLE 22–3 MEAN PRIMARY DMF TEETH PER CHILD OF CONTINUOUS
RESIDENCY IN SELECTED CANADIAN CITIES IN 1948, 1951, AND 1954

Year	1948		1951		1954	
AGE GROUPS	6-8	9-11	6-8	9-11	6-8	9-11
BRANTFORD*	4.95	2.37	3.58	2.25	2.76	1.93
STRATFORD**	2.20	1.66	2.62	1.76	2.63	1.58
SARNIA***	4.89	2.50	4.89	2.41	5.21	2.11

* BRANTFORD ADDED APPROX. 1.2 ppm F TO WATER IN 1946
** STRATFORD HAS   "   " " IN WATER NATURALLY
*** SARNIA   HAS NO F IN WATER

From Division of Medical Statistics, Ontario Department of Health: J. Canad. D. A.,
22, 1956.

drink fluoride-containing water while most of their permanent teeth were being
calcified. The former group had a reduction in dental caries in their permanent
teeth of 57.9 per cent when compared with control Kingston children. The latter
group had a reduction of 53.0 per cent under similar circumstances.

Selected findings from the Brantford study are presented in Tables 22–3 and
22–4. Although water fluoridation was begun in 1945, the summary data are taken
from the years 1948, 1951 and 1954. In addition to the caries experience of Brantford children who received the benefits of water fluoridation, information is
presented for children residing in the city of Stratford, where the same level of
fluoride is present naturally in the water. Both of these are contrasted with the
findings for children in Sarnia, where the water is almost fluoride free.

Table 22–3 affords an opportunity to compare water fluoridation and the susceptibility of the primary teeth to dental caries. In 1948 the average 6 to 8 and 9 to
11 year olds residing in Brantford had had the benefits of water fluoridation for
approximately three years. Their primary teeth had formed and erupted prior to
the addition of fluoride to the water. The Stratford children had had the benefit of
natural fluoridation during their total prenatal and postnatal lives. Whereas 6 to 8

TABLE 22–4 MEAN PERMANENT DMF TEETH PER CHILD OF CONTINUOUS
RESIDENCY IN SELECTED CANADIAN CITIES IN 1948, 1951, AND 1954

Year	1948			1951			1954		
AGE GROUPS	6-8	9-11	12-14	6-8	9-11	12-14	6-8	9-11	12-14
BRANTFORD*	1.41	4.07	7.68	0.93	2.85	6.10	0.44	2.27	4.89
STRATFORD**	0.41	1.13	2.55	0.75	1.76	3.12	0.47	1.46	3.02
SARNIA***	1.60	4.21	7.94	1.99	4.48	8.55	1.69	4.67	8.84

* BRANTFORD ADDED APPROX 1.2 ppm F TO WATER IN 1946
** STRATFORD HAS   "   " " IN WATER NATURALLY
*** SARNIA   HAS NO F IN WATER

From Division of Medical Statistics, Ontario Department of Health: J. Canad. D. A.,
22, 1956.

and 9 to 11 year old Brantford children under these conditions had showed no demonstrable benefits of water fluoridation, Stratford children had a significantly reduced caries experience. By 1954 the Brantford and Stratford children in these age groups had both had the benefit of drinking fluoride-containing water for comparable lengths of time. The caries experience, particularly in the 6 to 8 year olds, was quite similar in both cities. In each instance it was greatly reduced from that seen in the children of Sarnia of the same age ranges who drank fluoride-free water. It may be concluded that less than ten years after 1 ppm of fluoride is added to the drinking water the dental caries experience of the primary teeth of children ingesting such water will be reduced by about 50 per cent.

Table 22–4 presents the caries experience of the permanent teeth of children of continuous residency in Brantford, Stratford and Sarnia in 1948, 1951 and 1954. It will be noted that in 1948 the caries experience of Brantford and Sarnia children from 6 through 14 years of age was quite comparable. After ten years of water fluoridation, however, the caries experience of 6 to 8 year old Brantford children was comparable to that of Stratford children, and the 12 to 14 year olds in Brantford showed a caries attack rate that was approaching that of Stratford.

These data and those from Kingston and Newburgh support the belief that the addition of 1 ppm of fluoride to the drinking water will result in a maximal reduction in the permanent tooth caries experience of 6 to 8 year old children of continuous residency within ten years after water fluoridation. Under similar circumstances a significant but probably not complete reduction in the permanent tooth dental caries experience will be achieved in 12 to 14 year olds. For maximal reduction in the tooth decay liability of the latter group, it seems likely that water fluoridation must extend at least through the first 12 years of life. Published results of the effect of 12 years of water fluoridation in Evanston, Illinois, are shown in Figure 22–3.

More recent reports from the Brantford study indicate that the anti-caries effect of water fluoridation hae endured through age 17 years. Additional studies

Figure 22–3 Evanston fluoridation study: 12 year report. (From Hill et al.: D. Progress, *1*, 1961.)

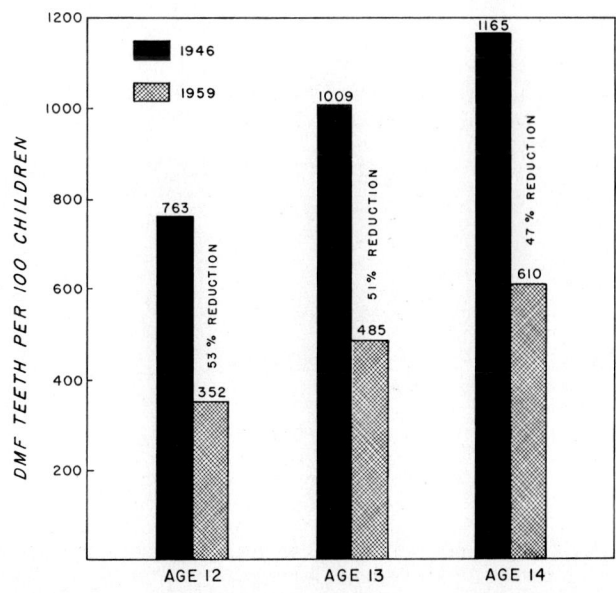

have documented the lasting anti-caries effect through the fifth decade of life. Other reports which involve studies on the effects of discontinuation of water fluoridation on dental caries would allow one to conclude that fluoride in communal water supplies continues to exert an appreciable influence even after the permanent dentition has completely erupted.

A community which used fluoridated water for 11 years discontinued the program for a period of four years. DMF studies at the end of that four year period indicated that the caries experience of children included in the study was similar to those of previously nonfluoridated cities. The authors concluded that exposure of teeth to fluoride during calcification and eruption provided protection against tooth decay. The protection persists as long as fluoride exposure is continued but will be slowly lost if exposure to fluoride is discontinued. Thus, periodic or continuous renewal of fluoride in the tooth enamel is mandatory for the greatest anti-caries effect.

Although the foregoing data give adequate testimony to the ability of fluoride-containing waters to effect an overall reduction in tooth decay, they do not indicate what specific types of tooth decay are inhibited by fluoride. Pertinent information on this subject is available. In the New York State study it was noted that the percentage of children 6 to 9 years old with caries-free primary cuspids and first and second primary molars was 25.5 in Newburgh, where the water had been fluoridated, as contrasted with 4.7 in the control city of Kingston.

The New York study also furnished information concerning the effects of water fluoridation on caries of the occlusal and proximal surfaces of posterior permanent teeth. The data suggest that optimal concentrations afford selective protection of the proximal surfaces in comparison with occlusal surfaces. Similar results were reported from the Evanston study.

A very early observation was made that the presence of fluorides in domestic water had a marked influence on the amount of proximal caries in the four permanent maxillary incisors. This is shown in Table 22–5. It is evident that when 1 ppm of fluoride is added to the drinking water, the caries liability of the proximal surfaces of the permanent maxillary incisors is reduced tenfold or more.

TABLE 22–5   DENTAL CARIES ON THE PROXIMAL SURFACES OF FOUR MAXILLARY PERMANENT INCISORS OF 12 TO 14 YEAR OLD CHILDREN

GROUP	NO. OF CHILDREN	CARIES PER 100 SURFACES
CITIES WITH LESS THAN 0.5 ppm F	386	10.17
CITIES WITH MORE THAN 1.4 ppm F	847	0.41
CITIES WITH BETWEEN 1.0 AND 1.4 ppm F	1403	0.87
CITIES WITH BETWEEN 0.5 AND 0.9 ppm F	1104	1.85

* CONTINUOUS RESIDENCE IN CITY OF BIRTH

From Dean et al.: in Moulton (ed.): Dental Caries and Fluorine. American Association for the Advancement of Science.

EFFECT ON DENTAL PRACTICE

It has been assumed that the anti-caries effect of water fluoridation would have significant effects on the structure of dental practice. In recent years several reports have become available which relate to this question. Additional reports from the Newburgh-Kingston study have shown that the average cost for dental care in 5 and 6 year old children from an optimally fluoridated community was approximately one-half of that necessary for similar children from a fluoride-deficient community. Less average time was required by dentists and their auxiliaries to treat children who had received the benefits of water fluoridation. These findings have been substantiated by other studies. In addition, fewer complex restorative procedures and extractions were necessary in children who lived in cities with fluoridated drinking water. Thus, dentists were able to carry a larger patient load than those in fluoride-deficient areas. However, the increased patient load in these areas does not seem to affect the demand for dental service or number of dentists needed, but does affect the number of patients which can be treated and the completeness of care for each patient.

Although some studies have reported a decrease in the prevalence of malocclusion and periodontal disease in optimally fluoridated areas, other reports have indicated that there is no effect. A recent survey of several pedodontists indicated that fluoridation had altered their practices to the extent that they were performing fewer reparative procedures and placing more emphasis on other aspects of their practice including office preventive procedures and interceptive orthodontics. They were also able to treat a larger number of patients. Of equal interest are the findings that dentists in optimally fluoridated areas receive a higher net income and work fewer hours than their counterparts in fluoride-deficient areas.

One slightly negative aspect of water fluoridation is that children who live in communities with fluoridated water tend to seek routine dental examination and care at a later age. In addition, dentists in such communities tend to assume that no other preventive measures are necessary and/or effective. While water fluoridation is extremely useful in combating dental caries, it must be complemented with early routine visits to the dentist. He, in turn, must recognize that caries reduction secondary to water fluoridation is not the complete answer, especially for an individual patient. Water fluoridation, and regular visits to the dentist to receive other preventive care and restorative treatment are important facets of a complete oral health program.

FLUORIDATION OF SCHOOL WATER SUPPLIES

Evidence exists to support fluoridation of school water supplies where it is not possible for the children attending the school to receive the benefits of fluoridated community water. Since the children would only be exposed to the fluoridated water for a limited period (5 days or 25 hours a week for approximately 9 months a year) 3 to 5 ppm of fluoride were added to the school water supply. Such an approach resulted in a significant decrease in dental caries with no associated mottling of the tooth enamel. It should be noted that while fluoridation of school water supplies is effective in the prevention of dental caries, especially in the permanent dentition, less benefit would occur in the primary dentition, since all these teeth would have developed and erupted before the children started to school and without the influence of the fluoridated school water.

PRENATAL EFFECTS OF FLUORIDE

The suggestion that fluoride should be administered to pregnant women was made well before the turn of the twentieth century. Much of the clinical data regarding fluoride and dental caries seem to indicate that the greatest benefit is derived when the teeth are exposed to fluoride during the calcification stage as well as during subsequent stages of development. Other data have indicated that maximum benefits can be achieved by exposure to fluoride during the last stage of calcification or during pre-eruptive maturation of the enamel. In addition, one group has said that almost complete protection is provided to smooth surfaces of teeth when they are exposed to fluoride two to three years before eruption, but pits and fissures must be exposed to fluoride during the very earliest stages of calcification.

These various reports make it difficult for one to determine just when fluoride therapy should be initiated to receive maximum protection against dental caries. In addition, unequivocal evidence still has not been presented to show that placental transfer of fluorides is in sufficient concentration to allow any significant uptake by the teeth, thus providing caries resistance. More recent studies in the area of tooth development have shown that, although some calcification of the primary and permanent dentitions does occur prenatally, the great majority of calcification in both dentitions occurs postnatally. Thus, it would appear that the question of placental transfer of fluoride might be more academic than practical as it affects caries resistance in teeth.

The rationale and impetus for past recommendations for prenatal usage of fluoride have come primarily from findings of water fluoridation trials. Investigators in both the Grand Rapids and Evanston studies indicated that children who had been exposed to fluoride from water supplies during both their prenatal and postnatal life exhibited greater protection against the ravages of dental caries than those children who had been exposed to fluoridated drinking water only during their postnatal life. However, a similar investigation related to the Newburgh-Kingston study indicated that little or no advantage was exhibited by children exposed prenatally to fluoridated drinking water.

A more recent study by Carlos utilizing a considerably larger sample of children has provided support for the Newburgh-Kingston group. A total of 2509 children, all approximately seven years old, but with different patterns of prenatal exposure to water fluoridation, were examined. The authors concluded "that the relation, if any, between prenatal exposure to fluoride and prevalence of caries in primary cuspids and molars and permanent first molars is of a very low degree and has no practical significance in the prevention of decay."

In light of the present evidence it appears that the administration of dietary fluorides to pregnant women cannot be justified on the basis of dental caries prevention for the developing child. The lack of sufficient evidence to support the effectiveness of prenatal fluoride therapy has prompted the Food and Drug Administration to ban the marketing of such products for use by pregnant women.

TOXIC EFFECTS OF WATER FLUORIDATION

Since the toxic effects of fluoride in large doses are known, opponents of water fluoridation have repeatedly questioned the advisability of adding even minimal quantities of the substance to communal water supplies. As a consequence, the New York State study and others have paid particular attention to the possible harmful effects of water fluoridation on the health of children. The ten year examinations of groups of children residing in the control and experimental cities are summarized as follows: "Each child was given a general medical examination by a qualified pediatrician. Height and weight were measured. Roentgenograms were taken of the right hand, both knees and the lumbar spine, and the bone density and bone age (maturation of the skeleton) were estimated. Laboratory examinations, including hemoglobin level, total leukocyte count and routine urine analysis, were also made. In addition, special studies were performed on smaller groups of children. These studies included detailed examinations of the eyes and ears, with determination of visual acuity, visual fields and hearing levels, and studies of the quantitative excretion of albumin, red blood cells, and casts in the urine." It was concluded that, "No differences of medical significance could be found between the two groups of children; thus further evidence was added to that already available on the safety of water fluoridation." Observation over a period of 25 years has resulted in little or no change in these conclusions.

The more rabid opponents of fluoridation have repeatedly voiced the opinion that the harmful effects of water fluoridation on older persons far outweigh the benefits of limiting tooth decay in children. These beliefs find no substantiation in a review,[12] wherein the available evidence concerning the effects of fluoride concentrations of the level presently being utilized in caries control is considered in terms of heart disease, kidney disease, cancer susceptibility, thyroid pathology, osteosclerosis, and a variety of other states. It is concluded: "When all the evidence is put together, it may be concluded that in water fluoridation adequate factors of safety exist against the known toxic effects of fluoride. . . . At present, the evidence does not justify the postponement of water fluoridation."

It is also pertinent to comment on two other possible dental effects of water fluoridation. The first of these is the possibility that it will produce disfiguring mottled enamel. In the entire Newburgh population only 46 of the 7 to 14 year old children had questionable fluorosis, 26 had very mild fluorosis, and 6 had mild fluorosis. No disfiguring mottled enamel was observed. Most investigators have observed that children who have received the benefits of water fluoridation have white or bluish-white teeth with a translucent quality. These "handsome teeth" are considered to be more esthetic than the yellowish-white teeth commonly found in fluoride-deficient areas. The second possibility, that water fluoridation promotes gingival disease, is contradicted by the findings in Canadian and American studies.

There have been a number of suggestions that substances other than the communal water supply be used as fluoridation vehicles. Consideration has been given to flour, milk, sugar and salt, to mention but a few. It would seem, however, that the individual variations in the ingestion of each of these foodstuffs are much greater than variations in water intake. As a consequence their benefits would not be as uniform as when water is fluoridated.

Despite a vigorous, organized opposition to the use of water fluoridation in caries prevention, by 1972 over 7400 communities in the United States with a population of almost 96,000,000 people, or 45 per cent of the total population, were using water containing added or natural fluoride as a means of combating tooth decay in children.

TOPICAL APPLICATION OF FLUORIDE

If all of the communal water supplies in the United States were to be supplemented with fluoride, more than a third of the population would not be benefited. These individuals reside principally in rural communities and obtain their drinking water from wells, cisterns, and springs. To them the benefits of fluoride action would seem to depend upon some other method of systemic therapy including fluoridation of school water supplies, fluoride tablets, or some form of topical fluoride therapy which might include office administration of fluoride by the dentist or dental auxiliary. Self administration with fluoride dentifrices and/or other fluoride compounds is another method of topical application. Beginning in 1942 with the report of Bibby, evidence has accumulated that the topical application of fluoride to the teeth is effective in limiting dental caries. Since that initial study more than 100 clinical studies have been reported in the intervening years relative to the effectiveness of various topical fluoride compounds in the prevention of dental caries.

In a 1952 summary of the literature it was noted that there had been more than twenty tests on more than 7000 patients in which different procedures of making topical applications had been employed. Although there are scattered negative findings reported, the results of the vast majority of controlled experiments are in general agreement. They give substance to the belief that, in children aged 4 to 14, topical fluoride medication will reduce tooth decay by 40 to 60 per cent. In support of this conclusion a summary of selected investigations is presented in Table 22–6.

Although it is most difficult to interpret the many variables involved in topical fluoride application, consideration must be given to a few pertinent observations. These involve (1) the nature of the fluoride, (2) the concentration of fluoride, (3) the number of applications and (4) the treatment procedures.

TABLE 22–6   EFFECT OF TOPICAL SODIUM FLUORIDE ON DENTAL CARIES IN CHILDREN

Investigator	Age Of Patients	No. Of Patients	% Conc. Of F	Duration Of Study	No. Of Applications Per Year	Spacing Of Applications	Control Method	Caries Reduction
BIBBY	10–13	90	0.1	1 year	3	4 mo.	Opposite Quadrants	46%
KNUTSON & ARMSTRONG	7–15	289	2	1 year	7–15	Within 8 Weeks	Opposite Quadrants	40%
FULTON & TRACY	4–14	69	2	1 year	2	6 mo.	75 Other Children	53%
SYRRIST	11–12	116	2	2 years	3	4 mo	Opposite Quadrants	42%
DAVIES	9–12	146	2	1 year	4	4 weeks	91 Other Children	58%

Bibby and Brudevold: in Shaw (ed.): Fluoridation as a Public Health Measure. American Association for the Advancement of Science, 1954.

TABLE 22–7   DENTAL CARIES INCREMENTS IN THE PERMANENT TEETH OF CHILDREN RECEIVING AN ANNUAL TOPICAL APPLICATION OF AN ACIDULATED FLUORIDE SOLUTION*

	MEAN DMFT INCREMENT	% DIFF.	MEAN DMFS INCREMENT	% DIFF.
12 month observation				
113 control cases	0.66	55	2.15	71
115 test cases	0.30		0.62	
24 month observation				
113 control cases	2.30	67	5.69	70
115 test cases	0.77		1.72	

* 1.23% NaF in 0.1 M phosphoric acid.
From Wellock and Brudevold: Arch. Oral Biol., 8, 1963.

NATURE OF THE FLUORIDE

Although numerous fluoride compounds have been subjected to laboratory and clinical tests to determine their possible usefulness in caries prevention, the compounds which have received the most attention to date are neutral sodium fluoride, acidulated sodium fluoride phosphate, and stannous fluoride. Studies have indicated that acidulated sodium fluoride phosphate and stannous fluoride provide consistently greater protection against caries than does neutral sodium fluoride.

In the past few years it has become apparent that acidulated solutions of sodium fluoride and stannous fluoride are even more effective than the earlier solutions. In a study by Wellock and Brudevold it was demonstrated that dental caries reductions of 70 per cent are possible with a single topical application yearly. These data are shown in Table 22–7. In a follow-up study using the 1.23 per cent NaF in 0.1 M phosphoric acid, the reduction obtained was about 70 per cent for subjects with good oral hygiene and 30 per cent for those with poor oral hygiene. Although the degree of protection varies with the particular study, most reports indicate a 30 to 45 per cent decrease in dental caries secondary to topical fluoride therapy.

CONCENTRATION OF FLUORIDE

Although the first study of the effect of sodium fluoride applications was carried out with 1:1000 sodium fluoride, most subsequent investigations have used solutions of a concentration of approximately 2 per cent. From the in vitro experiments there is evidence that the concentration of the sodium fluoride applied to the tooth is not, within a wide range, the limiting factor in determining its caries-reducing effect. Under suitable conditions an exposure of enamel to a 0.1 per cent sodium fluoride solution results in a reduction in acid solubility almost as great as a 4 per cent sodium fluoride solution. However, animal experiments have indicated that the concentration of fluoride in some preparations may be a significant factor in caries reduction even though it may not be important in the reduction of enamel solubility in acid.

Fairly concentrated aqueous solutions of the tin fluoride compounds can be prepared, and several large scale studies of stannous fluoride in 8 per cent and even more concentrated solutions have shown this to be an effective topical agent.

Very high concentrations of sodium fluoride in paste form have been used by Russian workers as is discussed later in this chapter. In the United States there have been attempts to formulate prophylaxis pastes with a high concentration of stannous fluoride. Some of these have had poor patient acceptance because of their bad taste. One paste which is more pleasant is prepared by mixing 10 cc. of an 8 per cent stannous fluoride solution and 1 to 2 drops of orange flavoring with 10 gm. of a stannous fluoride–compatible abrasive. There are now commercially available prophylaxis pastes incorporating acidulated sodium fluoride in an abrasive paste of zirconium silicate. Although this is a promising approach, there is not sufficient evidence at the present time to evaluate the merits of prophylaxis pastes containing fluoride.

NUMBER OF APPLICATIONS

The literature contains reports of experiments with sodium fluoride wherein the number of applications in a year varied from one to fifteen. When viewed collectively they support the belief that the maximal reduction in dental caries obtainable with a neutral solution of 2 per cent sodium fluoride is achieved with four treatments within a year. However, an acidulated fluoride solution seems to be more effective and requires only one application, either yearly or every six months.

Stannous fluoride has been used mostly as an 8 per cent solution applied to the teeth only once a year. More recently the suggestion has been made that stannous fluoride applied every six months is more beneficial. The average child patient should go to the dentist every six months for a dental check-up, and at that time the dentist will find it convenient to give the prophylaxis and fluoride treatment.

TREATMENT PROCEDURES

Knutson's technique is widely recommended for topical application of sodium fluoride to the teeth. On the first visit the teeth are carefully cleaned with pumice and a rubber cup. The mouth is then rinsed and the teeth isolated with cotton rolls. One satisfactory method is to isolate the maxillary and mandibular teeth on one side at a time. This is achieved with a cotton roll holder and a long cotton roll in the upper and lower buccal sulci and a short roll in the lingual area. A saliva ejector helps to keep the area dry. The teeth are then air dried and the 2 per cent sodium fluoride solution applied to each tooth surface, including the proximal surfaces, with a cotton applicator or spray. The solution is allowed to dry on the teeth for 3 to 5 minutes; then the teeth on the opposite side are treated.

On three subsequent visits, usually a week apart, the same procedure is repeated with the exception that the prophylaxis is omitted. It is customary to treat the teeth at 3, 7, 10, and 13 years of age to ensure that the erupting teeth receive the beneficial effect of the fluoride.

The recommended method for topical treatment of the teeth with stannous fluoride is the single application technique. This consists of a thorough prophylaxis using pumice to polish each tooth surface followed by stripping every proximal surface. The teeth are then isolated as described above, and a solution of 8 per cent stannous fluoride solution is applied to the dried teeth with a cotton applicator. In contrast to the Knutson technique the teeth are kept moist with the stannous fluoride solution for four minutes by applying the solution every 15 to 30 seconds. After all teeth have been treated, the patient is instructed not to eat, drink, or rinse the mouth for thirty minutes. The same technique can be used when applying acidulated sodium fluoride phosphate.

It has been observed that the fluoride incorporated in the outer enamel during topical treatments is progressively removed by the surface action of foods, by tooth brushing with a nonfluoride dentifrice, or by ionic transfer of the fluoride ion from the enamel to the environment. It is considered important that the fluoride content of the enamel be maintained at as high a level as possible, and for this reason it has been recommended that topical fluoride treatments be supplemented by regular tooth brushing with fluoride dentifrices. The data in support of this concept are considered further in Chapter 24, Prophylactic and Operative Techniques in Dental Caries Prevention. It has also been suggested that, following the topical application of fluoride, the fluoride retention in enamel is greater if the teeth are immediately covered by a layer of silicone grease. Petroleum jelly or cocoa butter is not effective.

The preparation of solutions of sodium and stannous fluoride for topical applications is simple. Sodium fluoride is prepared by mixing 2.0 gm. of sodium fluoride in 100 ml. of distilled water. The solution can be kept for a long period of time without deterioration. For the preparation of the stannous fluoride solution, the pharmacist can dispense 0.80 gm. of stannous fluoride into No. 0 gelatin capsules which are kept sealed until ready for use. When the prophylaxis is completed, the contents of one capsule are added to 10 ml. of distilled water and shaken. A 25 ml. polyethylene bottle is suitable for the preparation of the solution. Any solution not used during the treatment is discarded because it will develop a white precipitate which indicates that the stannous tin is not in active form.

It is unfortunate that stannous fluoride in solution has an unpleasant astringent taste, and as much care as possible should be taken to prevent excess solution from wetting the gingivae and the tongue. Another problem is that decalcified enamel will be stained dark by stannous fluoride. Both the child and his parents should be advised beforehand of the possibility of staining, with the suggestion that it shows the effectiveness of the treatment in preventing the progression of the lesion.

Acidulated fluoride solutions are more difficult to compound, and it is probably simpler for the dentist to purchase one of the solutions prepared by a manufacturer. These solutions are stable if stored in plastic containers.

It should be emphasized that there is ample evidence that neither sodium nor stannous fluoride will be very effective if they are carelessly applied to the teeth. Some practitioners have not been convinced that topical fluorides have been effective in their practice. However, it is only fair to consider that if a gold inlay does not fit the preparation, poor technique has been used, and this obviously does not detract from the merits of the gold. Likewise, if topical fluorides do not bring about a reduction in caries, probably the fault lies not in the fluoride but in the technique of the operator.

BERGMAN'S INVESTIGATION

Since the effectiveness of topical fluoride administration is questioned by some, it seems pertinent to review in this section the findings of Bergman in Sweden. They seem particularly conclusive because of the great care that was taken to minimize the effect of experimental variables. This investigator studied 114 children who were 11 to 12 years old at the beginning of the experiment. "One half of the dentition of these children was painted with a 2 per cent solution of sodium fluoride, using rubber dam. Each application lasted 5 minutes. Four such applications were made at intervals of 5, 4, and 3 months, and none during the second and third year. The caries development was followed over 3 years." His observations are shown in Table 22–8.

It will be noted that inhibitions of 61, 54 and 43 per cent were detectable after one, two and three years, respectively. It should be emphasized that great care was taken to set up this investigation so that the treatment and control tooth quadrants of the patient groups were comparable at the beginning of the experiment. It should also be remembered that "Linen thread passed between the teeth was used to apply the liquids to the proximal surfaces."

RUSSIAN STUDIES

Finally, it seems important to call attention to the work of Russian investigators as it relates to the control of dental caries with fluorides. As early as 1940 much of their research had been summarized in a monograph, "Fluorine and Medicine." It is interesting to note that even at this time they were unwilling to accept the explanation of some workers that fluoride reduced experimental rat caries by inhibiting the oral microbial fermentation of carbohydrates. Rather, they believed that the fluorides effected this by combining locally with the tooth to form a more caries-resistant structure. Subsequently, in the mid-1940's, they reported experimental findings wherein they gave three applications of a 75 per cent sodium fluoride in glycerin paste to the molars on one side of the arch of 188 children. The opposite molars served as a control. One year later they reported a caries reduction in the treated side in excess of 90 per cent.

TABLE 22–8   EFFECT OF TOPICAL FLUORIDE ON DENTAL CARIES IN
114 CHILDREN

| PERIOD | ACCUMULATED MEAN NO. OF NEW CARIES PER CHILD | | CARIES INHIBITION |
	TREATED SIDE	CONTROL SIDE	
1 Year	1.3	3.4	61%
2 Years	2.4	5.2	54%
3 Years	3.8	6.7	43%

* ALL CHILDREN WERE 11-12 YEARS OLD AT BEGINNING OF THE STUDY

From Bergman: Acta Odont. Scandinavica, *11*: Supp. 12, 1953.

As of 1954 there is evidence that these techniques are being used on a large scale in the prevention of dental caries. In one experiment it is indicated that a group of children treated semiannually with the 75 per cent fluoride paste had a caries incidence of 0.7 per cent in their 6 year molars after a three year period. A control group of similar age, not treated by fluoride, had 31 per cent caries in their first molars after three years. There is obvious need for confirmation of this finding by American investigators.

FLUORIDES IN DENTIFRICES

As has been noted previously, fluoride-containing dentifrices, mouth washes and pastilles were marketed for the control of tooth decay over fifty years ago. Presumably because of insufficient evidence of their effectiveness, their use was largely discarded in the early years of this century. It was only natural that the topical fluoride research should revive interest in this possibility. The initial attempts to reduce dental caries in children with a toothpaste containing 0.1 per cent fluoride gave negative results.

Since fluorides are highly reactive, their inclusion in a dentifrice is complicated by the possibility that they may combine with or be inhibited by some of the dentifrice ingredients, thereby being made unavailable to react with the enamel surface. Support for this contention was noted in early experiments in which radioactive fluoride was added to a liquid dentifrice that was later permitted to come in contact with enamel. Even under these favorable circumstances the uptake of fluoride by the tooth surfaces was reduced.

A large number of studies have been conducted with fluoride-containing dentifrices. A review of the present status of these dentifrices is presented in Chapter 24.

FLUORIDE TABLETS, DROPS, AND MOUTH WASHES

Until recently most of the claims that fluoride tablets, drops, and mouth washes reduce decay were not supported by scientific evidence. However, several experiments in Europe and the United States now seem to indicate that with these vehicles some of the beneficial effects of fluoride may be obtained by persons who, for various reasons, cannot have the maximum protection afforded by controlled fluoridation of the public drinking water supply.

Water fluoridation is the best way for the public to receive fluoride, but it should be realized that in the United States alone there are approximately 60 million people who do not have access to public water supplies which can be fluoridated. For the children in this group to receive the benefits of systemic fluoride the only answer at present is the daily ingestion of fluoride supplements from birth until the eruption of the teeth is completed.

Fluoride tablets have been evaluated in several studies. The results of one study in Germany indicated that, starting at 3 to 4 years of age, a 38 per cent reduction in dental caries in children was obtained after three years of daily use of a tablet containing 1.0 mg. of fluoride as sodium fluoride. In another study of 6 year old children in the same country, a 26 per cent reduction in DMF surfaces was observed at 12 years of age after six years of taking tablets daily at school. Another large study of first, second and third grade students showed a 20 per cent decrease in caries. In none of these studies was fluoride administered from birth onwards.

Arnold has recently reported that sodium fluoride tablets can bring about reductions in dental caries comparable to the results of public water fluoridation. The subjects who completed this study were 121 children living in and around Washington, D.C., and were somewhat unusual in that most were the children of dentists, physicians, and professional employees of the Public Health Service. Since this particular group was highly motivated to good dental health, and since it has been shown that the children of dentists have less caries than other children, it is likely that the excellent results in this study will be achieved only in groups that carefully follow the procedures used by Arnold. The absence of a true control group in this study makes it difficult to determine the actual caries reduction achieved. Briefly, Arnold's recommendations are: sodium fluoride tablets (2.21 mg. NaF, equivalent to 1.0 mg. of fluoride) are administered to different age groups of children as follows:

> Children 0 to 2 years — 1 tablet to a quart of water. All formula and drinking water to be obtained from this solution.
> 2 to 3 years — 1 tablet every other day crushed in water or fruit juice. Use a full glass and stir before drinking.
> 3 to 10 years — 1 tablet daily as for the 2 to 3 year olds.

The use of these tablets is not recommended where the public water supply contains more than 0.5 ppm of fluoride. The tablets should be stored in a safe place away from children.

Vitamin-fluoride combination tablets are widely prescribed by pediatricians, and reports on the effectiveness of these preparations are most encouraging. After three years of use, a group of preschool children had 55 per cent fewer decayed primary teeth and 66 per cent fewer decayed primary tooth surfaces than children who ingested vitamin tablets without fluoride. These results were obtained in an area without water fluoridation. This approach to systemic fluoride therapy is not yet endorsed by the Council on Dental Therapeutics of the American Dental Association, because no evidence exists to indicate that the vitamin-fluoride combination increases the effectiveness of the fluoride. In addition, the combination makes it more difficult to prescribe specific amounts of fluoride in areas where the drinking water contains substantial but insufficient levels of fluoride. The major advantage of vitamin-fluoride combinations is the added motivational factor that many people exhibit related to regular intake of vitamin supplements.

It has been suggested that fluoride lozenges be sucked to allow for a combined topical and systemic effect. This interesting approach will need further study to determine its value.

Fluoride drops usually consist of a solution of sodium fluoride which is added by dropper to the child's drinking water or fruit juice. Presumably this method of administering the fluoride should give results similar to fluoride tablets, but the chance of inaccurate dosage is increased. There is a lamentable tendency on the part of some mothers to think that if five drops are good, ten drops should be twice as good. Also, droppers vary in the volume of the drop they deliver. The pedodontist should emphasize the importance of giving the correct amount — no more and no less. Mottling of the teeth is a possibility where the intake of fluoride is higher than recommended.

Fluoride mouth washes have not been so widely studied as fluoride tablets. In a study of the effectiveness of a 0.25 per cent solution of sodium fluoride used twice daily as a mouth wash, Weisz has claimed a reduction of 80 to 90 per cent in dental caries in his pedodontic practice over a period of ten years. An editorial note accompanying Weisz's report points out that as little as 0.5 gm. of sodium fluoride ingested at one time could cause the death of a 5 to 8 year old child. It is estimated that 0.3 gm. of sodium fluoride is included in 4 fl. oz. of the mouth wash, and this approaches a potentially lethal dose. Other investigators have reported that 0.05 per cent sodium fluoride used daily as a mouth wash is more effective in preventing caries than fluoride dentifrices. Generally, it seems that the higher the fluoride concentration and the more often it is used, the higher will be the caries reduction.

A Swedish study recently considered the feasibility of using sodium fluoride solutions brushed on the teeth. During a two year period, 568 children brushed their teeth nine times with a 1 per cent sodium fluoride solution. The toothbrush was dipped in the solution and the teeth carefully brushed under supervision for four minutes. A reduction of caries was noted in comparison to 1116 untreated children, with the effects being more marked on maxillary teeth and on teeth which erupted during the experimental period. The reduction in caries on the maxillary teeth was between 25 and 30 per cent, whereas on the mandibular teeth the reduction was less. Following this approach it has been claimed that, where the water is fluoridated, brushing with a 6 per cent solution of sodium monofluorophosphate can reduce caries by an additional 40 per cent.

ACTION OF FLUORIDE IN LIMITING TOOTH DECAY

Since there is evidence that fluoride in the drinking water and in topical applications can inhibit dental caries, a consideration of the mechanism by which this is brought about seems pertinent. It must be recognized that in one instance the fluoride is being incorporated into the tooth at the time of calcification. This view finds support in animal experimentation wherein animals were fed fluoride during the period of tooth formation and placed on a low fluoride diet immediately after the teeth erupted. When these animals were placed on a caries-producing diet, they were shown to have a definite resistance to tooth decay. Similarly, it has been noted that persons who live in areas with optimal fluoride in the drinking water when their teeth are calcifying and who subsequently move to a section of the country that has fluoride-free water continue to have a reduced caries susceptibility. Both of these observations seem explainable on the basis that if substantial amounts of fluoride are present in the water at the time of tooth calcification, the teeth will have an increased fluoride content after they erupt.

It has also been demonstrated with radioactive isotopes that when dilute solutions of fluoride are brought in contact with fully calcified enamel, a union of the fluoride with the enamel results. It has been postulated that the nature of the reaction depends upon the concentration of the fluoride. One possibility is that the surface hydroxyapatite is converted in part to fluorapatite. Regardless of this void in our knowledge, there is ample evidence that teeth subjected to topical fluoride have a reduced acid solubility. It has also been reported that topical fluoride applications can decrease the permeability of the enamel and that tooth structure with adsorbed fluorides inhibits acid formation from carbohydrates by oral microorganisms.

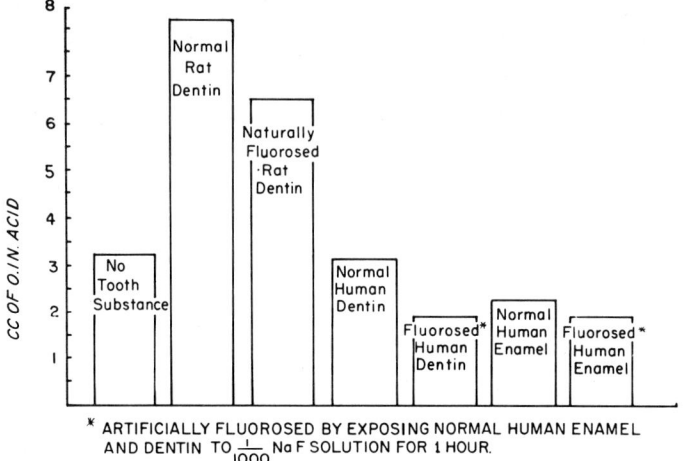

Figure 22–4 Twenty-four hour acid production by streptococci in the presence of normal and fluorosed enamel and dentin. (From Bibby: in University Bicentennial Conference: Dental Caries. University of Pennsylvania Press, 1941.)

It is of interest that tooth structures with substantial amounts of fluoride incorporated into them during calcification have a decreased acid solubility and also possess the ability to inhibit acid production by oral microorganisms from carbohydrate substrates. The latter property is illustrated in Figure 22–4.

There is laboratory evidence indicating that teeth may be softened by acid and then rehardened by solutions of salts of calcium phosphate. It has been observed that the rate of rehardening is greatly accelerated when the rehardening solution contains 1 ppm of fluoride. Similarly it has been shown that hydroxyapatite removes calcium and phosphate from solution much faster in the presence of fluoride. Such findings suggest an additional mechanism for the action of fluoride in limiting tooth decay. It may be that fluoride is able to alter the environment of the enamel surface so that the ionic transfer between saliva and the enamel is accelerated in the direction of enamel. This would account for the lower number of cavities where the fluoride is built into the calcifying tooth and would explain the arrest of caries observed in the use of topical fluoride treatments.

The dental plaque is known to have concentrations of fluoride often higher than 50 ppm. Since it has been shown in Britain that at 6 ppm and above fluoride begins to interfere with bacterial enzyme activity, it seems reasonable to suspect that this effect may be related to caries reduction in fluoridated communities.

SUMMARY

It has been established that fluorides are associated with the natural immunity of teeth to dental caries. This has been suspected for almost a hundred years but only within the last 20 years have researches established a sound basis for their use in preventive therapy. Several techniques for fluoride use in the limitation of dental caries have been developed: water fluoridation, topical fluoride applications, fluoride tablets, and fluoride dentifrices and mouth washes. Water fluoridation has been in effect in several controlled experiments for over 20 years. There is evidence that it results in greater than a 50 per cent reduction in the overall dental caries attack rate in children. Topical fluoride applications to the erupted tooth surfaces have been used for almost 25 years as a caries control measure. There is general agreement that when applied with the correct technique they effect an overall reduction in the caries attack rate approximating that of water fluoridation. More recently fluoride tablets, mouth washes, and dentifrices have been reported to limit dental caries. These developments may be presented chronologically as follows:

1800's

First Third of the Century
Fluoride noted as a component of calcified tissues.
Middle Third of the Century
Fluoride suggested as a limiting factor in enamel decalcification.
Last Third of the Century
Fluoride shown to combine with fully formed calcified tissue.
Increased fluoride content of caries-resistant teeth reported.
Fluoride made available in therapeutic form for caries control.

1900's

1900–1910
Mottled enamel described.
1910–1920
Resistance of mottled teeth to dental caries reported.
1930–1940
Fluoride shown to be the etiologic agent in mottled enamel.
Increased fluoride content in caries-resistant enamel reported.
Evidence accumulated that approximately 1 ppm of fluoride in communal water reduces dental caries in children without producing disfiguring mottled enamel.
Topical fluoride shown to be adsorbed on the enamel surface, changing its physical properties.
1940–1950
Topical fluoride applications shown to reduce dental caries in children.
Fluoridation of communal water supply shown to reduce dental caries in children.
1950–1960
Fluoride-containing dentifrices reported to reduce dental caries in children and adults.
Topical stannous fluoride treatment shown to be more effective when accompanied with regular use of a stannous fluoride dentifrice.
1960–1970
Fluoride tablets shown to reduce dental caries in children.
Fluoride shown to increase the rate of remineralization of the tooth surface.

Water fluoridation probably acts to control tooth decay by incorporating fluoride in the tooth structure during calcification. With the topical applications and dentifrices the fluoride seems to be effective because of posteruptive combination with the enamel surface. There is a possibility that the action of the fluoride in limiting dental decay in all three instances is similar. Present knowledge suggests that this is accomplished primarily by altering the physical and chemical properties of the tooth, but there are data that suggest an inhibitory action on the metabolism of the oral microflora.

It seems reasonable to conclude that at the present time the use of fluoride along with effective oral hygiene procedures is the most effective available means of combating tooth decay.

REFERENCES

1. Accepted Dental Therapeutics. Edited by Council on Dental Therapeutics, American Dental Association, 34th Ed., Chicago, Illinois, 1971–1972.
2. Arnold, F. A., McClure, F. J., and White, C. L.: Sodium fluoride tablets for children. D. Progress, *1*:8–12, 1960.
3. Ast, D. B., Cons, N. C., Pollard, S. T., and Garfinkel, J.: Time and cost factors to provide regular, periodic dental care for children in a fluoridated and nonfluoridated area: Final report. J.A.D.A., *80*:770–776, 1970.
4. Ast, D. B., Smith, D. J., Wachs, B., and Cantwell, K. T.: Newburgh-Kingston caries-fluorine study. XIV. Combined clinical and roentgenographic dental findings after ten years of fluoride experience. J.A.D.A., *52*:314–325, 1956.
5. Backer Dirks, O., Houwink, B., and Kwant, G.: Some special features of the caries preventive effect of water-fluoridation. Arch. Oral Biol., *4*(special supp.):187–192, 1961.
6. Berggren, H., and Welander, E.: Supervised tooth brushing with a sodium fluoride solution in 5000 Swedish school children. Acta Odont. Scandinavica, *18*:209–234, 1960.
7. Bergman, G.: The caries inhibiting action of sodium fluoride. Acta Odont. Scandinavica, *11*:Supp. 12, 1953.
8. Bibby, B. G.: The bacteriology of dental caries; in University of Pennsylvania Bicentennial Conference: Dental Caries. Philadelphia, University of Pennsylvania Press, 1941, p. 27.
9. Blayney, J. R., and Hill, I. N.: Fluorine and dental caries. J.A.D.A., *74*:233–302, 1967.
10. Brown, H. K., and Poplove, M.: Brantford-Sarnia-Stratford fluoridation caries study: Final survey, 1963. J. Canad. D.A., *31*:505–511, 1963.
11. Brudevold, F., and Messer, A. C.: Seeding effect of HA in calcifying solutions containing different levels of fluoride. J.D. Res., *40*:728, 1961.
12. Carlos, J. P., Gittelsohn, A. M., and Haddon, W., Jr.: Caries in deciduous teeth in relation to maternal ingestion of fluoride. Public Health Rep., *77*:658–660, 1972.
13. Denby, G. C., and Hollis, M. J.: Effect of fluoridation on a dental health public programme. New Zealand Dental J., *62*:32, 1966.
14. Diefenbach, V. L., Nevitt, G. A., and Frankel, J. M.: Fluoridation and the appearance of teeth. J.A.D.A., *71*:1129–1137, 1965.
15. Division of Medical Statistics, Ontario Department of Health: The Brantford fluoridation experiment. J. Canad. D.A., *22*:342–349, 1956.
16. Douglas, B. L., and Coppersmith, S. B.: The impact of water fluoridation on the practice of dentistry for children. J. Dent. Child., *33*:128–134, 1966.
17. Douglas, B. L., Wallace, D. A., Lerner, M., and Coppersmith, S. B.: Impact of water fluoridation on dental practice and dental manpower. J.A.D.A., *84*:355–367, 1972.
18. Englander, H. R., and Wallace, D. A.: Effects of naturally fluoridated water on dental caries in adults. Public Health Rep. (U.S.), *77*:887–892, 1962.
19. Englander, H. R., and White, C. L.: Periodontal and oral hygiene status of teen-agers in optimum and fluoride-deficient cities. J.A.D.A., *68*:173–177, 1964.
20. Gish, C. W., Howell, C. L., and Muhler, J. C.: The use of a stannous fluoride-containing prophylaxis paste. J.D. Res., *40*:711–712, 1961.
21. Goas, P. W., McElwaine, L. P., Biswell, H. A., and White, W. E.: Anticariogenic effect of a sodium monofluorophosphate solution in children after 21 months of use. J.D. Res., *45*:286–290, 1966.
22. Goddard, J. L.: Food and Drug Administration: Statement of general policy or interpretation, oral prenatal drugs containing fluorides for human use. Federal Register, Vol. 31, No. 204, Oct., 1966.
23. Grainger, R. M., and Coburn, C. I.: Dental caries of the first molars and the age of children when first consuming naturally fluoridated water. Canad. J. Public Health, *46*:354–357, 1955.

24. Hennon, D. K., Stookey, G. K., and Muhler, J. C.: The clinical anticariogenic effectiveness of supplementary fluoride-vitamin preparations. Results at the end of three years. J. Dent. Child., *33*:3–12, 1966.

25. Hill, I. N., Blayney, F. R., and Wolf, W.: Evanston fluoridation study. Twelve years later. D. Progress, *1*:95–99, 1961.

26. Hodge, H. C.: Fluoride metabolism, its significance in water fluoridation. J.A.D.A., *52*:307–314, 1956.

27. Horowitz, H. S., and Heifetz, S. B.: Effects of prenatal exposure to fluoridation on dental caries. Public Health Rep. (U.S.), *82*:297–304, 1967.

28. Horowitz, H. S., Heifetz, S. B., Law, F. E., and Driscoll, W. S.: School fluoridation studies in Elk Lake, Pennsylvania, and Pike County, Kentucky—results after 8 years. Am. J. Pub. Health, *58*:2240–2250, 1968.

29. Knutson, J. W.: Sodium fluoride solutions: technic for application to the teeth. J.A.D.A., *36*:37–39, 1948.

30. Koulourides, T., Cueto, H., Reed, J., Kim, M. S., and Pigman, W.: Studies on rehardening of artificially softened enamel. J. D. Res., *40*:698, 1961.

31. Kraus, B. S.: Calcification of the human dentition. J.A.D.A., *59*:1128–1136, 1959.

32. Lemke, C. W., Doherty, J. M., and Ara, M. C.: Controlled fluoridation: the dental effects of discontinuation in Antigo, Wisconsin. J.A.D.A., *80*:782–786, 1970.

33. Ludwig, T. G., Denby, G. C., and Struthers, W. H.: Caries prevalence among dentists' children. New Zealand D.J., *56*:174–177, 1960.

34. Magitot, E.: Treatise on Dental Caries. Trans. Chandler, T. H., Cambridge, Mass., Houghton, Osgood, and Company, 1878.

35. McClure, F. J. (ed): Water Fluoridation: The Search and the Victory. U.S. Department of Health, Education, and Welfare. National Institutes of Health, Bethesda, Maryland, 1970.

36. Moulton, F. R. (ed.): Dental Caries and Fluorine. Washington, D.C., American Association for the Advancement of Science, 1946.

37. Muhler, J. C.: Topical treatment of the teeth with stannous fluoride; single application technique. J. Dent. Child., *25*:306–309, 1958.

38. Muhler, J. C., Radike, A. W., Nebergall, W. H., and Day, H. G.: Effect of a stannous fluoride-containing dentifrice on caries reduction in children. J.D. Res., *33*:606–612, 1954.

39. Pelton, W. J., and Elasser, W. A.: Studies of dento-facial morphology III. The role of dental caries in the etiology of malocclusion. J.A.D.A., *46*:648–657, 1953.

40. Pollak, H.: Caries prevention by administration of Mulgatum F tablets. Deutsche Zahnärztebl, *14*:363–365, 1960.

41. Schlesinger, E. R.: Dietary fluorides and caries prevention. A.J.P.H., *55*:1123–1129, 1965.

42. Schlesinger, E. R., Overton, D. E., Chase, H. C., and Cantwell, K. T.: Newburgh-Kingston caries-fluorine study. XIII. Pediatric findings after ten years. J.A.D.A., *52*:296–306, 1956.

43. Schutzmannsky, G.: Dental findings after six years of caries prevention by fluoride tablets. Paper presented at O.R.C.A. meeting, London, 1961.

44. Shaw, J. H. (ed.): Fluoridation as a Public Health Measure. Washington, D.C., American Association for the Advancement of Science, 1954.

45. Stooky, G. K., and Katz, S. K.: Chairside procedures for using fluorides for preventing dental caries. Dent. Clin. N. Amer., *16*:681–692, 1972.

46. Tank, G., and Storvic, A.: Caries experience of children one to six years old in two Oregon communities (Corvallis and Albany). II. Relation of fluoride to hypoplasia, malocclusion, and gingivitis. J.A.D.A., *70*:100–104, 1965.

47. Terhune, R. C., and Muhler, J. C.: The influence of communal fluoridation upon dental practice. J. Dent. Child., *34*:228–236, 1967.

48. Torell, P., and Ericsson, Y.: Two-year clinical tests with different methods of local caries-preventive fluorine application in Swedish school-children. Acta. Odont. Scandinavica, *23*:287–322, 1965.

49. Volker, J. F.: The effect of fluorine on the solubility of enamel and dentin. Proc. Soc. Exper. Biol. Med., *42*:725–727, 1939.

50. Volker, J. F., and Bibby, B. G.: The action of fluorine in limiting dental caries. Medicine, *20*:211, 1941.

51. Weisz, W. S.: Reduction of dental caries through use of a sodium fluoride mouthwash. J.A.D.A., *60*:438–456, 1960.

52. Wellock, W. D., and Brudevold, F.: A study of acidulated fluoride solutions. II. The caries inhibiting effect of single annual topical applications of an acidic fluoride and phosphate solution. A two year experience. Arch. Oral Biol., *8*:179–182, 1963.

53. Wrzodek, G.: Ist eine kariesprophylaxe mit fluor-drages efolgnersprechend? Zahnärzl. Mitteilungen, *7*:1, 1959.

23

FOOD AND DENTAL CARIES

*by JOSEPH F. VOLKER
and SIDNEY B. FINN*

Since the words "nutrition," "diet" and "food" are often used incorrectly, the following definitions are included in the introduction of this chapter:

Nutrition is defined as "the sum of the processes concerned in the growth, maintenance, and repair of the living body as a whole or of its constituent parts."

Diet is referred to as "food and drink regularly consumed."

Food is taken to mean "any substance which when taken into the body of an organism may be used either to supply energy or to build tissue."

If we accept these definitions, we may say that we are primarily concerned with nutrition and subsequent liability to dental caries during that time the tooth is being formed, and with diet and dental caries susceptibility once the tooth has erupted. In both cases we are concerned with food.

PRE-ERUPTIVE NUTRITION AND DENTAL CARIES

In Chapter 21 it was noted that nutrition is most important during the period of time when teeth are undergoing matrix formation and calcification. It was further shown that these processes could be influenced by maternal, infant and childhood diet. Under such circumstances the physical and chemical properties of the enamel could be altered in the direction of increased dental caries susceptibility. Since the formation of the primary and permanent teeth begins in uterine life and continues until the twelfth year, the third molars excluded, it is the responsibility of the dentist to give adequate dietary advice regarding dental health in young children and pregnant women.

It is especially important to recommend foodstuffs rich in calcium, phosphorus, and vitamins A, C, and D. Under ordinary circumstances the ingestion of

518

TABLE 23–1 RECOMMENDATIONS FOR MINERALS AND VITAMINS IN
INFANTS, CHILDREN, AND PREGNANT AND LACTATING WOMEN

AGE	Ca GM.	P GM.	Vit. A IU.*	Vit. C Mg.	Vit. D IU.*
INFANT	1.0	1.5	2000	30	400 –800
1 To 3	1.0	1.5	2500	40	400 –800
4 To 6	1.0	1.5	3000	50	400 –800
7 To 9	1.0	1.5	3500	60	400 –800
10 –12	1.0+	1.5+	4000	70	400 –800
PREGNANT WOMEN 3rd. TRIMESTER	2.3	2.6	11,000	100	400 ADDED
LACTATING WOMEN	2.8	2.6	13,000	150	400 ADDED

*INTERNATIONAL UNITS

liberal amounts of milk, eggs, and citrus fruit will accomplish this objective, especially if the milk is fortified with vitamin D. The daily nutritional requirement of these substances for adequate health and presumably for tooth formation is shown in Table 23–1.

Although the adverse effects of carbohydrates on the erupted dentition are well known, only recently have we had evidence that excessive quantities of these materials in the diet when the teeth are being formed may increase their posteruptive caries susceptibility. It has been shown that when large quantities of sugar are present in the maternal diet of experimental animals, the teeth of the offspring have an increased susceptibility to tooth decay (see Table 23–2). It has been postulated that this phenomenon explains the "lag" in caries development in European children immediately following World War II. During the conflict these children had a rationed diet low in sugar. After the war the sugar consumption per capita increased rapidly but those teeth that formed when sugars were restricted showed a considerable resistance to tooth decay.

It should be emphasized that there is much evidence showing that people who have defective tooth formation may escape tooth decay provided that after their teeth erupt they subsist on diets with low fermentable carbohydrate content. However, there are a number of reports that such dentitions have a higher susceptibility

TABLE 23–2 EFFECT OF PRE-ERUPTIVE AND POSTERUPTIVE DIETARY
SUGAR ON HAMSTER CARIES

NUMBER OF ANIMALS	SUGAR PRESENT(+) OR ABSENT (−)		AVERAGE CARIES PER ANIMAL	
	DURING DEVELOPMENT	AFTER ERUPTION	MOLARS	SURFACES
28	−	−	0.9	1.0
17	−	+	4.5	7.9
8	+	+	7.3	20.0

From Sognnaes: J.A.D.A., *37*, 1948.

to tooth decay when they are exposed to an unfavorable oral environment. It is also pertinent that no substantial investigation has demonstrated that the physical and chemical nature of the enamel, dentin, or cementum can be influenced systemically once the tooth has erupted.

DIET AND DENTAL CARIES

The foods that are available to man are carbohydrates, fats, and proteins. The carbohydrates have been demonstrated to be important etiologic agents in dental caries. There is reason to believe that fats are associated with caries inhibition. It is only recently that any substantial scientific information has been accumulated showing a relationship between proteins and dental caries. The role of proteins, fats and carbohydrates will be discussed in sequence.

PROTEINS AND DENTAL CARIES

Although it is known that carnivorous animals rarely develop tooth decay and that persons ingesting high protein diets have no particular susceptibility to dental caries, there is very little information to indicate that the presence of protein in carbohydrate-containing diets may influence the caries-producing ability of the latter. It has been suspected by some that the quantities and physical properties of proteins in wheat flour are of importance in tooth decay. The proteins of wheat, gliadin and glutenin, possess the property of forming gluten when moistened with water. The gluten in turn largely determines the physical properties of the wheat dough. Whether or not these properties may alter the caries potential of baked goods is a matter of conjecture. It has been shown, however, that the addition of gluten to bread decreases the salivary sugar-enhancing effect of the bread.[20]

It has been reported that dental caries in the rat is accelerated when certain experimental diets are heat treated.[11] This phenomenon seems to be associated with the destruction of the amino acid lysine in the diet. The addition of lysine to these heat-treated rations reduces their cariogenicity. It is interesting that this effect has also been noted in experimental diets containing dried milk powder. Autoclaving of the dry milk powder destroys the lysine and increases the decay-producing capacity of diets that incorporate milk powder exposed to such treatment. The lysine possibly reduces the rate of enamel decalcification by forming a complex with the enamel surface, thus retarding the diffusion of acids to the enamel.[9] Although it is too early to assess the importance of this finding in terms of dental caries etiology, it does point to the possibility that under certain circumstances modification of the constituents of dietary proteins may affect caries initiation.

FATS AND DENTAL CARIES

Evidence that dietary fats have a limiting influence on dental caries has been noted in both human and animal studies. The observations on people, with few exceptions, have not been directed primarily toward an understanding of the relationship between fats and dental caries. Rather they have been incidental observations made in surveys of primitive peoples or noted in broad studies of the nutrition of institutional inmates.

In the former category, findings in the Eskimo are of interest. As long as he lived a primitive, nomadic life he had little or no tooth decay. When he adopted a civilized diet, dental caries resulted. Under primitive living conditions the Eskimo consumed diets that at times had as much as 65 per cent fat. Even when limited quantities of bread were available to him it was dipped into animal fat oil prior to ingestion. At least one observer has reported that dental caries does not occur in Eskimos to any considerable extent until the fat content of the diet is reduced to 25 per cent or less.

Indicative of the institutional studies are the reports of one investigator that high fat diets arrest tooth decay in children. The same worker later showed that caries inhibition could also occur with diets containing appreciable quantities of simple sugars. A common feature of his caries-arresting diets, however, was the inclusion of cod liver oil. In this connection it is interesting to note the report from other sources that when vitamin D was administered as a cod liver oil preparation to residents of a children's home, it was more effective in limiting tooth decay than similar or larger quantities of vitamin D given in the form of irradiated ergosterol. These findings indicated that the physical properties of cod liver oil, a fat, were responsible for the caries inhibition.

The experiments with animals are more conclusive. It has been observed that experimental dental caries decreases when increasing amounts of corn oil or lard are added to the diets of rats. This suggests that the inhibition mechanism is a local one, very possibly associated with an oil film on the tooth surface. This view has been supported by findings in studies of the effects of dietary fats on hamster dental caries. It has been noted, as seen in Fig 23–1, that the addition of 25 per cent fat in the form of several types of vegetable oil or lard makes for a substantial decrease

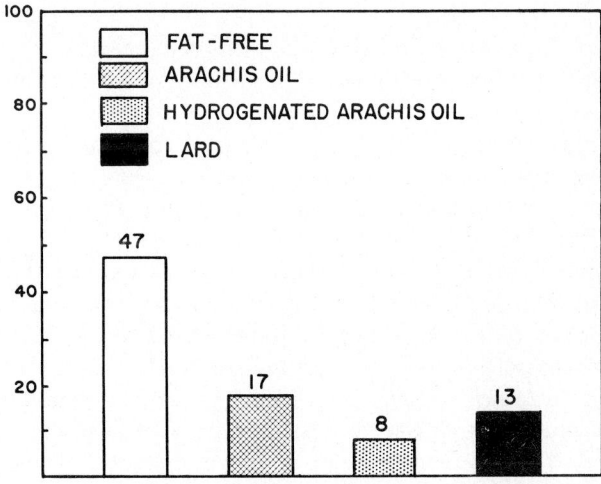

REPLACEMENT NUMBERS REPRESENT CARIOUS UNITS
ONE CARIOUS UNIT INDICATES THAT 1% OF THE TOTAL
AREA OF THE TOOTH IS INVOLVED

Figure 23–1 The effect of fat on hamster caries. (From Gustafsson et al.: Acta Odont. Scandinavica, *13*, 1955.)

in tooth decay. It has also been shown with in vitro tests that the solution of sucrose from a fat-containing diet is slower than from a fat-free diet.

The effects of fatty acids on the in vitro growth of oral lactobacilli, staphylococci, streptococci, and mixed oral flora from tooth plaques and saliva have been investigated. Fatty acids of 6 to 12 carbons in length showed inhibition of microbial growth, but the unsaturated fatty acids containing 18 carbons slightly stimulated the growth of some strains of lactobacilli.

The effects of fatty acids on the enamel surface have also been studied. It has been reported that when oleic acid is applied to a tooth surface prior to its exposure to an acid saliva mixture, it affords protection against decalcification.

From the above and other observations it may be tentatively concluded that dietary fats inhibit dental caries. This effect may be attributable to (1) alteration of the surface properties of the enamel, (2) interference with the metabolism of oral microorganisms and (3) modification of the oral physiology of carbohydrates.

CARBOHYDRATES AND DENTAL CARIES

In Chapter 21 the causative role of carbohydrates in dental caries was reviewed. Since it is our intention to discuss the prevention of tooth decay, it is pertinent to summarize our knowledge in this area. This may be done in a series of statements:

1. The carbohydrates must be in the mouth to initiate dental caries.

2. The carbohydrates must be susceptible to the action of oral microorganisms to the extent that products are formed that participate in the destruction of the enamel surface.

3. Many dietary polysaccharides, disaccharides, and monosaccharides have cariogenic properties, some more than others.

4. Natural as well as refined carbohydrates are capable of participation in caries initiation.

5. Those carbohydrates from which plaque forms readily appear to have the greatest potential for caries production. The carbohydrates that are slowly cleared from the mouth favor caries initiation.

6. The carbohydrates that are rapidly cleared from the mouth are of lesser significance in the causation of caries.

If we reflect on these statements it becomes apparent that three aspects of the oral physiology of carbohydrates are of major importance in caries etiology. They are (1) the chemical form of the carbohydrates eaten, (2) the rate at which carbohydrates are cleared from the oral cavity, and (3) the frequency with which carbohydrates are eaten. These principles have been adequately demonstrated by Swedish workers in experiments in which sugar was fed in such a form and manner that it was present in the oral cavity for varying portions of the day ranging from several hours to almost the entire day. Under these conditions tooth decay was found to increase to only a very limited extent in persons having sugar in their mouths for only a short time, and to occur with marked frequency in persons who had sugar in their mouths for many hours. These findings are presented in Fig. 23–2.

In the early attempts at dietary control of dental caries, the emphasis was placed primarily on the quantity rather than on the physical characteristics of the

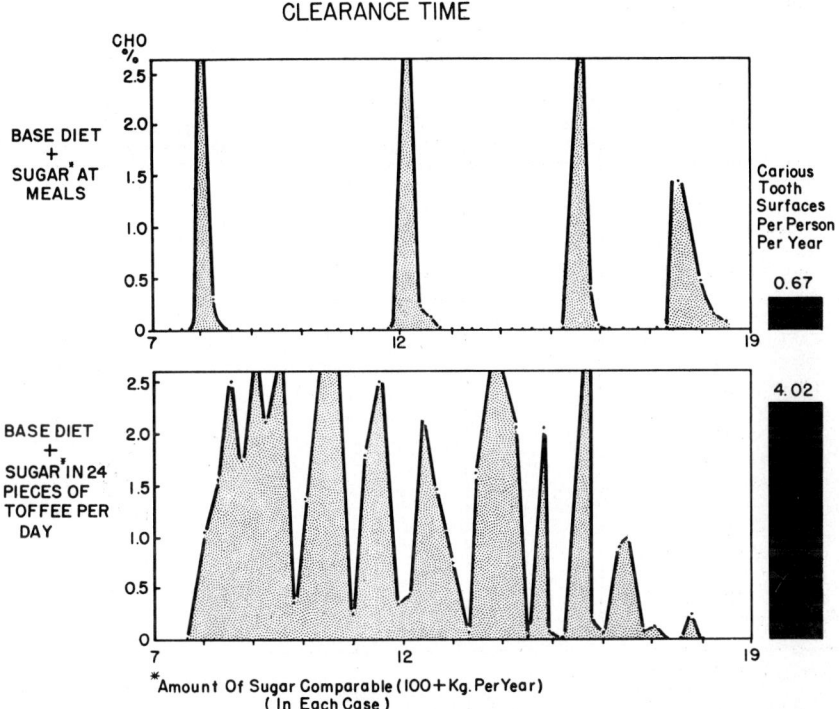

CLEARANCE TIME

Figure 23–2 Comparison of clearance time of sugar fed at meals with clearance time of sugar fed as toffee throughout the day. (From Gustafsson: Acta Odont. Scandinavica, *11*, 1954. Lundqvist: Odont. Revy, *3*:Supp. 1, 1952.)

carbohydrate present in the diet. Because of more recent knowledge this approach should be superseded by dietary corrections that take into account the ability of carbohydrate-containing foods to be retained in the mouth (see Appendix I and II) and to be converted into acid by oral microorganisms. Although it may be many years before detailed information is available on the oral physiology of all of the ordinary carbohydrate-containing foodstuffs, the findings reproduced in Table 23–3 deserve careful attention.

Decalcification Potential

In this study a variety of common foods was fed to clinical subjects, and the amount of food adhering to the teeth after eating was determined. Subsequently this amount of food was incubated with saliva and the quantity of 0.1 N acid formed in four hours was measured. The product of the quantity of food retained multiplied by the quantity of the acid formed after salivary incubation was designated as the decalcification potential. This was suggested as being a measure of the caries-producing ability of the particular foodstuff. It may be illustrated with white bread containing a total of 49 per cent carbohydrate and 13 per cent free sugar. One hundred eighty-eight mg. of food were retained after eating. When this was incubated with saliva for four hours, 1.8 cc. of 0.1 N acid were formed. The decalcification potential was calculated by multiplying 188 by 1.8. This gave a value of 338 (Table 23–3).

TABLE 23–3   FOOD RETENTION AND DECALCIFICATION POTENTIALS OF REPRESENTATIVE FOODS

Food	Total Carbohydrate %	Free Sugar %	Food Retained Mg.	4-Hour Acid Formation Ml. 0.1 Normal Sodium Hydroxide	Decalcification Potential
COOKIE (FIG)	70	27.6	678	1.2	814
DATE	77.5	33.8	507	1.6	811
CHOCOLATE	50	39	370	2.1	777
ICE CREAM	17	..	423	1.6	677
COOKIE (SHORTBREAD)	59.5	24.8	370	1.3	481
DANISH PASTRY	53.8	40	181	1.6	434
CRACKER (SALTED)	70	11.0	340	1.2	408
CARAMEL	56.8	43	219	1.8	394
CHOCOLATE PUDDING	35	18.5	300	1.3	390
CRACKER (OIL SPRAYED)	71	12.1	310	1.2	372
TOFFEE	90	..	266	1.3	346
WHITE BREAD	49	13.0	188	1.8	338
POTATO (BOILED)	18.2	4.0	128	2.4	307
COLA DRINK	10.5	10.5	237	1	237
APPLE	17.5	11.0	228	1	228
ORANGE SODA	10.5	10.5	219	1	219
ORANGE JUICE (FRESH)	8.5	..	177	1.2	212
POTATO CHIPS	48.2	12.7	61	1.9	116
CARROT (FRESH)	9.5	..	73	1.2	88
CARROT (COOKED)	8.3	6.8	2	1.5	3

From Bibby: J.A.D.A., *51*, 1955.

It will be noted that there is a ninefold increase in the amount of carbohydrate retained in the mouth after the ingestion of a fig cookie when compared with a fresh carrot. A similar difference exists between their decalcification potentials, since their four-hour acid formation values are similar.

The authors emphasize that this is probably a qualitative rather than a quantitative index of the caries-producing capacities of food. They point out that they are measuring mucous membrane retention as well as tooth surface retention. They state that "the retention of dates was about the same in the two regions, apples were retained almost entirely on the teeth, but only about 20 per cent of the retention of liquids was on the teeth and 80 per cent on the mucous membranes."

Caries Potentiality Index

The investigation of the Swedish group included the results of extensive sugar clearance studies with different foodstuffs in two clinical subjects. The original data accumulated included the foodstuff content of soluble carbohydrates, the weight of the foodstuff consumed, the total sugar and the reducing sugar content of the saliva after ingestion, and the time necessary for varying amounts of the sugar to be cleared from the saliva. These data permitted the tentative calculation of a caries potentiality index based on the rate of oral sugar clearance. This was done by observing the time in minutes after the food was ingested that the total sugar content in the saliva exceeded 0.02 per cent, 0.2 per cent, 2 per cent, and 20 per cent. These times were noted as a, b, c, and d, respectively. Their total $(a+b+c+d)$ was designated as the caries potentiality index. A specific example of how the caries potentiality index is calculated may be seen in the findings with caramels. They weighed 6.9 gm. each and had a sugar content of 64 per cent. One-half minute after their ingestion the total salivary sugar level exceeded 20 per cent. For $2\frac{1}{2}$ minutes after ingestion the total salivary sugar exceeded 2 per cent. For 5 minutes after ingestion the total salivary sugar exceeded 0.2 per cent and for 18.75 minutes it exceeded 0.02 per cent. Adding 0.5 of a minute, 2.5 minutes, 5 minutes and 18.75 minutes, we get the caries potentiality index of approximately 27 minutes.

In the original study nine fluids and a large number of solids were so tested. The solids included thirteen classified as flours and breads, six milk and egg products, seven meats, three fishes, eight fruits and berries, two honey combinations, and eleven candies. Only candy, honey, jams and certain types of bread were noted as having a caries potentiality index above 10. No fluid, meat, fish, fruit or berry had a caries potentiality index in excess of 6. Subsequently, representative foods were selected from this study and added to the dietaries of experimental groups. With certain exceptions the caries potentiality index of these additions, calculated from laboratory data, was predictive of the amount of tooth decay that developed in the experimental subjects. An abbreviated summary of the data is presented in Table 23–4. Although the original research is available now in several foreign journals in English, its obvious significance makes it advisable to include the complete table as an appendix (see pp. 686-688)

Modification of Carbohydrate Foodstuffs

There are several general possibilities that carbohydrate foodstuffs can be modified in such a fashion as to diminish their participation in caries initiation. Theoretically, this could be accomplished by changing the carbohydrate so as to

TABLE 23–4 CARIES POTENTIALITY INDEXES OF REPRESENTATIVE FOODS

Food	Total Sugar %	Sugar Concentration In Saliva		Caries Potentiality Index
		Maximum %	Av. Clearance Time (Min.) Above 0.2 %	
CARAMEL	64.0	18.8	5	27
HONEY + BREAD + BUTTER	19.0	4.6	7.5	24
CHOCOLATE, LIGHT	47.5	10.1	6.25	21
HONEY	72.8	5.6	5	18
SWEET COOKIES (BISCUITS)	9.0	1.9	5	18
DANISH PASTRY	30.0	2.4	2.5	13
WHEATEN BREAD	12.3	2.8	4	13
ICE CREAM	2.4	3.2	2.5	9
MARMALADE	65.3	3.5	3.5	10
MARMALADE + BREAD + BUTTER	16.3	1.8	2.5	9
POTATOES (BOILED)	0.8	1.6	2	7
POTATOES (FRIED)	3.9	0.4	2.5	7
WHITE BREAD + BUTTER	1.5	0.8	2	7
COARSE RYE BREAD + BUTTER	2.3	1.3	2	7
MILK	3.8	0.6	2	6
APPLE	7.5	0.4	1	5
ORANGE	6.5	0.3	1	3
FRUIT JUICE	11.5	1.2	1	3
LEMONADE	9.3	0.5	0.75	2
CARROT (BOILED)	2.4	0.1	..	1

From Lundqvist: Odont. Revy, *3*:Supp. 1, 1952.

make it less available for bacterial breakdown or by adding to the carbohydrate substances which would counteract the products of bacterial metabolism.

Illustrative of the first approach would be the conversion of glucose, the aldose hexose, to sorbitol. This merely involves the conversion of the terminal aldehyde group to a primary alcohol group. It has been shown that the sorbitol resists acid formation by oral microorganisms. There is also evidence that it does not cause appreciable caries in experimental animals, and this has been the basis for its inclusion in some confections. Although it is not broken down in the mouth, there is evidence that it is absorbed in the gastrointestinal tract and can be stored as glycogen. The ingestion of 10 gm. of sorbitol daily over a period of one month has not given evidence of causing pathology in man. It is not known at present to what extent sorbitol can be substituted for glucose in the diet, but even if this question is resolved, the problem of economics will arise since sorbitol is considerably more expensive than glucose.

The second approach is illustrated by recent reports that the addition of appreciable quantities of phosphates to carbohydrate-containing diets inhibits their cariogenic action. In many animal experiments it has been shown that dietary phosphate in different forms can bring about large reductions in experimental caries in rats. The relative solubility of the different phosphates is considered important in their action in altering caries rates, and it is likely that the cause of the change is not a major systemic effect, but rather an intra-oral mechanism. Equivocal results have been reported with dicalcium phosphate. In chewing gum base it appears to be effective, enhanced perhaps by the increased salivary flow. Other phosphates, such as sucrose phosphate, sodium trimetaphosphate, and calcium glycerolphosphate, have proved effective or are at present being clinically tested in humans.

Attempts to modify the diet by supplements of naringenin, an alkaloid found in chocolate, and protamine, found in a variety of foods, have been effective in limiting rodent caries.[4] Such modifications of the diet have reduced caries by over one third. Even larger caries reductions have been observed in hamsters when the diet was supplemented with cocoa.[13] The whole cocoa powder and defatted cocoa powder had strong caries inhibitory properties, but cocoa butter had no cariostatic action and seemed to increase caries.

DETERGENT FOODS AND THEIR POSSIBLE INFLUENCE ON DENTAL CARIES

It is generally believed that fibrous foodstuffs exert a detergent effect during mastication, resulting in improved oral hygiene. There is at least one study which supports this possibility. The study technique was to have the experimental subject chew a yeast cake. This test material has the advantage of resembling both microorganisms and foods, each of which has been generally associated with caries etiology. Since the relative numbers of yeast cells normally present in the mouth are minimal, salivary samples taken at an established interval after the ingestion of a yeast cake give some indication of the oral clearance pattern. Subsequently, various foodstuffs and therapeutic procedures can be tested for their ability to accelerate the normal clearance of the yeast. The findings reported in this study suggest that certain foods such as apples and oranges have detergent properties

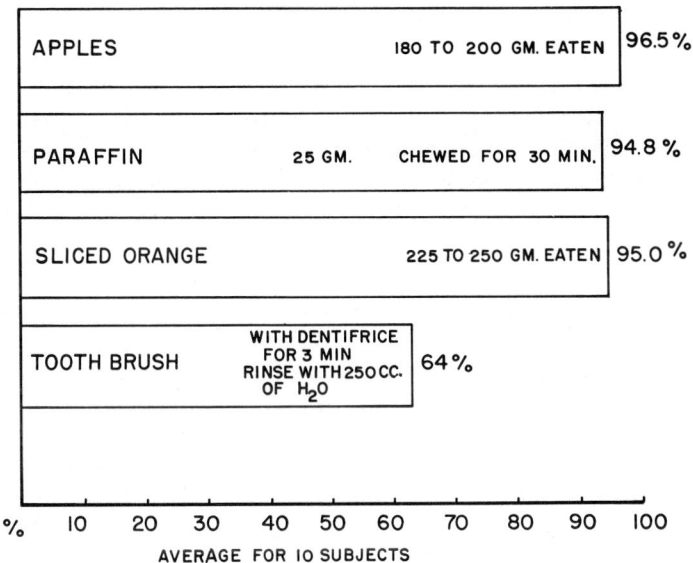

APPLES	180 TO 200 GM. EATEN	96.5%
PARAFFIN	25 GM. CHEWED FOR 30 MIN.	94.8%
SLICED ORANGE	225 TO 250 GM. EATEN	95.0%
TOOTH BRUSH	WITH DENTIFRICE FOR 3 MIN RINSE WITH 250 CC. OF H_2O	64%

% 10 20 30 40 50 60 70 80 90 100

AVERAGE FOR 10 SUBJECTS

Figure 23–3   The effect of various cleansing agents on reducing the number of oral yeast cells. (From Knighton: J.A.D.A., *29*, 1942.)

that approach or surpass the average variety of tooth brushing—at least under the conditions of this particular study. Representative data are presented in Fig. 23–3.

Foods such as apples, oranges, celery, and other fibrous foods are preferable to sticky foods at the end of a meal or between meals. The fibrous foods are retained on the teeth in smaller amounts and conceivably can dislodge some food sticking to the teeth. However, it does not seem that the plaque on teeth—at least the anterior teeth—is removed appreciably by chewing fibrous food. In a study which is easily repeated in the dental office, it was shown that chewing fibrous sugar cane, celery, an apple, crisp lettuce, and carrots consecutively over a period of three hours had very little effect on the plaque on anterior teeth as revealed by erythrosin disclosing wafers.[1a] Although children and parents should be advised to eat detergent foods in preference to sticky foods, it is important to avoid leaving the impression that these are a substitute for careful brushing and flossing of the teeth.

TRACE ELEMENTS AND DENTAL CARIES

Aside from fluorine, a number of trace elements have been implicated in the increased resistance or susceptibility to dental caries.

The elements molybdenum, vanadium, and strontium, among others, are thought to be cariostatic, while other elements such as selenium, magnesium, and cadmium are thought to be cariogenic.

The amounts needed to produce these results and the mechanism of action, whether local or systemic, have not been elucidated. A great deal of further work is necessary before any definitive conclusions can be drawn.

DIET HISTORY

The foregoing information may serve as a sound theoretical basis for the control of dental caries by diet. As the first practical step an adequate dietary history should be obtained from the patient. This history should cover a period of at least a week or ten days when the child is living under ordinary circumstances. If, for example, he is attending boarding school, it should not be taken at a time when he is home on a visit. Neither should it be taken when his normal eating habits are obscured, such as during a holiday season.

It is of great importance that no attempt be made to communicate to the child or his parents any information prior to the history-taking period that might influence the normal dietary pattern. If, for example, a subsequent recommendation is to be made for reducing between-meal eating, this should not be discussed when the patient is first interviewed. If it is, the chances are that the dietary history received will list a minimum of between-meal snacks even though this has been a regular feature of the patient's past dietary habits. It should be recognized that when one strives to influence food habits he must be aware that he is dealing not only with the dietary problem but with highly involved behavior patterns which unquestionably require an intellectual approach.

The following information should be readily available from the diet history: (1) the nature of the food eaten; (2) an estimate of the quantity of food eaten; (3) the approximate time at which the food is eaten; (4) the order in which the food is eaten; and, whenever possible, (5) information as to how the food was prepared. To facilitate patient cooperation it is best to make available a series of diet sheets with preprinted instructions. It is also wise to arrange for a review of the first-day dietary history so that omissions and inconsistencies receive prompt correction. If this is not done, the patient may present with a ten day history that is inadequate for analysis, and valuable time will be lost. A hypothetical diet sheet is presented in Figure 23–4.

In reviewing the diet report special attention should be paid to (1) the presence of retentive fermentable carbohydrates, (2) the frequency of carbohydrate ingestion, and (3) the presence and position of detergent foods in the diet. When checking for the presence of retentive carbohydrate it should be recalled that polysaccharides, monosaccharides and disaccharides are all potential caries-provoking agents. Special heed should be paid to products with refined flour, cane sugar, and syrups. The presence of foods with high natural sugar contents, such as honey and maple sugar, should be given the same prominence as refined sugars. In addition to noting the ingestion of snacks between the main meals, primary attention should be given to whether or not they contain appreciable quantities of fermentable carbohydrates. It is of special importance that eating before retiring be studied, since the clearance of these retained foods will not be assisted by salivary flow during sleep. The observations on detergent foods should include the presence or absence of salads and of raw fruit and vegetables.

After the dentist or dental hygienist has made the dietary analysis, the findings should be carefully reviewed and their significance explained to the patient if he is old enough to comprehend, or to his parents if he is not. Since both of these procedures are time consuming and require a high level of special knowledge, they should be done on a fee basis comparable to that for regular dental work. Obviously, this is an important diagnostic procedure and has a significance comparable to a roentgenographic examination and diagnosis.

<u>Instructions</u>

Please keep a detailed record of everything that you eat or drink for a ten day or two week period. Indicate (A) the nature of the food consumed, (B) an estimate of the quantity of food that is eaten, (C) the approximate time at which the food is eaten, (D) the order in which the food is eaten and, when possible, (E) information on how the food was prepared.

The following abbreviations are suggested for portion size:
L = large, M = medium, S = small, also T = tablespoon and t = teaspoon.

Name *John Jones* Address *56 Forrest Dr.* Date *June 6, 1956.*
Birmingham, Ala.

Age *12* Permanent DMF *13* SNYDER TEST *Positive in 24 hrs.*

Time	Food Description
7:50 a.m. (Breakfast)	Orange Juice S ✓ Oatmeal hot L + 4 t. sugar ✓ 2 Toast white + marmalade 2t
10:30 a.m. (Recess)	✓ 1 cookie M milk M ✓ 1 cookie M
12:30 P.m. (Lunch)	✓ 2 sandwiches white bread, strawberry jam 2T and peanut butter 2T milk M ✓ cake lemon icing M
3:30 P.m. (after school snack)	Milk L 1 Doughnut 1 Bread white + honey 1T
6:00 P.m. (Dinner)	Mashed Potatoes M. Green Peas S. } eaten together Hamburger L + Ketchup Milk L ✓ Apple pie L and ice cream S.
9:00 P.m. (Bed time snack)	Milk M ✓ Cake with lemon icing S. ✓ 2 caramels S

<u>Dental</u> <u>Notes</u> <u>and</u> <u>Comments</u>:

1. Fermentable carbohydrates taken 6 times in 13 hour period - discuss!
2. Cariogenic foods noted by check total to 11 - discuss!
3. Note particularly substances taken before retiring - discuss!
4. Note absence of detergent foods - discuss!

Figure 23-4 Diet sheet.

ADVICE TO THE PATIENT

It should be recommended that patients consume appreciable quantities of fermentable carbohydrates only at meal time. Despite the contrary opinion of some, the elimination of vegetables containing large amounts of starch is not advocated. To highlight this contention it should be noted that the inhabitants of the island of Tristan da Cunha had a very low caries experience even though potatoes were a staple in their diet. The use of nutritive foodstuffs containing carbohydrates in a liquid or semiliquid form should be encouraged. Soups are excellent examples.

If the person is particularly caries susceptible, sugar and baked goods additions to the major meals should be minimized. These meals should be limited almost completely to meat, fish, poultry and dairy products, vegetables and dark bread. Fresh fruit and salad are also advisable and whenever possible should be eaten at the end of the meal. Desserts, other than fresh fruit, are not recommended. Cakes, pies, pastries, preserved fruits and candies should be permitted only on the most special occasions.

The importance of between-meal eating should be discussed thoroughly. Since children in particular seem to need these dietary additions they should be restricted to milk, fresh fruit and sandwiches of dark bread with meat or cheese. White bread sandwiches with jams and jellies should be forbidden along with candy and cookies. Present evidence does not forbid such things as potato chips, peanuts, soft drinks and chewing gum. Since the available data suggest that ice cream has a substantial decalcification potential and caries potentiality index, it is not recommended as a dessert or for between-meal ingestion by caries-susceptible patients. The same source suggests that fruit juices can be taken without fear of harmful consequences.

A typical diet which on the basis of current information would be non-cariogenic is shown in Figure 23–5.

CARIES SUSCEPTIBILITY TESTS

It is reasonable to assume that if the patients are cooperative and follow the dietary regimes outlined above, dental caries will be controlled. It should be recognized, however, that it is most difficult to change the dietary habits of children. It should also be understood that human frailties being what they are, many patients will not adhere to the dentist's instructions. Even worse, they will not be honest about their indiscretions. This immediately raises the question whether or not there is any means whereby the dentist may determine the degree of cooperation he is getting from his patient in a dietary control program. The use of caries susceptibility tests would appear to offer this possibility.

The basis for such tests rests on a sound foundation. It begins with the assumption that oral microorganisms and fermentable carbohydrates are causative agents in dental caries. It further assumes that when diets high in fermentable carbohydrates are ingested, appreciable amounts of these foodstuffs are retained in and about the teeth. In these locations they are available to oral microorganisms for their maintenance and growth. Consequently, those oral microorganisms that have the ability to utilize fermentable carbohydrates in their growth processes are favored. Accordingly, their numbers grow and the quantity of end products resulting from their digestion increases. It is known that the growth of oral lactobacilli and

<u>Instructions</u>

Please keep a detailed record of everything that you eat or drink for a ten day or two week period. Indicate (A) the nature of the food consumed, (B) an estimate of the quantity of food that is eaten, (C) the approximate time at which the food is eaten, (D) the order in which the food is eaten and, when possible, (E) information on how the food was prepared.

The following abbreviations are suggested for portion size:
L = large, M = medium, S = small, also T = tablespoon and t = teaspoon.

Name *John Smith* Address *5 Oxmoor Place* Date *June 8, 1956.*
Birmingham 7, Ala.

Age _____ *13* _____ Permanent DMF _____ *3* _____ SNYDER TEST *Positive in 72 hrs.*

Time	Food Description
7:30 a.m. (Breakfast)	1 egg fried + 2 strips bacon + 1 Toast wholewheat and butter Orange L in sections
10:15 a.m. (Recess)	Apple L milk M
12:30 P.m. (Lunch)	Vegetable soup M Tunafish salad M Milk M Banana S
3:30 P.m. (After school snack)	Sandwich ham with rye bread milk L Celery stalk L
6:15 P.m. (Dinner)	Potatoes french fried M ⎫ eaten Chicken sliced M ⎬ together Lima Beans M ⎭ milk L Tossed green salad M Melon L
9:10 P.m. (Bedtime snack)	milk L Pear L

<u>Dental Notes and Comments:</u>

1. Note absence of fermentable carbohydrates.

2. Note presence of detergent foods such as fruits and salads.

3. Note pre-bedtime snack is not cariogenic.

4. Note frequency in eating same as in previous figure.

Figure 23-5 Diet sheet.

streptococci is particularly enhanced by fermentable carbohydrates. This is reflected in an increase in their number and an increase in their capacities to form organic acids from a carbohydrate substrate. Since this is the case, it may be reasoned that salivary samples taken from children ingesting excessive quantities of fermentable carbohydrates will have increased numbers of acidogenic bacteria and increased capacities for acid formation from sugar. By the same token, children ingesting diets low in fermentable carbohydrates will have a reduction in the number of acidogenic microorganisms in their saliva, and the quantity of acid formed when their salivary samples are incubated with sugar will be minimal. It should also be anticipated that if children with a high caries susceptibility are placed on a diet like the one in Figure 23–5, there will be a consistent reduction in the number of acidogenic organisms in their saliva and the acid-forming abilities of their saliva. If they do not cooperate in following the prescribed diet, the anticipated reduction should not be forthcoming. If they cooperate at first and then become lax, the criteria discussed above should show an initial decrease and a subsequent rise.

THE LACTOBACILLUS TEST

The first caries susceptibility test to be generally used was based on the quantitative detection of lactobacilli in saliva. It is believed that the number of these organisms in the mouth increases on high carbohydrate diets and decreases when low carbohydrate diets are consumed. Immediately after arising the child patient chews a small piece of paraffin. The saliva that accumulates in the following 3 minute period is collected in a sterile container. After vigorous shaking, 0.1 cc. samples are withdrawn. The undiluted and diluted samples are then spread evenly over a Rogosa's SL agar plate. The medium is available from several commercial sources. The plates are incubated for four days and the number of lactobacillus colonies that develop are counted. When multiplied by ten times the dilution factor, they are an estimate of the number of lactobacilli in a cubic centimeter of saliva. The significance of the lactobacillus count is summarized in Table 23–5.

THE SNYDER TEST

The Snyder test measures the ability of salivary microorganisms to form organic acids from a carbohydrate medium. The medium contains an indicator

TABLE 23–5 LACTOBACILLUS COLONY COUNTS IN SALIVA AS RELATED TO CARIES SUSCEPTIBILITY

NUMBER OF ORGANISM PER CC	SYMBOLIC DESIGNATION	DEGREE OF CARIES ACTIVITY SUGGESTED
0–1000	±	LITTLE OR NONE
1000–5000	+	SLIGHT
5000–10,000	++	MODERATE
MORE THAN 10,000	+++ OR ++++	MARKED

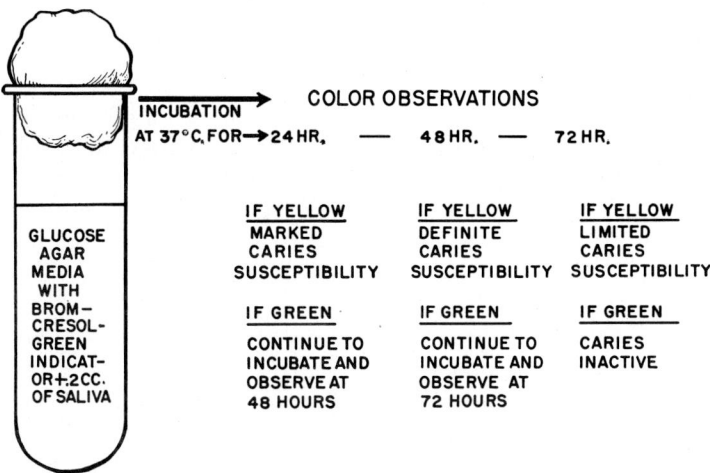

Figure 23–6 Snyder test and dental caries susceptibility. (From Snyder et al.: J. D. Res., *35*, 1956.)

dye, bromcresol green. This indicator dye changes from green to yellow in the range of pH 5.4 to 3.8. The prepared medium, with the dye included, is available from commercial sources. The salivary samples are collected in a manner similar to that used in the lactobacillus test. After the salivary sample is thoroughly mixed, 0.2 cc. of saliva is pipetted into the melted medium at 50° C. The inoculated medium is then incubated at 37° C. for periods up to 72 hours. The rate of color change from green to yellow is indicative of the degree of caries activity. If it occurs within 24 hours the child is considered to have a marked susceptibility to dental caries. If it is noted at 48 hours, he is classified as having a definite susceptibility to tooth decay. If the color change requires 72 hours, he is thought to have only a limited suscepti-bility to tooth decay. The absence of a color change at 72 hours places the child in a caries-inactive group. This is shown schematically in Figure 23–6.

There are numerous comparisons of the efficiency of the lactobacillus test and the Snyder test as measures of caries susceptibility. It is generally agreed that they are equally predictive. In one of them, the lactobacillus test, the increased number of organisms is the diagnostic yardstick; in the other, it is the increased acid production. The Snyder test lends itself more readily to office practice, since obser-vation of color change is much easier than counting the number of bacterial colo-nies. It also has the advantage that it can be noted by the child. As a consequence it has a value in patient education.

THE ENAMEL SOLUBILITY TEST

A third and more involved procedure is the enamel solubility test. Since this test is not generally suited for office procedure the details of its use are not presented here. It is based on the fact that when glucose is added to saliva contain-ing powdered enamel, organic acids are formed. These in turn decalcify the enam-el, resulting in an increase in the amount of soluble calcium in the saliva-glucose-enamel mixture. The extent of increased calcium is supposedly a direct measure of the degree of caries susceptibility.

THE SALIVARY REDUCTASE TEST

This is the newest test which has been devised.[16] The test measures the activity of the reductase enzyme present in salivary bacteria. A kit is available under the trade name Treatex. Saliva is collected in a plastic container, the subject chewing paraffin wax to stimulate salivary flow. The sample is then mixed with the dye diazoresorcinol, which colors the saliva blue. As the dye is reduced, the color changes, and the "caries conduciveness" reading is taken after 15 minutes, no incubation or other procedures being required. The results are obtained as shown in Table 23–6.

It should be recognized that none of the so-called caries susceptibility tests accurately predicts caries susceptibility for an individual. On the other hand, each test can be used as a patient education and motivation procedure. Patients are impressed by the ability of salivary microorganisms to ferment carbohydrate and by the reduction in their number that may be achieved by limiting the amount and frequency of eating of dietary carbohydrate.

PATIENT EDUCATION WITH METHYL RED

A simple but effective technique that may be of assistance in educating child patients to the problem of dental caries control involves the use of aqueous solutions of methyl red.[1] This indicator dye changes color in the pH range 6.3 to 4.2. At the former pH it is a distinct yellow, at the latter pH it is a decided red. One may easily demonstrate to child patients that the presence of a red color is indicative of acid formation by placing a drop of the indicator dye (0.1 to 0.02 per cent) in a Dappen dish and adding to it a drop of dilute lactic acid. If the latter is not available a drop of vinegar will suffice.

Plaque material removed from teeth or fresh sediment obtained from centrifuged saliva is placed in a Dappen dish or a spot plate and a drop of 5 per cent glucose solution is added. When a drop of the indicator dye is added to the mixture, the color change from yellow to red will appear in most instances within 15 minutes. Since in some cases, however, the color change may take 30 minutes or longer to develop, the test should be initiated at the beginning of the patient's appointment. The principle may be the subject of in vivo demonstration. The patient is scheduled for an early morning appointment with the advice not to brush his teeth prior to the office visit. If the aqueous methyl red solution is then applied to the surfaces of the teeth by dropper, the red color may develop immediately in the areas of plaque accumulation. This is interpreted to the patient as evidence of al-

TABLE 23–6   COLOR CHANGES IN SALIVARY REDUCTASE TEST AS RELATED TO CARIES CONDUCIVENESS

COLOR	CARIES CONDUCIVENESS
Blue in 15 minutes	Nonconducive
Orchid in 15 minutes	Slightly conducive
Red in 15 minutes	Moderately conducive
Red immediately on mixing	Highly conducive
Colorless in 15 minutes	Extremely conducive

From Rapp: Illinois D. J., *31*, 1962.

most continuous acid formation. If no acid formation occurs the patient is instructed to rinse his mouth thoroughly with a 1 per cent glucose rinse. Two minutes later the methyl red is reapplied to the tooth surfaces by dropper. Almost without exception acid formation will be demonstrable by an orange-red to an intense red color in the areas of plaque accumulation.

SUMMARY

Since the available evidence indicates that carbohydrates in the diet are essential agents in the production of tooth decay, dental caries may be minimized or prevented by intelligent dietary therapy. This demands an adequate knowledge of the subject by the dental practitioner or dental hygienist and a high degree of cooperation on the part of the patient. It should be remembered that the greatest reduction in tooth decay that can be anticipated through the use of fluorides is between 50 and 70 per cent. It is asking too much of fluorides to expect them to prevent dental caries in the child who consumes large amounts of fermentable carbohydrates at frequent intervals. In these patients we must of necessity depend upon dietary regulations to accomplish the objective.

It is the duty of the dental practitioner to suggest dietary revisions as the first step in tooth decay control. If the child cooperates, this in itself will effectively limit the disease. If the patient fails to follow the outlined regime, the program should be abandoned and techniques adopted that demand a smaller degree of cooperation.

It should be emphasized that the control of dental caries may be accomplished without the complete elimination of fermentable carbohydrates, sugars included, from the diet. We agree with Magitot[12] that "With the child, therefore, as with the adult, it is indicated to moderate or suppress the use of sugar; and here we speak of sugar that dissolves slowly or remains long in the mouth rather than the liquids or sweetened foods whose passage over the teeth is comparatively rapid. We do not proscribe sugar, an important element in our alimentation; we simply protest against its abuse."

REFERENCES

1. Arnim, S. S., and Harwick, J. L.: Clinical demonstrations of acid production by mouth organisms using aqueous methyl red. North-West Dent., *33*:147–154, 1954.
1a. Arnim, S. S.: The use of disclosing agents for measuring tooth cleanliness. J. Periodont., *34*:227–245, 1963.
2. Bibby, B. G.: Effect of sugar content of foodstuffs on their caries-producing potentialities. J.A.D.A., *51*:293–306, 1955.
3. Gustafson, G., Stelling, E., Abramson, E., and Brunius, E.: Experiments with various fats in a cariogenic diet. IV. Experimental caries in golden hamster. Acta Odont. Scandinavica, *13*:75–84, 1955.
4. Gustafsson, B. E., and Krasse, B.: The caries-reducing effect of naringenin and of protamine in hamsters. Acta Odont. Scandinavica, *16*:355–361, 1958.
5. Gustafsson, B. E., Quensel, C. E., Swenander Lanke, L., Lundqvist, C., Grahnen, H., Bonow, B. E., and Krasse, B.: The effect of different levels of carbohydrate intake on caries activity in 436 individuals observed for five years. Acta Odont. Scandinavica, *11*:232–364, 1954.
6. Harris, R. S.: Minerals, Calcium and Phosphorus in Dietary Chemicals vs. Dental Caries. Advances in Chemistry Series 94. Washington, D. C., Amer. Chem. Soc., 1970.
7. Jenkins, G. N.: Natural Protective Factors of Foods in Nutrition and Caries Prevention. Uppsala, Almquist and Wiksells, 1965.

8. Knighton, H. T.: Effect of various foods and cleansing agents on elimination of artificially in-oculated yeast from mouth. J.A.D.A., *29*:2012–2018, 1942.
9. Koulourides, T. A., and Bounocore, M. G.: Effect of organic ions on solubility of enamel and dentin in acid buffers. Jour. Dent. Res., *40*:578, 1961.
10. Lundqvist, C.: Oral sugar clearance: its influence on dental caries activity. Odont. Revy, *3*:Supp 1, 1952.
11. McClure, F. J., and Folk, J. E.: Lysine and cariogenicity of two experimental rat diets. Science, *122*:557–558, 1955.
12. Magitot, E.: Treatise on Dental Caries. Trans. Chandler, T. H. Cambridge, Mass., Houghton, Osgood & Company, 1878.
13. Nizel, A. E.: Nutrition in Preventive Dentistry: Science and Practice. Philadelphia, W. B. Saunders Co., 1972.
14. Nizel, A. E.: Protein nutrition and its interaction with infection. In: Nutrition in Preventive Dentistry: Science and Practice. Philadelphia, W. B. Saunders Co., 1972.
15. Pigman, W.: Carbohydrates, Fats and Dental Caries: Advances in Chemistry Series 94. Washington, D. C., Amer. Chem. Soc., 1970.
16. Rapp, G. W.: A fifteen minute caries test. Illinois D. J., *31*:290–295, 1962.
17. Snyder, M. L., Suher, T., Porter, D. R., Claycomb, C. K., and Gardner, M. K.: Evaluation of laboratory tests for the estimation of caries activity. J. D. Res., *35*:332–343, 1956.
18. Sognnaes, R. F.: The caries-conducive effect of a purified diet when fed to rodents during tooth development. J.A.D.A., *37*:676–692, 1948.
19. Strålfors, A.: Inhibition of hamster caries by cocoa. The effect of whole and defatted cocoa, and the absence of activity in cocoa fat. Arch. Oral Biol., *11*:149–161, 1966.
20. Swenander Lanke, L.: Influence on salivary sugar of certain properties of foodstuffs and individual oral conditions. Acta Odont. Scandinavica, *15*:Supp. 23, 1957.
21. Young, C. M.: Nutrition Counseling for the Pedodontic and Periodontic Patient. Workshop conference in Nutrition and Preventive Dentistry. Eastman Dental Dispensary, October, 1960.

24

PROPHYLACTIC AND OPERATIVE TECHNIQUES IN DENTAL CARIES PREVENTION

by JOSEPH F. VOLKER
and JOE PRICE THOMAS

In addition to the use of diet and fluoride in the control of tooth decay, the dental practitioner has available a variety of other prophylactic and operative procedures. These will be discussed in this chapter in three major sections, Oral Hygiene, Therapeutics, and Operative Dentistry. In some instances the reports available for analysis are fragmentary; in others they are controversial. These limitations should be kept in mind when the reader is making his evaluation of their possible place in a preventive program.

ORAL HYGIENE

The cleaning of teeth may be performed by the dental hygienist or the dentist as an office procedure or it may be done by the patient as a routine home treatment. In the former instance the technique involves the use of hand instruments and motor-driven brushes or cups with mild abrasives, at three to six month intervals. In the latter it includes the use of a toothbrush and dentifrice plus dental floss and oral rinsing. These procedures may be used in part or completely as many as four or five times daily. The effects of each of these procedures on dental caries will be discussed in sequence.

OFFICE PROPHYLAXIS

It is generally conceded that office dental prophylaxis is of little or no significance in the control of tooth decay and that its major contribution in dental health is in the prevention of periodontal disease. This view is supported by findings in over a thousand patients who received a prophylaxis and examination every three or four months for periods ranging from one to fifteen years.[27] Included in this study were 121 children of school age. No reduction in their dental caries pattern attributable to regular dental prophylaxis was observed.

TOOTH BRUSHING

There is considerable evidence that tooth brushing with a neutral dentifrice immediately after meals is an effective means of limiting tooth decay. In one investigation 702 individuals were studied for two years. Of these, 273 served as controls and 429 were test subjects. The persons in the experimental group were instructed to brush their teeth within ten minutes after the ingestion of food or sweets, and to rinse their mouths immediately after brushing. The control group were permitted to continue with their customary brushing procedures provided that this did not include tooth brushing immediately after food ingestion. The majority of the people in the control group brushed their teeth only on arising and retiring. Both clinical and roentgenographic methods were used in recording caries. The findings, shown in Table 24–1, support the belief that tooth brushing immediately after meals reduces tooth decay by approximately 50 per cent. Other studies with clinical subjects, although not showing as great an effectiveness, present the same trends. Experimental findings in animals also support this concept.

One of the greatest impediments to the effective utilization of tooth brushing in the control of dental caries is that it demands a high degree of patient cooperation. In one investigation,[62] where the tooth brushing habits of adults were studied, 405 persons were shown to use an average of 267 strokes in the brushing of their

TABLE 24–1   THE EFFECT OF TOOTH BRUSHING IMMEDIATELY AFTER MEALS WITH A NEUTRAL DENTIFRICE FOR TWO YEARS ON DENTAL CARIES INCIDENCE

Group and Instructions	No. of Subjects	Avg. No. of New Carious Surfaces by Clinical Examination	X-Ray Examination	% Decrease Over Control
Control (normal hygiene habits)	273	2.53	1.34	—
Experimental (brushing within 10 minutes after food ingestion)	429	1.49	0.53	41 (Clinical) 60 (X-ray)

From Fosdick: J.A.D.A., 40, 1950.

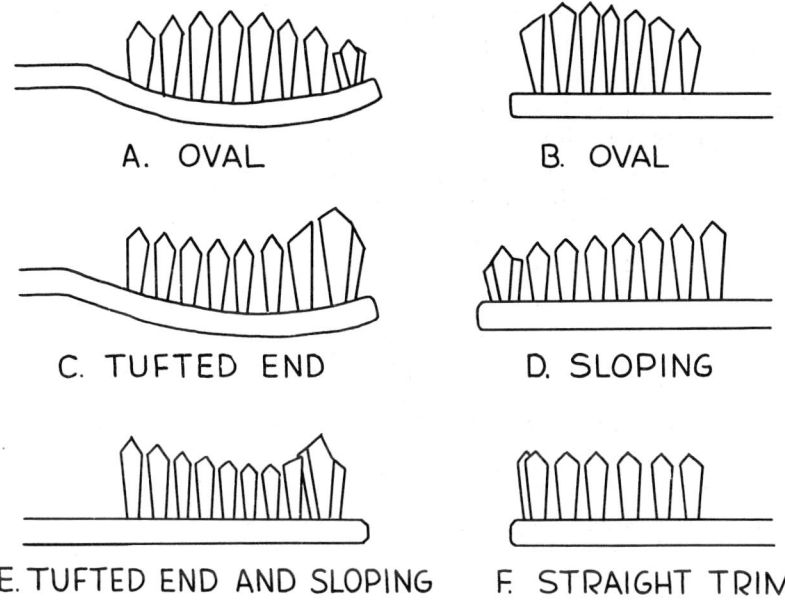

A. OVAL   B. OVAL

C. TUFTED END   D. SLOPING

E. TUFTED END AND SLOPING   F. STRAIGHT TRIM

Figure 24–1 Predominant toothbrush designs. (From McCauley: J.A.D.A., *33*, 1946.)

teeth. The entire procedure was accomplished in slightly more than a minute. Of the persons examined, 37 per cent used rotary brushing methods, 24 per cent used vertical brushing methods, and 36 per cent used the crosswise methods. Very few persons brushed surfaces other than the buccal and labial. It is notable that the average amount of time used for brushing teeth was only a third that usually recommended by the dental practitioner. The figures for children are even more discouraging. It has been shown that most children under age five brush less than 20 seconds, and the only brushing zones which are favored are the labial surfaces and the occlusal surfaces of lower molars.[44] It is interesting that the force applied by children is similar to that exerted by adults.

It is apparent that the effectiveness of tooth brushing in cleansing the dentition will be largely influenced by the design of the brush and the technique of brushing. At the present time the patient must choose between a variety of brush designs and brushing techniques. The predominant brush designs as listed by one source are shown in Figure 24–1.

The most recent research on designs of children's toothbrushes indicates that the most suitable brush tested had the following brush-head specifications: 1 inch long, 0.36 inch high, 11 triple rows with center row of 0.12-inch bristle diameter and each outer row of .008-inch bristle diameter.[45] It is generally suggested that medium bristle brushes be used since they clean the teeth better than hard or soft bristles and do not usually produce injury to the gingival tissues.

It is important to understand the reluctance of patients to discard distorted and worn-out brushes. The findings of one study indicate that less than 20 per cent of the toothbrushes in use in American homes are suitable for mouth hygiene. Consequently, patients should be instructed to replace their brushes at frequent intervals. If children are being seen by the dentist on a 3 or 4 month visit schedule it is wise to ask them to bring their toothbrushes for his inspection and approval.

Several different types of electrically powered toothbrushes have come into use. Most clinical studies indicate that they are of value. For handicapped children or adults who have difficulty cleaning their teeth, this type of brush would seem more effective than a conventional type. Hall and Conroy[29] found that, when used by preschool children, the automatic toothbrush was superior to the hand brush for removing plaque and debris. These investigators also reported that the parents of preschool children cleaned their children's teeth better by either method than could the children themselves. Conroy and Melfi[15] stated that in a group of children aged 5 to 12 the electric brushes were more effective than the manual. In a well controlled study, Owen[54] reported no significant differences between the effectiveness of manual or electric brushes.

There are numerous techniques of tooth brushing currently in use. A recent review lists six major techniques.[51] Many of them are so involved that they cannot be adequately mastered by young children. Accordingly, it is recommended that a simple technique be taught to young children. One such method is the Fones technique, the general details of which are illustrated in Figure 24–2. In this method, with the teeth in occlusion, the buccal and labial surfaces are brushed with a large circular motion. The lingual and occlusal surfaces are brushed with an in-and-out horizontal brushing action.

Kimmelman[44] has reported that a scrubbing action is best for dislodging debris from all surfaces and that the arch form and tooth forms in the primary dentition are well suited to horizontal scrubbing strokes. It is also considered unlikely that the gingivae will be damaged by such a technique. Until the child can tell the time from a clock, a three minute sandglass timer is useful to indicate how long to brush.

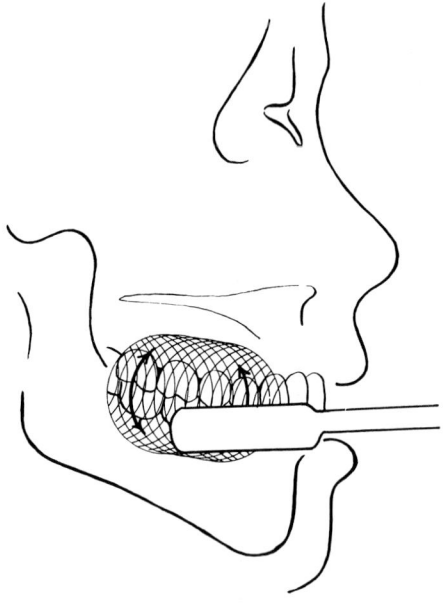

Figure 24–2   Fones method of tooth brushing.

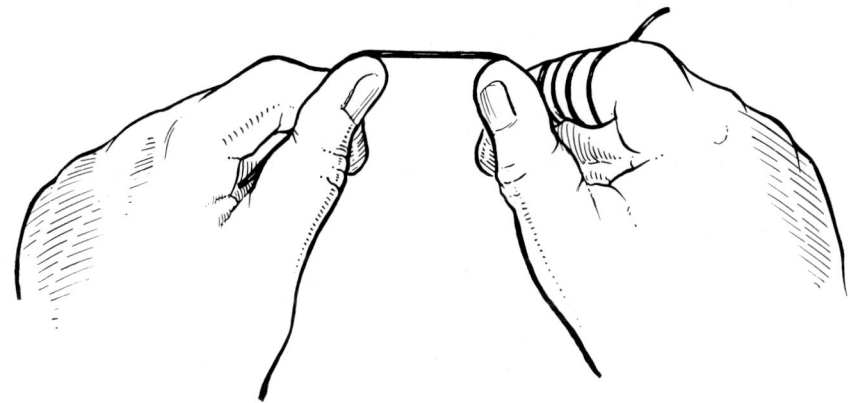

Figure 24–3 The position of dental floss for lower molar cleansing. (From Bass: J. Louisiana Med. Soc., *106*, 1954.)

The very young child cannot be expected to master an effective tooth brushing technique, so it is best to have the parent do the brushing for the child. Starkey[68] has described a technique whereby the child stands in front and leans the head back against the parent. The parent uses one forearm to cradle the head for support and uses the fingers of that hand to retract the lips, leaving the other hand free to do the brushing. Looking over the child gives a good view of the teeth, and the teeth can be easily cleaned, using a scrubbing action on all surfaces.

USE OF DENTAL FLOSS

It is suggested that in certain cases tooth brushing should be supplemented with effectively used dental floss. It has been stated that the best dental floss is that which consists of a large number of unwaxed microscopic nylon filaments having a minimum of twist. To be of any value this material should be used systematically, the floss being passed through the contact point and being drawn along both the mesial and the distal surfaces of the interproximal area. Immediately thereafter the loosened debris should be removed by rinsing the mouth vigorously with water. Although it is recognized that this is a fairly involved procedure, in older children at least it should be included in the hygiene pattern even if it is confined to the mesial and distal interproximal areas of the first permanent molars.

For the best results a length of floss about 18 inches long is cut. One and one-half inches of this is held between the index fingers and thumbs, the excess being wound around the index finger of one hand. After each molar interproximal area is cleaned the used floss can be twisted around the opposite index finger and clean floss can be unwound for use at the new site. This is illustrated in Figure 24–3. If the benefits of this procedure are questioned it should be remembered that Bergman's investigations with topical fluoride showed the improbability of consistently reaching interproximal sites by any other means.

DISCLOSING WAFERS

Many dentists and hygienists use disclosing wafers as an aid in home care instruction. The tablets contain a red vegetable dye (F.D.C. Red # 3 [erythrosin]). After the patient chews the tablet and swishes the saliva between and around the teeth for half a minute, the bacterial plaque is stained bright red. The patient is shown the stained areas and advised that he is brushing but not cleaning the teeth. Instruction is then given on how to position the brush during brushing so that every available surface is cleaned. This is followed by dental flossing. The patient is given a supply of tablets for use in the home to check periodically on the efficiency of the oral hygiene technique. (See Figs. 24–4 and 24–5.)

ORAL RINSING

The use of tooth brushing and dental floss will loosen many particles of food and tooth plaque bacteria. These can be removed by vigorous rinsing with water. The same procedure will, in addition, do much to speed the oral clearance of semifluid carbohydrates. This possible advantage has been explored in considerable detail by one group of investigators. They had 50 test subjects eat a piece of toffee candy in order to saturate the oral cavity with sugar. Six and one-half minutes later, at which time the toffee was dissolved, the mouth was rinsed with water. Analyses for salivary sugar were performed at stated intervals before and after water rinsing. The relative effect of one to three rinsings was observed and the quantity of water used per rinsing was varied from 5 to 15 ml. Repeated rinsings resulted, as might be expected, in a rapid lowering of the salivary sugar level. They did not, however, except in a few cases, bring about a complete elimination of sugar from the oral cavity.

As part of this study, information was accumulated as to the average amount of water selected for oral rinsing in varying age groups. It was found that children 3 to 4 years old use approximately 5 ml. of rinse water. Those in the 5 to 8 year age range were found to choose between 10 and 12 ml. of rinse water. Children in their tenth year used between 15 and 20 ml. of water for oral rinsing. This is comparable to the figure for adults. With this as background information, the effect of a single oral rinsing of 20 ml. of water on salivary sugar was studied in adults. It was found that whereas half of the test subjects had sugar-free saliva within 16 minutes after mouth sugar saturation, all of the control nonrinsing group were positive for sugar at this time. This is illustrated in Figure 24–6. These findings suggest that oral rinsing is of considerable benefit. It is recommended, therefore, that, following the ingestion of carbohydrate snacks, children be instructed to rinse their mouths vigorously two or three times with as much water as can be adequately held in the mouth. It is especially important to do this if it is impractical to brush the teeth at such a time.

Use of a pulsating device for oral irrigation seems to have a place in the oral hygiene program, particularly for patients who wear orthodontic appliances and those who have physical or mental handicaps that would interfere with their effective handling of other oral hygiene devices.

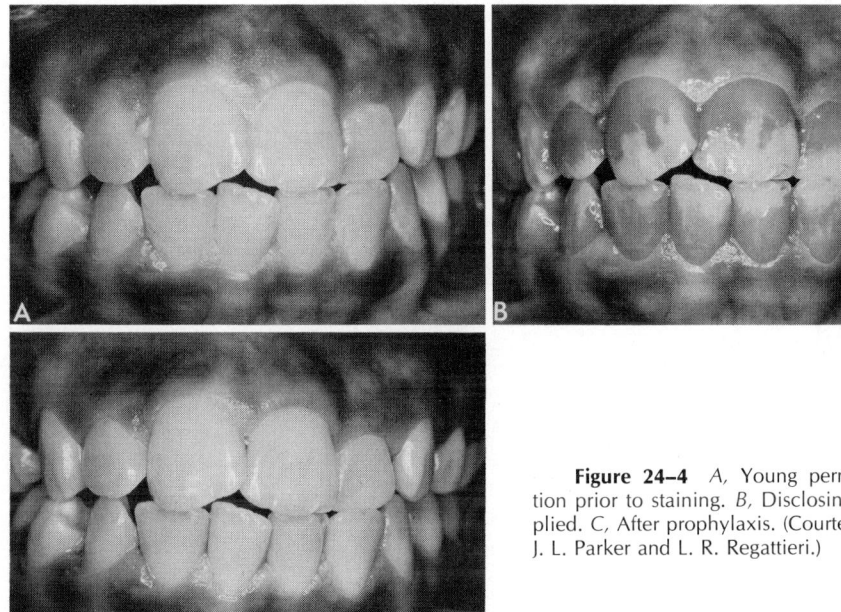

Figure 24–4   *A,* Young permanent dentition prior to staining. *B,* Disclosing solution applied. *C,* After prophylaxis. (Courtesy of Doctors J. L. Parker and L. R. Regattieri.)

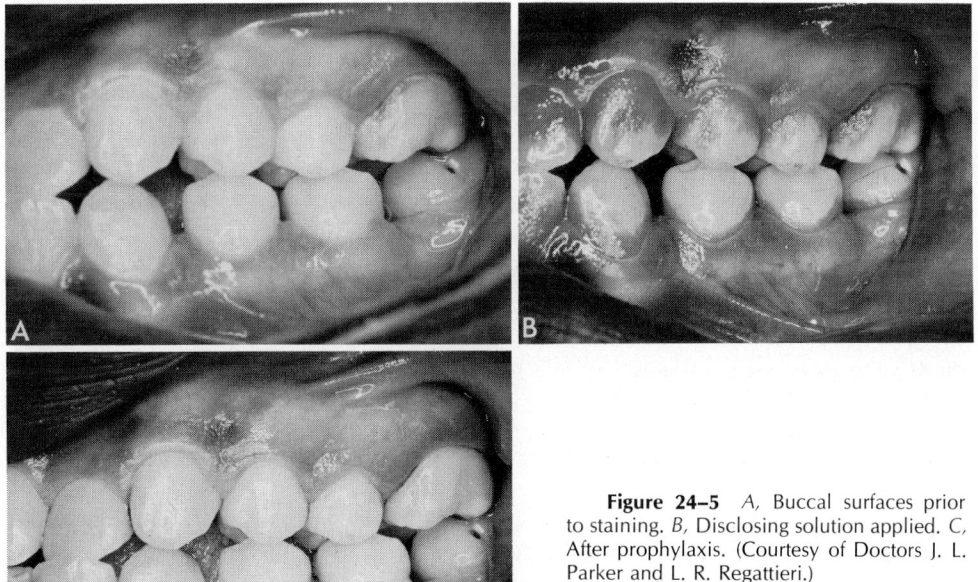

Figure 24–5   *A,* Buccal surfaces prior to staining. *B,* Disclosing solution applied. *C,* After prophylaxis. (Courtesy of Doctors J. L. Parker and L. R. Regattieri.)

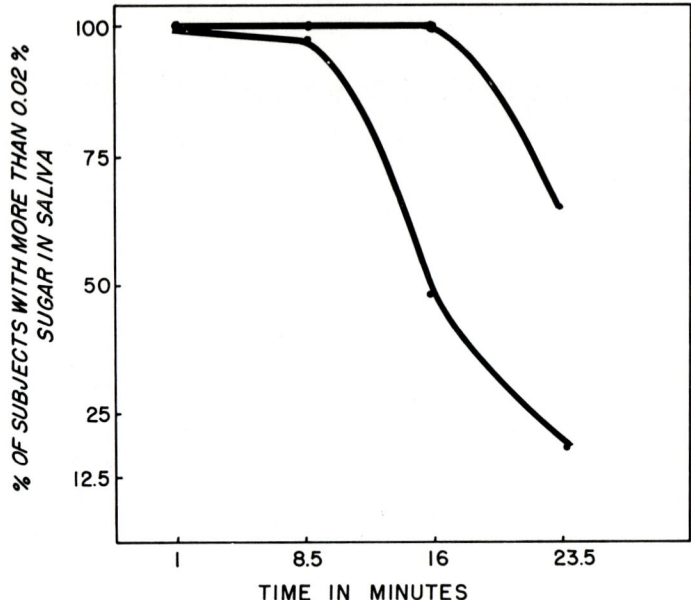

Figure 24–6   The effect of rinsing with 20 ml. of water on oral sugar clearance. (From Lundqvist: Odont. Revy, 3: Supp. 1, 1952.)

THERAPEUTICS

In the preceding section particular attention was paid to techniques that would accelerate the removal of carbohydrate foodstuffs and plaque bacteria from the mouth. It is not only apparent that these techniques are time consuming but even under ideal conditions they do not completely accomplish their objective. This has stimulated a continuing interest in the development of therapeutic dentifrices, mouth washes, and chewing gums. Theoretically, such vehicles would have the usual oral hygiene benefits of removing carbohydrates and bacteria. In addition they might introduce into the mouth agents that inhibit the growth of oral microorganisms or increase the resistance of the dental hard tissues to the products of bacterial fermentation. The reported effects of therapeutic dentifrices, mouth washes and gums will be presented in turn. It should be noted that therapeutic fluoride dentifrices were also discussed in Chapter 22.

AMMONIATED DENTIFRICES

In the early 1930's it was reported that rinsing the mouth with a 0.006 per cent aqueous solution of ammonium hydroxide effectively cleaned the teeth. The same investigators presented evidence that the ammonia content of the saliva of caries-resistant persons was consistently higher than that of caries-susceptible patients. This led the investigators to the conclusion that tooth cleansing by ammonia was brought about by its solvent action on salivary mucin plaque. Some time later an inhibitory effect of urea both on acid formation by glucose-saliva mixtures in the test tube and on tooth plaque carbohydrate fermentation was reported. Since urea could serve as a source of ammonia, these findings also focused attention on a possible therapeutic use of ammonium compounds in dental caries control.

Ultimately, the continuing studies in this field resulted in the development of ammoniated dentifrices. These products were thought to inhibit tooth decay by preventing the breakdown of glucose by oral microorganisms. Since the laboratory tests showed the combination of 5 per cent dibasic ammonium phosphate and 3 per cent urea to have a maximal effect, these were the quantities used in a popular dentifrice formula. A two year test in 341 10 to 11 year olds, however, resulted in only a very slight reduction in tooth decay in an experimental group using the ammoniated dentifrice when compared with the control group who used a comparable dentifrice without the ammonium phosphate and urea. Another study reported shortly thereafter gave essentially negative findings. Both sets of findings are shown in Table 24–2. Although these data indicate that dentifrices of this composition are of no great significance in caries control, there is a possibility that toothpastes with much greater amounts of ammonia compounds and urea may have value in inhibiting tooth decay. Some very limited experimental evidence supports such an opinion. Before this point can be resolved there is need for controlled clinical research in the matter.

PENICILLIN DENTIFRICES

It is of interest that Fleming, the discoverer of penicillin, appreciated the potential use of this antibiotic in preventing tooth decay. It was not, however, until the drug became available for general therapeutic purposes that its action on dental caries was explored. The original studies were quite encouraging. It was noted that when penicillin was applied to the molar teeth of hamsters by daily brushing they developed almost no dental caries even when they were maintained on a highly

TABLE 24–2   AMMONIATED DENTIFRICES AND DENTAL CARIES
IN CHILDREN

INVESTI-GATORS	No. of Subjects		AGES	DURA-TION OF STUDY	SUPER-VISION	DETAIL	RESULT
	EXPERI-MENTAL	CONTROL					
Kerr and Kesel[42]	170	171	10–11 yrs.	2 yrs.	Yes	5% dibasic ammonium phosphate and 3% urea as powder 2x's per day in school 2x's per day at home advised	Slight reduction, 10–20%
Davies and King[18]	171	168	12–18 yrs. 19–31 yrs.	9 mos.	No	5% dibasic ammonium phosphate and 3% urea as powder No supervision	No significant reduction

TABLE 24–3 PENICILLIN DENTIFRICES AND DENTAL CARIES IN CHILDREN

INVESTI- GATORS	No. of Subjects		AGES	DURA- TION OF STUDY	SUPER- VISION	DETAIL	RESULT
	EXPERI- MENTAL	CONTROL					
Hill and Kniesner[33]	108	68	8-15 yrs.	1 yr.	None	Penicillin powder 1000 units per gram; instructed to brush twice each day	No signif- icant reduc- tion in caries
Zander[74]	174	235	6-14 yrs.	2 yrs.	Partial	Penicillin powder 500 units per gram; brushed once each day in school; in- structed to brush morn- ing and night at home	50-60% reduc- tion in caries inci- dence

cariogenic diet. Comparable findings were noted in rats. It was also shown that when students with high oral lactobacillus counts were placed on a dentifrice containing 1000 units of penicillin per brushing a marked reduction in these organisms was achieved within a few weeks. Finally, it was observed that for several hours after the use of a penicillin mouth wash the ability of saliva to ferment carbohydrates was almost completely lost.

As a result of these experiments the action of penicillin dentrifices on dental caries in children was investigated by several researchers. In one carefully controlled study children brushed their teeth with a penicillin powder at school once a day and were instructed to do the same at home in the morning and at night. A 50 to 60 per cent reduction in caries incidence over a suitable control group was reported after two years. In a one year study, however, where children of a comparable age range were instructed to brush their teeth twice a day, but were not subject to any supervision, no significant reduction in tooth decay was noted. These findings are illustrated in Table 24–3. From these studies the tentative conclusion may be drawn that penicillin dentifrices can inhibit dental caries in children provided that their use is closely supervised. If this is not done we are not justified in expecting them to be of any value.

The prolonged use of a penicillin dentifrice has been shown to cause an increase in the number of penicillin-resistant bacteria in the mouth. There is also the possibility of inducing penicillin sensitization in patients. In view of such hazards it is questionable whether penicillin dentifrices should be recommended.

CHLOROPHYLL DENTIFRICES

These materials were used rather extensively in dentifrices some years ago. Although more extravagant claims have been made for their benefits in reducing mouth odors and controlling periodontal disease, some statements have been issued as to their caries-inhibitory properties. These stem from observations that sodium copper chlorophyllin reduces dental caries in hamsters from 67 to 93 per cent when administered at 1:500 and 1:100 concentrations in the drinking water. It has been further noted that chlorophyllin in a 1:400 concentration inhibits acid production in saliva-carbohydrate mixtures. There are also reports that the use of water-soluble chlorophyll results in a reduction in oral lactobacillus counts. Since there is no substantial evidence, however, that chlorophyll dentifrices have a limiting effect on human dental caries, their use by children for these purposes is unwarranted.

SARCOSINATE DENTIFRICES

When the penicillin dentifrices were being developed, evidence was accumulated that they had an extended oral effect. This raised the possibility that penicillin and other compounds entered into at least a temporary combination with tooth plaques where they adversely influenced bacterial metabolism for long periods of time. As a consequence a laboratory test was devised for establishing whether or not therapeutic substances possessed this property.

As a first step the protein casein is exposed to a solution of the test substance. After the experimental solution is removed the treated casein is thoroughly washed with water. Next, it is incubated in a Snyder tube inoculated with saliva from a caries-susceptible individual. If after 72 hours the Snyder tube remains green (no appreciable acid production) it is presumed that the test substance has adsorbed on the protein film and has resisted removal with water but has retained its ability to inhibit acid formation by salivary microorganisms.

Promising compounds are further screened by the same procedure except that salivary proteins are substituted for the casein. If results under these conditions are also favorable, the compound's ability in oral rinse form to inhibit tooth plaque acid formation in the mouth is observed. The overall screening technique is presented in Figure 24–7.

TECHNIQUE OF SCREENING PROMISING SUBSTANCES FOR THEIR
POSSIBLE USE AS CARIES INHIBITORS

1. Casein exposed to solution of test substance
   ↓
2. Casein washed thoroughly with water
   ↓
3. Washed casein added to Snyder tube with saliva from caries active person
   ↓
4. If color change does not occur agent is held for further screening. If color
   ↓   changes study of the substance is discontinued   →
5. Salivary protein substituted for casein and test repeated
   ↓
6. If color change does not occur agent held for further study. If control change
   ↓   occurs   →
7. Agent tested for ability to inhibit acid formation in tooth plaques. If it does
   it is ready for clinical test

Figure 24–7   (From King et al.: J. D. Res., 34, 1955.)

Among the compounds shown to have promise in these tests was lauroyl sarcosinate, which has been popularly designated as an "antienzyme" substance. Fosdick reported in 1956 that in young adults a dentifrice containing 2 per cent sodium N-lauroyl sarcosinate caused about a 50 per cent reduction in caries over a two year period.[25] More recently, several studies have yielded less encouraging results. In two studies, in Holland[4] and the United States,[31] it was shown that the dentifrice caused no practical reduction in dental caries. In another[47] it was shown that a sodium fluoride-sodium N-lauroyl sarcosinate dentifrice likewise was ineffective in preventing caries. Consequently, at the present time such "antienzyme" dentifrices are unlikely to play a major role in caries prevention in children or young adults.

FLUORIDE DENTIFRICES

Extensive investigations of the effects of dentifrices containing fluoride compounds of various types have yielded some encouraging results. Those attracting the most interest at this time are stannous fluoride, sodium monofluorophosphate, acid phosphate-fluoride, and amine fluoride.

After the evaluation of numerous clinical studies, the Council of Dental Therapeutics has rated two dentifrices as Group A: Crest (which contains stannous fluoride-calcium pyrophosphate) and Colgate with MFP (which contains sodium monofluorophosphate and insoluble metaphosphate as the abrasive). This endorsement is qualified by the statement that these dentifrices afford caries protection if a program of good oral hygiene is practiced.

Various experimental designs have been used with different age groups for the study of the two Group A dentifrices, and, in general, results from these studies have upheld the value of their overall effectiveness in a caries preventive program. Some test groups who used the stannous fluoride dentifrice exhibited more dental pigmentation than their controls.

Since stannous and fluoride ions are highly reactive, it has been difficult to formulate a dentifrice to deliver these ions in a reactive state to the tooth surface. A major problem has been that of preventing the fluoride ion and the calcium of the abrasive from forming a relatively insoluble compound. Stannous fluoride calcium pyrophosphate has been reported as a compatible and clinically effective compound. However, in some studies, it has been found that both aging and storage at elevated temperatures have decreased the availability of the fluoride ion. In the search for an improved stannous fluoride dentifrice, an insoluble sodium metaphosphate (IMP) is being tested in three dentifrices: Cue, Tact, and Superstripe. Laboratory tests of these formulas showed stabilization of the soluble fractions of fluoride and tin. The classification of these dentifrices as Group B indicates that studies verifying their effectiveness have been limited in number and that more research is needed to substantiate the current findings.

MULTIPLE PRINCIPLES OF PREVENTIVE DENTISTRY

It has been suggested that the optimal influence of fluorides occurs when a combination of several different procedures is used to combat dental caries.

Muhler[53] has demonstrated that, even in areas where there is a sufficient quantity of fluoride in the drinking water, topical application of stannous fluoride can produce an added beneficial effect. Neutral sodium fluoride topicals, apparently, have no such additive effect.

Despite some variation in the findings of different studies, several investigators have shown that acidulated phosphate fluoride solutions and gels are cariostatic. In a review of the current status of topical fluorides, Horowitz and Heifitz concluded that, in the form of solutions, gels, and pastes, such fluoride treatment is beneficial; and they found that, in communities with and without fluoridated water supplies, a combination of two or more methods of fluoride treatment had reduced dental caries experience by as much as 70 per cent.

In communities without a fluoridated water supply, an effective anticariogenic program might consist of semiannual topical application of either stannous or acidulated-phosphate fluoride in conjunction with the daily use of a fluoride dentifrice. During the developmental period of the teeth, fluoride tablets should also be considered in nonfluoridated areas.

MOUTH WASHES

The mechanical abilities of oral rinsing to remove foodstuffs and bacteria have been discussed in the first section of the chapter. It is obvious that, as in the case of therapeutic dentifrices, there is the possibility of adding bacteriostatic agents to rinse material. In all probability the action on dental caries of substances such as urea, dibasic ammonium phosphate, chlorophyll, penicillin, and sarcosinate in mouth rinse form should be similar to that observed when they are used in a dentifrice. It has been claimed that a mouth wash of sodium p-hydroxymercuribenzoate is particularly effective as a cariostatic agent. Although this has not been extensively tested in controlled human experimentation, it has been shown to be ineffective in limiting caries in the hamster. There also have been studies of the effects of hexylresorcinol, sodium ricinoleate, and sodium alkyl sulfate solutions on the oral flora. Although these and other agents cause a rather substantial immediate decrease in the numbers of oral microorganisms, two hours after their use the numbers of mouth bacteria have usually increased to where they exceed the original level. These findings fail to support the belief that ordinary antiseptic mouth washes are of benefit in the control of tooth decay.

Early animal studies concerning the effects of dextranase on plaque and dental caries in hamsters showed it to have promise as a plaque reducing agent. Molars of hamsters treated with dextranase had a significantly smaller accumulation of coronal plaque than molars of the controls. In the plaque matrix, dextranase was able to degrade microbially produced, extracellular polysaccharides of the dextran type. In recent short-term human studies, dextranase mouth rinses used in an effort to prevent the formation of plaque, or to remove previously formed plaque, have been less effective than was hoped. Long-term human tests will be necessary before it is possible to determine the effect of this enzyme on dental caries and periodontal disease.

Fluoride mouth washes have been shown to be effective. These are discussed in Chapter 22, The Prevention of Dental Caries with Fluoride.

GUM CHEWING

It is well established that the chewing of paraffin and nonflavored, nonsweet-ened gum base will remove considerable numbers of microorganisms and debris from the mouth. This effect results from the normal detergent action of these materials and is enhanced by the increased salivary flow that accompanies their use. The addition of a flavoring agent to the gum base will, it is generally agreed, elicit a further increase in salivary flow. It is argued, however, that when sugar is added to flavored gum base these advantages are minimized or counteracted because the added carbohydrate is cariogenic.

The available evidence does not support this contention. In one study of dental students extending over 18 months, the chewing of four sections of gum for a minimum of 20 minutes a day resulted in no increase in dental caries. It was noted, however, that under standardized conditions this degree of gum chewing could remove an average of 80 per cent of residual oral debris. Attempts have been made to limit dental caries by incorporating bacteriostatic substances in the gum base. In one instance 0.75 mg. of 2-methyl-1,4-naphthoquinone was added to a commercial chewing gum containing calcium carbonate. A substantial reduction in dental caries was described. Similarly, a chewing gum containing 7+ mg. of a furan deriva-tive, furadroxyl, has been reported to reduce significantly the incidence of new caries in subjects highly susceptible to tooth decay. These findings are shown in Table 24–4.

From these observations it may be tentatively concluded that the chewing of gum assists in the removal of oral debris and does not ordinarily increase caries sus-ceptibility.

The use of chewing gum as a vehicle for the administration of fluoride has been investigated by Emslie.[20] Using F^{18} he reported that 80 to 90 per cent of the fluoride, as sodium or stannous fluoride, was released within 10 to 25 minutes of chewing. There was also evidence of the uptake of fluoride by enamel, suggesting that this approach may afford an additional means of administering fluoride to the

TABLE 24–4   EFFECT OF CHEWING GUM ON DENTAL CARIES

TYPE OF GUM ADDITIVE	TYPE OF SUBJECTS	DURATION OF STUDY	CARIES REDUCTION
None[12]	Dental students	18 mo.	13-80%
None[70]	Age 18-32	18 mo.	None
None[19]	Age 8-35	12 mo.	None
None[69]	Primary school	12 mo.	None
Synthetic vitamin K[12]	Dental students	18 mo.	60-90%
Furadroxyl[19]	Age 6-38	12 mo.	80%
Chlorophyll[28]	Adults (bakers)	12 mo.	20% (approx.)
Potassium fluoride[48]	Age 11	12 mo.	None
Dicalcium phosphate[22]	Age 12	30 mo.	52-62%

teeth. Phosphate-containing gums may also prove to be effective anticariogenic agents.

REMINERALIZATION

There is much evidence that the first step in tooth decay is a decalcification of the enamel surface. In the incipient carious lesion there is a loss of translucency without a break in surface contour. This can be duplicated in vitro and in vivo by the careful use of organic acids. The subsequent application to these areas of a complex solution of soluble mineral salts will return the surface to its normal appearance, presumably by remineralization. With the introduction of relief adhesion replica techniques and electron microscopy, additional evidences of microscopic and submicroscopic enamel repair have been noted. These and similar observations have served as a basis for attempting caries prophylaxis with remineralizing powders. Several such preparations are available commercially in a dentifrice powder form. It is usually recommended that they be applied by brushing but that their application not be followed by oral rinsing. It should be emphasized that there is no controlled clinical experimentation that confirms the hypothesis. However, a recent investigation with the artificial mouth has shown that enamel which has undergone extraordinary softening can be rehardened under special circumstances. Also, a clinical study of a mouth wash containing ionic calcium, phosphate, and 3 ppm fluoride has given promising results.[52]

ENAMEL IMPREGNATION

In most instances the loss of enamel translucency is followed by the definite breakdown of the tooth structure. This may be of a very limited magnitude and detectable only with a very sharp explorer point. In the event the change is in the interproximal area a precise bite-wing roentgenogram may be needed to confirm the diagnosis. Although most clinicians advocate cavity preparation at this stage of carious development, there are those who feel the lesion may be arrested by selected therapeutic treatments.

There is also a group of dental clinicians and researchers who believe that the initial point of caries attack is not the mineral components of the enamel. They are convinced that the decay process begins with an invastion of the organic "roads" of the enamel by oral microorganisms. They point to histologic evidence supporting the presence of organic pathways extending from the enamel surface into the underlying enamel or even into the dentin. They also call attention to the presence of bacteria in many of these structures. In their concept of tooth decay the organic structure of enamel is the weak point in caries defense. They believe that it is invaded by and partially destroyed by the oral bacteria. In turn, the products of the interaction of bacteria and the organic matrix weaken and destroy the mineral portion of the enamel. In this view of caries etiology the initial disease mechanism is proteolysis. It should also be noted that even in the more widely accepted concept of dental caries, proteolysis is assumed to play a secondary but important role in dentin decay.

This type of reasoning has been responsible for the use of protein precipitants in caries prevention. The theoretical basis for this therapy is that these agents combine with the structural tooth proteins, making them unavailable for oral microorganism utilization. Two such techniques have staunch advocates. In one of these techniques, the active material is ammoniacal silver nitrate. In the other, it is zinc chloride. In both instances, the active agent is applied to the dry tooth surfaces, with particular care being taken that it reaches the highly caries-susceptible interproximal surfaces. Immediately thereafter formalin is applied to the silver nitrated teeth and potassium ferrocyanide to the zinc chloride treated teeth. The successive use of these reagents results in tooth protein modification. Despite rather extravagant claims for the benefits of these procedures, the preponderance of evidence accumulated in controlled clinical experiments does not support their continued use in caries prevention. The more pertinent findings are summarized in Table 24–5.

It will be noted that in most of the studies an ideal control mechanism has been utilized, namely, the treatment of the teeth in one quadrant, with the dentition in the opposite quadrant remaining untreated. In at least one instance the effectiveness of therapeutic silver nitrate applications has been studied in experimental animals. They were found to be ineffective in both rats and hamsters.

The entire theoretical basis for the therapy has been questioned. Experimentally it has been shown that samples of dentin must be partially decalcified before the organic material can be digested by proteolytic enzymes. Treatment of the partially decalcified dentin with zinc chloride and potassium ferrocyanide prior to its exposure to proteolytic enzymes affords it no protection from destruction.

TABLE 24–5   ENAMEL IMPREGNATION AND DENTAL CARIES IN THE MOLAR TEETH OF CHILDREN

INVESTIGATORS	AGENT	No. of EXPERIMENTAL SUBJECTS	AGES	DURATION	CONTROL	RESULT
Klein and Knutson[46]	Ammoniacal silver nitrate	700	5-12	3½ yrs.	Opposite molars	No reduction in caries
Younger[73]	Ammoniacal silver nitrate	83	8-13	1 yr.	12 subjects	Marked reduction in caries
Ast, Bushel and Chase[3]	Zinc chloride, potassium ferrocyanide plus aqueous silver nitrate	179	12-15	1 yr.	Opposite quadrant	No reduction in caries
Pelton[57]	Zinc chloride, potassium ferrocyanide	100	8-14	1+ yr.	Opposite quadrant	No reduction in caries
Anderson and Knutson[2]	Zinc chloride, potassium ferrocyanide	299	7-15	1 yr.	Opposite quadrant	No reduction in caries

OPERATIVE DENTISTRY

The techniques presented in the earlier part of this chapter have not involved the use of dental instruments. They have been advocated for the prevention of the disease or for its very early treatment. The procedures herein described will be concerned primarily with operative procedures, restorative materials, and surgical procedures. They have been included in this chapter because there is at least some evidence that they may be of benefit in preventing disease extension.

PROPHYLACTIC ODONTOTOMY

"Prophylactic odontotomy" designates a technique popularized by Hyatt and his co-workers.[38] It consists of the removal of defective parts of the tooth so that the tooth is protected from the threatened onset of decay. Those who advocate these procedures point out that the pit and fissure areas of the posterior teeth have a great susceptibility to dental decay. Under the usual circumstances it may be anticipated that they will become carious within a reasonable time after eruption. In the event of rapid progress of the lesion it may involve a great portion of the tooth tissue. This in turn will endanger the pulp and make mandatory extensive restorative work. Both of these possibilities may be minimized by removing caries prone areas such as pits and fissures on posterior teeth, particularly the 6 year molars, and restoring them with amalgam fillings. In a few selected cases in which the defect does not involve the entire thickness of enamel, Hyatt recommends "immunization." This consists of using round burs and stones to convert the defect into a shallow, smooth, rounded fossa or groove that will not retain food debris.

The statistical basis for these beliefs is found in clinical examination of over 12,000 persons 16 to 60 years of age. It was noted that over 52 per cent of the cavities were found on the occlusal surfaces of premolars and molars. Approximately 6 per cent were found on the buccal surfaces of the lower molars, and 5 per cent were observed on the lingual surfaces of the upper molars and lateral incisors. The remaining 37 per cent of the lesions were distributed over the other 130 surfaces of all the permanent teeth. Although comparable data for the primary dentition are not available, observations in 150 school children are of interest. It was found that 9 months after the first examination, 568 out of 616 precarious fissures had developed into cavities. As a consequence of these studies, it became rather standard procedure to practice prophylactic odontotomy in the pits and fissures of the primary molars and permanent premolars and molars of children. The advantages have been summarized by Hyatt:[38]

> "a. Small fillings, hence the minimum possibilities of pulp irritation.
> b. Relatively painless operations, as most of the excavation is within the enamel. This results in the early establishment of confidence between patient and operator.
> c. Extension for prevention is not necessary.
> d. Small and well-finished pit and fissure fillings confer immunity for many years.
> e. The serious injury of deep decay is prevented. The danger of recurrent decay is lessened."

In considering the problem of caries susceptibility it seems probable that the aforementioned data were accumulated in areas of high caries incidence. There is every reason to believe they are higher than would normally be expected in areas where the communal water supply is fluoridated. Since fluoridation is being made available to increasing numbers of children it seems pertinent to consider factors which might modify judgment as to whether tooth structure in a suspected fissure area should be removed and restored by a filling.

Very possibly the researches of Bossert[8, 9] have bearing on this question. This investigator has taken a group of 300 children, 2 to 8 years of age, and has studied the relationship between primary molar cusp height and fissure depth. This has permitted him to place teeth into shallow and deep fissure groups. Subsequently, the caries susceptibility of the shallow and deep fissured molars was noted, and the deep fissured teeth were found to be more prone to decay. Similar observations have been made on the first permanent molar. These data are found in Figure 24–8. From a practical point of view we may say that serious consideration should always be given to prophylactic odontotomy in teeth having high cusps and deep grooves. In posterior teeth with low cusps and shallow grooves the practice of prophylactic odontotomy may be premature.

Modification of Carious Lesions

In discussing prophylactic odontotomy, the high degree of caries susceptibility of the occlusal surfaces of the primary and permanent molars was described. In many instances caries begins in the fissures and quickly undermines almost all of the occlusal surface before it is seen by the dentist. It is not unusual to find first permanent molars one year after eruption with such extensive involvement that they seem indicated for extraction. Even if these teeth can be saved they require exten-

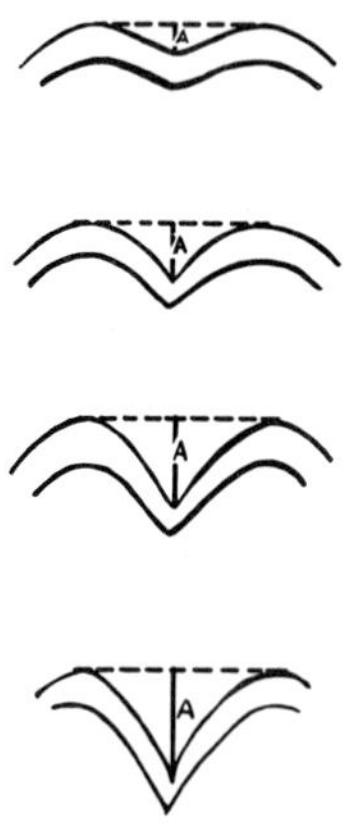

		NO. OF TEETH STUDIED*	% CARIOUS	% NON-CARIOUS
Shallow Fissure		25	20	80
Medium Deep Fissure		25	26	74
Deep Fissure		25	46	54
Very Deep Fissure		25	60	40

DEPTH OF CENTRAL PIT REPRESENTED   *ALL THE PATIENTS WERE 7–12 YRS. OF AGE
   BY VERTICAL LINE A   (AVERAGE 7.5)

Figure 24–8   The relation of upper first molar central pit depth to caries susceptibility. (From Bossert: J. D. Res., *13,* 1933; *16,* 1937.)

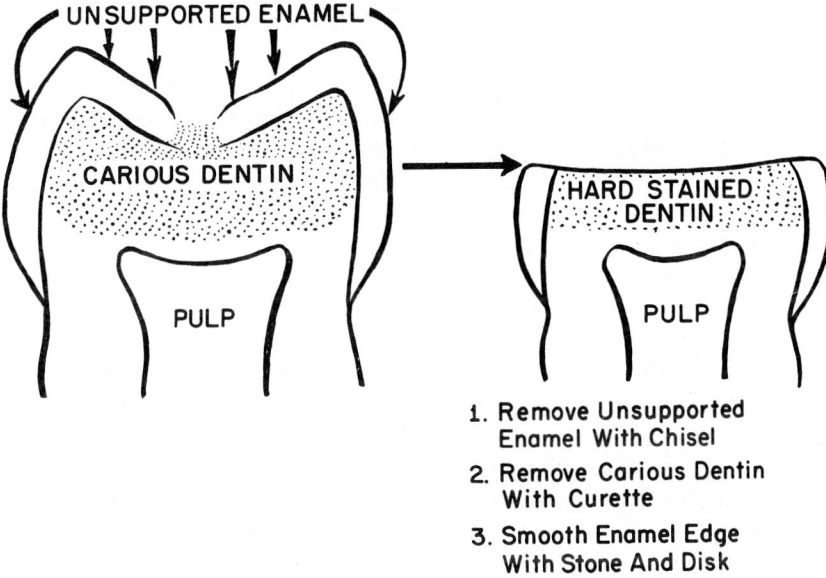

Figure 24-9   Technique for arresting acute dental caries in molars. (From Anderson: J. D. Res., *17*, 1938.)

sive restorative treatment. This in a limited number of instances may not be economically feasible.

In these cases it may be pertinent to consider caries-arresting procedures that do not require extensive restorative work. These are particularly indicated in lesions that have been called "acute dental caries." These involve most of the pits and fissures of the molar occlusal surfaces, in which comparatively little of the enamel structure is lost. In one study 20 of these permanent molars in children and young adults were treated by removal of the overhanging enamel to the level of solid dentin with a mallet and chisel, curetting away most of the mass of necrotic dentin, and finally, smoothing the enamel margin with stones and disks. Follow-up observations from six months to three years later indicated that all treated teeth had either a partial or a complete arrest of the caries process. This was characterized by a hardening and dark staining of the exposed dentin and a disappearance of its sensitivity to thermal changes, mastication, and explorer probing. It seems probable that these changes are attributable to environmental alterations. The surfaces so treated do not favor the accumulation of carbohydrate foodstuffs and may possibly be remineralized by salivary constituents. Dentists contemplating such procedure should recall the possibility of extrusion of teeth in the opposite arch. The steps in the technique are shown in Figure 24-9.

Recently, the value of burring and disking proximal caries in primary molars followed by silver nitrate treatment has been studied. In a group of 7- to 9-year-old children it was noted that one year after such therapy 111 of the 136 teeth had arrested caries. Of the 93 control teeth subjected to the operative procedures without silver nitrate only 16 showed caries arrest. It was concluded that the aforementioned operative procedures followed by silver nitrate application were a suitable preventive treatment for primary molars approaching exfoliation.[65]

FISSURE SEALING

Buonocore has recently proposed a promising approach to the problem of fissure caries. His studies show that caries may be averted if, prior to the initiation of a lesion, the collection of bacteria and food in deep fissures is prevented by the use of resin fillings. The technique is currently undergoing active clinical investigation with good results. Although the procedure requires no conventional preparation in the enamel, successful long-term retention of the adhesive does depend on following the meticulous directions.

The effectiveness of this technique in preventing dental caries was reported by Cueto and Buonocore.[16]

A study of first and second permanent molars and premolars of 269 children aged 5 through 17 years (Figs. 24–10 and 24–11) showed that after one year the treated teeth had 86.3 per cent less caries than control teeth in the same mouth. In this study a loss of the adhesive occurred in 20 per cent of the cases. Parkhouse and Winter used a similar technique and material. In their study, the sealant was not retained and their results were negative. Buonocore later tested an improved adhesive that hardens when exposed to ultraviolet light. One year after application of this adhesive, 200 primary and permanent teeth had been completely protected from caries. These teeth, in the mouths of 60 children, aged 4 to 15 years, were matched with contralateral teeth which developed caries in 42 per cent of the cases.

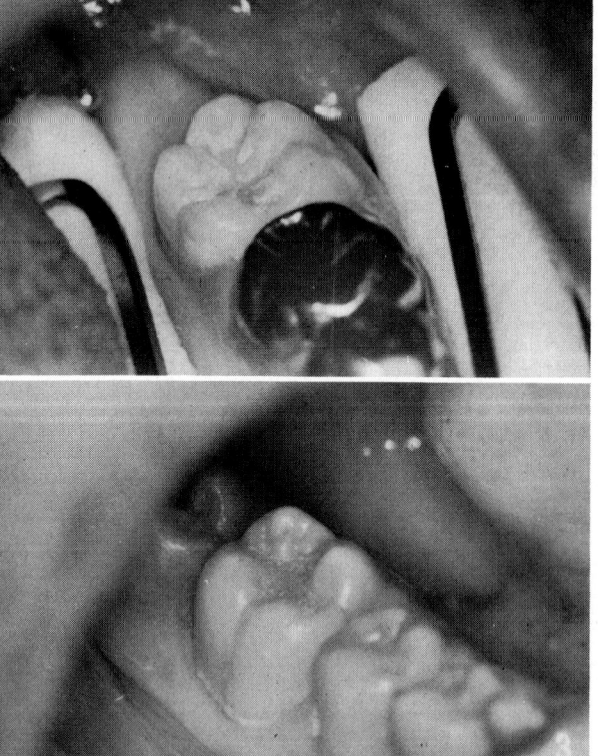

Figure 24–10 Adhesive material remaining on occlusal surfaces after 6 months. (Courtesy of Dr. E. I. Cueto.)

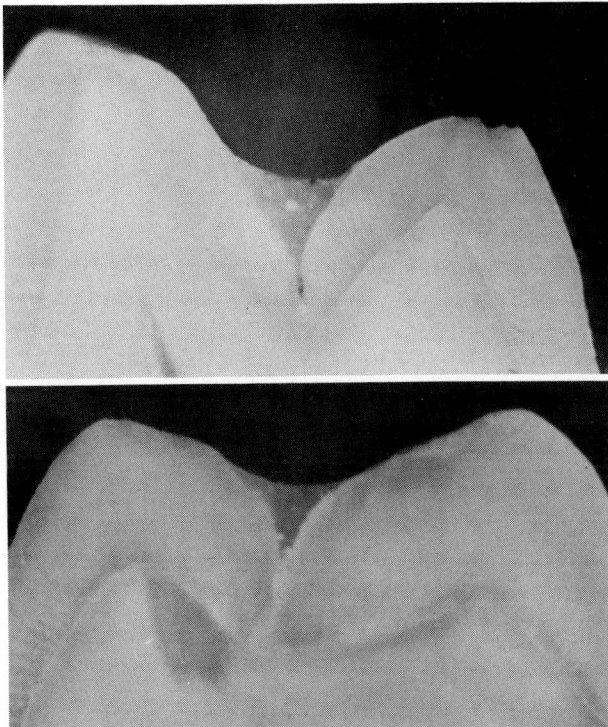

Figure 24–11 Cross section of a molar and a bicuspid showing two types of fissures filled by adhesive resin. (Courtesy of Dr. E. I. Cueto.)

This high level of protection was still in effect after one and one-half and two years. At the end of this two year study, 99 per cent of the permanent and 87 per cent of the primary teeth were still protected from caries. After two years, the sealant had been lost from 13 per cent of the permanent teeth and from 50 per cent of the primary teeth. Success in the use of this technique, like that in other aspects of operative dentistry, is contingent upon strict adherence to the prescribed procedure which, in this case, is as follows: (1) application of the etching solution; (2) application of the conditioning solution; (3) washing with water, keeping saliva contamination to a minimum; (4) drying with warm air for 10 to 20 seconds; and (5) applying the adhesive so as to avoid bubbles.

In 1968, Roydhouse[63] selected 130 children whose molars were judged to be caries free. Half the molars were treated with an adhesive and the remainder served as controls. In this study, protection from caries exceeded 30 per cent. For a period of 2 years, the sealant appeared to protect the teeth and the retention was better in fissures of the maxillary molars.

Pugnier used a fluorocyanoacrylate resin as a sealant for caries reduction in the teeth of children aged 8 to 13 years. Prior to sealant placement, prophylaxis and a subsequent four minute topical fluoride treatment were performed on both treated and control teeth. After two years the treated teeth had 53.5 per cent fewer decayed occlusal surfaces than the controls. This resin required no acid etch or pretreatment to increase adhesion, nor was there need of an external catalyst to expedite setting time. The sealant, however, was not retained after three months. Sealant loss in this study probably resulted from the application of a topical fluoride prior to resin application. In a recent laboratory experiment, the use of acid-etched bovine enamel indicated that bond strength was significantly reduced by applying a topical fluoride before applying the sealant; therefore, it appears clinically advisable to apply sealants prior to routine fluoride topical application.

DETERMINATION OF CARIES-SUSCEPTIBLE AREAS ON THE SMOOTH SURFACES OF TEETH

In many instances the dental practitioner in his oral examination may note unusual tooth surface alterations, particularly in the cervical and interproximal areas. Although it is advantageous for him to know whether these are sites of potential tooth decay, it is a difficult decision to make. From a consideration of the chemobacterial theory of dental caries it would appear that this question could be partially answered if there were evidence of decalcification and food accumulation at the site.

A technique has been proposed to answer this question.[23] It involves the staining of the teeth with a solution of gentian violet saturated in absolute alcohol. Selected segments of the jaw are isolated and thoroughly dried. The test solution is applied to all the surfaces of the teeth with cotton pellets, after which the tooth surfaces are dried with warm air. After mouth rinsing the patient is dismissed with instructions to return in one week. In the interim period he is advised to continue his normal hygiene routine. Areas retaining the stain after the seventh day are thought to be incipient caries and should be considered for restoration. The presence of the stain is indicative of enamel decalcification and insufficient cleansing.

RESTORATIVE MATERIALS AND THE CARIOUS PROCESS

This is largely an unexplored field but the possibilities are worth considering. It seems reasonable to anticipate that new materials will be developed to restore lost tooth structure and thereby tend to limit the recurrence of the caries around margins and on proximal tooth surfaces. Support for this belief has been accumulated in a clinical and laboratory study in which a detailed record was made as to how frequently caries recurred around the margins and underneath inadequate silicate restorations, and whether the nearest surface of the adjacent tooth became carious. It was found that, despite any defects in the restoration, there was little or no evidence of caries in the sites mentioned. Soluble fluorides from the silicate restorations adsorb to the tooth surfaces adjacent to the filling, making them caries resistant. It is known that this restorative material is irritating to the dental pulp, but its use in anterior, proximal, and cervical restorations seems warranted as a measure of caries prevention, provided the pulp is adequately protected with a base.

SUMMARY

Since the carious process is associated with the retention of refined carbohydrates on specific tooth surfaces, good oral hygiene should limit the disease. There is evidence that oral rinsing and the correct use of the toothbrush and dental floss are of benefit in this regard. To be effective, however, they demand a high degree of patient cooperation.

A considerable number of attempts have been made to supplement the detergent properties of dentifrices and mouth washes with therapeutic agents that have bacteriostatic properties. Although extravagant claims have been made for some of these substances, there is need for repeated clinical confirmation before they are endorsed for routine use. Fluoride dentifrices seem to offer the best possibility of reducing caries at the present time. The belief that dental caries can be controlled by topical applications of impregnating and remineralizing materials has not been substantiated. There is need for research evaluating the effectiveness of operative and restorative techniques that have been recommended in the prevention of dental caries.

REFERENCES

1. Anderson, B. G.: Clinical study of arresting dental caries. J. Dent. Res., *17*:443–452, 1938.
2. Anderson, R. W., and Knutson, J. W.: Effect of topically applied zinc chloride and potassium ferrocyanide on dental caries experience. Pub. Health Rep., *66*:1064–1066, 1951.
3. Ast, D. B., Bushel, A., and Chase, Helen C.: A clinical study of caries prophylaxis with zinc chloride and potassium ferrocyanide. J.A.D.A., *41*:437–442, 1950.
4. Backer-Dirks, O., Kwant, G. W., and Starmans, J. L. E. M.: Effect of a sodium lauroyl sarcosinate dentifrice: A clinical investigation. D. Abstr., *5*:371, 1960.
5. Bass, C. O.: An effective method of personal oral hygiene. Part II. J. Louisiana Med. Soc., *106*:100–112, 1953.
6. Berdon, J. K., and Griffin, J. A.: A survey of the toothbrushing habits of dental school students. West Virginia Dent. J., *42*:6–10, 1968.
7. Bixler, D., and Muhler, J. C.: Effect on dental caries in children in a nonfluoride area of combined use of three agents containing stannous fluoride: a prophylaxis paste, a solution and a dentifrice. II. Results at the end of 24 and 36 months. J.A.D.A., *72*:293–396, 1966.
8. Bossert, W. A.: The relation between the shape of the occlusal surfaces of molars and the prevalence of decay. J.D. Res., *13*:125–128, 1933.
9. Bossert, W. A.: The relation between the shape of the occlusal surfaces of molars and the prevalence of decay II. J.D. Res., *16*:63–67, 1937.
10. Buonocore, M. G.: Caries prevention in pits and fissures sealed with an adhesive resin polymerized by ultraviolet light: A two-year study of a single adhesive application. J.A.D.A., *82*:1090–1093, 1971.
11. Buonocore, M.: Adhesive sealing of pits and fissures for caries prevention, with use of ultraviolet light. J.A.D.A., *80*:324–328, 1970.
12. Burrill, D. Y., Calandra, J. C., Tilden, E. B., and Fosdick, L. S.: The effect of 2-methyl-1,4-naphthoquinone on the incidence of dental caries. J. D. Res., *24*:273–282, 1945.
13. Caldwell, R. C., Sandham, H. J., Mann, W. V. Jr., Finn, S. B., and Formicola, A. J.: The effect of a dextranase mouthwash on dental plaque in young adults and children. J.A.D.A., *82*:124–131, 1971.
14. Caldwell, R. C., and Thomas, J. P.: Application of chemical agents for the control of dental caries. Advances in chemistry, No. 94, Dietary chemicals vs. dental caries, American Chemical Society, 1970.
15. Conroy, C. W., and Melfi, R. C.: Comparison of automatic and hand toothbrushes: Cleaning effectiveness for children, J. Dent. Child., *33*:219–225, 1966.
16. Cueto, E. I.: Adhesive Sealing of Pits and Fissures for Caries Prevention. Thesis, The University of Rochester, Rochester, New York, 1965.
17. Cueto, E. I. and Buonocore, M. G.: Sealing of pits and fissures with an adhesive resin: Its use in caries prevention. J.A.D.A., *75*:121–128, 1967.
18. Davies, G. N., and King, R. M.: The effectiveness of an ammonium ion toothpowder in the control of dental caries. J. D. Res., *30*:645–655, 1951.
19. Dreizen, S., and Spies, T. D.: Effectiveness of a chewing gum containing nitrofuran in the prevention of dental caries. J.A.D.A., *43*:147–153, 1951.
20. Emslie, R. D., Veall, N., and Duckworth, R.: Chewing gum as a vehicle for the administration of fluoride: Studies with 18 F. Brit. D. J., *110*:121–127, 1961.
21. Fanning, E. A., and Henning, F. R.: Toothbrush design and its relation to oral health. Aust. Dent. J., *12*:464–467, 1967.

22. Finn, S. B., and Jamison, H. C.: The effect of a dicalcium phosphate chewing gum on caries incidence in children: 30 month results. J.A.D.A., *74*:987–995, 1967.

23. Fisher, W. S.: Determination of individual caries-susceptible areas with a classification of carious patients. J.A.D.A., *21*:1790–1804, 1934.

24. Fosdick, L. S.: The reduction of the incidence of dental caries. 1. Immediate tooth-brushing with a neutral dentifrice. J.A.D.A., *40*:133–143, 1950.

25. Fosdick, L. S.: Clinical experiment on the use of sodium N-lauroyl sarcosinate in the control of dental caries. Science, *123*:988–989, 1956.

26. Frandsen, A. M., Barbano, J. P., Suomi, J. D., Chang, J. J., and Houston, R.: A comparison of the effectiveness of the Charters', scrub and roll methods of toothbrushing in removing plaque. Scand. J. Dent. Res., *80*:267–271, 1972.

27. Garvin, M. H.: A practical analysis of regular dental prophylaxis. J.A.D.A., *20*:27–34, 1933.

28. Gerke, J., and Klimt, W.: Prevention of "baker's caries" through chewing gum medicated with chlorophyll. D. Abstr., *2*:56–57, 1957.

29. Hall, A. W., and Conroy, C. W.: Comparison of automatic and hand toothbrushes: Toothbrushing effectiveness for preschool children. J. Dent. Child., *38*:309–313, 1971.

30. Handelman, S. L., Mills, J. R., and Hawes, R. R.: Caries incidence in subjects receiving long-term antibiotic therapy. J. Oral Therap. Pharm., *2*:338–345, 1966.

31. Hayden, J., and Glass, R. L.: Relative efficacy of sodium N-lauroyl sarcosinate in reducing dental caries. J. Dent. Res., *38*:671–672, 1959.

32. Heifitz, S. B., and Horowitz, H. S.: An appraisal of therapeutic dentifrices. J. Public Health Dent., *30*:206–211, 1970.

33. Hill, T. J., and Kneisner, A. H.: Penicillin dentifrice and dental caries experience in children. J. D. Res., *28*:263–266, 1949.

34. Hine, M. K.: The tooth brush. Internat. D. J., *6*:15–25, 1956.

35. Horowitz, H. S., and Doyle, J.: The effect on dental caries of topically applied acidulated phosphate-fluoride: Results after three years. J.A.D.A., *82*:359–365, 1971.

36. Horowitz, H. S., and Heifetz, S. B.: The current status of topical fluorides in preventive dentistry. Council on Dental Therapeutics. J.A.D.A., *81*:166–177, 1970.

37. Hurst, J. E., and Madonia, J. V.: The effect of an oral irrigating device on the oral hygiene of orthodontic patients. J.A.D.A., *81*:678, 1970.

38. Hyatt Study Club: Prophylactic Odontotomy. New York, The Macmillan Co., 1933.

39. Johnson, R., and Albertson, D.: Plaque control for handicapped children. J.A.D.A., *84*:824–828, 1972.

40. Jordan, W. A., and Peterson, J. K.: Caries-inhibiting value of a dentifrice containing stannous fluoride: final report of a two year study. J.A.D.A., *58*:42–44, 1959.

41. Keller, S. E., and Manson-Hing, L. R.: Clearance studies of proximal surfaces. Parts III and IV: *In vivo* removal of interproximal plaque. Alabama J. Med. Sci., *6*:399–405, 1969.

42. Kerr, D. W., and Kesel, R. G.: Two-year caries control study utilizing oral hygiene and an ammoniated dentifrice. J.A.D.A., *42*:180–188, 1951.

43. Keyes, P. H., Hicks, M. A., Goldman, B. M., McCabe, R. M., and Fitzgerald, R. J.: 3. Dispersion of dextranous bacterial plaques on human teeth with dextranase. J.A.D.A., *82*:136–141, 1971.

44. Kimmelman, B. B., and Tassman, G. C.: Research in designs of children's toothbrushes. J. Dent. Child., *27*:60–64, 1960.

45. King, W. J., Manahan, R. D., and Russell, K. L.: Methods for screening possible inhibitors of dental caries. J. D. Res., *34*:703, 1955.

46. Klein, H., and Knutson, J. W.: Studies on dental caries. XIII. Effect of ammoniacal silver nitrate on caries in the first permanent molar. J.A.D.A., *29*:1420–1426, 1942.

47. Kyes, F. M., Overton, N. J., and McKean, T. W.: Clinical trials of caries inhibitory dentifrices. J.A.D.A., *63*:189–193, 1961.

48. Lind, V., Stelling, Em., and Nystrom, S.: Experiment with chewing gum containing fluorine. D. Abstr., *7*:456, 1962.

49. Lobene, R. R.: 2. A clinical study of the effect of dextranase on human dental plaque. J.A.D.A., *82*:132–135, 1971.

50. Lundqvist, C.: Oral sugar clearance. Odont. Revy, *3*:Supp. 1, 1952.

51. McCauley, H. B.: Toothbrushes, toothbrush materials and design. J.A.D.A., *33*:283–293, 1946.

52. McCormick, J., and Koulourides, T.: A study of neutral calcium, phosphate, and fluoride remineralizing mouthwashes. I.A.D.R. Abstracts, 43rd Annual Mtg., #402, p. 138, 1965.

53. Muhler, J. C.: The anticariogenic effectiveness of a single application of stannous fluoride in children residing in an optimal communal fluoride area. J.A.D.A., *61*:431–438, 1965.

54. Owen, T. L.: A clinical evaluation of electric and manual tooth brushing by children with primary dentitions. J. Dent. Child., *39*:15–21, 1972.

55. Parkhouse, R. C. and Winter, G. B.: Fissure sealant containing methyl-2-cyanoacrylate as a caries preventive agent: clinical evaluation. Brit. D. J., *130*:16–19, 1971.

56. Peffley, G. E., and Muhler, J. C.: Effect of a commercial stannous fluoride dentifrice under con-

trolled brushing habits on dental caries incidence in children; preliminary report. J. D. Res., *39*:871–874, 1960.

57. Pelton, W. J.: Effect of zinc chloride and potassium ferrocyanide as a caries prophylaxis. J. D. Res., *29*:756–759, 1950.

58. Pickel, F. D., and Bilotti, A.: The effects of a chewing gum containing dicalcium phosphate on salivary calcium and phosphate. Alabama J. Med. Sci., *2*:286–287, 1965.

59. Pugnier, V. A.: Cyanoacrylate resins in caries prevention: A two-year study. J.A.D.A., *84*:829–831, 1972.

60. Richardson, A. S., Hole, L. W., McCombie, F., and Kolthammer, J.: Anticariogenic effect of dicalcium phosphate dihydrate chewing gum: Results after two years J. Canad. Dent. Assoc., *38*:213–218, 1972.

61. Ripa, L. W., Buonocore, M., and Cueto, E.: Adhesive sealing of pits and fissures for caries prevention: Report of two year study. I.A.D.R. Abstracts, 44th Annual Mtg., #247, p. 100, 1966.

62. Robinson, H. B. G.: Toothbrushing habits of 405 persons. J. D. Res., *33*:1112–1117, 1946.

63. Roydhouse, R. H.: Prevention of occlusal fissure caries by use of a sealant: A pilot study. J. Dent. Child., *35*:253–262, 1968.

64. Roydhouse, R. H., and Richardson, A. S.: The current clinical status of fissure sealants. J. Canad. Dent. Assoc., *38*:219–220, 1972.

65. Schultz-Haudt, S., Taylor, R., and Brudevold, F.: Silver nitrate treatment of proximal caries in primary molars. J. Dent. Child., *23*:184–186, 1956.

66. Scola, F. P., and Ostrom, C. A.: Clinical evaluation of stannous fluoride when used as a constituent of a compatible prophylactic paste, as a topical solution and in a dentifrice in naval personnel. J.A.D.A., *73*:1306, 1966.

67. Sheykholestam, Z., Buonocore, M. G., and Gwinnett, A. J.: Effect of fluorides on the bonding of resins to phosphoric acid-etched bovine enamel. Arch. Oral Biol., *17*:1037–1045, 1972.

68. Starkey, P.: Instructions to parents for brushing the child's teeth. J. Dent. Child., *28*:42–47, 1961.

69. Toto, P. D., Rapp, G., and O'Malley, J.: Clinical evaluation of chewing gum in gingivitis and dental care. J. D. Res., *39*:750–751, 1960.

70. Volker, J. F.: The effect of gum chewing on the teeth and supporting structures. J.A.D.A., *36*:23–27, 1948.

71. Volker, J. F., Belkakis, E., and Melillo, S.: Some observations on the relationship between plastic filling materials and dental caries. Tufts D. Outlook, *18*:4–8, 1944.

72. Year Book of Dentistry, 1972. Chicago, Year Book Medical Publishers Inc.

73. Younger, H. B.: Clinical results of caries prophylaxis by impregnation. Texas D. J., *67*:96–98, 1949.

74. Zander, H. A.: Effect of a penicillin dentifrice on caries incidence in school children. J.A.D.A., *40*:569–574, 1950.

25

TREATMENT OF THE HANDICAPPED CHILD

by PALMI MOLLER

During the last 20 to 30 years a tremendous change has evolved in the general attitude toward individuals born with physical or mental disabilities. Through the tireless efforts of the medical profession and various health agencies the shroud of superstition and shame formerly attached to the handicapped has been virtually eliminated, and the fact that these unfortunate individuals are human beings with special habilitative requirements is now generally accepted.

Today, parents are aware of the need for expert preventive and restorative dental care for their handicapped children. The dental profession has expended great effort toward fulfilling this need. Dental school curriculums include instruction in special treatment techniques for the handicapped, and a vast amount of research in this field is in progress.

The dental condition of handicapped children may be directly or indirectly related to their physical or mental disabilities. The child born with cleft lip or palate, or both, may suffer also from dental problems of great complexity and severity. Mentally retarded children and those with cerebral palsy, heart disease, and bleeding disorders may not have specific dental problems but their physical or mental handicaps often hinder good oral hygiene and dietary habits, thereby creating a serious threat to their oral health.

The dental treatment of the majority of handicapped children requires no singular effort on the part of the dentist. The dental care of these children can generally be accomplished by the procedures utilized for the normal child. The more severe and complex dental problems afflicting some of the handicapped individuals can be solved by the dentist if he possesses the knowledge, patience, and understanding required for clinical treatment of these children

Despite recognition of the important role the dental profession can and should play in the habilitation of handicapped children, many dentists display a reluctance to accept these children as patients. This reluctance may arise from the dentist's lack of knowledge about the particular disabilities afflicting the children and his unfamiliarity with the various precautions and techniques required for their dental care. For the dentist who recognizes the need in this field and develops the appropriate skills, dental service to the handicapped can be a gratifying experience.

It is our aim to present the salient features of some of the more commonly encountered physical and mental pediatric disabilities, the specific dental problems that often accompany these disorders, and the precautions and clinical management needed to solve these problems. This chapter also includes discussions on the use of both nitrous oxide analgesia and general anesthesia for the handicapped child.

Premedication, which is routinely indicated in the dental treatment of many handicapped children, requires no detailed description here since the use of drug therapy for premedication and sedation of the child patient is discussed in another chapter of this book.

CLEFT LIP AND CLEFT PALATE

Cleft lip and cleft palate are among the most common congenital malformations occurring in man. These structural defects of the facial-oral complex may vary from a slight notching of the lip or a small cleft of the uvula to a complete separation of the lip and absence of the partition between the oral and nasal cavities. In the majority of cases individuals born with cleft lip and/or palate develop various associated defects, such as malformed teeth, malocclusion, impairment of speech, middle ear infections, and a high susceptibility to upper respiratory infections.

With the ever expanding participation of dental specialists in the rehabilitation of individuals with these malformations, it has become mandatory for the dentist to be familiar with the state of knowledge concerning this complex problem.

CLASSIFICATION

Despite a great need, an unambiguous, standardized classification of structural defects of the lip and palate has not been established. A number of classifications have been proposed but none has been universally accepted.

In 1958 Kernahan and Stark proposed a classification of cleft lip and palate founded on morphological and embryological patterns. This classification appears to be the most widely accepted and utilized by researchers concerned with the problem. The basic principles of this classification are listed below:

Group I.   *Clefts of the primary palate.* Within this group are all clefts lying anterior to the incisive foramen, i.e., all forms and degrees of cleft lip, and combinations of cleft lip and cleft alveolar process (usual abbreviation: CL) (Figs. 25–1 and 25–2).

Group II.   *Clefts lying posterior to the incisive foramen.* This group embraces all degrees of clefts of the soft and hard palates (usual abbreviation: CP). (Figs. 25–3 and 25–4).

Group III.   *Combinations of clefts of both primary and secondary palates.* This group involves combination of Groups I and II (usual abbreviation: CLP) (Figs. 25–5 through 25–8).

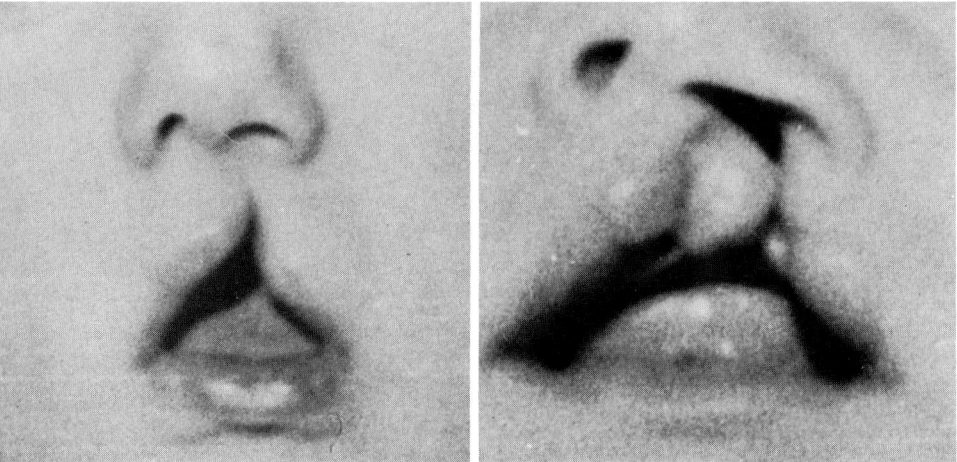

Figure 25–1.   **Figure 25–2.**

Figure 25–1 Unilateral cleft lip — incomplete — (Group I).

Figure 25–2 Unilateral cleft lip — complete — (Group I).

Any of the three major groups described above can be subdivided for more detailed description of the defect. For example, a case of unilateral complete cleft of the right side of the lip with a cleft of both the soft and hard palate would belong to Group III (CLP), and could be further designated as follows: CL-right, complete + CP (S + H).

Since there are embryologic and genetic similarities between Groups I (CL) and III (CLP), most authors have presented data on these two groups in the combined form, as cleft lip with or without cleft palate. This combination is usually abbreviated as CL(P).

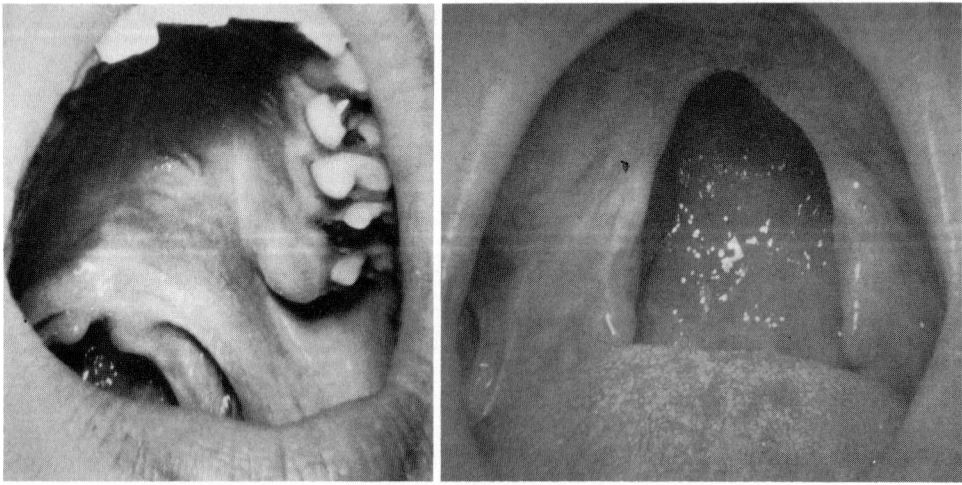

Figure 25–3.   **Figure 25–4.**

Figure 25–3 Cleft palate, involving the soft palate only (Group II).

Figure 25–4 Cleft palate, involving the soft palate and portion of the hard palate (Group II).

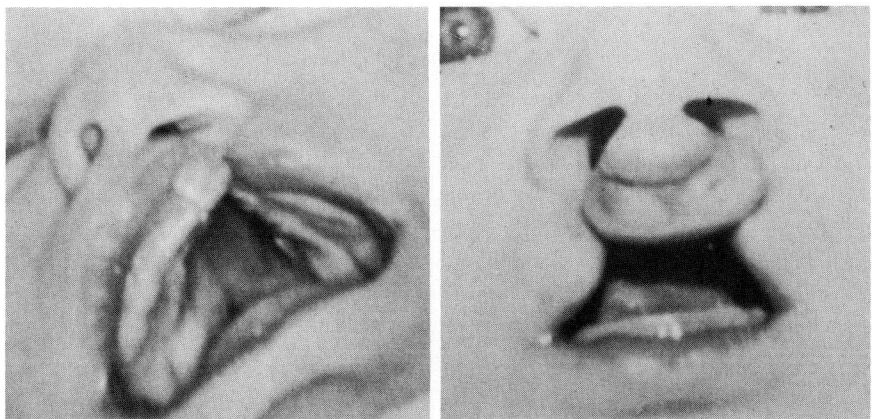

Figure 25–5.   Figure 25–6.

Figure 25–5 Unilateral cleft lip with complete cleft of soft and hard palate (Group III).
Figure 26–6 Bilateral cleft lip with complete cleft of soft and hard palate (Group III).

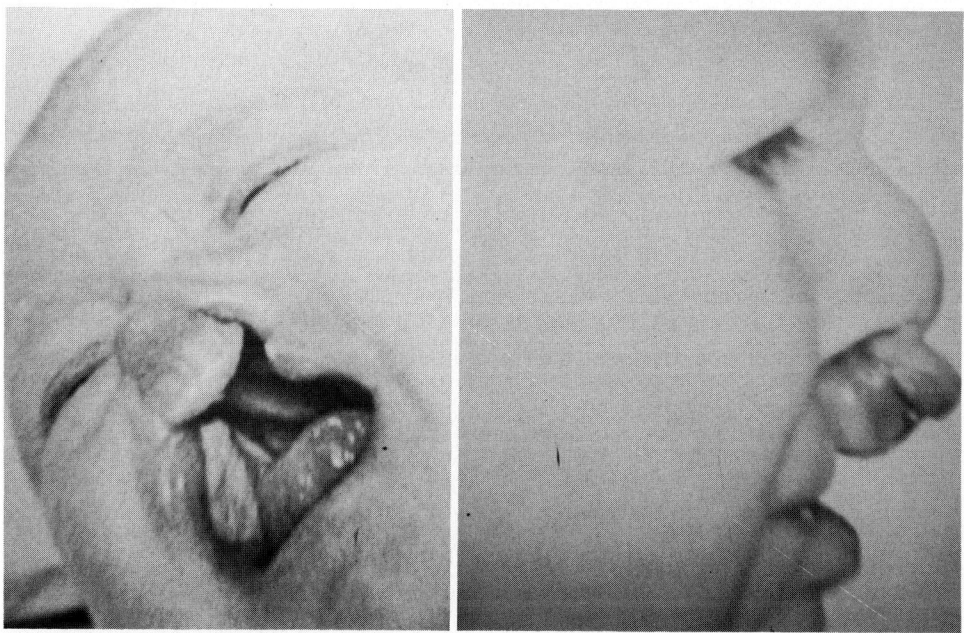

Figure 25–7.   Figure 25–8.

Figure 25–7 Bilateral cleft lip with complete cleft of soft and hard palate (Group III). Note width of palatal cleft.

Figure 25–8 Bilateral cleft lip with complete cleft of hard and soft palate (Group III). Note labial displacement of premaxilla.

PATHOGENESIS

Cleft Lip

Though numerous scientists have sought to explain how clefts of the primary palate develop, it is still a poorly understood problem and the available information is limited and conflicting.

The nonfusion explanation for the occurrence of cleft lip has been virtually abandoned by most students of the pathogenesis of this anomaly. Presently, the "mesodermal deficiency" theory is the most widely accepted as a plausible explanation. This theory suggests that the lip and premaxilla exist in their early forms as an ectodermal hood in which three masses of mesoderm are present. Normally, these masses of mesoderm grow and unite to form the upper lip and premaxilla, but, should they fail to grow and infiltrate the ectodermal hood, a consequent weakening of this delicate membrane induces a rupture of the hood and a cleft lip results.

Cleft Palate

The embryological mechanisms that bring about clefts of the secondary palate are better understood than those leading to clefts of the lip. It is commonly accepted that cleft palate results from failure of the palatal shelves to meet and fuse in the midline. Movement of these shelves from vertical positions on either side of the tongue to eventual fusion in a horizontal position above the tongue, entails a complicated process that could encounter much interference.

Following are some factors demonstrated in animal experiments as possible obstacles to normal movements and fusion of palatal shelves.

    a. Failure to displace the tongue from between the shelves may prevent closure.

    b. Fusion may be prevented because shelves are too narrow to meet in the midline, or because of other structural defects.

    c. Normal palatal shelves may not meet in the midline if an individual has an unusually wide head.

EPIDEMIOLOGY

Incidence

Studies related to the frequency of cleft lip and palate have been conducted in many countries and have generally produced creditable estimates of the incidence of these anomalies.

Based on the available information it can be estimated that one out of every 750 infants, or approximately 6000 to 7000 children with cleft lip and/or palate are born each year in the United States.

A slightly higher incidence for cleft lip and/or palate has been reported for a number of European countries. Reports from Denmark and Iceland have demonstrated a slight increase in the annual incidence of these malformations. This yearly increase may be attributable to the enhanced chances of survival of cleft individuals, or to advances in cosmetic surgery, or both, with a resultant improved likelihood of marriage and reproduction for affected persons.

Of the three major cleft groups, cleft lip with cleft palate (CLP) has highest incidence, accounting for 45 per cent of all clefts, cleft palate (CP) accounts for 30 per cent, and cleft lip (CL) for 25 per cent.

Race

A notable difference in the frequency with which these malformations appear in Negroes, Caucasians, and Japanese has been observed in a number of studies. Negroes were affected least frequently and the Japanese most frequently.

Sex Distribution

The total incidence of clefts is substantially higher among males than among females. Considered by sex and cleft group it is evident that cleft lip (CL) and cleft lip with cleft palate (CLP) are more frequent among males than among females, but cleft palate (CP) is notably more prevalent in females than in males.

Parental Age

The association of parental age with the occurrence of cleft lip and/or palate has been considered in several studies. Although the evidence is scanty, there appears to be a slight increase in the frequency of cleft lip with or without cleft palate (CLP) with advancing parental age, particularly of the father.

Associated Malformations

A number of studies have shown that, in individuals born with cleft lip and/or palate, there is an increased likelihood of other congenital malformations.

Approximately 10 to 20 per cent of the individuals with clefts of the lip and/or palate have one or more other congenital anomalies. Additional malformations are found more frequently in the isolated cleft palate (CP) group than in the other groups.

Associated anomalies most commonly noted are defects of the extremities (Figs. 25–9 and 25–10) and congenital heart disease.

ETIOLOGY

The exact etiology of cleft lip and/or palate is still unknown; however, recent research has shed new light on the possible causal factors of such malformations.

Generally accepted information on the etiology of these malformations are briefly summarized as follows:

1. Exogenous Factors

In only a few isolated cases, in which the syndromes resulted from rubella or thalidomide, have clefts of the lip and/or palate been proved attributable to a specific environmental agent.

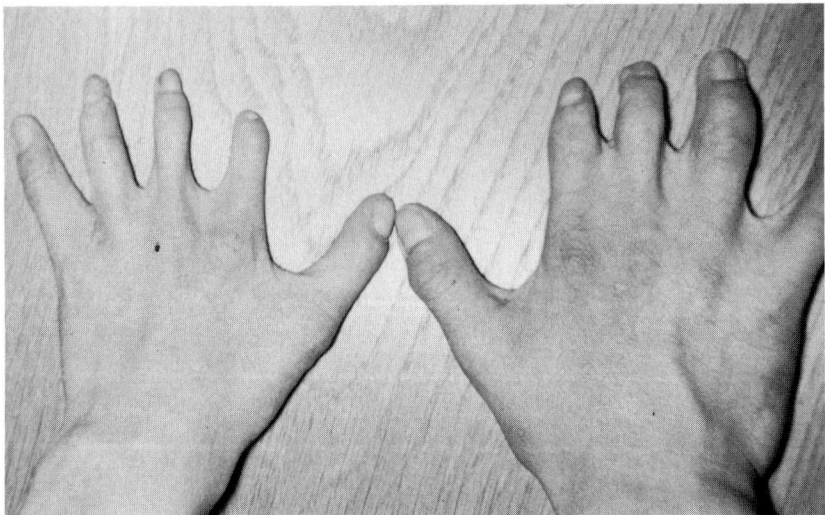

Figure 25–9 Syndactyly (webbed fingers) in a patient with cleft palate.

2. Mutant Genes and Chromosomal Aberrations

Clefts of the lip and/or palate occur as one of the features in a number of the rare syndromes that have been ascribed to (1) mutant genes, such as cleft lip and palate with ectodermal dysplasia, and (2) chromosomal aberrations, such as D-trisomy and E-trisomy.

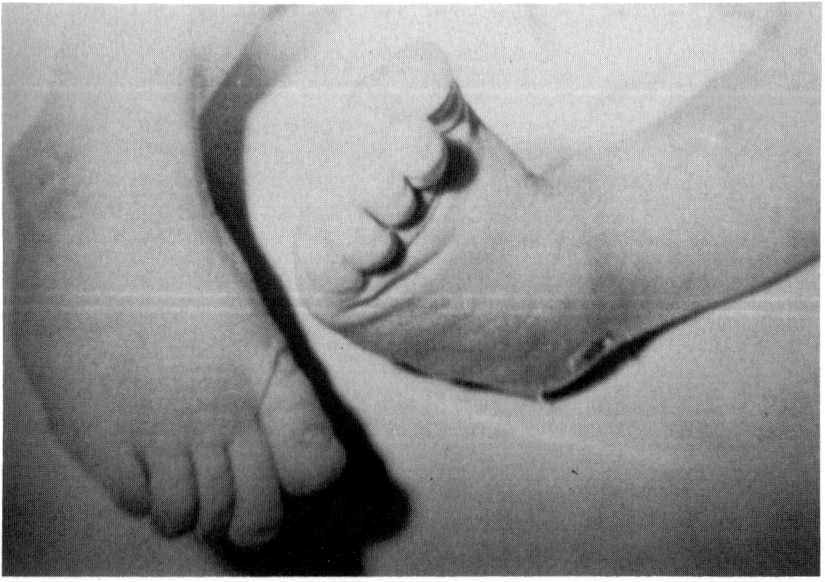

Figure 25–10 Malformation of lower extremities in a patient with unilateral cleft lip with cleft palate.

3. MULTIFACTORIAL CAUSES

It is considered most likely that the majority of clefts of the lip and/or palate are caused by a combination of exogenous factors and a gene-pattern that is predisposing to these malformations. Heredity is now commonly credited with playing a major role in the etiology of cleft lip and/or palate. Though several modes of transmission have been suggested, the theory with the most widespread support from researchers in the field is that of polygenic inheritance, wherein inheritance is believed to be determined by the effects of many genes, each with a relatively small influence.

Risk Figures

The manner of inheritance has not been fully clarified; however, information from a number of detailed family studies provided a basis for some empiric risk figures. It must be remembered that these figures represent averages and are applicable only when known chromosomal and genetic syndromes have been eliminated as a possible cause of the malformations in the patient.

The dental practitioner should not be expected to undertake the often delicate procedure of genetic counseling. Nevertheless, he should be aware of the available information concerning the risk of recurrence in some of the more common situations that are briefly described below:

1. If unaffected parents have a child with a cleft lip with or without cleft palate (CL(P)), the risk of recurrence of the defect in each subsequent child is approximately 4 per cent, or 1 chance in 25. With cleft palate (CP) the risk figure decreases to approximately 2 per cent.
2. If one parent is affected, the risk that his offspring will be similarly affected is 4 to 6 per cent. If an affected parent has an affected child, the risk for any subsequent children rises to about 1 chance in 6.

TREATMENT

Because of the complexity of congenital malformations of the lip and/or palate, the "team approach" has been recognized as the only intelligent method of treatment and rehabilitation of the unfortunate persons born with these anomalies. Recognition of this need for concerted action by representatives of various specialties for diagnosis and planning treatment of cleft lip and/or palate has, in many countries, led to the establishment of numerous cleft palate clinics staffed by highly skilled plastic surgeons, pediatricians, pedodontists, orthodontists, prosthodontists, speech and hearing specialists, and sociologists.

In most instances the primary functions of the cleft palate clinics are the evaluation and planning of the habilitative needs of the patients. The responsibility of fullfilling these needs eventually rests with the practicing members of the various specialties involved. To obtain optimal rehabilitation of the cleft lip and/or palate patient, it is imperative that each member of the disciplines involved have at least a general concept of the problems and procedures faced by other members of the "treatment team."

Surgical Treatment

The fundamental principles of the surgical procedures consist of repositioning and suturing the cleft parts. It is not within the scope of this textbook to dwell on an extensive and detailed description of the surgical treatment of cleft lip and/or palate; therefore, only the general aspects of the surgical procedures will be touched upon.

Surgical closure of the cleft lip is usually performed between 2 and 12 weeks of age. Several techniques are available for accomplishing this surgery. The choice of a method is dictated by the surgeon's experience with the various techniques and the morphological conditions of the cleft. It is readily understandable that a different approach is indicated with an uncomplicated unilateral cleft lip than that required with the complex problem of a complete bilateral cleft of the lip with a grossly displaced premaxilla and associated nasal deformity.

The optimal age of the patient at which closure of the cleft palate should be attempted arouses some controversy. However, most surgeons favor performing this operation when the patient is 18 to 24 months old.

The ultimate goal of cleft palate surgery is the provision of a mechanism that adequately separates the patient's oral and nasal cavities so as to cause no interference with the growth of the facial bones or with the development of normal speech, hearing, and dental occlusion.

Of the several accepted operative techniques for closing a cleft palate, the basic principle in most involves the use of mucoperiosteal flaps, which are obtained from the bony palatal shelves and brought together in the midline. Frequently the surgeon combines this midline closure with a so-called push back of the flap, a procedure for providing adequate length of the soft palate to permit velopharyngeal closure during speech and swallowing.

If the surgeon judges that adequate velopharyngeal closure cannot be obtained by this method he may create a tissue bridge between the pharynx and the soft palate. This is accomplished by dissecting a flap from the posterior wall of the pharynx, extending it forward, and suturing it to the denuded posterior border of the soft palate.

The last two or three decades have witnessed tremendous improvements in the cosmetic and functional results of cleft lip and palate surgery. Despite these advances we occasionally encounter cleft individuals whose surgical results appear far from satisfactory. Persons who are inclined to classify these cases as surgical failures might well reconsider their judgment had they the opportunity of observing and evaluating the magnitude of the facial and oral defects with which the surgeon is confronted in many of these cases.

Dental Treatment

The presence of clefts of the lip and/or palate in the newborn may give rise to various dental problems. Many dentists admittedly are apprehensive of accepting as patients persons with these congenital malformations. This apprehension possibly arises from a tendency to label these individuals as problem patients and the failure to realize that people born with cleft lip and/or palate are human beings with some special dental problems.

Many of these patients are understandably sensitive and depressed, but, with a little extra patience and understanding, the dentist can usually overcome these barriers to cooperation. In most instances he is deeply rewarded by the gratitude expressed for his efforts to improve the person's oral health and appearance.

Although the magnitude and severity of dental problems associated with clefts of the lip and/or palate may demand extra skill and patience of the dentist, he can realize tremendous satisfaction from the knowledge that he has fulfilled his important role in the overall habilitation of these patients.

The extent of dental care needed by these patients may vary considerably and is usually dictated by the severity of the original malformation. Some patients, such as those born with cleft of the soft palate only, may need only the routine dental care extended to all dental patients. With increased severity of the original cleft the number and severity of the patient's dental problems increases. None of the problems is insurmountable and most do not require the services of specialists.

In some cases the dentist may become involved in the habilitation process immediately after the birth of the patient. The dentist may be called upon to fabricate an appliance resembling an upper denture base. This appliance serves two purposes: (1) it facilitates the feeding of the cleft palate infant, and (2) it prevents the collapse of the maxilla. The appliance is processed in acrylic resin on a cast of the child's palate. An impression tray is made from baseplate wax that is softened in warm water and adapted against the child's palate and musculature. After smoothing and reinforcing the tray, an impression is obtained by using a thin film of alginate impression material. A wax pattern is fabricated on a stone cast obtained from the impression. The wax pattern is then processed in clear acrylic resin, trimmed, and polished.

As a rule, the initial visit to the dentist is made when the patient is between 2 and 3 years old. At this time the deciduous dentition is developing and surgical closures of the clefts have been completed. On the first few visits the child should be examined, receive light prophylaxis, and be allowed to familiarize himself with the dentist and his surroundings. Because of the shape of the surgically treated palate, some difficulty may arise in taking radiographs. However, it is essential that these diagnostic aids be obtained, at approximately four years of age, for detection of caries and determination of supernumerary, congenitally missing, or malformed teeth.

Cavity preparations in the cleft lip and/or palate patient do not vary from the accepted procedures used for the normal child. Topical and local anesthesia should be used, whenever indicated. Many of these children are mouth breathers because of a deviation of the nasal septum that is frequently associated with the facial-oral clefts. Interference with their breathing during operative procedures may create a high degree of anxiety in these patients. Usually the dentist can overcome this problem by reassuring the patient, by limiting the use of cotton rolls, or by the use of a rubber dam with large air holes.

Patients with cleft lip and/or palate frequently have supernumerary teeth in both the deciduous and permanent dentitions. In the former, such teeth are either allowed to exfoliate naturally, or extraction may follow loss of adjacent teeth. The majority of supernumerary teeth in the permanent dentition are removed at the earliest convenient time.

Congenitally missing teeth are seen in approximately 50 per cent of cleft lip and/or palate patients. The space normally occupied by congenitally missing teeth, or by teeth lost prematurely, must, in the majority of cases, be carefully maintained. Teeth missing in the anterior area should be replaced, primarily for esthetic reasons. The artificial teeth can be attached to an acrylic plate, which the children usually retain in the mouth with no difficulty.

Dental enamel hypoplasia is often seen in the cleft lip and/or palate patient. This defect occurs most frequently on the central and lateral permanent incisors immediately adjacent to the cleft site. Whenever possible these teeth should be restored even if this demands the placement of stainless steel crowns. Preservation of these teeth is of vital importance for their eventual use as abutments for individual crowns or dental bridges.

Orthodontic problems are usually associated with all clefts that involve the alveolus or the hard palate, or both. While the family dentist or pedodontist can in many instances utilize his training in preventive orthodontics in the care of these patients, the majority of these problems need evaluation and treatment by a well trained orthodontist.

Special prosthetic appliances are sometimes required for optimal habilitative results of the cleft lip and/or palate patients. These appliances may be needed to improve the patient's speech or appearance and sometimes both. The improvement of the appearance of individual teeth and the replacement of missing teeth by the fabrication of crowns or dental bridges can be successfully accomplished by most dentists (Fig. 25–11). On the other hand, the often delicate and painstaking procedures involved in the fabrication of speech appliances should be referred to a prosthodontist with special training in this field.

Most of these speech appliances consist of a partial denture framework with an extension of the metal frame into the cleft area. This extension, which is covered with processed acrylic, provides adequate closure of the velopharyngeal space during speech and swallowing (Fig. 25–12).

In cleft palate patients in whom the maxilla is markedly underdeveloped in relation to the mandible, fabrication of an overlay denture may be necessary for improved occlusion and appearance (Fig. 25–13).

Since retention of prosthetic appliances presents a major problem in an edentulous cleft palate patient, preservation of teeth for eventual retention of these appliances is of the utmost importance. When teeth are used as abutments for dental prostheses, they should be restored with crowns or copings to prevent possible future breakdown by dental caries, as well as to provide ideal retention for the prostheses.

Speech and Hearing Treatment

It has been estimated that, of the individuals with clefts involving the hard and/or soft palate, approximately 50 per cent suffer from some type of speech impediment.

One of the primary goals of all treatment procedures previously described in this section is to create a mechanism that will allow the patient to attain normal speech. Most of these procedures could not achieve this goal without special speech training of the patient. The complexity of speech pathology and its treatment is discussed in a special chapter in this book.

Hearing problems are often associated with clefts of the palate. These problems are usually caused by middle ear infections, which are, in turn, due to the increased exposure of the Eustachian tube to bacteria and food in the patient with cleft palate. While it is not within the compass of the dental profession to treat these

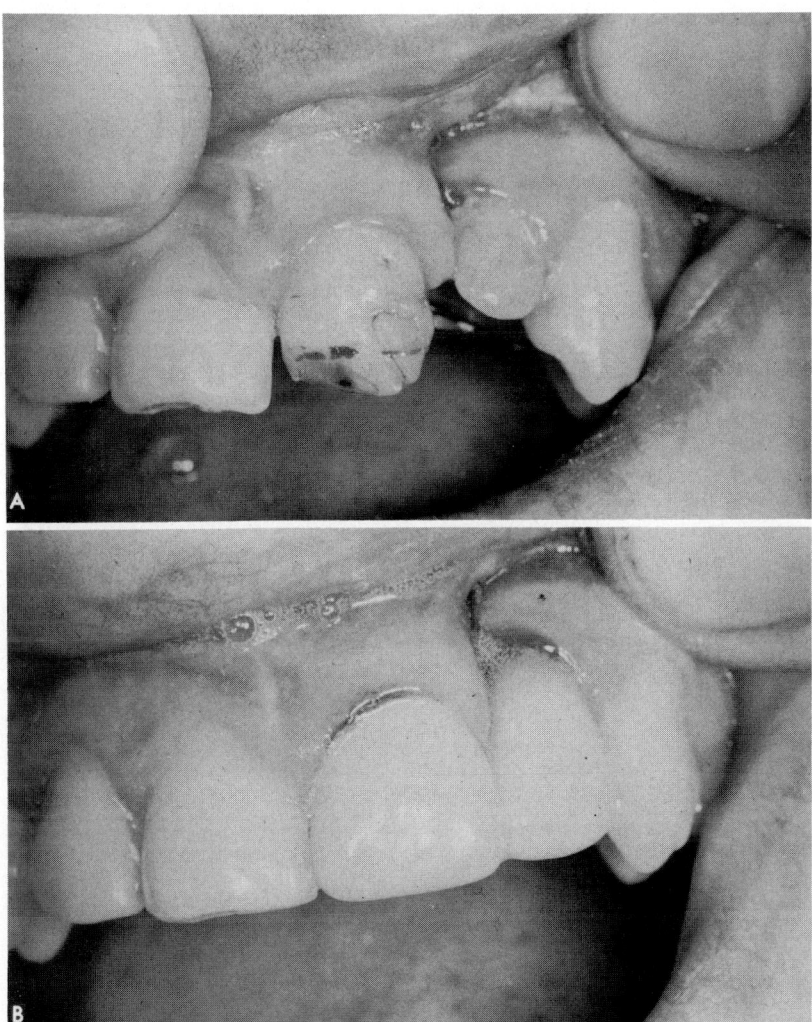

Figure 25–11 Anterior bridge for a patient with cleft lip. *A,* Enamel hypoplasia of maxillary central and displacement of maxillary lateral. *B,* Maxillary central and lateral restored with a two unit bridge (porcelain-on-gold). The crowns were splinted for stabilization. (Courtesy of Dr. W. Powell.)

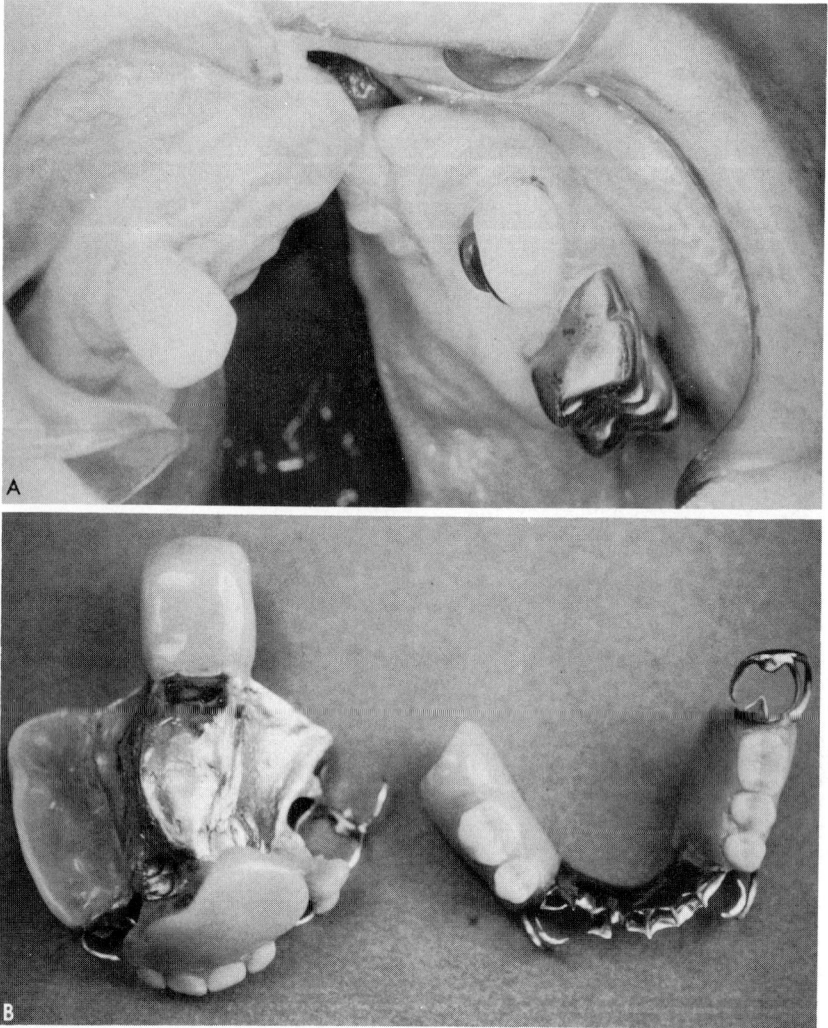

Figure 25–12 Prosthetic appliances for a patient with cleft palate. *A,* Abutment teeth restored with crowns for protection against future caries attack and retention for prosthetic appliance. *B,* Maxillary and mandibular removable prosthesis. Note extension of obturator into velopharyngeal area on maxillary appliance. (Courtesy of Dr. D. Castleberry.)

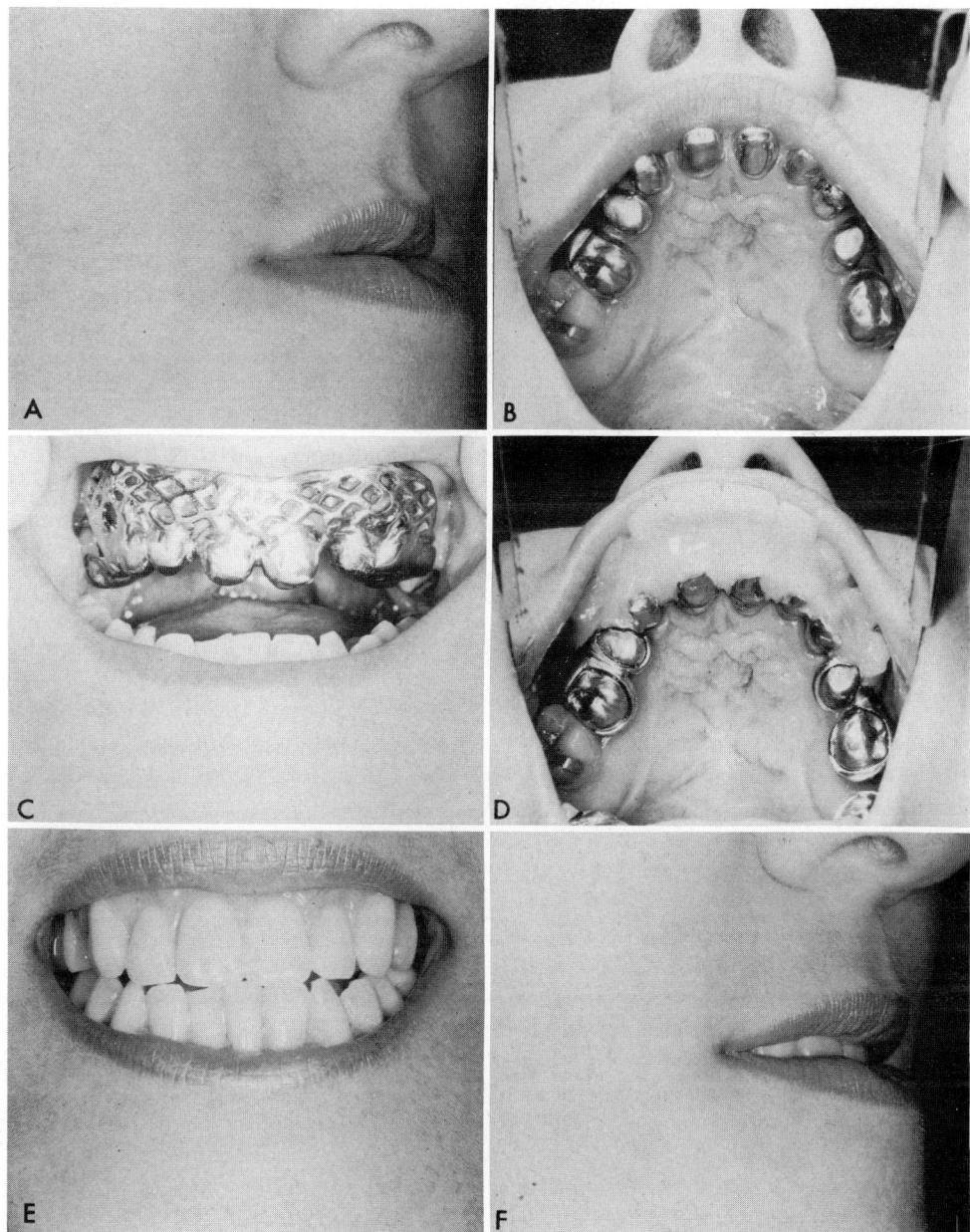

Figure 25–13 Overlay denture for a patient with cleft palate. *A,* Side view of patient. Note underdevelopment of maxilla. *B,* Teeth restored with copings and crowns. *C,* Metal framework for overlay denture. *D,* Palatal view of denture. *E,* Anterior view of prosthesis. *F,* Side view of patient after insertion of denture. Note improvement in appearance. (Courtesy of Dr. D. Castleberry.)

problems, the dentist caring for the cleft lip and/or palate patient must be aware of the possibility that the patient may be suffering from a serious loss of hearing, which can hinder the necessary dentist-patient communication and cooperation.

CEREBRAL PALSY

Cerebral palsy is the most severely handicapping problem affecting the new-born. Approximately 50 per cent of cerebral palsied children either die in infancy or are so damaged as to require institutional care.

This disease is a central nervous system disorder which manifests itself as various types of neuromuscular dysfunctions such as spasticity, athetosis, ataxia, rigidity, or tremor.

Since each type poses a somewhat different challenge, the dentist should familiarize himself with the main aspects of the various neuromuscular disorders and ascertain the type with which his patient is troubled before any treatment is planned for the child. The three most common types of neuromuscular dysfunctions are spasticity, athetosis, and ataxia.

Spasticity, observed in approximately 40 per cent of children with cerebral palsy, is characterized by hypercontractility of the muscles and a general stiffness in the affected parts. This stiffness may be so pronounced that the extremity cannot be moved passively.

Athetosis, characterized by purposeless, involuntary muscular contractions, is observed in approximately 45 per cent of children with cerebral palsy.

Ataxia, or loss of muscle coordination, is characteristic of approximately 10 per cent of cerebral palsied children. This loss of muscular coordination produces a lack of balance and an unsteady gait.

For further classification the area affected by this disorder may be described by the following terms:

Hemiplegia—involvement of one half the body
Quadriplegia—involvement of all four limbs
Paraplegia—involvement of the legs only
Monoplegia—involvement of one limb

Children with cerebral palsy have a high incidence of mental retardation. It has been estimated that 36 per cent have IQ's below 50, and 21 per cent have IQ's between 50 and 70. The highest incidence of mental retardation has been observed in the spastic group and the lowest in the athetoids. Despite this high incidence of mental retardation among cerebral palsied children, and because of those whose abnormal facial and physical postures leave the impression of retardation, the dentist must recognize that the degree of achievement and cooperation of which each patient is capable varies greatly and must be evaluated individually.

ETIOLOGY AND INCIDENCE

Cerebral palsy is caused by brain lesions that may result from prematurity, anoxia, toxemia of pregnancy, traumatic injuries, or they may be of unknown etiology. The location of the brain lesion determines the type of neuromuscular dysfunction by which the disorder manifests itself. Lesions of the cerebral cortex are manifested by spasticity; damage to the basal ganglion results in athetosis; and ataxia is caused by lesions of the cerebellum.

Cerebral palsy is the most common of all the central nervous system disorders. Recently, it was estimated that 200,000 children in the United States suffer from this disability.

DENTAL PROBLEMS

Most cerebral palsied children have a higher caries rate than normal children. This increase can be attributed to their inability to maintain good oral hygiene, to their parents' tendency to indulge them with soft and cariogenic food, and to the increased prevalence of enamel hypoplastic defects of their teeth.

The poor oral hygiene and soft diet also contribute to a significant increase and severity of periodontal disease in the cerebral palsied as compared with normal children.

Many investigators have reported a higher evidence of malocclusion in these children, which can be attributed to the abnormal muscle function and the unnatural tongue position that is characteristic of the cerebral palsied.

Most children with cerebral palsy can be provided with satisfactory dental care in the routinely equipped dental clinic, if the dentist is cognizant of their mental and physical limitations and of the precautionary measures needed for their dental treatment. Only a small percentage of these children will require general anesthesia to make it possible for the dentist to treat them.

Dental Treatment

With the exception of increased rates of caries and periodontal disease, the majority of children with cerebral palsy exhibit no specific dental problems. The chief concern of the dentist responsible for their dental care is a matter of adjusting his procedures of management to the physical and mental condition of the individual patient. Success is possible if the dentist secures a thorough personal history of the child prior to his initial visit to the dental clinic. This information must be gathered from the parents or custodians and from the attending physician.

The dental care of the handicapped child can be accomplished only through the well coordinated teamwork of the dentist and his auxiliary personnel. To achieve the needed cooperation, the dentist must make available to his dental assistant all of the pretreatment information regarding the patient, so she can prepare adequately for her important role in the dental treatment of the child.

After obtaining all available information regarding the physical and mental characteristics of the cerebral palsied child, the dentist should make his own evaluation when the patient first visits the dental clinic. This visit should also be utilized for treatment planning and to afford the patient an opportunity to get acquainted with his surroundings and with the people who will participate in his dental care.

Because many of these children lead a sheltered life and are unaccustomed to strangers, the dentist may anticipate that they will be highly apprehensive. In cases in which use of drug therapy for *premedication* purposes is indicated, the child's physician should be consulted regarding the choice of premedication. Chlordiazepoxide hydrochloride (Librium) is the drug most widely used for reducing both anxiety and muscle spasm.

The handicapped child should be made as comfortable as possible in the dental chair. A chair adjusted to a tipped back position gives more support and a feeling of security to the patient, which is especially important to the child with ataxia. The spastic child may need even more support and control of a type that can best be given by the dental assistant. *Restraining* procedures such as the use of straps are rarely necessary and may hinder rather than aid in management of the child, since excessive restraint may provoke extreme involuntary muscle spasm.

If it can be safely administered, there are no contraindications to the use of *local anesthesia* for the cerebral palsied child. The dentist must be prepared for sudden movements of the patient's head and the syringe must be firmly supported while the injection is being made.

Mouth props are routinely indicated during restorative procedures, since they will prevent injury to the patient or to the dentist should the jaws suddenly be clenched. Props should be removed from the patient's mouth for frequent rest periods as the child's muscles tire easily.

Any small supplies, such as mouth props, cotton rolls, and rubber dam clasps, which might be easily dislocated in the child's mouth, should be securely attached to a length of dental floss for quick removal to prevent their aspiration by the patient. The cough reflex is frequently delayed in these children, therefore liberal use of aspirating equipment is essential for removal of any debris in the oral cavity.

The importance of preventive dentistry for the handicapped child cannot be overemphasized. Satisfactory dental service to those individuals necessitates that the dentist spend much time in making their parents or custodians aware of the available measures for preventive dentistry. The proper tooth brushing techniques must be repeatedly demonstrated, and the importance of limiting the use of cariogenic food must be stressed. If the child is living in an area where the drinking water is not fluoridated, the use of fluoride tablets should be recommended.

EPILEPSY

The term epilepsy, which refers to a symptom, not to a disease, is of Greek origin and means "to seize." Various disorders may cause abnormal neuronal discharge in the brain that may induce a seizure. If these seizures are recurrent, the condition is termed epilepsy, and may affect a person by a change in the state of consciousness, an abnormal sensory experience, tonic or clonic muscle contractions, or a disturbance in behavioral functions.

ETIOLOGY AND INCIDENCE

Epileptic disorders can be divided into two etiological groups: idiopathic and symptomatic. In the *idiopathic* group the epilepsies cannot be attributed to a demonstrable structural lesion of the brain, and are frequently of genetic origin. Epilepsies in the *symptomatic* group are associated with pathology of the brain due to developmental anomalies, injury, or disease.

Epilepsy is one of the most prevalent chronic disorders. It has been estimated that there are approximately 17 million epileptics in the United States.

DENTAL PROBLEMS

With the exception of the typical fibrous hyperplasia of the gingiva produced by the anticonvulsant drug Dilantin, the epileptic patient has no dental problems peculiar to his condition. In the majority of cases the gingival hyperplasia can be surgically removed and then controlled with good oral prophylactic measures. If the periodontal problem tends to recur, the child's physician should be consulted regarding the possibility of changing the patient's drug regime.

Dental Treatment

The dentist should familiarize himself with the type and frequency of the epileptic child's seizures before dental treatment is started. As previously mentioned, the disorder may manifest itself in various forms of seizure, two of which should be recognized by the dentist so that he will be prepared to cope with the problem.

Petit Mal Seizure

This type of seizure is characterized by episodes of abrupt, momentary loss of consciousness. The child has a blank expression and discontinues any voluntary activities he is engaged in at that time. Rhythmic jerking of head and arms may be associated with loss of consciousness. The duration of each attack is approximately 10 seconds, and the child recovers quickly.

Because of its brevity, this type of seizure presents little difficulty in the dental management of the patient.

Grand Mal Seizure

As the name implies, the classical grand mal seizure is of much more violent nature than the petit mal attack. Typically the eyes roll up, the pupils dilate, and the face becomes either flushed or pale. Consciousness is lost and the body is seized by a tonic spasm that arrests the respiration, and the child becomes cyanotic. After 10 to 30 seconds, the tonic spasm is followed by a clonic phase of possibly several minutes duration when the muscles are violently contracted with possibly profuse salivation, perspiration, and involuntary bladder and bowel evacuation. The muscle contractions become gradually less violent and then cease. Usually the child remains stuporous after the attack and sinks into a deep sleep, which may last an hour or more. When the patient awakens, he may have a severe headache and show signs of restlessness for a period of variable duration.

When his patient has a grand mal seizure, the dentist is primarily concerned with preventing the child from injuring himself. A rubber or plastic mouth prop should be inserted in the oral cavity to avert tongue biting, and the patient should be put in a position where he cannot harm himself. An open space on the floor is probably the safest and most convenient place.

MENTAL RETARDATION

The terms mental retardation or mental subnormality refer to the subaverage intellectual functioning characteristic of children suffering from developmental defects such as feeblemindedness, idiocy, imbecility, mongolism, hypo- or oligophrenia and moronism. All these unfortunate children characteristically have an IQ below 70.

The World Health Organization recommends the division of the mentally subnormal into three broad categories:

1. Mild subnormality—with IQ of 50 to 69 and a mental age in the adult of 8 to 12 years.
2. Moderate subnormality—with IQ of 20 to 49 and a mental age in the adult of 3 to 7 years.
3. Severe subnormality—with IQ of 0 to 19 and a mental age in the adult of 0 to 2 years.

ETIOLOGY AND INCIDENCE

Mental retardation has been attributed to numerous etiologic factors, such as heredity, prenatal influences, prematurity, anoxia or injury at birth, malnutrition, encephalitis, and cerebral palsy.

Mental retardation, which affects more children than any other congenital disease, occurs in approximately 3 per cent of the population of the United States. It has been estimated that every year, 126,000 mentally retarded children are born in this country.

DENTAL PROBLEMS

With the exception of mongoloids, the mentally retarded experience no characteristic dental problems. However, because of poor oral hygiene and cariogenic dietary habits, they may show a higher rate of dental caries and periodontal disease than normal children.

Dental Treatment

Before formulation of a rational plan for treating the mentally retarded patient, the dentist must be aware of the child's mental level to assess the degree of cooperation to be expected and to make any necessary adjustments in management procedures.

The majority of the mentally retarded who are brought for dental care are in the category referred to as mild subnormality and most of these children can be managed with the blend of kindness and firmness needed for the successful management of the normal 8 to 10 year old child. With understanding and patience the dentist can usually gain the confidence of these children. Should he fail to attain the level of cooperation necessary for routine restorative work, or should the handicapped child be in need of extensive habilitative dental care, the use of general anesthesia for the patient may be the only hope of achieving successful treatment.

CONGENITAL HEART DISEASE

Congenital heart disease is due to structural abnormalities of the heart and these anomalies are commonly divided into two groups:

1. ACYANOTIC CONGENITAL HEART DISEASE

Patients in this group have a left-to-right shunt and suffer from a number of heart defects, such as atrial septal defect, ventricular septal defect, congenital aortic stenosis, patent ductus arteriosus, and pulmonary stenosis.

2. CYANOTIC CONGENITAL HEART DISEASE

Patients in this group are born with defects that cause right-to-left shunt, and they become cyanotic upon exertion. Transposition of the great vessels, tricuspid valve atresia, and tetralogy of Fallot are examples of the heart defects included in this group.

ETIOLOGY AND INCIDENCE

The exact etiology of congenital heart disease has not been established. Heredity and environmental factors during pregnancy, such as German measles and anoxia, have been recognized as plausible etiologic factors.

The incidence of congenital heart disease has been estimated at 6 to 8 per 1000 live births. About one third of this group dies in the first year of life, and 70 per cent of these within the first month.

DENTAL PROBLEMS

Congenital heart disease appears frequently as an associated anomaly in mongoloids and children born with cleft lip and/or palate. Most children afflicted with these developmental disorders also suffer from numerous dental problems of varying complexity and severity. With these exceptions, children with congenital heart disease do not exhibit any specific dental problems beyond the increased rate of caries and periodontal disease that is commonly encountered in most handicapped children.

Dental Treatment

Before the dentist initiates any dental treatment for a child with heart disease, whether congenital or acquired, it is essential that he obtain a thorough history of the child's heart defect. The family physician and the attending cardiologist must be consulted regarding any questions concerning the child's ability to tolerate the planned dental treatment, the possible complications that may arise, and all precautionary measures that may be needed.

In treating children with heart disease, one of the primary concerns of the dentist is the prevention of bacterial endocarditis. This serious complication is generally caused by *Streptococcus viridans*, which is commonly found about the teeth. Many dental treatments, such as deep scaling and extractions, are followed by bacteremia, which may cause endocarditis in a child with a heart defect. It is essential that prophylactic antibiotics be used before and for at least 48 hours after starting this type of treatment. Oral potassium penicillin is the medication most often used; however, the patient's physician should be consulted regarding the choice of antibiotic for each case.

If precautionary measures are followed, most children with congenital heart disease can be treated safely in the conventional dental clinic. Patients suffering from severe, handicapping heart defects or patients in need of extensive dental service are best treated in a hospital under general anesthesia.

HEMOPHILIA

Several inborn abnormalities of metabolism, which manifest themselves as hemostasis disorders, have been given the collective name *hemophilia*. These disorders may result from lack of any one of the substances necessary for normal thromboplastic activity.

The most common hemophilic condition is the disorder caused by deficiency of factor VIII (antihemophilic globulin). This condition is transmitted as an X-linked mendelian recessive and occurs exclusively in males. Although children born with factor VIII deficiency are potential "bleeders" from birth, excessive bleeding may not be observed until increased activity begins, at about 6 months of age. Bleeding may occur from any site, but is most common in the muscles, kidneys, mouth, and joints. The knee joints of the infant who is beginning to walk are especially vulnerable.

DENTAL PROBLEMS

Although the hemophiliac has no characteristic dental problems, any dental treatment these children require must be considered as serious because of the grave risks involved. The necessity for good oral care and prevention of dental disease for the hemophiliac cannot be overemphasized, since preventive dentistry for these children minimizes the need for the hazards of restorative treatment.

Dental Treatment

Even during the most routine dental treatment for the hemophilic child, the dentist must exercise extreme caution to prevent tissue lacerations. Scaling and polishing, reduction of subgingival tooth structure, and adaptation of matrix bands must be managed with great care to maintain the integrity of the periodontal tissues. Should minor bleeding problems occur, they can usually be controlled by pressure packs in conjunction with hemostatic agents such as thrombin.

The use of local anesthesia is contraindicated for these children except when pain is extreme and then it should be used with caution. The mandibular block should be avoided, because this form of injection may cause hemorrhage into the lateral pharyngeal spaces, where it is difficult to apply controlling measures.

A carefully placed rubber dam will serve a twofold purpose in the dental treatment of the hemophiliac. Besides securing a dry field for the placement of restorative materials, it also will help protect the soft tissues from accidental lacerations.

Tooth extraction for the hemophiliac should be considered only as a last resort, after the possibility of maintaining the teeth by conventional pulpectomy or root canal therapy has been rejected.

Extreme precautionary measures should be practiced for *all* patients suffering from any type of hemorrhagic disorder, as for example with the so-called *pseudo-hemophiliac,* who may be a male or a female with a characteristically prolonged bleeding time.

Removing Teeth

When extractions or other surgical procedures are unavoidable and excessive bleeding is anticipated, the patient should be hospitalized for more adequate handling of any complications that might arise.

Prior to the patient's admission to the hospital, the dentist should organize a plan for dental treatment. This plan, in conjunction with the patient's medical history, should be discussed by the dentist, the physician, and the hospital staff to outline a medical work-up that will include a detailed blood analysis for determining the type of bleeding problem, the coagulation and bleeding time, and the platelet count. After these steps are completed, the hematologist should coordinate the medical management for the child.

Premedication of the hemophiliac is indicated when lengthy procedures are planned or when the patient is apprehensive or unruly. Preoperative plasma transfusion may be recommended if excessive bleeding is anticipated.

As mentioned earlier, local anesthesia is usually contraindicated for a child with hemophilia. A general anesthetic, administered by a trained anesthesiologist, who is cognizant of the bleeding problem, should be a relatively safe procedure for the hemophiliac patient.

Before surgical treatment is attempted, all necessary restorative procedures should be completed with strict adherence to the precautionary measures already described. The extractions and other surgical treatment must be performed with the least possible trauma. Use of pressure packs for the initial control of hemorrhage should be followed by packing the socket with Gelofoam or some other hemostatic agent that can be held in place by gauze impregnated with petrolatum to prevent the incorporation of the gauze in the blood clot.

A follow-up transfusion schedule should be planned by the hematologist and the dentist. The duration of this therapy depends on the approximation of the healing time for the surgical wounds. The patient should receive nothing by mouth for 4 hours after the operation and should receive only liquids for the subsequent 24 hours. The importance of the patient's diet and postoperative home care must be carefully explained to his parents.

NITROUS OXIDE ANALGESIA

With the handicapped child, inhalation analgesia with nitrous oxide can be a safe and effective method of decreasing apprehension or resistance to dental treatment. Except for children who have severe mental retardation or emotional disturbance, there are few contraindications to its use.

A dentist experienced in administering nitrous oxide analgesia can combine this procedure with premedication and local anesthesia to overcome many of the problems associated with handicapped children. Nitrous oxide analgesia decreases the muscular spasticity and the uncoordinated movements of the cerebral palsied child and lessens the physical stress and discomfort, thereby making it possible for him to tolerate longer periods of treatment.

Nitrous oxide analgesia for the handicapped child should be limited to the stage of *relative analgesia*, by the use of relatively low nitrous oxide and high oxygen flows, safely below the excitement level. The major purpose of a relative analgesia level is to relax the patient and increase his cooperation. During the most painful periods of the dental treatment, this analgesia level can be supplemented by the use of local anesthesia when the patient's condition permits.

Careful consideration and management of the introduction of nitrous oxide analgesia and its initial administration to the handicapped child are the governing factors for a successful utilization of the procedure. For most handicapped children, premedication is needed to allay the apprehension that frequently accompanies their first experience with analgesia. The attending physician should be consulted regarding the choice of drug therapy for each patient.

Particular patience and understanding is imperative at the initial administration of nitrous oxide analgesia. The child must have time to adjust to this new experience; the use of the nosepiece should be demonstrated and the flow of gases can be played on the child's hands and cheeks before placement of the nosepiece. Resistance may be countered with gentle physical restraint and flow of 50 per cent nitrous oxide directed close to the nostrils. This mixture may have a mild euphoric effect and relax the patient sufficiently to permit seating of the nosepiece, after which the concentration of nitrous oxide should be reduced to the appropriate level, usually a 10 to 15 per cent flow.

Since verbal communication with the handicapped child is frequently difficult and unreliable, the dentist must be able to evaluate the level of analgesia from the physical and behavioral changes in the patient. When the appropriate level of analgesia has been reached, the dentist can begin the treatment. Operative procedures in these cases vary little from those routinely employed. The rubber dam and a mouth prop are helpful; however, it is important to remember that the use of the rubber dam lessens the dilution effect that is created when the mouth is open, thereby necessitating a decrease in the proportion of nitrous oxide.

GENERAL ANESTHESIA

Risks of vomiting, spasm, and apnea invariably exist in association with the use of a general anesthetic; therefore, it is expedient that milder, though possibly less potent, measures be considered when an anesthetic is in order.

A child's response, especially with the aid of premedication, is usually cooperative when the dentist exercises patience and understanding. This is true even with children who may appear incapable of the mental and physical control needed for successful dental treatment. Should these patient management procedures fail, or if a severely handicapped child needs extensive dental care, the use of general anesthesia offers a possible solution for the problem.

Indications for General Anesthesia

Children in one of the following categories usually require general anesthesia:
1. The uncooperative child who resists treatment after all conventional management procedures have been tried.
2. The child with a hemostasis disorder who needs extensive dental service.
3. The mentally retarded child so severely handicapped that dentist-patient communication is impossible.
4. The child suffering from central nervous disorders manifested by extreme involuntary movements.
5. The child with severe congenital heart disease who is considered incapable of tolerating the excitement and fatigue of extensive dental service.

Preoperative Procedures

Although the utilization of a general anesthetic in the dental office is acceptable, provided the essential equipment and a qualified anesthesiologist are available, the safest place for dental treatment under general anesthesia is undoubtedly the hospital.

When a child's dental treatment requires hospitalization and a general anesthetic, the best way to insure cooperation from the parents is to orient them as to the program planned for their child and their responsibilities concerning his hospitalization. A useful chart outlining the essential parental instructions is illustrated in Figure 25–14.

THE CHILDREN'S HOSPITAL OF BIRMINGHAM, ALABAMA
DENTAL CLINIC OPERATING ROOM
PARENT INSTRUCTIONS

The following instructions are prepared to aid you when you bring your child to CHILDREN'S HOSPITAL to have necessary dental work in the outpatient Dental Operating Room.

YOUR APPOINTMENT IS: _____, _____, at _____
                             DAY   MONTH   TIME

1. Your child must have a physical examination and laboratory work completed not more than 48 hours before the day of his appointment. This information should be recorded on the accompanying form by your physician and should be brought with you on the day of your appointment.
2. Do not let your child eat or drink anything the day of the appointment (not even water). If you have an afternoon appointment, an early liquid breakfast is permitted. This is very important to avoid nausea after the operation.
3. Call CHILDREN'S HOSPITAL DENTAL CLINIC—323-8901, ext. 235, if the appointment cannot be kept, at least *24 hours in advance*.
4. If your child develops cold, fever, or any illness, please notify the Dental Clinic two days before appointment as it may have to be changed.
5. After the dental procedure the patient may go home, usually within a period of 1 to 2 hours.

Figure 25–14 Parent instruction sheet.

THE CHILDREN'S HOSPITAL OF BIRMINGHAM, ALABAMA
DENTAL CLINIC
PREANESTHETIC EXAMINATION

NAME_____AGE_____WEIGHT_____

ADDRESS_____PHONE_____

PHYSICIAN: Dear Doctor_____,

I plan to do the following dental procedure under general anesthesia

at THE CHILDREN'S HOSPITAL:_____

_____

_____

Please complete the following examination and hemoglobin determination.

_____
Attending Dentist's Signature

Heart:_____

Lungs:_____

Past Pertinent Illness:_____

_____

_____

Present Medications:_____

_____

Allergies:_____

_____

LABORATORY:

Hemoglobin_____Grams_____

Urinalysis (report abnormalities)_____

OK for general anesthesia: Yes_____No_____
M.D.

_____
Examining Physician's Signature

Figure 25–15 Form for physician's preanesthetic examination.

The family physician, who should be consulted regarding the hospitalization procedures, should examine the child and submit a written confirmation that a general anesthetic is not contraindicated. The physical examination and the laboratory analysis to be requested are indicated in the chart illustrated in Figure 25–15.

Since considerable paper work is associated with any hospitalization, the dentist should familiarize himself with accepted hospital protocol before a definite admission date is arranged for his patient.

Treatment Procedures

After the patient's hospital admission, the dentist should discuss plans for the treatment with the anesthesiologist, who determines the tolerance limit of each patient for the general anesthetic; with this as a guideline, the dentist can then set up a rigid time schedule for treatment.

After evaluating the patient's medical history and determining the extent of the required treatment, the most suitable premedication and anesthetic can then be chosen. Since it was first tried in pediatric anesthesia, some 15 years ago, Fluothane (halothane) has gained wide acceptance because of its low irritant quality, nonflammability, and the rapid awakening of a patient who has received it.

Nasal endotracheal intubation, where the tube is out of his way, simplifies the treatment procedures for the dentist. After intubation, the patient's eyes should be covered with damp gauze for protection against dental and material debris. Great care must be taken to prevent blood or any type of debris from entering the patient's throat. After complete anesthetization a throat pack of moist gauze should be laid over the pharyngeal opening, across the tonsillar area, and under the tongue (Fig. 25–16). For its easy, safe removal, the end of the throat pack, with a string securely attached to it, should extrude from the oral cavity.

Efficient use of aspiration equipment (Fig. 25–17) facilitates dental procedures for the anesthetized child. A mouth prop may be used, when needed, to keep the child's mouth open. For any restorative treatment on the anesthetized patient, use of the rubber dam provides the dentist with a dry field and better visibility, and serves as an adjunct to the throat pack in preventing debris from entering the patient's throat. Prior to extractions or other surgical treatment, all restorative procedures should be finished; with this done, the mouth should be cleaned, the throat pack replaced with fresh gauze, and the surgical procedures initiated.

Upon completion of the planned treatment, any hemorrhage must be controlled and all debris carefully evacuated from the oral cavity; after this, the throat pack can be removed and the child taken to the recovery room.

Before hospital dismissal, an appointment should be set up for a postoperative

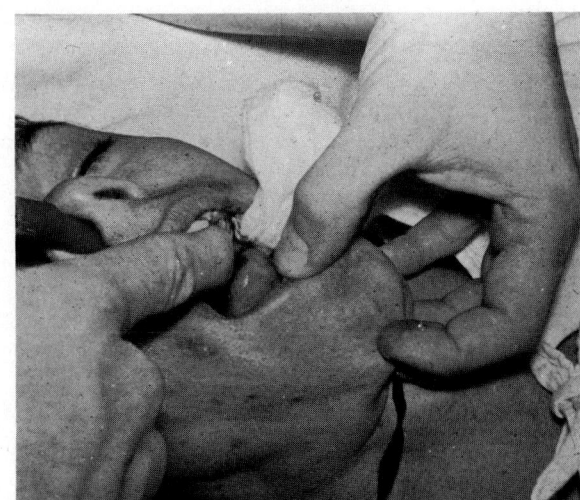

Figure 25–16 Gauze pack being inserted.

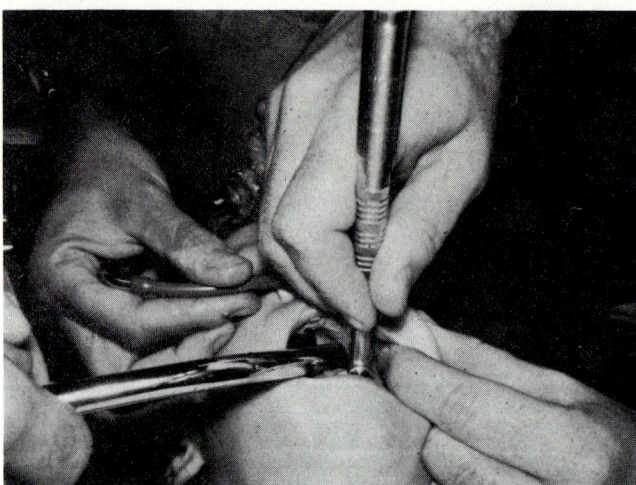

Figure 25–17 Cavity preparation under general anesthesia. Observe the use of aspiration equipment.

check on the patient within the following two weeks. On this visit, the parents must be impressed with the urgency for careful oral home care for their child and the exigency of reducing his intake of cariogenic food as a means of avoiding the ordeal of repetitive dental treatment.

SUMMARY

In this chapter the more commonly encountered handicapping pediatric problems were discussed. The dental problems associated with these disorders were described, as well as the precautionary measures and the management procedures indicated for dental treatment of children suffering from these handicaps.

Though premedication and anesthetic agents are valuable aids in the dental treatment for these children, the dentist should realize that these management aids cannot replace the essential patience and understanding he must exercise while treating the handicapped. Accepting the fact that the dental procedures for these children may demand more time than those for normal children, the dentist can experience tremendous personal satisfaction from his contribution to the habilitative process of these unfortunate individuals and from an awareness of their deep appreciation for his services.

REFERENCES

1. Adisman, I. K.: Cleft palate prosthetics. *In* Cleft Lip and Palate. Grabb, W. C. Rosenstein, S. W., and Bzoch, K. R. (eds). Boston, Little, Brown, and Co., 1971.
2. Arena, J. M.: Davison's Compleat Pediatrician. Philadelphia, Lea & Febiger, 1969.
3. Barnett, H. L.: Pediatrics. New York, Appleton-Century-Crofts, 1968.
4. Fogh-Andersen, P.: Inheritance of Harelip and Cleft Palate. Copenhagen, Nyt Nordisk Forlag, Arnold Busck, 1942.
5. Fogh-Andersen, P.: Incidence of cleft lip and palate: Constant or increasing. Acta Chir. Scand., *122*:106-111, 1961.

6. Fraser, F. C.: Cleft lip and cleft palate. Science, *158*:1603-1606, 1967.

7. Fraser, F. C.: The genetics of cleft lip and cleft palate. Am. J. Hum. Genet., *22*:336-352, 1970.

8. Gullikson, J. S.: Oral findings of mentally retarded children. J. Dent. Child., *36*:133–137, 1969.

9. Hooley, J. R.: Hospital Dentistry. Philadelphia, Lea & Febiger, 1970.

10. Jacobson, B. N. and Rosenstein, S. W.: The dentist and the cleft palate patient. Schweiz Mschr. Zahnheilk., *80*:507-517, 1970.

11. Kernahan, D. A., and Stark, R. B.: A new classification for cleft lip and cleft palate. Plast. Reconstr. Surg., *22*:435–441, 1958.

12. Kroll, R. G.: The effects of premedication on handicapped children. J. Dent. Child., *36*:103–114, 1969.

13. Langa, H.: Relative Analgesia in Dental Practice. Philadelphia, W. B. Saunders Co., 1968.

14. Moller, P.: Dentofacial deformities: Cleft lip and palate. *In* The Epidemiology of Oral Health. Pelton, W. J. (ed.). Cambridge, Harvard University Press, 1969.

15. Moller, P.: An Epidemiologic and Genetic Study of Cleft Lip and Cleft Palate in Iceland. (Dissertation). June, 1971.

16. Olsen, N. H.: Pediatric dentistry. *In* Cleft Lip and Palate. Grabb, W. C., Rosenstein, S. W., and Bzoch, K. R. (eds.). Boston, Little, Brown and Co., 1971.

17. Parkin, S. F., Hargreaves, J. A., and Weyman, J.: Management of children in the dental surgery. Brit. Dent. J., *129*:82–85, 1970.

18. Parkin, S. F., Hargreaves, J. A., and Weyman, J.: Dental care of physically and mentally handicapped children. Brit. Dent. J., *129*:515-518, 1970.

19. Parkin, S. F., Hargreaves, J. A., and Weyman, J.: Dental care of medically handicapped children. Brit. Dent. J., *129*:573-576, 1970.

20. Smith, R. M.: Anesthesia for Infants and Children. St. Louis, C. V. Mosby Co., 1968.

21. Winer, R. A.: Dental care for the handicapped. J. Dent. Child., *36*:449–451, 1969.

22. Young, W. O., and Shannon, J. H.: Providing dental treatment for handicapped children. J. Dent. Child., *35*:225-240, 1968.

26

COMMUNICATIVE DISORDERS IN CHILDREN

by GWENYTH R. VAUGHN,
H. PERRY HITCHCOCK, and
JOHNNYE AKIN

The oral cavity is intimately involved in the speech process, both normal and abnormal. The dentist who treats children in his practice should be familiar with the physiology of speech and some of the causes and means of correcting speech defects. Since he may be the first professional to see a child with a communicative disorder, the dentist who is concerned with the effects of disordered communication upon children, their families, and their communities can provide valuable service to his patients through appropriate referrals. Many dental/speech pathophysiologies may be prevented, corrected, or minimized when the dentist and speech pathologist work cooperatively in identification, diagnosis, and treatment of speech disorders.

Of all human capabilities, verbal communication is one of the most valued and one of the most complex. In order to understand the functional and optimal levels of human communication systems, the dentist needs to be aware of the linguistic, physiological, and acoustic aspects of speech production. He should be conversant with the concepts involving expressive, central, receptive, and sensor feedback processes. The structural and physiological changes in the oral cavity effected by growth and development are well known to dentists; knowledge on the part of dentists of the psychological, social, and educational implications of normal and abnormal development of speech and language can provide a dimension crucial to quality patient care.

HUMAN COMMUNICATION SYSTEMS

Human communication systems use verbal and nonverbal codes. Some of the verbal forms were defined by the 1968 *Rehabilitation Codes* in the following manner:

1. *Speech* implies the vocal and verbal expression of language appropriate to the environment of speaker and listener.
2. *Voice* function implies the auditory experience of phonation which is culturally appropriate for human communication.
3. *Language* is a system of communication among human beings who comprehend and use symbols possessing arbitrary conventional meanings.
4. *Hearing* function implies reception and recognition of sounds within appropriate environmental limits.

In addition to the systems described above, *reading* and, perhaps to a lesser degree, *writing* are verbal systems critical for optimal educational achievement, personal-social adjustment, and vocational placement.

LEVELS OF HUMAN COMMUNICATION

The oral/aural system of communication, consisting of speech production and reception, is of mutual interest to dentists and speech pathologists. Communication from the mind of the speaker to the mind of the listener, by the means of speech, requires that language be codified in different forms and at various levels.

Linguistic Levels.   The activities of integration and interpretation — the coding and decoding of language within the brain — are carried on by the central processes and are governed by linguistic rules that include the selection of vocabulary and the arrangement of words and phrases according to the grammar and syntax of the specific language the speaker is using.

Physiological Levels.   Physiological levels consist of programmed neural impulses necessary to the initiation and coordination or respiration, phonation, resonation, and articulation processes. Neural activity continues as the spoken message is perceived and interpreted, and a reply is formulated.

Acoustic Levels.   The acoustic, or physical, levels include the transmission of the spoken message to the listener and the auditory feedback to the speaker. "Speakers do not generally produce identical sound waves when they pronounce the same words on different occasions. The listener, in recognizing speech, does not rely solely on information derived from the speech wave he receives. He also relies on his knowledge of an intricate communication system subject to the rules of language and speech, and on cues provided by the subject matter and the identity of the speaker" (Denes and Pinson, 1966, p. 8).

HUMAN COMMUNICATION PROCESSES

In spite of the apparent ease with which the majority of children learn to speak, human communication consists of very complex and exacting processes: (1) expressive, or signal output processes, (2) central, or symbol integrative and interpretative processes, (3) receptive, or signal input processes, and (4) sensor feed-back processes.

EXPRESSIVE PROCESSES

The expressive, or signal output processes include speech, writing, gesturing, and other communication systems. Speech is a distinctly human achievement. The development, maturation, and maintenance of good speech depends greatly upon the integrity of the structural, neurological, physiological, psychological, social, and cultural processes.

Vocal Organs

The vocal organs are the *lungs*, the *trachea*, the *larynx*, which houses the *vocal folds*, the *pharynx*, and the *oral* and *nasal* cavities. The articulators — the *velum*, *tongue*, *lips*, and *vocal folds* — act as valves, or valve contacts, that approximate the fixed surfaces — *teeth*, *alveolar ridges*, and *hard palate*. Those areas lying above the larynx are generally referred to as the *vocal tract*. Adjustments and movements of the articulators change the resonating chambers, thus altering the acoustic proper-ties of the vocal tract.

Neuromuscular Systems

The neuromuscular systems coordinate all the communicative mechanisms. The phenomenology of speech production includes four mutually dependent divi-sions: (1) respiration, (2) phonation, (3) resonation, and (4) articulation. Speech is often described as "an overlaid process," secondary to vegetative functions. Some scholars hold, however, that man is specifically endowed with mechanisms pre-destined to produce verbal communication.

1. Respiration. The first step in the speech producing process is respiration, or the power division. The exhaled air stream causes the vocal folds to vibrate, moves through the resonating cavities, and is shaped into discrete sounds.

2. Phonation. The second step is that of phonation. The power or breath stream is emitted from the lungs and strikes the vocal folds which are housed in the larynx. An important event occurs: on sounds such as *b* and *d*, the vocal folds vibrate, thus causing the sounds to be voiced. This is a characteristic that disting-uishes them from their *voiceless* equivalents, *p* and *t*. Paired sounds such as *b* and *p* or *d* and *t* are called *homorganic* equivalents because the two sounds are produced in approximately the same manner. The distinguishing characteristic is that the vocal folds are vibrating on *b* and not on *p*.

3. Resonation. The resonance system is the division that gives a distinguish-ing quality, or timbre, that is characteristic of each voice. The fundamental sound that is produced in the larynx through the vibration of the vocal folds is unidenti-fiable; for example, *Middle C*'s of the human voice, of a saxophone, a piano, or a violin, are indistinguishable. As the glottal tone is resonated in the constantly changing supralaryngeal structures — the laryngopharynx, oropharynx, naso-pharynx, oral cavity, and nasal cavities — the sounds begin to assume discrete char-acteristics, such as *p, b, t*, or *d*, according to the size, shape, and degree of participa-tion of various resonating cavities.

Palatal defects and velopharyngeal incompetence interfere with the control of the air stream in the production of speech. Even with improved techniques for studying palatal movement by cineradiography, the degree of closure and the degree of nasality often appear incompatible. Some individuals with what appears to be inadequate closure, produce acceptable speech quality; others, with what seems to be good closure, exhibit excessive nasality. The ultimate tests of surgical technique, prosthetic design, and speech therapy are the intelligibility and acceptability of the speech product. This concept does not underestimate the psychological and vocational importance of cosmetic appearance nor the vital function of a mechanism capable of good mastication.

4. Articulation. The fourth step in the speech producing sequence is articulation. The vocal organs responsible for this act are called the *articulators;* the places at which the air stream is modified to produce the speech sounds are referred to as *articulatory valves.* When the articulatory organs assume a certain position, a phoneme, or speech sound, may be produced in isolation. After the sound is put back into context, slight changes in the acoustic characteristics and in the articulatory placement may occur through *phonotactics:* the influence of stress, rate, pitch, and other adjacent or distant phonemes.

The vocal organs capable of forming the articulatory valves stop, constrict, and narrow the air stream, thus producing speech sounds. The articulatory mechanism directs the air stream through varying combinations of resonating cavities. The placements of the articulators, or valving mechanisms, provide the speech sounds with oral topographical names: *bilabial, labiodental, linguodental, linguo-alveolar, linguopalatal, linguovelar, nasal,* and *glottal.* This descriptive terminology does not preclude the possibility of other articulatory positions that produce acceptable sounds. For instance, an *s* sound is generally described as a linguoalveolar sound, but it may be made by placing the tongue tip at the base of the lower incisors. The body of the tongue is then used to form a groove through which the breath stream is emitted. Friction is produced because of the proximity of the two organs—incisors and tongue. If the *s* produced in this manner is intelligible, is comfortable for the speaker, and is pleasing to the listener, there is no need to change to another articulatory position.

Table 26–1 lists the divisions of the speech production systems and their respective functions.

Sound Categories

The sounds of English are roughly divided into the following categories: *vowels, diphthongs,* and *consonants.* A few sounds are classified as *semi-vowels* or *glides.*

Vowels. There are seventeen vowel sounds that are represented by only five vowel letters in English, *a, e, i, o,* and *u.* The semi-vowels are *w, l, r,* and *j.* The vowel sounds are divided into front vowels, central vowels, back vowels, and semi-vowels.

Front Vowels	Central Vowels	Back Vowels	Semi-Vowels
/i/ be	/ʌ/ cup	/u/ booT	/w/ we
/ɪ/ it	/ə/ sofa	/ʊ/ foot	/r/ rat
/e/ vacation	/ɝ/ bird	/o/ obey	/l/ let
/ɛ/ bet	/ɚ/ sister	/ɔ/ saw	/j/ yet
/æ/ at	/ɜ/ bird (as	/ɒ/ (infrequently	
/a/ (infrequently	pronounced in certain	used)	
used)	areas)	/ɑ/ calm, lot	

TABLE 26–1   DIVISIONS OF SPEECH PRODUCTION SYSTEM AND THEIR
RESPECTIVE FUNCTIONS FOR SPEECH*

I. Respiratory Mechanism

A. Structures	*B. Functions*
1. Thoracic cavity	1. Generates expiratory air pressures and flows required at the larynx for phonation.
2. Lungs and tracheo-bronchial tree	2. Generates oral air pressures required for consonant articulation.
3. Neuromuscular systems which control the volume of the thoracic cavity	3. Participates in control of pressure and flow required for regulation of vocal pitch and intensity and to divide speech into syllables, phrases, etc.

II. Laryngeal Mechanism

A. Structures	*B. Functions*
1. Larynx (cartilages, folds, membranes, ligaments, etc., both intrinsic and extrinsic).	1. Vocal fold vibrations provide quasi-periodic sound source during voice production.
2. Neuromuscular systems for controlling adduction-abduction, lengthening-shortening, stiffening (tensing) and relaxing of vocal folds and for controlling gross movements of the larynx as a whole.	2. Laryngeal adjustments coordinate with intratracheal air pressure regulation to control voice pitch and vocal intensity.
	3. Vocal fold action determines input acoustic spectrum to vocal cavities thus setting basic voice quality characteristics.
	4. Valving action assists in regulation of air flow during both consonants and vowels.

III. Vocal Cavity System

A. Structures	*B. Functions*

1. Pharyngeal, oral and nasal cavities.
  a. Pharyngeal walls
  b. Epiglottis
  c. Tongue, jaw, lips, hard and soft palate
  d. [Teeth] etc.
	1. Articulation of vowels by
	  a. Shaping of oral-pharyngeal tract to regulate resonance properties of tract.
	  b. Controlling coupling to nasal cavities.

2. Neuromuscular systems controlling movements of the tongue, jaw, lips, soft palate, pharyngeal walls, etc.	2. Articulating consonants by
	  a. Generation of continuous spectrum noise by constricting air flow at various locations in oral tract.
	  b. Generation of transient noises by stopping and sudden release of air flow at various oral cavity locations.
	  c. Regulating coupling to nasal cavities.
	  d. Controlling shaping of oral-pharyngeal tract to regulate resonance properties

	3. Assists in regulations of air flow through valving actions.
	4. Participates in regulation of voice quality and vocal intensity.

*Adapted from a report, Human Communication and Its Disorders: An Overview, Monograph No. 10, by the Subcommittee on Human Communication and Its Disorders, of the National Advisory Neurological Diseases and Stroke Council (1969, p. 145).

The two most important factors for the *front vowels* are the position of the lips and tongue, and the depression of the mandible. The apex of the tongue is below and distal to the mandibular incisors; the body is arched anteriorly and flattens as the mandible is progressively depressed.

The lips, tongue, and mandible continue to be the principal factors in the positioning of the *back vowels*. The movements are reversed so that the mandible progresses superiorly from the lowest, unstrained position to the rest position. The tongue body moves to a posterior-superior position; the apex of the tongue is no longer important and is pulled distally from the position it assumed for the front vowels.

For the *central vowels*, the tongue obliquely crosses from the occlusal portion of the posterior maxillary molars to the gingival portion of the first molar. In the production of the stressed /ɝ/ (b*ird*) and unstressed /ɚ/ (sist*er*), the tongue apex is curled to a superior retroflex position. The mandible is depressed slightly from a rest position. In /ɜ/ and /ə/, the tongue apex is not in a retroflex position, thus the *r*-quality is only slight. The latter holds for the stressed /ʌ/ (c*u*p). In the central vowels, the unrounded lips play no important role and remain in neutral position. The mandible is depressed to approximate the position of the mid-front vowels. The semi-vowels, by definition, are also semi-consonants.

Diphthongs.   There are six diphthongs: /eɪ/ g*a*te, /aɪ/ m*i*ce, /ɔɪ/ b*o*y, /oʊ/ g*o*, /aʊ/ cow, and /iu/ (music). The diphthongs are made by combining two of the vowel sounds.

Vowels and diphthongs impart much of the tonal quality to speech; consonants provide some tonal quality, but their main function is to give clarity and understandability.

Consonants.   Consonant quality is determined by whether it is: *voiced* or *voiceless, fricative* or *non-fricative, nasal* or *non-nasal.* The point of articulation determines the organic description while the durational value gives the sound a distinctive characteristic of a *stop* or *continuant*. A *fricative* sound results when the air is forced through a small aperture. The *nasal* sounds *m*, *n*, and *ng* are produced with the nasal port open. The *l* has the distinction of being a *lateral* or *bilateral* sound. The tongue apex makes contact with the alveolar ridge in a position back of the upper incisors. The air is emitted through lowering one or both sides of the tongue, depending upon the habit of the individual.

Stops, such as *p* and *b*, are sounds that are initiated and terminated almost instantaneously. These sounds are also called *plosives* or *explosives*. The terminology is interchangeable. These terms simply mean the air must be impounded and then exploded.

A *continuant*, for example, *m*, can be continued as long as the speaker has breath. *Glides* are sounds in which the tongue tends to move away from the initial position and "glide" into the following vowel. Glides do not usually have such fixed positions as other isolated sounds. The *glottal stop* may be used between two vowel sounds not appearing in the same syllable. Thus, *being* may become /biʔɪŋ/ or /bijɪŋ/, both of which are acceptable. The glottal stop in standard American English is not used in the medial position as a substitution for a *t* as in *dentist* /dɛnʔɪst/. This substitution is sometimes heard in areas of Scotland and in Brooklynese.

Table 26–2 is a consonant chart that groups the sounds according to several characteristics.

TABLE 26–2 CONSONANT CHART

	Bilabial	Labiodental	Lingua-dental	Lingua-alveolar	Lingua-palatal	Lingua-velar	Glottal
Stops	p-b* /p-b/			t-d* /t-d/	ch-j* /tʃ-dʒ/	k-g* /k-g/	
Nasals	m* /m/			n* /n/		ng* /ŋ/	
Laterals				l* /l/			
Fricatives	wh /hw/	f-v* /f-v/	th-th* /θ-ð/	s-z* /s-z/ r* /r/	ch-j* /tʃ-dʒ/ sh-zh* /ʃ-ʒ/		h /h/ /ʔ/
Semivowels	w* /w/			l* /l/ r* /r/	y* /j/		

*These sounds are voiced.
(The symbols between the virgules are from the International Phonetic Alphabet.)

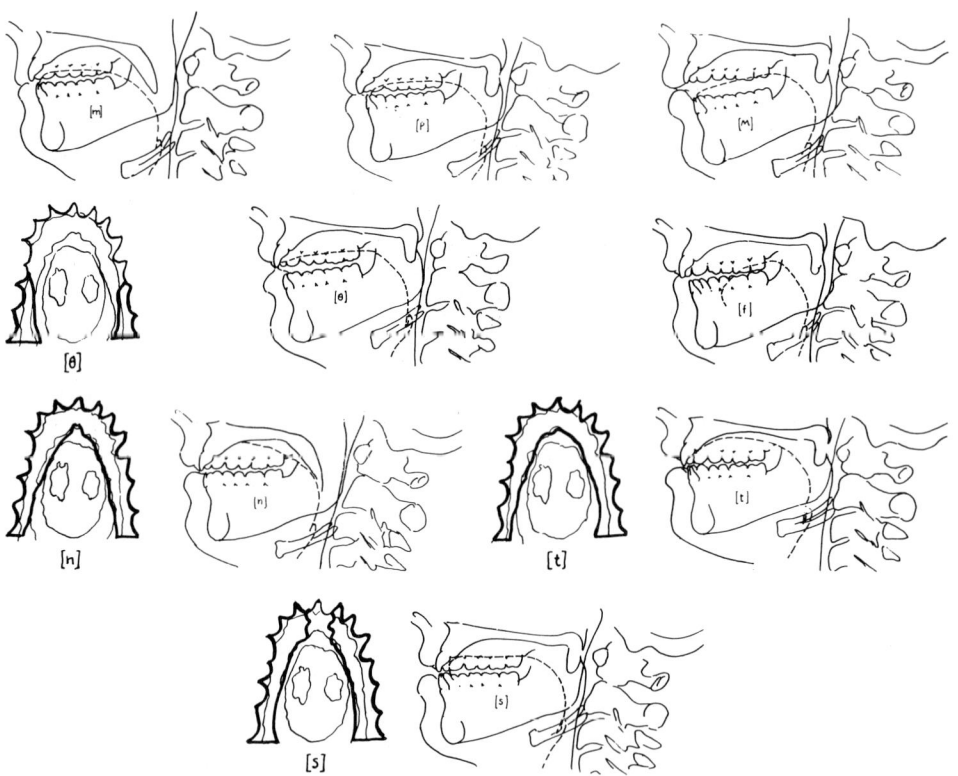

Figure 26–1 Palatograms and x-ray tracings. The palatograms of this figure present a topographical record of the informant's palate. The contour lines are 5 millimeters apart in vertical dimension. The height of the palatal vault, the angle of slope, and the area of the successive planes are to be interpreted in the same manner as a contour map of the earth's surface. Starting with the gingival border of the palate as a zero line, this palate is slightly over 15 millimeters high (p. 613).

(*Fig. 26–1 continues on the opposite page.*)

In Figure 26–1, the articulatory valves and co-articulatory mechanisms may be seen. The palatograms and X-ray tracings are of the same subject during a distinctive moment in the production of certain consonants. These studies are taken from a chapter by H. Harlan Bloomer in the Handbook of Speech Pathology and Audiology by Lee E. Travis, (1971, pp. 715–766).

CENTRAL PROCESSES

Language Processes

Integration. Integration, the internal monitor of communication processes, consists of encoding and decoding of verbal and nonverbal messages. Addi-

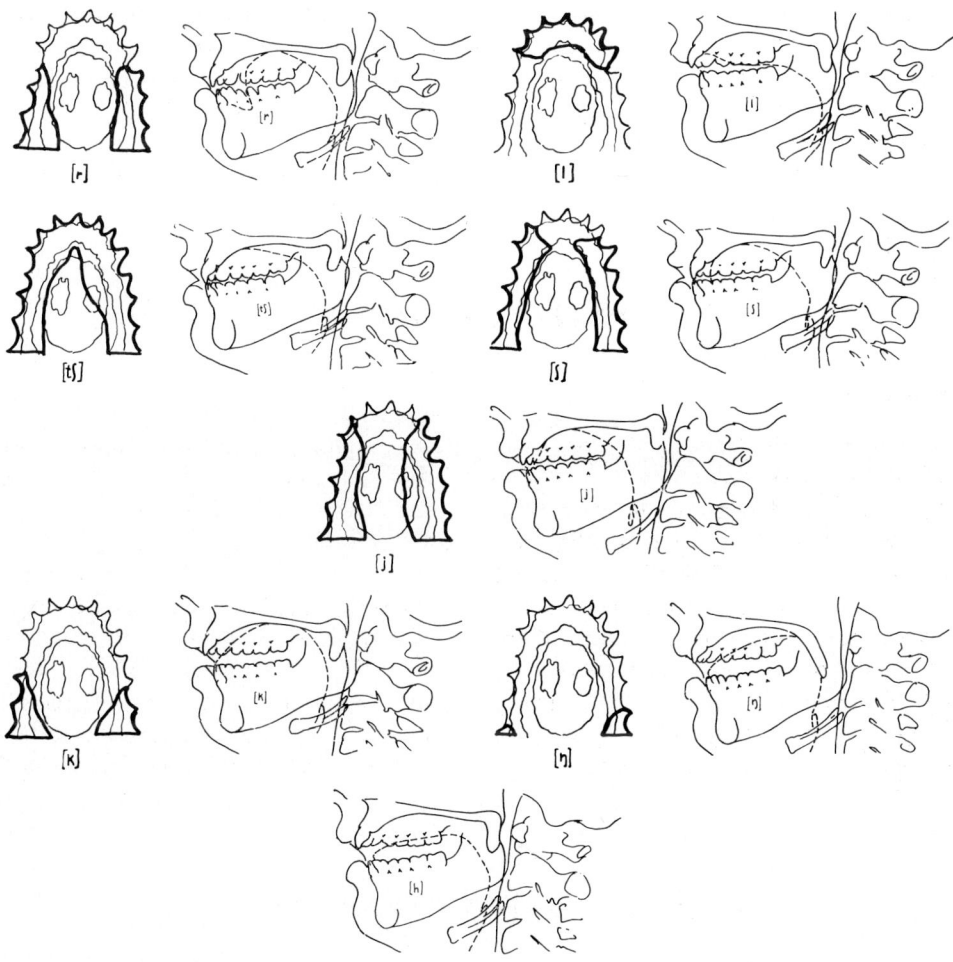

Figure 26–1 *(Continued).* Further appreciation of the interrelationship of oral structures in speech can be obtained from lateral x-ray films of the head during the "contact" phase of consonant articulation (p. 615).

tional central process functions are concerned with conscious perception, symbol integration and interpretation, assignment of meaning, establishment of relationships, and mediation of linguistic competence.

Prenatal rubella, trauma at birth or from accident, kernicterus, disease, and cerebral vascular accidents are some of the causes of severe sensory, motor, and language disorders. Problems may take the form of: dysphasia, learning disabilities, behavioral aberrations, and visuomotor and perceptual problems, such as reading, writing, and spelling disabilities. Often, minimal damage to the central processes requires extensive study before one or more of the defects can be identified.

Studies have indicated that the language functions, in most individuals, are located on the left hemisphere, even in persons who are left handed. If the damage to the language areas occurs early in life—prior to eight years of age—it has been reported that language may be established on the opposite hemisphere. Children who have had early damage and have not learned to talk may have suffered bilateral lesions or an interference below the cortex in the brain stem. For children with damage to both language centers, the implications for treatment and education involving the nonverbal areas of the nondominant hemisphere deserve attention. Consideration should be given to the use of nonverbal communication systems for these children, instead of restricting them exclusively to the use of verbal communication.

RECEPTIVE PROCESSES

Hearing

Learning to speak depends greatly upon auditory input—the majority of human beings speak *as* they hear and *because* they hear. Without adequate function of the auditory avenue, children may become strangers in their own families, failures in school, and, ultimately, seek friends *only* with other deaf adults. Most adults who became deaf at birth, or before development of speech and language, live as a minority group and are unemployed, or underemployed, because they lack *functional* receptive and expressive communication.

In the above instance, the term *functional* refers to communication that permits the person to *function* satisfactorily in an educational, social, or vocational milieu. A *functional* speech disorder usually refers to a communication deficit that is *nonorganic* in etiology, therefore, possibly of psychological or environmental origin.

SENSOR FEEDBACK PROCESSES

Sensor feedback might be described as the intrapersonal communication monitoring process. This self-monitoring includes the auditory, visual, tactile, kinesthetic, and proprioceptive mechanisms. The integration of cutaneous and kinesthetic information is sometimes referred to as "haptic perception."

James C. Chalfant and Margaret A. Scheffelin (1969), in a review of research, *Central Processing Dysfunctions in Children*, relate the disturbances of the sensor feedback systems to speech disorders through a disturbance of the kinesthetic basis of speech. They classify this condition as an afferent kinesthetic motor aphasia. The disruption of the coordinated movements essential for the kinesthetic basis of motor acts results in failure to organize and execute articulation in speech (Liepmann, 1913). Lesions of the inferior divisions of the postcentral region of the left hemisphere have also been found to result in *apraxia* of the tongue, lips, and palate (Luria, 1966). While the subject can produce sounds, he is unable to select the correct positions of lips, tongue, or palate.

In contrast to apraxia, the condition of dysarthria may display defective sounds as well as slurred speech and monotonous speech patterns. Entire phrases may be produced easily while some individual sounds may be articulated with difficulty.

COMMUNICATION CODES AND CHARACTERISTICS

Communication implies language—a set of symbols that must be understood by at least two persons: the sender and the receiver. Language may be expressed in analogic or digital form. Digital codes use abstract oral and graphic symbols; analogic codes provide communication through objects, pictures, movements, and other nonverbal stimuli.

Analogic Codes

Early in life, the child learns to interpret hostile or affectionate nonverbal cues through the manner in which he is touched, fed, bathed, or diapered. In turn, he transmits nonverbal messages—messages that may not be comprehended or may be left unanswered by parents and professionals. Conscious verbal assurances are easily contradicted by unconscious rejection made evident through gestures, facial expressions, posture, movements, and other nonverbal means.

The verbal and nonverbal contradiction was clearly illustrated in the case of a four-year-old boy who was brought by his mother to the speech pathologist because he had developed very little speech. The mother insisted that ankyloglossia was the reason for the delay. During the taking of the case history, it became evident that the mother rejected the boy and resented the fact that he did not speak well. Despite opinions to the contrary given by an oral surgeon and a speech pathologist, the mother insisted upon a frenectomy and searched until she found a surgeon willing to undertake the procedure. In most cases, speech pathologists do *not* feel that ankyloglossia is the cause of speech delay or articulation defects.

Analogic codes assume many forms, such as: signs; signals; gestures; actions; facial expressions; postures; motions; body language, including posture and gait; objects; pictures; chemical, thermal, and mechanical reactions; colors; shapes; textures; noise; biological codes of insects, birds, and animals; and the genetic codes of inheritance.

Dentistry is replete with nonverbal cues: *gestures* are used to show the child where to sit; *demonstration* facilitates opening and rinsing the mouth; *sounds* of dental equipment may be frightening unless accompanied by *verbal* explanations or analogic demonstrations; *pictographs,* in the form of X-rays are used to record caries; and traces of *action language* are left in the oral cavity by mouth breathing, tongue pressure, fingernail biting, thumb or object sucking, and bruxism.

Object and *color* language may induce fear if the dentist is not skillful in keeping instruments and evidence of bleeding out of sight. Some children may become conditioned to white jackets and relate them to unpleasant experiences.

Digital Codes

Digital representations are used for speaking, reading, writing, and mathematics. Special adaptations include finger spelling for the deaf and braille for the blind. Commerical and military digital codifications include the Morse Code and flag and lantern alphabets. Digital symbols are combined to form words, phrases, and sentences, all subject to rules of logic, syntax, and grammar. These combinations provide human beings with communication systems capable of transmitting abstract ideas, interpreting nonverbal detail, and insuring continuity of cultures.

Orthographic Symbols.   English orthographic symbols, the letters used in printing and writing, are inconsistent with acoustic symbols, the sounds used in speaking. The verbal skills of reading, writing, and spelling are complicated because they lack a direct relationship to spoken language. One of the examples of orthographic confusion is found in the variability of pronunciation given the series of graphic symbols, *ough*. In the following words, *ough* is pronounced in a different manner in each word: t*ough*, b*ough*, thr*ough*, th*ough*, th*ough*t.

Phonetic Symbols.   A more consistent relationship between spoken and written or printed symbols can be achieved through the use of the International Phonetic Alphabet (IPA). Speech sounds, phonemes, the sound blocks of which spoken words are built, are assigned separate graphic symbols, each phonetic symbol representing one sound. Anyone capable of interpreting the phonetic symbols can produce words from any language, even though he may not know the meaning of the words. A phonetic transcription of the example of the orthographic system contrasts the ambiguity of the orthographic symbols with the clarity of the phonetic symbols: *tough* /tʌɬ/, *bough* /baʊ/, *through* /θru/, *though* /ðoʊ/, *thought* /θɔt/.

GROWTH AND DEVELOPMENT OF SPEECH AND LANGUAGE

Communication is one of the most complex biosocial achievements of the human organism. Delayed and disordered communication skills often forecast disrupted personal maturation and social development, poor educational achievement, and restricted vocational opportunity. The importance placed by society upon early development of communication skills is reported in the following paragraph:

> No child is fully adopted into human society unless and until he makes progress in picking his way through the labyrinth of language. Of all the achievements of the infant, none is more commented upon, at least in our civilization, than the first intelligible sounds and the subsequent acquisition of language skill. From the earliest days, our proficiency in speech not only serves the simple utilitarian end of signalling for food or protection; it is a measuring stick constantly applied to our personality as a whole. Language facility usually carries with it a stream of indulgence from members of the home circle and beyond, while failure shrivels the self (Lasswell & Leietes, 1949, pp. 5–6).

Developmental Sequences. All areas of growth, including speech and language, are subject to individual variation. The chronological scales for language, adaptive, motor, and personal-social behavior appear in Table 26–3. These are useful as measuring devices by which comparisons between actual and expected levels of development can be obtained. In addition, inter-sequence relationships provide a comprehensive view of the "whole child" so that discrepancies in any one of the areas can be identified. Such discrepancies may alert the clinician to the need for referral to other health professionals.

Language, in the broad linguistic sense and in contrast to *speech* — an articulatory act — is basic to the development of all verbal skills, including speaking, reading, writing, speech reading, and finger spelling. The child acquires linguistic skills in accordance with his need, his opportunity, and his environmental model. Some of the influences that may interrupt progress are illness, physical or emotional trauma, lack of stimulation or motivation, and organic, physiological, or neurological abnormalities.

Table 26–4 presents speech and language development: the time individual sounds usually appear, the numerical size of vocabulary at certain ages, the word type most common at each age, sentence length in words, and percentage of in-

TABLE 26–3 DEVELOPMENTAL SEQUENCES

Age	Language Behavior	Adaptive Behavior	Motor Behavior	Personal-Social Behavior
5	Speaks without infantile articulation. Asks "Why?"	Counts 10 pennies.	Skips on alternate feet.	Dresses without assistance. Asks meaning of words.
4	Uses conjunctions. Understands prepositions.	Builds gate of 5 cubes. Draws "man."	Skips on one foot.	Can wash and dry face. Goes on errands. Plays cooperatively.
3	Talks in sentences. Answers simple questions	Builds bridge of 3 cubes. Imitates cross.	Stands on one foot. Builds tower of 10 cubes.	Uses spoon well. Puts on shoes. Takes turns.
2	Uses phrases. Understands simple directions.	Builds tower of 6 cubes. Imitates circular stroke.	Runs. Builds tower of 6 cubes.	Verbalizes toilet needs. Plays with dolls.
18 mos.	Jargons. Names pictures.	Dumps pellet from bottle. Imitates crayon stroke.	Walks without falling. Seats self. Tower of 3 cubes.	Uses spoon with moderate spilling. Toilet regulated.
12 mos.	Says 2 or more words	Releases cube in cup.	Walks with help. Cruises. Prehends pellet with precision.	Cooperates in dressing. Gives toy. Finger feeds.
40 wks.	Says one word. Heeds his name.	Combines 2 cubes.	Sits alone. Creeps. Pulls to feet. Crude prehensory release.	Plays simple nursery games. Feeds self cracker.
28 wks.	Crows. Vocalizes eagerness. Listens to own vocalizations.	Transfers cube from hand to hand.	Sits, leaning forward on hands. Grasps cube. Rakes at pellet.	Plays with feet and toys. Expectant in feeding situations.
16 wks.	Coos. Laughs. Vocalizes socially.	Competent eye following. Regards rattle in hand.	Head steady. Symmetrical postures.	Plays with hands and dress. Recognizes bottle. Poises mouth for food.
4 wks.	Small throaty sounds. Heeds bell.	Stares at surroundings. Restricted eye following.	Head sags. T-n-r. Hands fisted.	Regards faces.

--- BIRTH ---

Adapted from Developmental Diagnosis (Second Ed.) by A. Gesell & C. S. Amatruda. New York: Paul B. Hoeber, 1956, pp. 11–14.

TABLE 26–4 LANGUAGE DEVELOPMENT OF THE CHILD*

(AGE IN YEARS)

MEASURE OF DEVELOPMENT	1	1½	2	2½	3	3½	4	4½	5	5½	6	6½	7	7½	8
(AGE IN MONTHS)	12	18	24	30	36	42	48	54	60	66	72	78	84	90	96
APPEARANCE OF INDIVIDUAL SOUNDS	(The indicated age of appearance of the individual sounds represents the upper limit of normality. Any sound may—and frequently does—appear before the age indicated.)					[m], [b], [p], [h], [w]. All Vowels of English		[k], [g], [t], [d], [n], [ŋ], (ng), [j] (y)		[f]		[v], [ʃ] (sh), [ʒ] (zh), [l], [θ] (th)		[s], [z], [r], [hw] (wh), [θ] (th), [tʃ] (ch), [dʒ] (j)	
NUMERICAL SIZE OF VOCABULARY	First Word	20 to 100 Words	200 to 300 Words		900 Words		1500 Words								
WORD TYPE (EACH TYPE APPEARS WITH THE MOST COMMON AT THE TOP.)	Nouns	Nouns and some Verbs and Other Parts	Nouns Verbs, and Other Parts		Verbs, Nouns, Pronouns, and Adjectives		Verbs, Pronouns, Nouns								
SENTENCE LENGTH IN WORDS		Single Word Sentences	Two Word Sentences		Three Word Sentences										
PERCENTAGE OF INTELLIGIBILITY OF CHILD'S SPEECH		25%	66%		90%				100%						
ERUPTION OF DENTITION**	12 mos. Mandibular first molar; 6–9 mos. All incisors	18 mos. Maxillary cuspid; 16 mos. Mandibular cuspid; 14 mos. Maxillary first molar	24 mos. Maxillary second molar; 20 mos. Mandibular second molar								6–7 yrs. Mandibular central incisor; Mandibular first molar; Maxillary first molar (permanent dentition)			7–8 yrs. Mandibular lateral incisor; Maxillary central incisor (permanent dentition)	

*From: Speech Disorders; Principles and Practices of Therapy. By M. F. Berry and J. Eisenson. Copyright © 1956. By permission of Appleton-Century-Crofts, Educational Division, Meredith Corporation.

**From R. C. Wheeler, A Textbook of Dental Anatomy and Physiology. Philadelphia: W. B. Saunders Co., 1950, p. 32.

telligibility of the child's speech. Although a number of the speech sounds are listed under seven-and-one-half years of age, most speech pathologists feel that a child should be able to produce most of the sounds correctly before entering school. Defective articulation has been shown to have adverse effect on reading achievement.

Boys are usually slower than girls in language and speech maturation. If there are older siblings who do most of the talking, younger children may have no adequate opportunity for "practicing" expressive skills. Structural anomalies, neurological defects, illness, trauma, and lack of opportunity for interpersonal communication may delay the growth and development of speech and language.

Correct articulation of speech sounds is related to memory span for individual and clustered sounds, to specialization in motor performance, and to adequate sensory feedback. Children with delayed or defective speech and language should be referred to a speech pathologist. After proper evaluation and arrangement for medical and dental treatment, a speech pathologist will place a child in a speech improvement or speech correction program. With young children, the preferred treatment may be parent counseling and a home language development program. Parents, especially among the affluent and professional groups, often appear to have unrealistic expectations concerning speech and language development for their children. By calling attention to what are "felt" to be inadequate communication patterns, parents, relatives, and friends may cause the child to be concerned about his speech and, in some instances, the conditions are set for the evolvement of more serious speech disorders. If there is some question concerning the "normalcy" of speech, language, or hearing functions, children should be referred to speech pathologists and audiologists, rather than being admonished to "slow down, speak right, or speak up."

One of the greatest services the speech clinician can provide for other health professionals is to coordinate referral procedures essential to differential diagnosis and comprehensive treatment for children with communicative disorders.

Multimedia Influence.   Today's child is bombarded with multimedia communication. He is provided with vast auditory and visual stimulation that, of itself, provides no opportunity for interpersonal communication. The mass media input through radio and television has created a modern troubadour civilization. Worldwide reporting may bring a sense of responsibility, a feeling of anxiety, and an awareness of up-to-the-minute happenings, but young viewers need more than to just listen, they need to ask questions and express their thoughts. This multipersonal communication practice can only be accomplished through the involvement of parents, teachers, siblings, and peers. Marshall McLuhan and Quentin Fiore, in *The Medium is the Massage,* describe the impact of multimedia:

> All media work us over completely. They are so pervasive in their personal, political, economic, aesthetic, psychological, moral, ethical, and social consequences that they leave no part of us untouched, unaffected, unaltered. The medium is the massage. Any understanding of social and cultural change is impossible without a knowledge of the way media work as environments (p. 28):

CLINICAL COMMUNICOLOGY

Communicative disorders in children have multiple etiologies. Disturbances in sensorimotor and central processes are likely to affect the human communication systems of speech, voice, language, and hearing, singly or in varying combinations. The time, nature, site, and degree of damage caused by the disturbances are reflected in the severity, type, and performance of the disorder. Verbal behavior, as one of the highest levels of human behavior, is particularly vulnerable to emotional impact, and, as a result, "functional" or nonorganic communication disorders may become manifest. Optimal habilitation and rehabilitation consists of not only physical restoration but also the achievement of maximal levels of communication. *Truly functional speech must be comfortable for the speaker, intelligible and pleasing to the listener, and appropriate to the occasion.* The term *functional*, in the area of communication disorders, is often used to denote a disorder that is *nonorganic*, is psychogenic, or is without a definitive diagnosis. In terms of educational, social, and vocational application, however, *functional* describes a level of usage—one that is satisfactory, even if it is not optimal.

Diagnosis by Symptom. Professionals in clinical communicology generally categorize communicative disorders into four major areas: *articulation, phonation, rhythm,* and *symbolization,* or as a complex disorder with multiple symptoms. Communicative disorders are described by the outstanding symptom and, if multiple symptoms are present, according to the primary, secondary, and tertiary involvement.

Almost every communicative disorder has an articulatory component, even though the outstanding symptom may be defective rhythm or language. Hearing loss may be a single factor in causing speech and language delay, or it may be one component of complex disorders such as cleft palate, cerebral palsy, and mental retardation. Other complex problems are foreign dialect and aphasia.

Articulation Disorders

Defects of articulation are usually described as substitutions, omissions, distortions, or additions. Most patients exhibit more than one error and may be inconsistent in the production of all the defective sounds. Articulation disorders have both kinesiologic and acoustic aspects. Sounds used for substitution are usually those most similar in topographical placement, articulatory movement, or acoustic similarity. Thus, voiced and voiceless sounds may be interchanged: one bilabial sound may be substituted for another, and a high frequency sound may be used to replace another of high frequency. Articulatory defects in adults may have their origins in childhood. Open bites and temporary hearing losses are problems that have contributed to sound substitutions or distortions early in life, and the improper habits have never been corrected.

Orofacial Abnormalities. Speech defects associated with malocclusions and related abnormalities are described by H. Harlan Bloomer (1971). He states:

> Defective sounds are produced if the essential valves...are not properly created because of abnormal oral structures or maladaptive patterns of articulatory movement. The nature of the articulatory defects thus caused is usually one of distortion rather than complete omission or substitution, although almost any form of defective articulation can occur. Some of the distortions are esthetically displeasing; others will interfere seriously with intelligibility. In most instances, some improvement can be achieved (p. 736).

Bloomer has originated a system of articulatory malphones that may be used during examination of a patient. The pictographic diacritics help the clinician identify not only what articulatory distortion exists but also what form of abnormal valving produced the defective consonant.

Cleft Palate and Cleft Lip. Cleft palate and cleft lip are conditions causing multiple symptomatology, including defective articulation and resonation and the possibility of hearing loss. Rhythm may also be disrupted because of the nasal leakage of air that makes speaking in phrases or sentences on a single breath of air very difficult.

When there is velar insufficiency, there is no distortion of the nasal sounds, *m, n, ng,* because of their normal nasal resonance. Some children display "cleft palate speech" without organic abnormality. This is sometimes the result of imitating parents with cleft palate speech.

In some cases of severe nasal obstruction, the bilabial plosive *b* will be replaced by the *m,* thus making *me* become *be.* The voiced, linguoalveolar *d* will be substituted for *n* making *no* become *doe.* The voiced velar *g* will be substituted for the linguovelar *ng,* thus *ring* might become *rig.* Hypernasality may appear after removal of nasal obstructions. It is usually recommended that the child be seen by a speech pathologist so the child can be assisted in making an adequate adaptation to the newly opened nasal passages before he establishes poor speech habits.

The diagnoses and treatment of cleft palate patients clearly call for interdisciplinary cooperation. The health team includes not only dentists and surgeons but also the speech pathologist, audiologist, psychologist, and social worker. The special education teacher and the vocational rehabilitation counselor may eventually be needed in order to assist the child in achieving optimal habilitation as an adult.

Infantile Perseveration. Infantile perseveration, or baby talk, is a carryover from early stages of speech development, usually characterized by the *w* substituted for the *r,* the *y* for the *l, t* for *k,* and *f* for *th.*

Lalling. Lalling is usually ascribed to sluggish tongue movement and is characterized by defective *s, z, t, d, r,* and *l* sounds. Many children with mental retardation, cerebral palsy, and certain glandular diseases exhibit lalling.

Lisping. The sounds usually defective in lisping are the *s, z, sh,* and *zh.* *Sigmatism* is a term used for the *s* phoneme. Closely associated with the sibilant mentioned above are the fricatives, or affricates, *ch* /tʃ/ and *j* /dʒ/. Affricates have the characteristics of both a stop and a fricative. J.L.M. Trim (1953, pp. 21–24) annotated 18 different kinds of lisps through use of the International Phonetic Alphabet. The following are the most usual classifications of lisp:

Central, frontal, lingual, protrusion or substitution	*th* substituted for *s* or *z*
Unilateral or bilateral	"voiceless *l*" for *s, z, sh, zh, ch* or *j*
Occluded	*t* or *d* for *s* or *z;* sometimes for *sh* or *zh*
Nasal (cleft palate snort)	airstream channeled through nose instead of oral cavity

Cerebral Palsy. The effects of a poorly functioning neuromuscular system may be quickly identified in the child with cerebral palsy. Voice, rhythm, resonation, and articulation disorders occur. In some cases, hearing loss and mental retardation or aphasia are present. Poor control of the air supply may result from poor valving by the laryngeal and articulatory mechanisms.

Foreign Dialect. The illogical acoustic and graphic relationships confront the foreigner wishing to become fluent in the English language. Sound substitutions and distortions are common in foreign dialects. Intonational patterns may be noted as "different" from those of the native speaker.

Local Dialects. Place of birth or residence was long identifiable because of a particular dialect of that region. Children acquire the speech of parents and peers. With the increased mobility of the general population throughout the United States, and with the inundation of multimedia communication, the dialectal borders are being erased and judgment of "good speech" has shifted from the *cultivated* pronunciation of the past to the *functional* communication demanded by modern marketing.

The "second language" dilemma of the native Hawaiian storekeeper who chooses to employ clerks from the Mainland because their "business English" is superior to that of many of the Hawaiian-born young people illustrates the emphasis on functional communication. A similar problem faces the children of certain minority or central city groups who use a "second language" that may be appropriate for home use but not acceptable in business and professions.

A study by Charles G. Hurst (1968) discusses some of the attitudes of young people concerning their inadequate speech and language. The participants in the study indicated that they felt their communication patterns were the result of (1) poor speech models when they were children, (2) a lack of speech improvement courses in high school, and (3) a resistance on their part to being taught standard speech. Hurst also stated that more than 85 per cent of the high school graduates from the slum areas use nonstandard language.

Voice Disorders

Voice quality may be thought of as the "personality of the voice." This, in turn, reflects the personality of the speaker. The quality may be nasal, hoarse, breathy, harsh, husky, guttural, or have too much vibrato and other undesirable attributes. Like other aspects of speech, dysphonia may be the result of organic, psychological, or functional disorders. A voice that is too loud or too soft for the occasion is usually the result of personality maladjustment and is not an organic problem.

The normal pitch of the voice is dependent on age. If there is a physical difficulty such as malformation of the larynx, vocal folds, or other structures there will be a pitch problem. Psychological pitch problems may be manifested in the pitch of an adult male if he has been surrounded by female voices, especially as a child.

Acceptable variations in voice appear to be wider than that of articulation.

> With some important exceptions, the voice may be viewed as the carrier wave; articulations as the message carried. We ordinarily pay more attention to the message we receive than to the vehicle bearing that message. We read the script rather than look at the paper or the ink; we listen to the speech sounds more closely than we do the tones of the voice. Perhaps it is for this reason that, according to the last White House Conference Report, there are fifteen times as many individuals who have articulation defects as there are those who have voice problems. Another reason why variant voice is judged more leniently than articulation is that the average parent has

less reason to worry about the appearance of voice in his first-born than he does about the acquisition of phonemes. Most babies come complete with a voice that varies in its pitch, intensity, and quality characteristics. The correct articulation of standard speech sounds must be learned. And so our society tends to become more concerned over deviant articulation than it does over deviant voice (Van Riper and Irwin, 1958, pp. 164–165).

Any hoarseness, or other voice abnormality, that persists should be referred to a medical specialist. Speech pathologists accept voice cases only upon medical referral.

Quality Disorders

The quality disorders most frequently noted by dentists are probably those of hypernasality and denasality. These disorders may be caused by misplaced articulators, cleft palate, or malformations that alter the size and shape of the resonating cavities. For example, nasality may be the result of assimilation—the process of one sound influencing the other. *Place* assimilation often occurs, for instance, when an *a* is adjacent to an *n* or an *m*. Nasalization becomes even more apparent when the *a* is between two nasal sounds as in *man*.

Rhythm Disorders (Time)

Speech is sequential, and time and rhythm are important to good communication patterns. The rate of speech is the speed at which a person speaks. In English, there is no standard rate for the number of syllables or words per second. The social and linguistic situations determine the rate. The sports announcer at a hockey game will, by necessity, use a more rapid rate than the speaker in a more deliberate situation. The layman often blames slovenly speech on such qualities as rapid rate, when the problem actually results from slovenly articulation. The speaker with a normal oral architecture may have poor speech because of too rapid a rate and distinct articulation, or he may have the reverse, either one of which would result in communication problems.

Early nonfluency is to be expected as a child "practices" his speech skills. If no attention is called to his easy repetitions and hesitancies, he most likely will progress to the normal rhythms of mature speech. Primary stuttering may lead to secondary complications, if the child becomes anxious concerning his speaking patterns. Tenseness and prolongations, in addition to tics and spasms of the vocal mechanism, cause fear and frustration. Thus, the vicious circle of secondary stuttering is initiated—the worse the speech, the greater the fear; and the greater the fear, the worse the speech.

Cluttering should not be confused with stuttering. Both are rhythm disorders, but the clutterer, as opposed to the stutterer, uses "pell-mell" speech, is not aware of his problem, and does not struggle as he speaks.

Symbolization Disorders (Language)

Most of the disorders included under symbolization are complex. Articulatory defects are common in these disorders.

Deafness. Speech and language are generally delayed in congenitally deaf children, since they have no acoustic patterns to aid them in developing their vocabulary, linguistic concepts, and the articulatory patterns of their environment.

Hard of hearing children usually display some articulation defects. They often experience difficulties in achieving optimal educational levels.

Mental Retardation. The speech of the mentally retarded child exhibits infantile perseveration of sounds as well as language delay and other complications.

Developmental Aphasia. Children who have suffered anoxia, trauma, meningitis, or jaundice often show symptoms of developmental or congenital aphasia. These children vary in types and degrees of language disabilities.

Psychogenic Retardation. In psychogenic retardation, speech and language difficulties are related to emotional problems.

Deafness, mental retardation, developmental aphasia, and psychogenic retardation are often confused. Without a differential diagnosis, suitable therapeutic and educational programs cannot be planned.

PREVALENCE OF SPEECH DEFECTS

An estimated prevalence of speech defects in the United States is shown in Table 26–5. The numbers of cases are based on an estimated population of 50,000,000 between the ages of 5 and 21 years and a total population of 200,000,000. The grand totals show that 8,500,000 Americans have either bilateral or unilateral hearing impairments, another 2,100,000 have central communicative disorders, and 10,000,000 have speech disorders. Even if a modest overlap is assumed in the totals, it appears that approximately 20,000,000 persons in the United States have communicative handicaps worthy of concern.

Summary

Many of the communicative disorders in adults could be prevented or partially alleviated by treatment during childhood. Such disorders commonly require com-

TABLE 26–5 ESTIMATED PREVALENCE OF SPEECH DEFECTS IN THE UNITED STATES*

Type of Speech Problem	Ages 5–21 Years		All Ages	
	Percent	Number	Percent	Number
Functional articulatory	3.0	1,500,000	3.0	6,000,000
Stuttering	.7	350,000	.7	1,400,000
Voice	.2	100,000	.2	400,000
Cleft palate speech	.1	50,000	.1	200,000
Cerebral palsy speech	.2	100,000	.2	400,000
Retarded speech development	.3	150,000	.3	600,000
Impaired hearing (with speech defect)	.5	250,000	.5	1,000,000
	5.0	2,500,000	5.0	10,000,000

*From Human Communication and Its Disorders—An Overview. Monograph No. 10. A Report prepared and published by the Subcommittee on Human Communication and Its Disorders of the National Advisory Neurological Diseases and Stroke Council, NIH. Bethesda, Md.: U.S. Dept. of Health, Education, and Welfare, 1969, p. 18.

prehensive evaluation and care from medical doctors, dentists, and specialists in speech, language, and hearing disorders.

Lead time in the application of present knowledge is being lessened as interdisciplinary research and experience are being applied to the diagnosis, prognosis, and treatment of children with speech, voice, language, and hearing disorders.

All who work in the many related areas of health, education, and welfare have long been aware of the tremendous achievements of the medical and dental disciplines in attaining the virtual elimination of many of the diseases that have plagued man throughout his history. These accomplishments have given impetus to preventive procedures and drawn attention to the importance of speech functionalism as an additional goal in health habilitation and rehabilitation. Speech that is comfortable for the speaker, intelligible and pleasing to the listener, and appropriate to the occasion has become a new measure of effectiveness in the delivery of health care.

REFERENCES

American Speech and Hearing Association Committee on the White House Midcentury Conference. Journal of Speech and Hearing Disorders. *17*:129–137, 1952.

Berry, M. F., and Eisenson, J.: Speech Disorders. New York, Appleton-Century-Crofts, 1956, p. 85.

Bloomer, H. H.: Speech defects associated with dental abnormalities and malocclusions. *In* Handbook of Speech Pathology, Travis, L. E. (ed.). New York, Appleton-Century-Crofts, 1957, pp. 613–616.

Bloomer, H. H.: Speech defects associated with dental malocclusions, *In* Handbook of Speech Pathology and Audiology, Travis, L. E. (ed.). New York, Appleton-Century-Crofts, 1971.

Chalfant, J. D., and Scheffelin, M. A.: Central Processing Dysfunctions in Children: A Review of Research. National Institute of Neurological Diseases and Stroke, Public Health Service, National Institutes of Health. Bethesda, Md., U.S. Dept. of Health, Education, and Welfare, 1969, pp. 40, 45, 46.

Denes, P. B., and Pinson, E. N.: The Speech Chain. (Produced and distributed by Bell Telephone Laboratories.) Baltimore, Md., Waverly Press, Inc., 1966, pp. 4, 8.

Gesell, A., and Amatruda, C. S.: Developmental Diagnosis (2nd Ed.). New York, Paul B. Hoeber, 1956, pp. 11–14.

Human Communication and Its Disorders—An Overview. Monograph No. 10. (A Report prepared and published by the Subcommittee on Human Communication and Its Disorders of the National Advisory Neurological Diseases and Stroke Council, National Institutes of Health, Public Health Service. Bethesda, Md., U.S. Dept. of Health, Education and Welfare, 1969, pp. 18, 145.

Hurst, C. G., Jr.: Higher Horizons in Speech Communication. Boston, General Electronic Laboratories, 1968.

Lasswell, H. D., Leietes, N., et al.: Language of Politics: Studies in Quantitative Semantics. New York, George W. Stewart, 1949, pp. 5–6.

Liepmann, H.: Motorische Aphasie und Apraxie. Monatsschr. Psychiat. u. Neurol., 34, 1913.

Luria, A. R.: Human Brain and Psychological Processes. New York, Harper & Row, 1966.

McLuhan, M. and Fiore, Q.: The Medium is the Massage. New York, Bantam Books, 1967, p. 28.

Rehabilitation Codes. Special Project RD-788, Office of Vocational Rehabilitation, 1961–1964. New York, Rehabilitation Codes, 1790 Broadway.

Trim, J. L. M.: Some suggestions for the phonetic notation of sounds in defective speech. Speech (London), *17*:21–24, 1953.

Van Riper, C., and Irwin, J. V. Voice and Articulation. Englewood Cliffs, N.J., Prentice-Hall, 1958, pp. 164–165.

Wheeler, R. C. A Textbook of Dental Anatomy and Physiology. Philadelphia, W. B. Saunders Co., 1950, p. 32.

27

HEREDITARY FACTORS IN PEDODONTICS

by SIDNEY B. FINN

In studying variations in growth and development and the physiology of the oral cavity in children, the determinative role played by heredity is all too frequently overlooked. Yet no book of children's dentistry should be considered complete without some thought being given this neglected subject. The study of genetics will not only provide an insight into what is considered normal, but it will also help us to understand a great many of the deviations seen in the oral cavity in children which cannot be attributed to local or systemic environmental factors.

Our knowledge of human heredity is based on several types of studies:

1. The study of genealogies, i.e., the study of the occurrence and prevalence in certain families of specific variations from the norm or average. Comparisons may be made with the population in general.

2. The study of identical twins to make comparisons of specific traits in these individuals. In identical twin studies the relative influences of heredity and environment can be compared with those in fraternal twins or with a like sample of the general population.

3. Animal experimentation and breeding.

Each of these methods of obtaining data is important and offers much valuable information. In studying alterations in oral tissues, each of these three means will be utilized. Genealogies will be presented as well as twin studies. Animal studies and human studies indicate that the susceptibility to dental caries may have a hereditary basis. Chromosomal aberrations will be described in Chapter 28.

610

MODES OF INHERITANCE

Every child is a biologic unit and is subject to the biologic laws which govern or regulate the orderly processes of nature. The most important of these from a developmental viewpoint are the mendelian laws of heredity. These are the basis of the science of genetics.

Genetics deals in part with the inheritance of characteristics which may account for differences and similarities in living things that are related by descent. Heredity also has a far greater implication. It is the stabilizing force in the evolution of species. Without the definite regulatory process of inheritance, one could not presume that members of a given species would reproduce their own kind.

CHROMOSOMES

All living organisms, whether plant or animal, from the most minute viruses to the largest trees, conform to the mendelian laws of heredity. The simple principles of inheritance in humans will be considered in this chapter as well as deviations from the normal observed in the oral cavity.

The characteristics for similarity or dissimilarity are handed down from parent to offspring in the chromosomes, which are a constituent of the germ plasm found in both the ovum and the sperm. The number of chromosomes varies in different species. In humans there normally are 23 pairs; 23 are handed down through the female ovum, or egg, and 23 through the male sperm. One of each pair of homologous chromosomes is received from each parent.

GENES

Within the chromosomes are smaller units called genes. The genes are masses of protoplasm, arranged in characteristic order along the length of the chromosome. Each gene occupies a specific position or locus. The genes are segments of deoxyribonucleic acid (DNA), which is the true hereditary material. The DNA molecule is composed of two very long chains coiled around a common axis to form a double helix. The important constituent of each chain consists of alternations of nucleic acid, sugar, and phosphate groups. The sugar is deoxyribose and is attached to purines and pyrimidines bound together by a hydrogen bonding. One can envisage the many permutations which can occur in the splitting and crossing over of these long chains. Any expressed characteristic may be inherited through a single pair of genes or through multiple gene pairs. When both genes of a given pair, one from each parent, are similar, we speak of the individual as being homozygous for this characteristic. When a given pair of genes from the same locus (alleles) are dissimilar, the individual is said to be heterozygous for the characteristic. Since human beings are hybrid for a great many characteristics, heterozygosity is common. When multiple pairs of genes are involved in transmitting a hereditary factor, the gene combinations can become extremely complex with various similar and dissimilar genes entering into the process.

DOMINANCE

When a character is expressed when the genes are dissimilar, or heterozygous, the factor is dominant. When both genes are required to be similar before the character is expressed, the factor is recessive. In order for a recessive character to appear in the offspring it must be present in both parents and must be handed down from both parents. A dominant factor, however, may be received from only one parent and be manifest in the offspring. If one of the parents is homozygous for this factor, all offspring in the first generation will be affected even though the other parent is heterozygous or negative for the factor. The dominant character should show up in every generation and in considerable numbers. Recessive variants may not show up for many generations, and then only in very limited numbers. The recessive inherited aberrations are therefore less common in the population and are generally more extreme and destructive to the species. The dominant characteristics are generally less destructive; otherwise the entire species might be jeopardized.

X-LINKAGE

There are certain variants which are transmitted as X-linked recessive, a trait which is manifest in the male while being handed down through the unaffected opposite sex. These are designated sex-linked characteristics. Human beings have sex chromosomes which are, among other things, the determinants of the sex of the offspring. Each woman has a pair of these X (or sex) chromosomes, having received one from each parent in addition to the other 22 pairs. Each man, however, has only one X chromosome and one Y chromosome, in addition to the other 22 pairs of autosomal chromosomes. Femaleness is determined by the presence of two X chromosomes, maleness by the presence of only one X chromosome.

The Y chromosome is shorter than the X chromosome and does not have a full complement of genes although it may contain genes not present on the X chromosome. This lack of genes on the Y chromosomes is significant in such hereditary diseases as hemophilia. A true hemophilia appears only in males but is carried by the unaffected females. This X-linked recessive blood abnormality is of special interest to the dentist because of the danger of uncontrolled hemorrhage. The mode of inheritance can be explained in the following manner: Since the male inherits from his parents an X and a Y chromosome and the female receives two X chromosomes, each male sperm may have either an X or a Y chromosome while each ovum contains an X chromosome. The four possible unions of sperm and ovum can give only two different combinations of sex chromosomes, with theoretically equal numbers of males and females. These are depicted in Figure 27–1.

The X chromosome in the sperm (X_H) carries the characteristic for hemophilia, but since that characteristic is recessive it will not be expressed if the X_H chromosome is paired with a normal X chromosome. Thus, both females with $X_H X$ will carry the characteristics for hemophilia but they will not be affected by the disease. However, if these $X_H X$ females mate with XY males, the next generation would have the four possibilities shown in Figure 27–2. The male $X_H Y$ combination contains the chromosome for hemophilia, and since the Y chromosome does not carry a corresponding gene for this factor, the single X_H is manifest in its haploid or

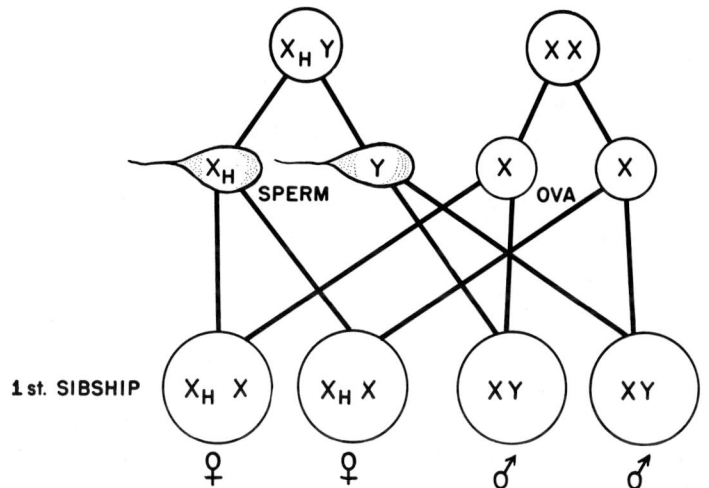

Figure 27–1 The mode of transmission of hemophilia through the first generation.

single state and the male individual bearing this combination has inherited hemophilia.

CROSSING OVER

Crossing over is a normal process in meiosis and is one of the mechanisms for assuring germ cells with different genetic factors.

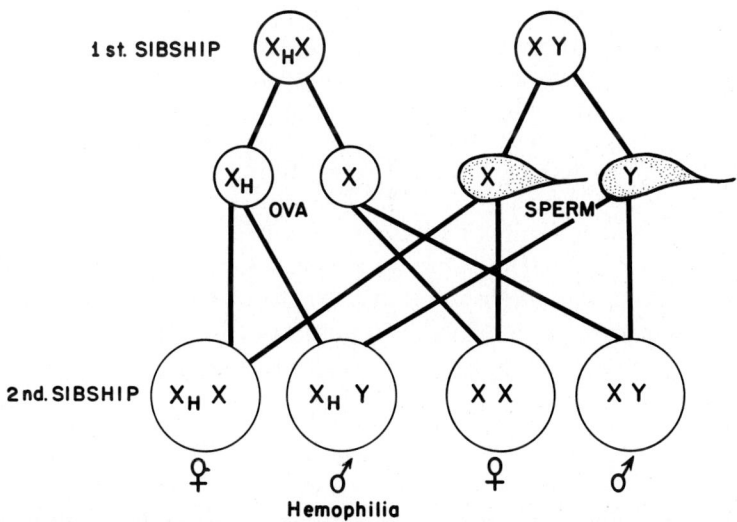

Figure 27–2 The mode of transmission of hemophilia through the second generation.

PENETRANCE

Another complicating factor is the possibility of the incomplete penetrance of the germ plasm to reduce the frequency of occurrence of the expressed variable. One may find a dominant characteristic completely skipping a generation. Osteogenesis imperfecta appears to be inherited in this manner. In certain other dominant inheritance, a particular trait may be expressed in varying degrees of intensity. This variable expressivity may account for the degrees of severity of certain manifest aberrations seen in the oral cavity.

In certain aberrations, the same alterations may be produced by different sets of gene patterns. As an example, susceptibility to dental caries may be produced by a gene combination making for a less resistant tooth structure, or by one reducing the salivary flow. In both instances, the end result might be the same.

One also finds in human genetics that the same pathologic aberration may be dominant in one family and recessive in another.

MUTATIONS

Occasionally one finds differences or anomalies which cannot be accounted for by environmental or previously observed hereditary influences in the family. These are called mutations. The gene is a stable body of protoplasm replicating at each cell division with amazing exactness. Occasionally, however, due to thermal, radiational or as yet undiscovered causes, the gene undergoes a sudden change producing a mutation. These mutations or changes then continue their replication so that the mutation persists through continuing generations.

Radiation, regardless of its source, whether it be x-ray or atomic radiation, can produce serious damage to the individual receiving it. One way is by altering the gene chemistry, another by the actual fragmentation of the chromosomes, and the production of mutations which are generally harmful. These mutant forms produced by the energy from the radiation persist from one generation to the next. The acquired mutant genes are almost always detrimental to the individual or his offspring; they may be expressed as an undesirable abnormality, as an inability to reproduce, or even by an early death. Even the less deleterious mutations, being more general and less evident, may in the final reckoning result in serious damage to the species. Being less evident they will not be bred out of the families and thus will persist longer and harm greater numbers of people.

The mutant gene characteristics are rarely fully expressed in the first generation in the person receiving the radiation. The mutant gene, being recessive, may be masked by a normal dominant gene for a number of generations, and the offspring may appear normal. However, even when the recessive mutant is dominated by a dominant gene, the abnormality may be expressed in an attenuated form, perhaps physically unrecognizable but still somewhat detrimental to the individual.

Any radiation dose, even in small quantity, can induce some mutation. There is no minimal radiation dose required for harmful mutations to occur. However, it appears that the number of gene mutations is directly proportional to the total dosage of radiation received by the reproductive cells. It is the sum total dosage of radiation that is all important, since radiation damage to the reproductive cells is cumulative. It is understood that increased amounts would produce a greater number of, but not more destructive, mutants. There appears to be no specific rate at which radiation can be received without producing harm. From a genetic viewpoint, it is the total accumulated dose received during the development of the parent up to the time the child is conceived that is harmful. What is most important to the offspring is the total radiation received by both of his parents.

Roughly, in about 2 per cent of the total live births there are hereditary defects which appear before sexual maturity, such as morphologic anomalies, mental defects, neuromuscular defects, blood defects, etc. If one were to receive double the normally received background radiation (cosmic rays, etc.), which has been estimated to be from 5 to 150 roentgens, then the number of genetic abnormalities would be doubled.

It has been reliably estimated that 10 roentgens is a reasonable but not altogether harmless additional dosage for the gonads to receive from conception to age 30, an age when half of the parents' children will have been born.

To keep this additional radiation at a minimum, it has been suggested that medical and dental x-rays be limited to the barest necessity, especially in the region of the reproductive organs. The operators of these machines should be well shielded from any direct or indirect rays. In addition, all radiation from other sources such as radioactive "fallout," atomic piles, atomic power plants, etc., should be avoided as much as possible. (See Chapter 6, Roentgenography.)

HEREDITY AND DENTAL CARIES

The relatively important role heredity plays in the susceptibility or resistance of an individual to dental caries has been of interest to a great many investigators. They have approached the subject from three different aspects: (1) animal breeding studies; (2) human family studies; (3) twin studies.

By selective breeding caries-resistant and caries-susceptible strains of hamsters and rats have been developed. Even when exposed to a caries-conducive oral environment, caries-resistant animals still are more resistant to caries than the caries-susceptible strains. Although the critical importance of oral environmental factors such as the substrate and oral flora does outweight to a substantial degree the hereditary disposition, it does not do so entirely.

Human family studies both in this country and in Sweden indicate that children of caries-free parents have less dental caries in general than a sample of unselected individuals of the general population, indicating a family predisposition to caries susceptibility. It must be borne in mind that individual families may have similar eating habits and diets, which could account for family similarities and differences.

Twin studies on humans with reliable statistical evaluation have been conducted by a number of investigators both in this country and abroad. These studies indicate that identical twins tend to have less intrapair difference in caries experience than do fraternal twins, although the difference may or may not be statistically significant depending upon the study. Since identical twins are formed from the splitting of the fertilized ovum, genetically they should be more similar than fraternal twins who develop from two individual fertilized ova. Because the parentage is the same regardless of the type of twin, one would expect less intrapair difference than between paired unrelated children of the same age and sex even though they may be on the same diet. Present day evidence indicates that this is so.

HEREDITARY ANOMALIES OF TOOTH NUMBER, STRUCTURE, AND FORM

A great many anomalies of tooth number, structure, and form have a hereditary basis. The nature of the anomaly depends largely upon the embryologic time of manifestation, the germ layer involved, and the effect of various modifying factors. The frequency of occurrence is governed by the mode of inheritance and other probability factors.

A number of these tooth anomalies appear independently as the only evident hereditary alteration. Others represent only one of a group of anomalies which comprise a genetic syndrome or disease complex. As an example, missing teeth and tooth buds with a hereditary history may exist as the only abnormality observable in that individual. In others, however, this absence of teeth may be linked with alterations of other ectodermal tissues such as hair, skin, and mucous membranes; the syndrome may then be referred to as hereditary ectodermal dysplasia.

HEREDITARY ANOMALIES OF TOOTH NUMBER

Missing Teeth

Many reports have appeared in the dental literature on the subject of congenitally missing teeth, many of which are shown to have a hereditary basis. In children, the most frequently missing permanent teeth are the second premolars; these are followed in frequency by the upper lateral incisors. Congenitally missing primary teeth occur with much less frequency. Congenital absence of teeth usually occurs bilaterally but may occur unilaterally. One explanation that has been offered for missing lateral incisors is that the hereditary tendency is atavistic and reverts back to the time in evolution when a diastema existed between the central incisors and posterior teeth. Whether congenitally missing teeth are an incomplete expression of ectodermal dysplasia or are an independent gene aberration is unknown.

One must differentiate in these cases between the actual absence of tooth germs and the delay or inhibition of eruption which may occur in certain cases of glandular malfunction or disease entities such as cleidocranial dysostosis. In the latter conditions, the teeth form but may fail to erupt into the mouth.

The hereditary absence of teeth and the formation of supernumerary teeth are the result of a genetic variable being manifested during the developmental stages of initiation and proliferation.

Ectodermal Dysplasia

One of the hereditary syndromes in which missing teeth are characteristic is ectodermal dysplasia. The disease involves more or less the tissues of ectodermal origin. The degree of involvement depends upon the differences of expression of the same genetic variation, although it is possible that different genetic mutations are involved in different intensities of the disease.

Ectodermal dysplasia is arbitrarily divided into two categories, depending upon whether the sebaceous and sudorific glands are involved. Ectodermal dysplasia of the anhidrotic type is the more severe manifestation. The syndrome is characterized by sparse, fine hair on the scalp, absence of eyebrows, a flat broad saddle nose, atrophic rhinitis, pouting and everted lips, protruding ears, a dry encrusted skin, an inability to perspire, and a complete (anodontia) or partial absence (oligodontia) of teeth (Figs. 27–3 and 27–4).

Because of the absence of sweat glands, the body cooling apparatus is impaired; these children show an inability to tolerate heat and are prone to develop markedly elevated temperatures with otherwise mild infections. Convulsions during infancy are not uncommon because of excessive body temperatures. Because of the absence of mucous glands in the nasal mucosa, this membrane is constantly infected, and is marked by the presence of dry encrustations and ozena. The number of teeth present varies among the individuals. The author reviewed 82 cases of anhidrotic ectodermal dysplasia and found that 63.5 per cent of the individuals had more maxillary teeth than mandibular teeth while only 5.4 per cent had more mandibular teeth than maxillary. The same number of teeth appeared in both jaws in 8.1 per cent, and 23.1 per cent were completely edentulous. A mere 2.7 per cent had posterior teeth only, while 31.5 per cent had anterior teeth only. Some anterior and posterior teeth occurred in 42.5 per cent. Many of the teeth were conical in shape (Fig. 27–5).

Ectodermal dysplasia has been reported as a straight dominant and as a sex-linked recessive. Figure 27–6 presents a genealogy of ectodermal dysplasia.

HEREDITARY ANOMALIES OF TOOTH FORM AND TIME OF CALCIFICATION

Although all tooth form is inherited as are all other body characteristics, mutations do occur which alter the tooth form or the time of beginning calcification.

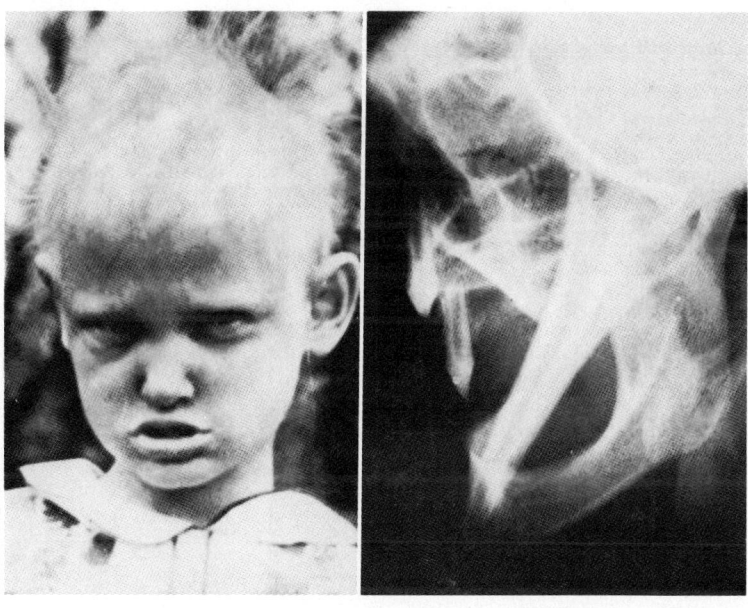

Fig. 27–3   Fig. 27–4

Figure 27–3   Female age 6 with ectodermal dysplasia of the anhidrotic type.
Figure 27–4   A lateral skull roentgenogram reveals only two conical teeth in the cuspid region of the maxilla.

These mutations, which have occurred over a long period in the evolution of mankind, have modified the original single-cusped molar tooth observed in man today. Mutations through the ages will change man's dentition perhaps even more than it has changed to the present time. These mutations will be transmitted through the germ plasm to future generations.

Many mutations of tooth form have been observed. Moody and Montgomery,[21] for instance, have a genealogy of a family with females in four generations showing gemination in the lower primary incisors.

Korkhaus[16] states that tooth form, size, and color are inherited as well as the Carabelli cusp.

Peg-shaped teeth have been observed as a hereditary anomaly. That this is an incomplete expression of missing teeth seems a reasonable possibility. These anomalies are manifest during the developmental period of initiation and differentiation.

Garn, Lewis, and Shoemaker[7] have observed that the order of beginning calcification of the teeth varies among families. In 21.9 per cent of the 359 children studied, the lower second permanent molars began to calcify before the lower second premolars. This variation of calcification time occurred more frequently in siblings than in the general population. The authors hypothesize that this varied eruption of the premolar may be a partial expression of a genetic mutation which, when completely expressed, might result in the congenital absence of the premolars. This is certainly an interesting observation.

Most of the studies that have been conducted on the hereditary aspects of tooth morphology, eruption time, and general arch size and relationships have been performed on twins, both fraternal and identical. A composite of the literature indicates quite definitely that tooth size and arch dimensions are hereditary and that crowding and spacing, although they may be strongly influenced by heredity, are not entirely responsible for certain types of malocclusion.

Harelip and cleft palate tend to be inherited. Refer to Chapter 25, Treatment of the Handicapped Child.

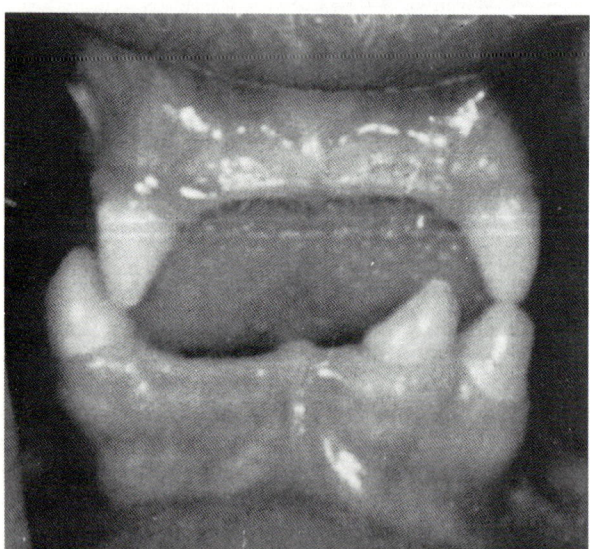

Figure 27–5 Ectodermal dysplasia. Typical conical teeth are common in the anterior of the mouth.

HEREDITARY ECTODERMAL DYSPLASIA

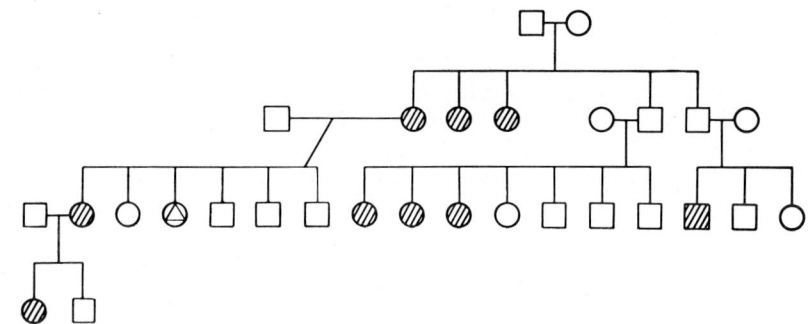

Figure 27–6 Genealogy shows 9 affected siblings and 12 unaffected siblings in 3 generations.

Supernumerary Teeth

Although supernumerary teeth may be found in any region of the dental arch, there are certain sites of predilection. One of the commonest sites is between the maxillary central incisors. In this position, the supernumerary tooth is referred to as a mesiodens. Other common sites are in the region of the central and lateral incisors and the bicuspid area. There has been some question as to the hereditary nature of the condition.

HEREDITARY ANOMALIES OF TOOTH STRUCTURE

Hereditary Amelogenesis Imperfecta

Amelogenesis imperfecta is an anomaly in the structure of the enamel and can be differentiated into two distinct types.

Hereditary Enamel Hypoplasia.   In this type the enamel is normal in structure but aborted in amount. Clinically, the crowns are yellow, smooth, glossy, and hard, although in certain cases there may be severe pitting or striations. The enamel is markedly reduced in thickness, giving the crown a conical or cylindrical shape, and often there is no contact between the teeth. Because of the normal high inorganic content of the enamel, it is soluble in acid to the same degree as the enamel of normal teeth. The extreme thinness of the enamel makes its presence on the teeth difficult to detect roentgenographically when the hypoplasia is severe.

Because of the thinness of the enamel (Fig. 27–7), excessive attrition is observed even in children. When the teeth are worn level with the gum line, it is frequently impossible to determine by clinical observation whether the dystrophy exists in the enamel or in the dentin. The worn, exposed dentin, heavily stained with friable enamel which may or may not be present about the crevices of the teeth, is common to anomalies of both the enamel and the dentin. It therefore becomes essential for diagnostic purposes, when the teeth are severely worn, that one obtain other diagnostic information such as roentgenograms or histologic sections. It is unfortunate that case reports in the earlier literature were deficient in this respect and the exact interpretation of the dystrophy was left to the imagination of the reader.

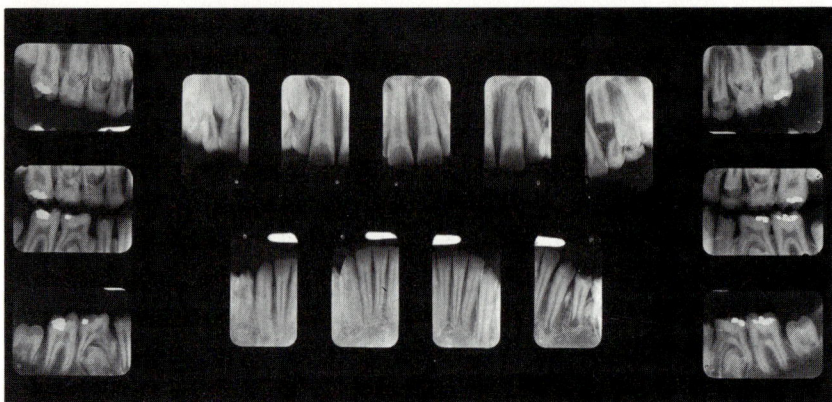

Figure 27–7 Amelogenesis imperfecta of the hypoplastic type. Newly erupted bicuspids show a complete absence of enamel, as do all teeth. Unerupted upper right cuspid crown is almost completely resorbed.

The genetic variable lies in faulty matrix formation (appositional stage). Since the matrix is laid down from the dentino-enamel junction peripherally, the thickness of the enamel would depend upon the period of ameloblastic growth in which the genetic factor became manifest.

Hereditary Enamel Hypocalcification. In this second type of amelogenesis imperfecta the enamel matrix is normal but hypocalcified. The enamel is of normal thickness throughout its substance, but it is of poor quality and sometimes appears soft and cheesy because of a cessation of function in the early stages of maturation. As a result, clinically the teeth absorb stain readily and turn from a dull opaque white to dark brown (Figs. 27–8 and 27–9); the color change results from the absorption of pigments from food and liquids, made possible by the low mineral and high water content of these teeth. The surfaces of the teeth appear dull and lusterless but the enamel is of normal thickness and the crowns of normal shape. Because of the low inorganic content, the enamel is insoluble in acid and does not appear as a distinct layer in a roentgenogram, as the enamel and the dentin are of about the same density. The enamel abrades easily and the crowns wear rapidly, frequently to the level of the margins of the gingiva. The exposed dentin stains heavily brown to black. The enamel on the anterior teeth frequently appears normal. Both dentitions are affected. (See Figure 27–9.) The scalloping of the dentino-enamel junction is normal in both types of amelogenesis imperfecta, as are the pulp chambers and canals.

Both types of amelogenesis imperfecta appear to be dominant and heterozygous with about equal numbers of affected and nonaffected offspring. There appears to be no sex linkage.

Hereditary Dentinogenesis Imperfecta (Odontogenesis Imperfecta, Opalescent Dentin)

Hereditary dentinogenesis imperfecta is a hereditary anomaly of the dentin and is the most prevalent hereditary dystrophy affecting the structure of the teeth. In a survey of over 96,000 school children in Michigan, Witkop[22] found the prevalence to be one affected child in 8,000 children. It is found in diverse nationalities throughout the Caucasian race. These teeth possess a high degree of translucency and their peculiar refractive property, which frequently displays a play of colors by by transmitted light, suggested to the author[5, 13] the alternate title of opalescent dentin. The teeth may appear gray to bluish brown in reflected light (Fig. 27–10). The dentin is soft, making the teeth subject to rapid and excessive wear, quite often level with the gingival margin. The dentino-enamel junction may lack the microscopic scalloped effect of normal teeth although not necessarily. The smooth junction allows for easy fracturing of the enamel and thus aids in the rapid attrition of the teeth. In areas denuded of enamel, the dentin, which is markedly

Fig. 27–8

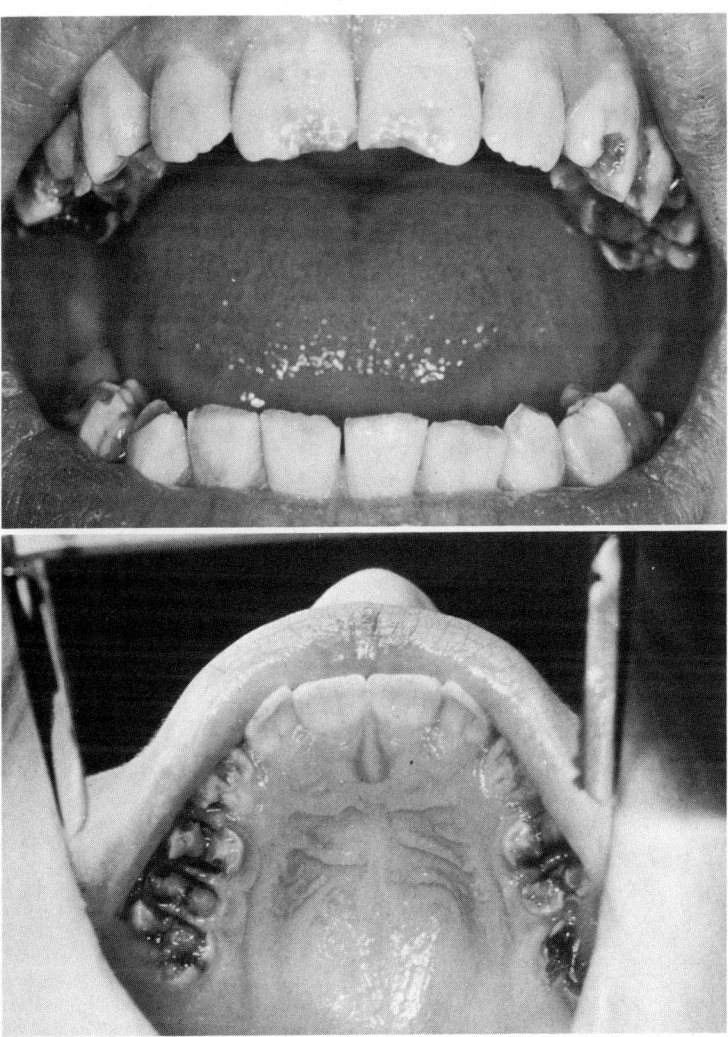

Fig. 27–9

Figure 27–8 Amelogenesis imperfecta showing hypoplasia of the maxillary incisors as well as hypocalcification of all teeth.
Figure 27–9 Amelogenesis imperfecta of the hypocalcification type; posterior teeth are markedly worn and stained in child age 12.

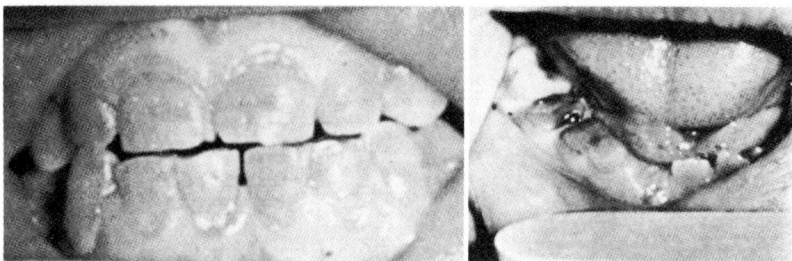

Fig. 27–10   **Fig. 27–11**

Figure 27–10   Dentinogenesis imperfecta. The teeth appear worn, translucent, and of a grayish color.
Figure 27–11   Dentinogenesis imperfecta. The teeth show early and rapid attrition. Caries becomes arrested.

hypoplastic, varies in color from yellow to deep brown, depending upon extrinsic staining. These teeth have a low caries susceptibility although the mass destruction of the crown closely simulates rampant caries. Because of the rapid attrition of the teeth, any caries that does develop generally becomes arrested (Fig. 27–11). The oral mucosa is normal in appearance. Because of the softness of the dentin the dentist often hesitates to place jacket crowns on the anterior teeth. The author has observed a patient with four such teeth which have had jacket crown restorations for 16 years. The teeth were removed with crowns intact to make way for full dentures.

Roentgenographically the crowns, before attrition, are of average size. There is a definite and characteristic decrease in root size. Pulp chambers may be absent and the pulp canals partially or completely obliterated (Fig. 27–12). This may be observed in unerupted teeth in Figure 27–13. The cementum, periodontal membrane, and alveolar bone all appear normal.

Histologic ground sections show a more or less structureless dentin and normal-appearing enamel. The dentin has a varied structural pattern, from complete absence of tubules and an irregularly granular matrix to relatively normal-appearing dentin with a normal tubule pattern in the mantle layer. The course of the tubules varies greatly and has no definite oriented direction. The

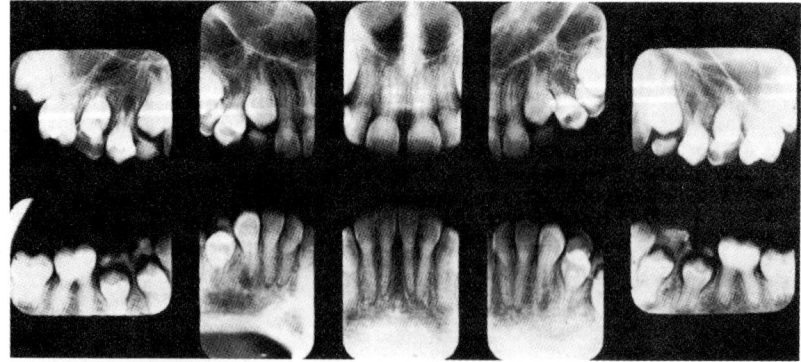

Figure 27–12   Roentgenograms in dentinogenesis imperfecta reveal the shortened roots and occasional absence of pulp chambers and canals.

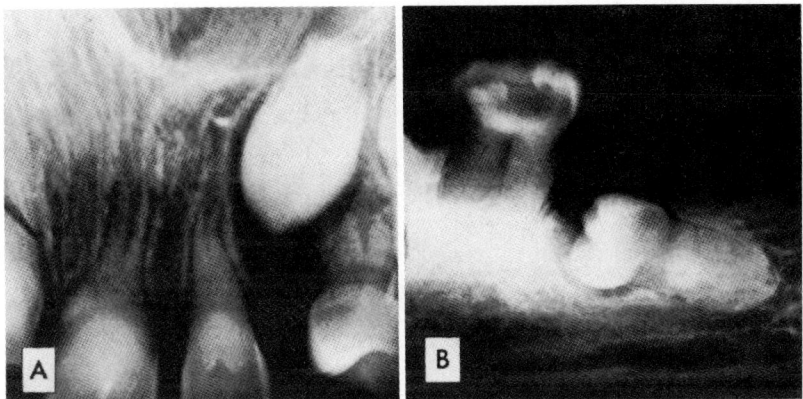

Figure 27–13 Dentinogenesis imperfecta. *A*, Developing cuspid tooth shows no evidence of a pulp chamber. *B*, Impacted premolar tooth shows an absence of pulp chamber and canal.

obliterated pulp chambers and canals are occupied instead by greatly enlarged, sagittally placed tubules. These sometimes appear as pulpal inclusions rather than tubules. The dentin has a high moisture and organic content and a decreased inorganic content.

Dentinogenesis imperfecta is inherited as a conditional dominant with no sex linkage (Fig. 27–14). In certain instances there is incomplete penetration of the germ plasm, which accounts for the occasional skipping of a generation. There also appear to be other modifying genes which account for the observed differences in intensity of the anomaly among different individuals. Dentinogenesis imperfecta is manifest during the developmental period of histodifferentiation.

Dentinogenesis imperfecta is frequently observed in cases of osteogenesis imperfecta, although the reverse need not be true.

Dentinal Dysplasia. The second anomaly of dentin which can be considered a separate genetic entity is dentinal dysplasia. This aberration is relatively rare and is much less prevalent than dentinogenesis imperfecta. The anomaly is transmitted as an autosomal dominant characteristic. Dentinal dysplasia in many respects resembles dentinogenesis imperfecta and the two diseases could be easily confused.

Roentgenographically the permanent teeth have very little root substance. In the posterior teeth the roots are short and bifurcations are near the root apices with the root tips either bunched together or assuming a configuration resembling a W. There are frequently large areas of rarefaction about the apices, resulting in drifting and early loss of the teeth. The general clinical picture of the teeth is normal with not-unusual crown contour. There is an absence or near absence of pulp chambers and canals. When chamber areas do exist, they generally assume the appearance of a half moon.

Histologic examination of the dentin shows a large number of spherical masses of collagenous matrix which produce a severe disarrangement in the structure of the dentin as the odontoblasts advance from the dentino-enamel junction inward. The differential characteristic of dentinal dysplasia from dentinogenesis imperfecta is the presence of these collagenous masses which continually interrupt the course of the tubules, producing a characteristic picture. There is no reduction in

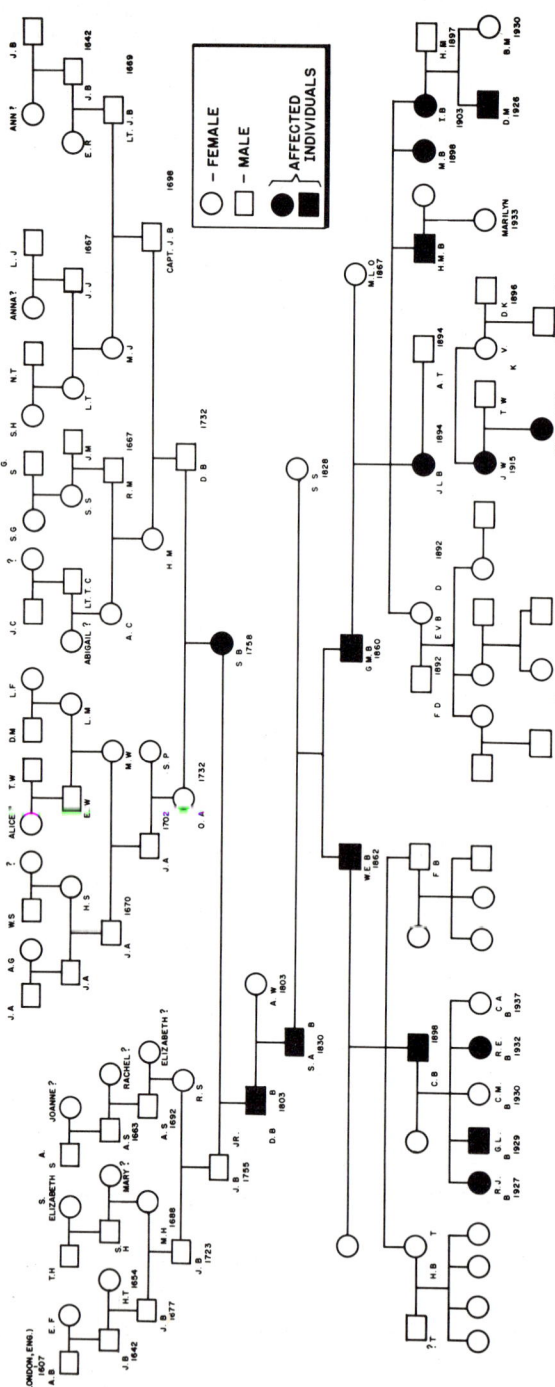

Figure 27–14 Dentinogenesis imperfecta in a family with a history of affected individuals dating back to 1758.

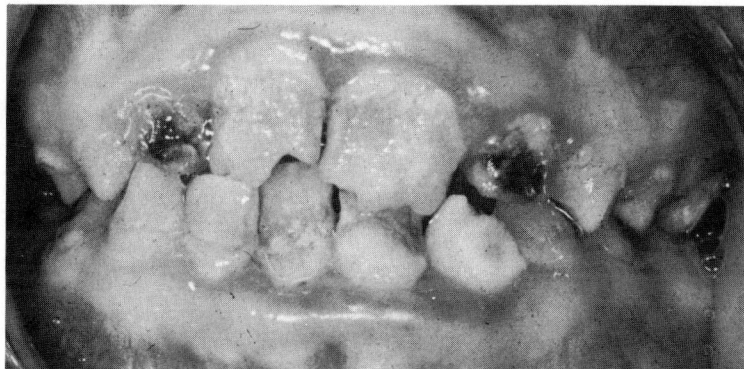

Figure 27–15 Nine-year-old child with amelogenesis imperfecta (hypoplasia type).

the number of odontoblasts which in dentinogenesis imperfecta is characteristic. These are dispersed in a matrix of deficient collagenous fibers with little orientation as they approach the pulpal area.

The treatment of the teeth is young individuals with either hereditary amelogenesis imperfecta or dentinogenesis imperfecta involves either the placing of crowns, or if there is little tooth structure remaining, extraction of the teeth and the construction of dentures. This will aid in maintaining proper vertical dimension as well as arch length. It will also produce a marked improvement in the esthetics of the individual (Figs. 27–15 and 27–16).

Hereditary General Syndromes Involving Either Enamel or Dentin

Included in this category are osteogenesis imperfecta, vitamin D resistant rickets, the Fanconi syndrome, hypophosphatasia, and pseudohypoparathyroidism.

Osteogenesis Imperfecta. This is a mesodermal syndrome involving not only the bones and teeth, but also the skin, ligaments, tendons, fascia, sclera, and inner ear. Functionally the most important defects are brittle bones and deafness. The occurrence of blue sclera and dentinogenesis imperfecta, although frequently found associated with the syndrome, may occur independently of it, and osteogenesis imperfecta may be present without any defect of the teeth or blue sclera. Figure 27–17 is of a patient 12 years of age with osteogenesis imperfecta. His mother was similarly affected and had had all her teeth extracted at an early age. The teeth show the characteristics of dentinogenesis imperfecta.

Two types of osteogenesis imperfecta are recognized: osteogenesis imperfecta congenita, in which the child is stillborn or dies soon after, and osteogenesis imperfecta tarda, which manifests itself later, and, although crippling, may not be fatal. McKusick[20] is of the opinion that the diseases are similar and differ only in severity, the tarda designate being less severe and in many instances recognized clinically only by the presence of blue sclera.

This author questions whether there is any significant difference between the dentinogenesis imperfecta observed in osteogenesis imperfecta and that observed as an independent dystrophy. Since there are many degrees of severity among fam-

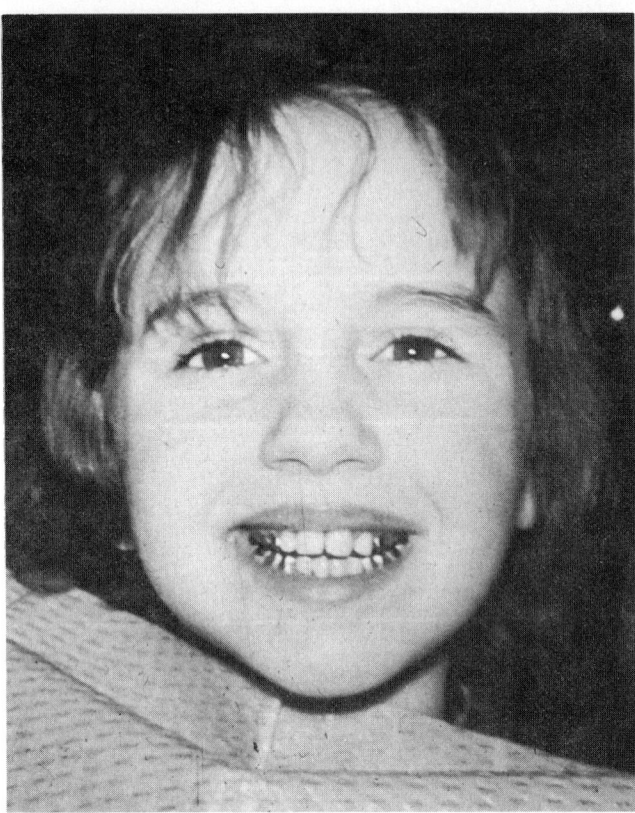

Figure 27–16 The same child with teeth restored with chrome steel crowns (Courtesy of Drs. Helmers and Finn).

ilies and even among members of the same family, severity itself is not a valid criterion for differentiating the two types of dentinal dystrophy. Both conditions may be due to the same gene. The condition is inherited as an autosomal dominant characteristic. The clinical appearance of the teeth (Figs. 27–18 and 27–19) is similar to that found without osteogenesis imperfecta.

Roentgenograms of the teeth (Fig. 27–20) show the characteristic worn crowns, the complete or partial absence of pulp chambers and canals and the short stubby roots. Histologically the dentin appears granular and deficient in tubules.

It is interesting that the characteristic changes that occur in the bones also occur in the dentin of the teeth if one can make comparisons between these two tissues. In the bone one finds a reduced number of osteoblasts and in the dentin one finds a decrease in the number of odontoblasts, their counterpart. In the bones there is also defective conversion of the argyrophilic staining fibrils of developing bone into true collagen. A similar observation has been made in the developing dentin matrix. Therefore, the defect apparently is of the organic portions of the dentin, resulting in a secondary decrease in mineralization.

Hereditary Vitamin D Resistant Rickets.   This condition is probably transmitted as a sex-linked dominant characteristic. The clinical appearance and roentgenographic appearance of bones and teeth are similar to that observed in vitamin D deficiency rickets. There are high blood alkaline phosphatase levels and hypophos-

Fig. 27–17   Fig. 27–18

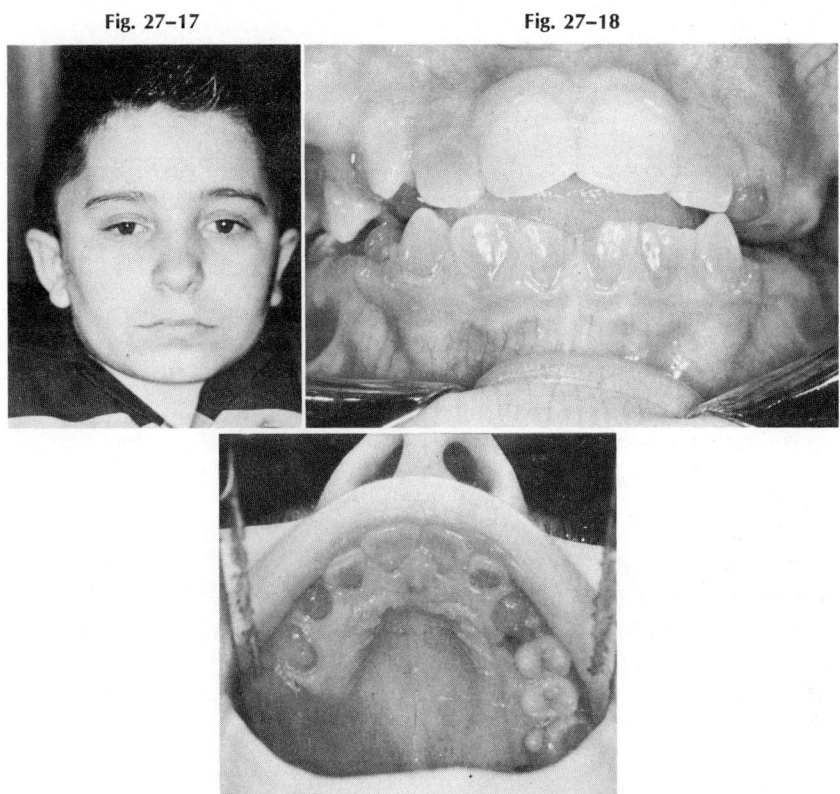

Fig. 27–19

Figure 27–17   Patient with osteogenesis imperfecta presenting the characteristic short neck and lateral compression of the skull.
Figure 27–18   Osteogenesis imperfecta. The teeth show the characteristic translucency of dentinogenesis imperfecta.
Figure 27–19   Osteogenesis imperfecta. The posterior deciduous teeth show marked wearing down of the crowns level with the gingival margin.

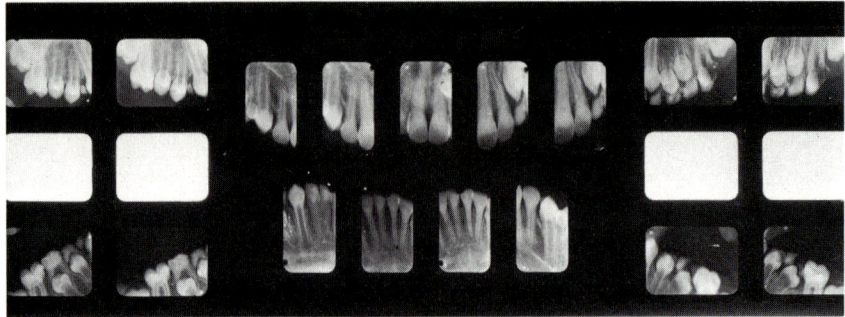

Figure 27–20 Osteogenesis imperfecta. The absence of pulp chambers in the anterior teeth and the peculiar shape of the roots are characteristic of a mild form of dentinogenesis imperfecta.

phatemia levels, although the calcium level may be normal. The basic metabolic defect is as yet undetermined.

The teeth on roentgenographic examination display large pulp chambers and canals. The dentin is poorly calcified with large interglobular spaces. The predentin zone is wide, and the enamel may be hypoplastic with openings from the enamel surface to the pulp.

Fanconi Syndrome.   This syndrome is transmitted as a rare recessive abnormal gene. It is characterized by low plasma inorganic phosphate, amino acid, glucose, phosphate, bicarbonate and perhaps potassium levels. The syndrome is associated with vitamin D resistant rickets and the dental aberrations are similar to those found in this disease. The defect is in the proximal convoluted renal tubules resulting in imperfect resorption.

Hypophosphatasia.   This disease was first reported by Rathbun[22] in 1948. In many respects the condition resembles rickets but is identifiable by a marked reduction in serum alkaline phosphatase, and does not respond to vitamin D therapy. Teeth are hypoplastic and have a tendency to shed prematurely. The early loss of the teeth is reminiscent of what occurs in dentinal dysplasia. The syndrome is transmitted as a recessive characteristic with perhaps more than one gene involved.

Pseudohypoparathyroidism.   This condition, first described in 1942, is a rare disease characterized by a general demineralization of bone and teeth. The defect appears to be a failure of the body to respond to the parathyroid hormone which is produced by the body in sufficient quantity. The syndrome is possibly genetic in origin involving three genes.

All the teeth show a marked hypoplasia of the enamel. Roentgenograms reveal resorption of the apical ends of several teeth (Fig. 27–21).

Diseases Associated with Blood Antigen-Antibody Reactions or with Blood Metabolism Resulting in Discoloration of the Teeth

Rh Incompatibility.   Erythroblastosis fetalis is a syndrome produced by a specific blood antigen-antibody reaction which may be fatal to the offspring unless the newborn receives an exchange transfusion. When an Rh positive child is born to a previously sensitized Rh negative mother and Rh positive father, there results hemolysis of the infant's blood and a breakdown into pigments producing icterus gravis neonatorum or jaundice of the newborn. These pigments may stain the teeth green or blue. The stain is intrinsic and cannot be cleaned through external means. Watson[27] has discussed the production of a typical enamel hypoplasia associated with this condition (Fig. 27–22). The enamel formed in utero is defective, but after birth it develops normally, producing an enamel shelf or hump and an exaggerated neonatal line. Rh incompatibility may be an etiological factor in certain cases of cerebral palsy.

The presence of Rh antigen is produced by a dominant gene. An Rh negative individual results when a homozygous recessive exists. Therefore, when both

Fig. 27–21

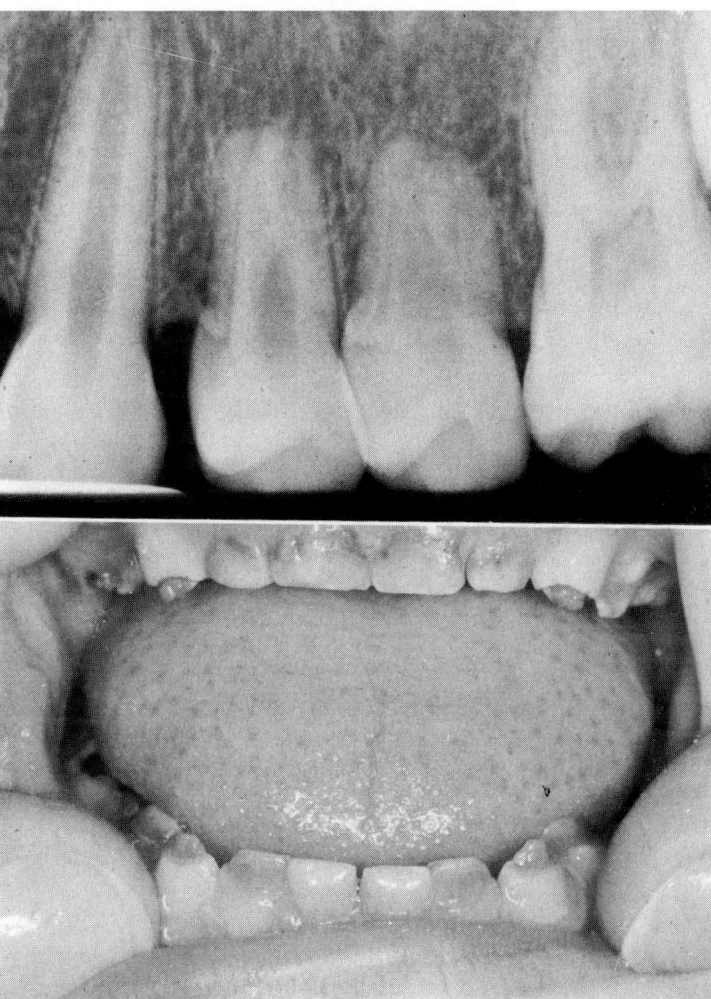

Fig. 27–22

Figure 27–21 Pseudohypoparathyroidism. The bicuspids show blunting and resorption of the roots at their apical ends.

Figure 27–22 Rh incompatibility. The teeth are stained a bluish green. The enamel hump or shelf may be observed on the primary cuspids and lateral incisors and molars.

parents are negative (homozygous) for the recessive factor, there can be only Rh negative offspring. Rh positive parents (heterozygous) can have both Rh positive and Rh negative children.

Congenital Porphyria. This is a rare disease characterized by an extreme photosensitivity. Exposure to sunlight results in an erythema, bulla formation and ulceration of the skin which may result in severe scarring and in some instances ulcerative destruction of bone. Figure 27–23 shows the hands of an individual with porphyria. Scarring and pigmentation of the skin and distortion of the fingers is evident.

In this disorder there is some abnormality of red cell formation and an increased rate of hemolysis resulting in increased quantities of free porphyrins, probably formed in the bone marrow and distributed throughout the body, producing pigmentation of the bones and teeth. There is an excretion of porphyrins in the urine, producing a red wine color.

There is probably a genetically determined abnormality in the enzymatic conversion of porphobilinogen to types I and III porphyrins. In this disease greater quantities of type I are produced which are not in the normal chain of metabolism to heme. This disease is transmitted as a rare autosomal recessive gene.

The teeth are pigmented dark brown to reddish brown and show the characteristic red fluorescence in ultraviolet light. Figure 27–24 presents the face and teeth of a female age 19 with this condition. Diagnosis of this case was first made at one year of age because of the discoloration of the teeth. Figure 27–25 shows a close-up of the anterior teeth of a child age 12 years.

There are a number of hereditary defects of a generalized nature that affect the oral structures but not the teeth. These are condensed in Table 27–1.

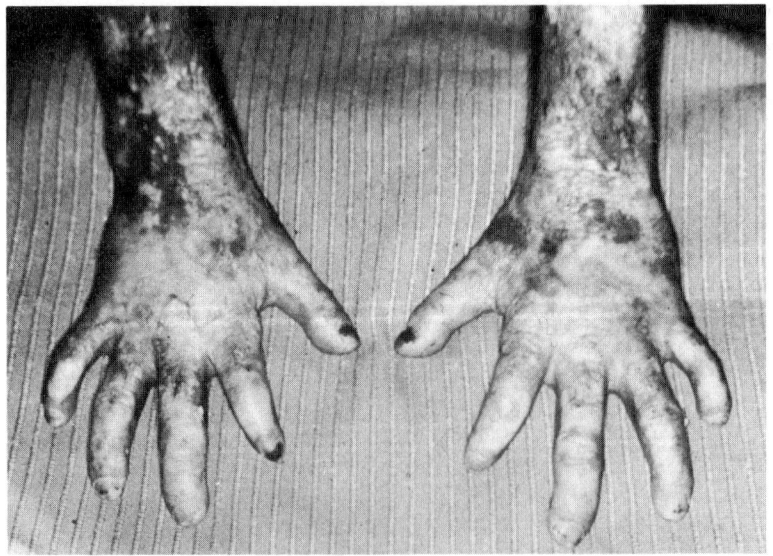

Figure 27–23 Porphyria. The hands and fingers show marked scarring with large areas of pigmentation.

Fig. 27–24

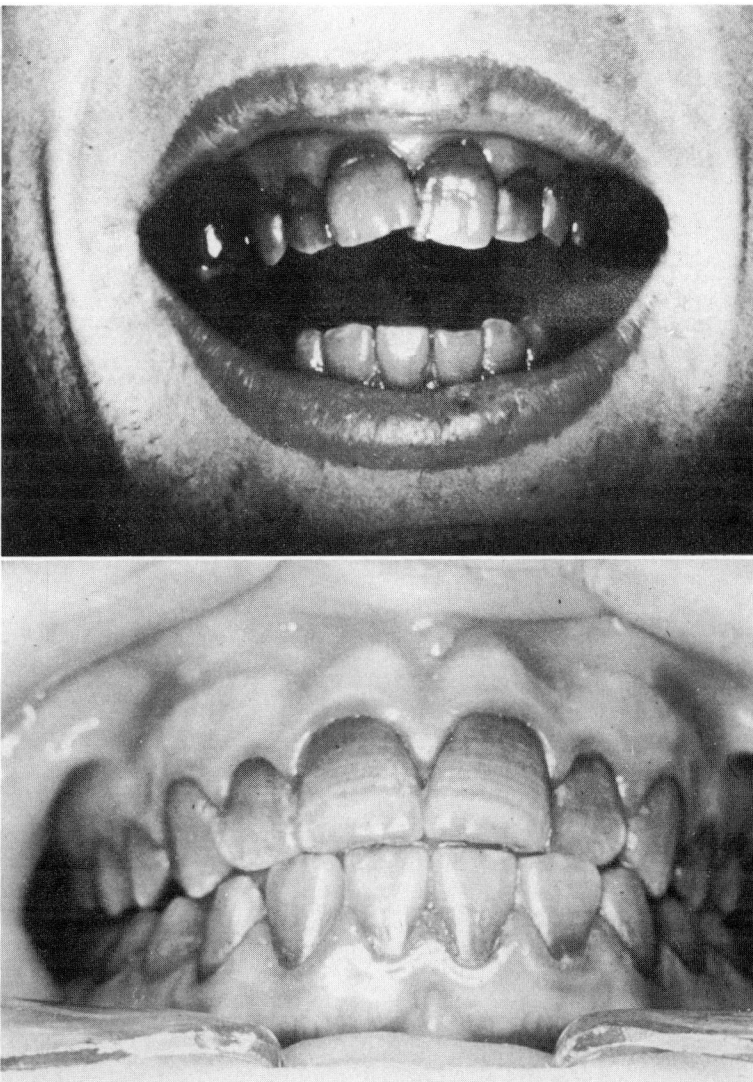

Fig. 27–25

Figure 27–24 Porphyria. The marked reddish brown stain of the teeth is evident by contrast with the face and gingiva. The face shows scarring.

Figure 27–25 Porphyria. The staining of the teeth in this disease shows up the imbrication lines in the enamel. The dark teeth contrast with the lighter gingiva.

TABLE 27–1 HERITABLE DEFECTS OF ORAL STRUCTURES WITH GENERALIZED DEFECTS

The following table of hereditable diseases (modified slightly from Witkop: Eugenics Quart., 5:15, 1958) which affect oral structures other than the teeth.

Disease	Oral Manifestation	How Inherited
Aetalasemia (Noma)	Gangrenous stomatitis	Recessive
Agammaglobulinemia	Periodontitis	Sex-linked recessive
Thalassemia major (Cooley's anemia)	Periodontitis and osteoperosis of jawbones	Recessive
Sickle cell anemia	Alveo ar bone changes (infarcts)	Recessive
Hemophilia and Christmas disease	Gingival and post-operative hemorrhage	Sex-linked recessive
Hemorrhagic telangiectasia (Osler)	Mucosal hemorrhages	Dominant
Sturge-Weber's disease	Gingival angiomatosis	Dominant (irregular)
Ehlers-Danlos syndrome	Oral hematomas and hemorrhage	Dominant
Gargoylism	Deformed face, enlarged tongue	Recessive (recessive sex-linked)
Mandibulo-facial dysostosis (Franceschetti)	Facial deformity	Dominant (irregular)
Cranio-facial dysostosis (Crouzon)	Facial deformity	Dominant (irregular)
Pierre Robin syndrome	Micrognathia	Recessive (incomplete dominant)
Achondroplasia	Hypoplasia of maxilla	Dominant
Multilocular cystic fibrous dysplasia of jaws and face (Jones)	Hypoplasia of maxilla	Dominant
Albers-Schönberg disease	Osteosclerosis	Dominant (irregular)
Generalized hyperostotic bone disease (Witkop)	Hyperostosis of jaws	Recessive
Neurofibromatosis (Von Recklinghausen's disease)	Neurofibroma and pigmentation	Dominant
Gastrointestinal polyposis (Peulz's syndrome)	Circumoral pigmentation	Dominant
Xeroderma pigmentosum	Facial pigmentation and carcinomas of lip	Recessive or incomplete sex-linked recessive
Benign intraepithelial dyskeratosis	Dyskeratosis of mucous membranes	Dominant
Familial amyloidosis	Gingival and lingual amyloid deposits	Dominant
White spongy nevus and mucous membranes	Gingival and lingual amyloid deposits	
Epidermolysis bullosa	Vesicles and bullae on oral mucous membranes	Probably recessive

REFERENCES

1. Albright, F., Burnett, C. H., Smith, P. H., and Parsons, W.: Pseudohypoparathyroidism; example of Seabright; bantam syndrome; report of three cases. Endocrinology, 30:922, 1942.
2. Bernard, W. V.: Roentgenographic and histologic differentiation of dentinogenesis imperfecta and dentinal dysplasia (abst.). J. D. Res., 39:674, 1960.
3. Chandry, C. P., Johnson, O. N., Mitchell, D. F., Gorlin, R. J., and Bartholdi, W. L.: Hereditary enamel dysplasia. J. Pediat., 54:776, 1959.
4. Finn, S. B.: Hereditary ectodermal dysplasia of the anhidrotic type; review of the literature and case report. J. D. Res., 23:214, 1944.
5. Finn, S. B.: Hereditary opalescent dentin. I. Analysis of the literature on hereditary anomalies of tooth color. J.A.D.A., 25:1240–1249, 1938.
5a. Finn, S. B.: Heredity in relation to caries resistance. Caries-Resistant Teeth, A CIBA Foundation Symposium. London, J. & A. Churchill, Ltd., 1965.
6. Follis, R. H.: Osteogenesis imperfecta: A connective tissue diathesis. J. Pediat., 41:713, 1952.
7. Garn, S. M., Lewis, A. B., and Shoemaker, D. W.: The sequence of calcification of the mandibular molar and premolar teeth. J. D. Res., 35:555, 1956.
8. Gates, R. R.: Human Genetics, vol. I. New York, The Macmillan Co., 1946.
9. Gorlin, R. J., and Pindborg, J. J.: Syndromes of the Head and Neck. New York, McGraw-Hill Book Co., 1964.
10. Grahnen, H.: Hypodontia in the permanent dentition. Odont. Revy (Lund), 7:1, 1956.
11. Harris, H.: Human biochemical genetics. London, Cambridge University Press, 1959.
12. Helmers, G. B., and Finn, S. B.: Treatment of Dentitions Affected by Hereditary Amelogenesis and Dentinogenesis Imperfecta. D. Clin. N. America, July, 1966, pp. 437–447.
13. Heys, F. M., Blattner, R. J., and Robinson, H. B. G.: Osteogenesis imperfecta and odontogenesis imperfecta: Clinical and genetic aspects in 18 families. J. Pediat., 56:234, 1960.
14. Hodge, H. C., Finn, S. B., Lose, G. B., Gachet, F. S., and Bassett, S. H.: Hereditary opalescent dentin. II. General and oral clinical studies. J.A.D.A., 26:1663, 1939.
15. Hodge, H. C., Finn, S. B., Robinson, H. B. G., Manly, R. S., Manly, M. L., Huysen, G. V., and Bale, W. F.: Hereditary opalescent dentin. III. Histological, chemical, and physical studies. J. D. Res., 19:521, 1940.
16. Hursey, R. J., Jr., Witkop, C. J., Jr., Miklashek, D., and Sackett, L. M.: Dentinogenesis imperfecta in a racial isolate with multiple hereditary defects. Oral Surg., Oral Med. & Oral Path., 9:641–658, 1956.
17. Johnson, O. N., Chaudry, A. P., Gorlin, R. J., Mitchell, D. F., and Bartholdi, W. L.: Dentinogenesis imperfecta. J. Pediat., 54:786, 1959.
18. Korkhaus, G.: Anthropologic and odontologic studies. Internat. J. Orthodont., 16:640, 1950.
19. Lundstrom, A.: An investigation of 202 pairs of twins regarding fundamental factors in the etiology of malocclusion. D. Record, 69:251, 1949.
20. McKusick, V. A.: Heritable disorders of connective tissue. St. Louis, C. V. Mosby Co., 1956.
20a. McKusick, V. A.: Human Genetics. Englewood Cliffs, N.J., Prentice-Hall, Inc., 1964.
21. Moody, E., and Montgomery, T. B.: Hereditary tendencies in tooth formation. J.A.D.A., 21:1774, 1934.
22. Rathbun, J. C.: "Hypophosphatasia," new developmental anomaly. Am. J. Dis. Child., 75:822, 1948.
23. Shafer, W. G., Hine, M. K., and Levy, B. M.: A Textbook of Oral Pathology. 2nd ed. Philadelphia, W. B. Saunders Co., 1963.
24. Shulze, C.: Erbliche Structuranomalien menschlicher Zahne. Proc. First International Cong. Human Genetics, Acta genet., 7:231, 1957.
25. Sobel, E. H., Clark, L. C., Fox, R. P., and Robinow, M.: Rickets, deficiency of "alkaline" phosphatase activity and premature loss of teeth in children. Pediatrics, 11:309, 1953.
26. Toller, P. A.: A clinical report of 6 cases of amelogenesis imperfecta. Oral Surg., Oral Med., Oral Path., 12:325, 1959.
27. Watson, A. O.: Infantile cerebral palsy: a survey of dental conditions and treatment emphasizing the effect of parental Rh incompatibility on the deciduous teeth. D. J. Australia, 27:6–14, 72–83, 93–102, 1955.
28. Weaver, W.: Genetic effects of atomic radiation. Science, 123:1157, 1956.
29. Weinman, J. P., Svaboda, J. F., and Woods, R. W.: Hereditary disturbances of enamel formation and calcification. J.A.D.A., 32:397, 1945.
30. Whyte, R.: Human inheritance. D. Record, 72:341, 1953.
31. Witkop, C. J.: Dental Genetics, 1959. J.A.D.A., 60:564, 1960.
32. Witkop, C. J., Jr.: Genetics and dentistry. Eugenics Quart, 5:15, 1958.
33. Witkop, C. J., Graham, J. B., and Rucknagel, D. L.: Hereditary benign intraepithelial dyskeratosis. II. Oral manifestations and hereditary transmission. A.M.A. Arch. Path., 70:696, 1960.

28

CHROMOSOMAL DISORDERS

by SARA C. FINLEY
and WAYNE H. FINLEY

Genetic disorders account for a significant amount of morbidity and mortality in man and many of them are of primary interest to the dentist. Other genetic diseases involve multiple organ systems and the dental problems may assume a secondary role to some of the more disabling facets of the disease.

Genetic diseases may be classified into three major groups: (1) Gross chromosomal aberrations in which there is either a structural or numerical abnormality of the chromosome; (2) single gene abnormalities which are transmitted in an autosomal dominant, autosomal recessive, or X-linked pattern; and (3) polygenic disorders in which environmental interaction may play a significant role. It is estimated that 0.5 per cent of newborns will have a gross chromosomal aberration, that approximately 1 per cent will have a single gene disorder, and that approximately 10 per cent will have a polygenic disorder.[1]

The chromosomal aberrations can be detected by examining the chromosomes of cells derived by culture of peripheral leukocytes or other tissues. The presence of single gene or polygenic disorders cannot be detected through direct examination of the chromosomes, but the pedigree and classification into mode of transmission can be very useful in genetic counseling. Accurate risk figures are available if the disorder is recognized as following the autosomal recessive, dominant, or X-linked recessive or dominant pattern; examples of single gene disorders which involve the oral cavity are given in Chapter 27.

In polygenic disorders, the chromosomal pattern in cells from the patient is normal and no mendelian pattern of inheritance can be established, although there is evidence of a genetic predisposition. The interaction of genetic and environmental factors in these cases is not understood. In these situations, the best risk figures available are empiric ones obtained by observing families to determine the risk for subsequent children being affected. These figures can be helpful and are often

634

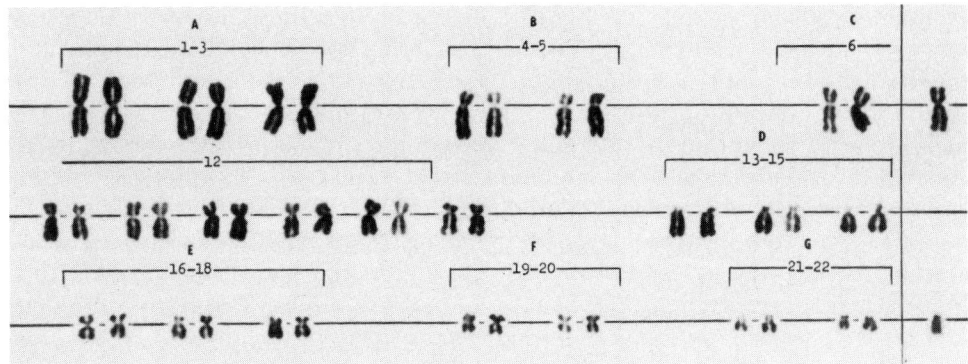

Figure 28–1 Normal male karyotype (46, XY).

encouraging to a couple who fear that any subsequent child born to them will also be affected. For example, in cleft lip, the overall recurrence rate is approximately 4 per cent; after bilateral cleft lip and palate, the risk of recurrence is approximately 6 per cent; and after unilateral cleft lip without cleft palate, it is approximately 2½ per cent. The recurrence risk after two affected siblings is approximately 12 per cent, as it is when one parent and one child are affected.[2]

The developments in cell culture techniques and the hypotonic treatment of cultured cells arrested in metaphase permitted the clear visualization and accurate counting of the human chromosomes in 1956.[3] Further developments led to the utilization of cells derived by culture of peripheral leukocytes to provide metaphase plates which can be photographed and arranged according to accepted nomenclature into a *karyotype*. The 46 chromosomes normally present in a karyotype of a human diploid cell are divided into 22 pairs of *autosomes* and one pair of *sex* chromosomes. Each parent normally contributes 22 autosomes and one sex chromosome to the zygote. A normal male karyotype, 46/XY, is shown in Figure 28–1. A normal female karyotype, 46/XX, is shown in Figure 28–2.

Various numerical and structural abnormalities in chromosomes are found in association with congenital malformation syndromes. The presence of an abnormal number of autosomes, if compatible with live birth, is found in several clinically rec-

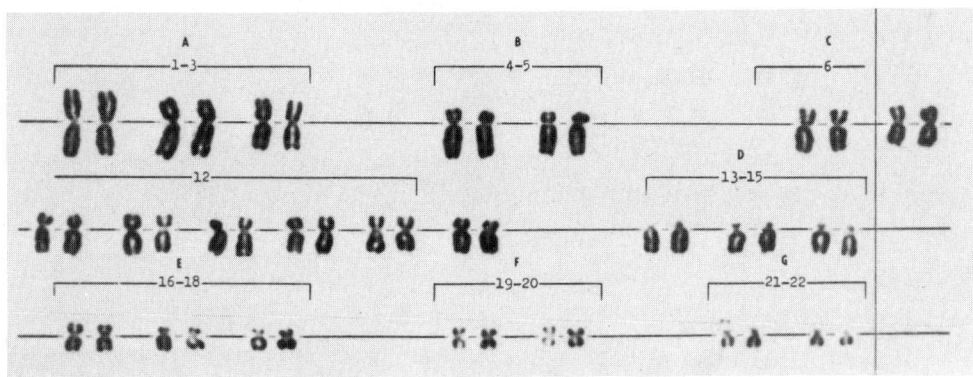

Figure 28–2 Normal female karyotype (46, XX).

ognizable syndromes. An extra chromosome results in a *trisomy* instead of the usual pair, and the absence of a chromosome results in a *monosomy*. The trisomy and monosomy conditions are thought to result from an unequal division of the chromosomes (nondisjunction) during the process of meiosis in either the father or mother. Some patients are found to have two different types of cells with regard to chromosomal pattern and this condition called *mosaicism* is considered to result from nondisjunction during mitotic cell division after fertilization. The sex chromosomes are often involved in mosaic patterns. Autosomal monosomy is considered lethal since few cases have survived the pregnancy but monosomy involving the sex chromosomes is not unusual in liveborns. It is of interest that any autosomal trisomy is associated with severe physical malformations and mental retardation whereas the presence of an extra chromosome or even the presence of several extra sex chromosomes produces less deleterious effects.

Structural chromosomal aberrations, although not as frequent as the numerical anomalies, involve both the autosomes and the sex chromosomes. Aberrations found in patients include deletions of chromosome parts following breakage, ring formation following breakage of both ends of the chromosome, translocation between two chromosomes which have been broken, and isochromosome formation. The reader is referred to a more detailed text on cytogenetics for information on these mechanisms in the production of congenital malformations.

AUTOSOMAL TRISOMY SYNDROMES

Trisomy 21 (Down's Syndrome)

Down's syndrome, or mongolism, is one of the most common recognizable malformation syndromes and has an incidence of approximately one in 600 newborns.

The chromosomal aberrations of trisomy, translocation, and mosaicism have all been found in patients with Down's syndrome. The vast majority of patients with this syndrome have 47 chromosomes and the 21-trisomy karyotype (Fig. 28–3), whereas approximately 5 to 10 per cent have a translocation chromosome involving

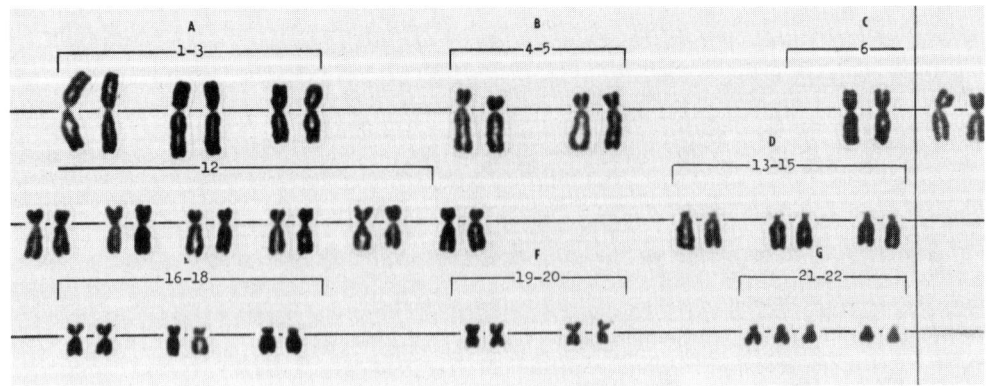

Figure 28–3   21-trisomy karyotype (47, XX, 21+).

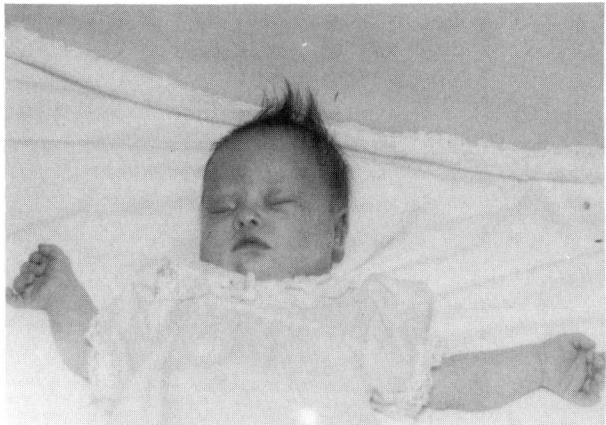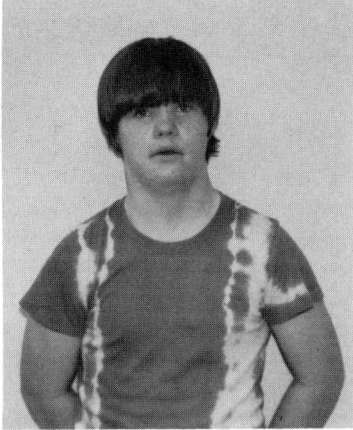

Figure 28–4 Patients with Down's syndrome.

extra chromosome 21 material and another 5 per cent have a mosaic karyotype.[4] A number of physical features are recognized as occurring with increased frequency in patients with Down's syndrome (Fig. 28–4), and these include short stature, flat occiput, epicanthic folds, broad nasal bridge, folded ears, small maxilla, protruding tongue, short hands and fingers, clinodactyly, simian line, distal triradius, congenital heart disease, and a gap between first and second toes. These patients have hypotonia and mental retardation.

Some of the dental findings commonly found in Down's syndrome patients are late eruption of deciduous teeth, early shedding of deciduous teeth, defective or absent upper lateral incisors, anomalies of tooth shape, periodontal disease, malocclusion, and prognathism.[5, 6] Periodontal disease is a more prevalent problem in Down's syndrome than is that of dental caries.

The different chromosomal types seen in Down's syndrome cannot be detected clinically; thus, laboratory studies are indicated for diagnosis as well as to provide information for genetic counseling. Infants with Down's syndrome are born to mothers of all ages; however, the risk of birth of such a child increases with advanced maternal age. If on karyotype analysis, a translocation type of abnormality is found in which an extra number 21 chromosome is attached to another chromosome, it is important to determine if one of the parents is a balanced carrier of the translocation. If so, the risk of having another mongoloid child in a subsequent pregnancy is high (perhaps as high as 33 per cent). Prenatal karyotype analysis is indicated in this familial type of Down's syndrome. While the couple would probably elect to have a therapeutic abortion if the fetus is found to have the karyotype diagnostic of Down's syndrome, the procedure may permit the birth of a normal infant when ordinarily, the couple would not risk having a child without benefit of prenatal chromosome studies.

Trisomy 18

The 18-trisomy patient, a more seriously affected child than one with Down's syndrome, usually does not live longer than a few months. These children[7] have marked retardation in growth and development, and other features including low

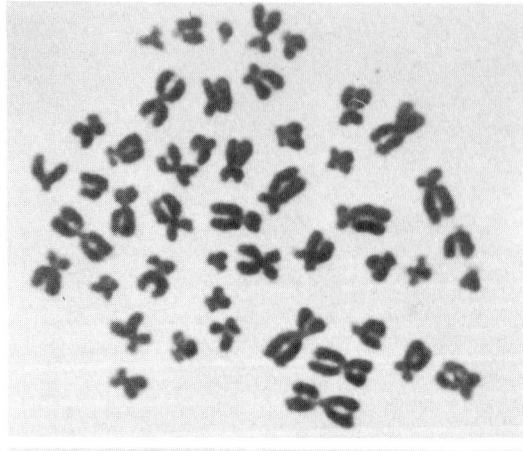

Figure 28–5   18-trisomy karyotype (47, XX, 18+).

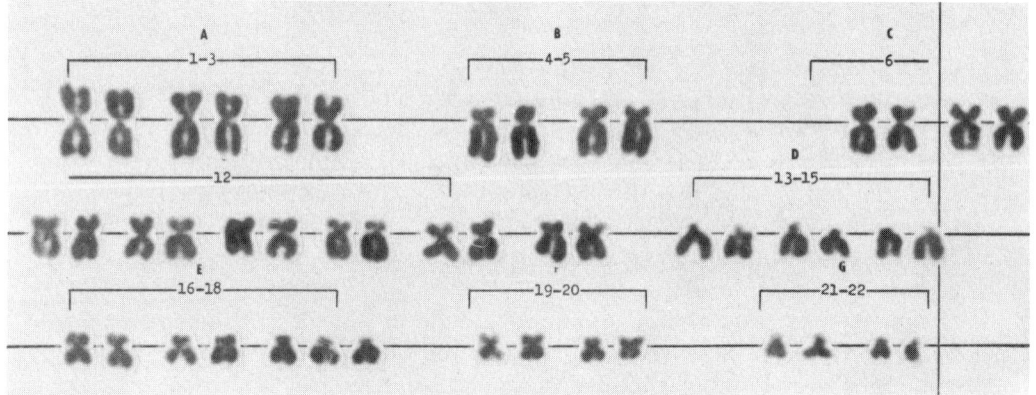

birth weight, epicanthic folds, small mouth, micrognathia, low-set ears, flexion and overlapping of fingers, congenital heart disease, and rocker bottom feet. Fig. 28–5 indicates the extra chromosome 18 in comparison to the other E chromosomes. This syndrome is associated with the presence of 47 chromosomes and a trisomy presumably caused by a meiotic error although translocation can be involved.

Trisomy 13 (D₁)

The individual with the D_1 trisomy syndrome has a short life expectancy and will only rarely survive infancy. Prominent physical features, some of which are demonstrated in the patient shown in Figure 28–6, include cleft lip and palate, a large bulbous nose, abnormal ears, microcephaly, microphthalmia and other eye defects, scalp defects, polydactyly, congenital heart disease, and holoprosencephaly type defect of the brain.[8] These infants have severe mental retardation. Until recently it has not been possible to distinguish between the three pairs of D chromosomes but with new cytological techniques, better identification of the specific chromosome involved is available. A karyotype of the D chromosomes of a patient with this syndrome which should be recognizable clinically is illustrated in Figure 28–7. Because of the multiple handicaps, including the severe mental retardation and usual short life expectancy which accompany this syndrome, the

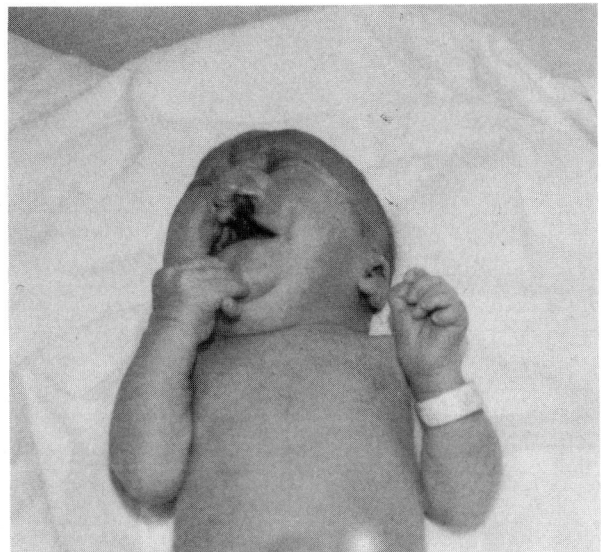

Figure 28–6 Patient with D₁-trisomy syndrome (47, XY, D₁+).

parents of a child with these defects should realize the prognosis in this syndrome before vigorous surgical repair of some of the defects such as the cleft lip and cleft palate are begun.

Rarer Trisomies

On rare occasions, an individual may have 48 chromosomes with a double trisomy. Triploidy is another type of rare chromosomal abnormality and in this situation the individual has an extra set of chromosomes with a total number of 69 chromosomes (Fig. 28–8). Children found to have this chromosomal pattern without mosaicism and a normal cell line in at least some cells have survived for only a few hours. The clinical features of low birth weight, retardation in growth and development, abnormal digits, and syndactyly have been present in patients with triploidy and one case has been reported to have cleft lip and palate.[9]

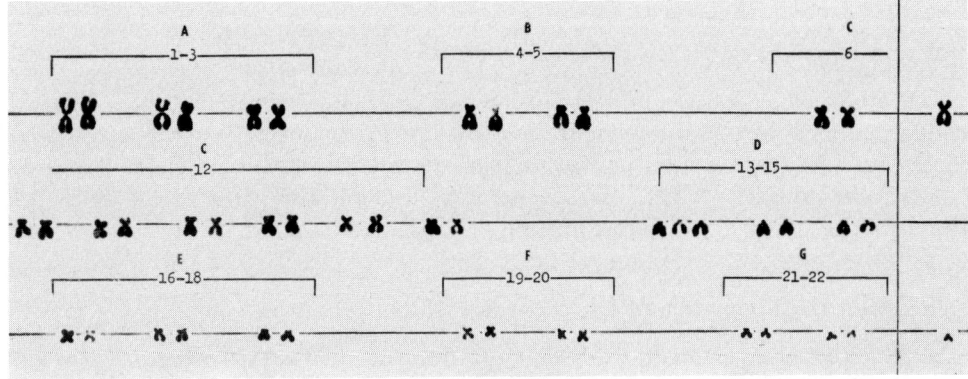

Figure 28–7 D₁-trisomy karyotype (47, XY, D₁+).

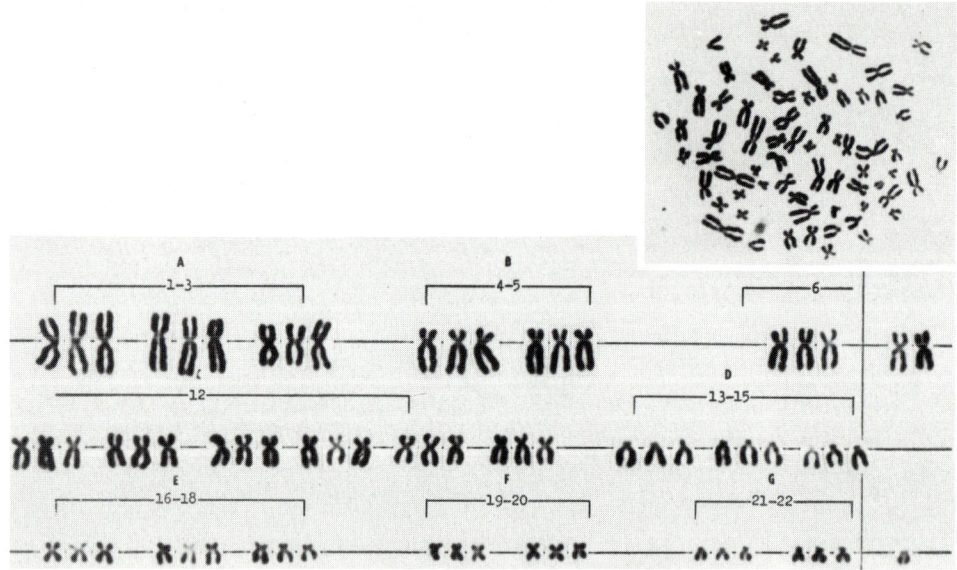

Figure 28–8 Triploidy karyotype (69, XXY).

AUTOSOMAL DELETION SYNDROMES

Cat Cry Syndrome

The cat cry or cri-du-chat syndrome was described in 1963[10] and is associated with a partial deletion of the short arm of one of the B group chromosomes which has been further identified as chromosome 5. Children with this syndrome may survive to reach adulthood. The name of the syndrome is derived from the fact that they have an abnormal cry early in life due to an abnormality of the larynx. Physical features include the abnormal cry, mental retardation, hypotonia, microcephaly, downward slanting of the palpebral fissures, hypertelorism, and epicanthic folds. Cleft lip and cleft palate have been reported in some of the patients having this syndrome and a bifid uvula is not uncommon. For purposes of genetic counseling, it is important to confirm the diagnosis with chromosomal analysis since in a few cases a familial translocation has been reported.

Deletion of the Short Arm of Chromosome 4

Partial deletion of the short arm of chromosome 4 may be suspected on clinical examination because of the presence of the following features: marked retardation in growth and development, mental deficiency, eye abnormalities, cleft lip and/or palate, downturned mouth, short upper lip, and midline scalp defect. Some of these children have been found to survive childhood.

Deletion of the Long Arm of Chromosome 18 (18q–)

The syndrome involving deletion of the long arm of chromosome 18 was described in 1964[11,] and enough cases have now been described to permit a strong suspicion of the disorder on clinical grounds. This syndrome varies in the degree of severity of involvement but survival to childhood or adulthood may be expected. Physical features include mental deficiency, hearing loss, microcephaly, hypoplasia of the midface, abnormally narrow ear canals, foot anomalies, epicanthic folds, and cleft palate in some cases. This syndrome is usually of sporadic occurrence although a few familial cases have occurred.

Deletion of the Short Arm of Chromosome 18 (18p–)

Physical features of this syndrome may not be diagnostic of the syndrome but suggest a chromosomal abnormality. These physical features include short stature, mental retardation, minor malformations including micrognathia, strabismus, and a general appearance which may suggest the presence of Turner's syndrome. Dental caries have been reported to be prevalent in this syndrome.[12]

Ring Chromosome 18 Syndrome (18r)

The ring chromosome is presumably formed when parts of both the short arm and long arm of a chromosome are broken and the broken ends attach to form the ring. Features of both short arm and long arm deletion are present in this syndrome and should suggest the possibility of this diagnosis.[13]

SEX CHROMOSOME ABNORMALITIES

As with the autosomes, there may be numerical or structural abnormalities of the sex chromosomes but these abnormalities usually do not exert as much detrimental effect upon the individual's growth and development as do the autosomal aberrations. Screening techniques are helpful in evaluating many of the patients suspected of having an abnormality of sexual differentiation or development. One of these is the sex chromatin determination which can be done by examining human interphase cells for the presence of a darkly staining chromatin mass near the nuclear membrane, the sex *chromatin body* or *Barr body*. Cells from individuals having at least two X chromosomes, as seen in the normal human female, will show the presence of one sex chromatin body. Cells most frequently used for this sex chromatin determination are those obtained by scraping the buccal mucosa. The number of sex chromatin bodies is expected to be one less than the number of X chromosomes, so that a normal human male with XY sex chromosome pattern is sex chromatin negative, whereas the normal human female with the XX sex chromosome pattern is sex chromatin positive. A newer screening technique also involves the use of the interphase nuclei stained with quinacrine mustard.[14] Cells containing a Y sex chromosome, using this technique, show a brightly fluorescent area which has been interpreted to be a Y chromosome. Both of the above tests are helpful not only in the workup of patients with disorders of sexual differentiation or development but also in prenatal sex determination. They are screening techniques, however, and usually need to be corroborated by study of the metaphase chromosomes.

Turner's Syndrome (Gonadal Dysgenesis)

A phenotypic female, with monosomy for the X chromosome (Fig. 28–9), 45/XO, usually has some or all of the following features: short stature, primary

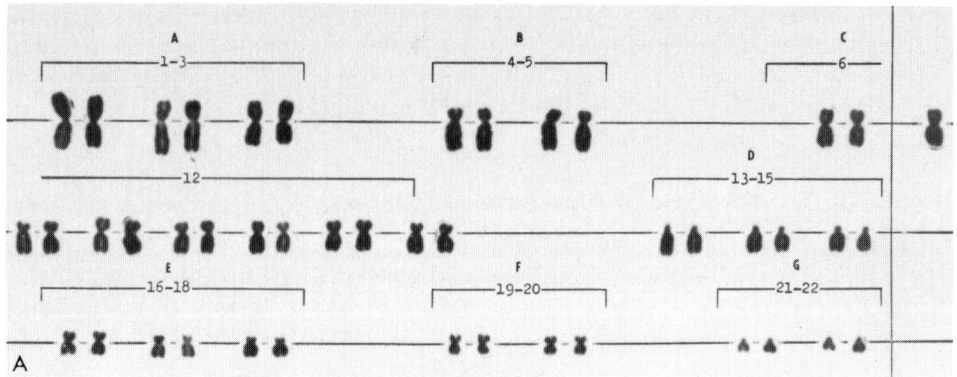

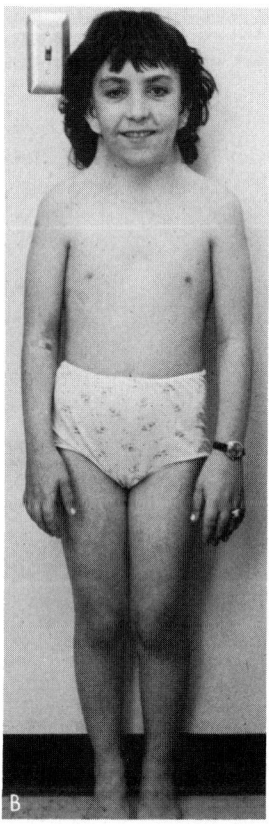

Figure 28–9   *A,* XO karyotype (45, XO). *B,* Patient with Turner's syndrome.

amenorrhea, poor development of secondary sexual characteristics, webbed neck, low set ears, high arched palate, cubitus valgus, hypoplastic fourth metacarpal, coarctation of the aorta, hypertension, low hairline on the neck, and streak gonads. Some of the dental findings include high arched palate and hypoplastic mandible.[6]

   Not all patients with these features will have a monosomy of the X chromosomes in all of their cells. Some have a mosaic pattern with part of their cells 45, XO and part of their cells normal 46/XX. Others will have a structural abnormality of one of the X chromosomes such as deletion of either the long or short arm or isochromosome formation. These females may have a good prognosis if therapy is instituted to provide exogeneous hormones to promote development of secondary sex characteristics. Short stature and sterility are permanent effects but often the mental ability is normal.

The Turner's syndrome patient with the XO karyotype will have a negative sex chromatin, whereas those patients with structural abnormalities of one of the X chromosomes may have positive sex chromatin even though their physical features suggest Turner's syndrome.

Females with an extra X chromosome (47/XXX) do not have distinctive clinical features and are fertile.

Klinefelter's Syndrome

Klinefelter's syndrome patients[15] most often have the karyotype, 47/XXY (Fig. 28–10), but variants are 48/XXXY, 49/XXXXY, and various mosaic patterns. Among chromosomal aberration syndromes, Klinefelter's is common and occurs in one of 400 newborn males. Physical features found in these patients are eunuchoid proportions, small testes, absence of spermatogenesis, gynecomastia, and reduced body hair. Behavioral problems are frequent and the presence of breast tissue may be significant enough to warrant surgical removal. These males will be sterile but may function sexually and with reassurance may assume a normal male role although mental retardation may be present in some. A positive sex chromatin is found. In those variants with three or more X chromosomes the number of sex chromatin bodies observed in some cells is one less than the total number of X chromosomes. Sex chromatin determination for screening and subsequent karyotype interpretation is indicated in those males with hypogonadism.

XYY Syndrome

The exact phenotype of males with the karyotype 47/XYY is not known at this time. It may be very common in our population and go undetected since there are no specific recognizable findings. These patients are sexually normal but the extra

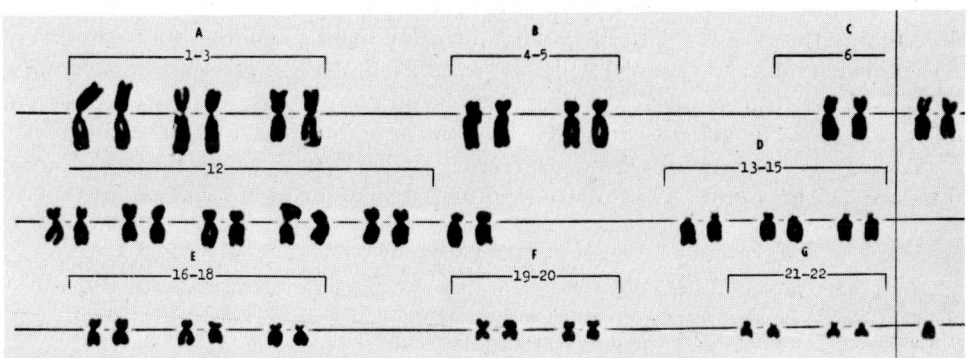

Figure 28–10   XXY karyotype (47, XXY).

Y chromosome seems to predispose them to the development of tall stature and antisocial behavior.[16]

Problems of Sexual Differentiation

Cytogenetic studies are most important in the evaluation of patients with sexual ambiguity. In beginning the clinical evaluation of patients presenting with ambiguity, the sex chromatin determination is helpful in suggesting other tests. Female pseudohermaphrodites have a positive sex chromatin and a normal female karyotype. Congenital adrenal hyperplasia, an autosomal recessive genetic disorder, is the most common cause of female pseudohermaphroditism.

Male pseudohermaphrodites have a negative sex chromatin and a normal male karyotype. Patients with the hereditary testicular feminization type of male pseudohermaphroditism are phenotypic females. There is normal growth, breast development, scant body hair, and abdominal testes in these genotypic males. Other forms of male pseudohermaphrodites have partial feminization as represented in those patients reported by Lubs, Gilbert-Dreyfus, and Reifenstein as reviewed by Federman.[15]

True hermophrodites usually have had 46/XX karyotypes and have both male and female gonads. Surgical exploration may be required to make the diagnosis.

GENETIC COUNSELING

The detection of patients with chromosomal aberration syndromes is of prime importance for genetic counseling, which is becoming more exact as new developments in medical genetics occur.

If the disorder is associated with a gross chromosomal aberration certain families will have an indication for prenatal karyotype analysis. Many others can be reassured to have a positive approach to planning other children without fear of being at high risk.

The use of mendelian laws permits accurate risk figures in the several hundred single gene disorders. Empiric risk figures can often reassure couples who have a history of one of the many polygenic disorders.

Genetic counseling requires that an accurate diagnosis be established. Because of the frequent involvement of the oral cavity in the congenital malformation syndromes, the dentist can be very helpful in detection of genetic disorders, in description of newly recognized familial disorders, and in genetic counseling.

Genetic counseling involves the use of clinical, cytogenetic, biochemical and other evaluations to establish the diagnosis. From these data, risk figures are often made possible. The genetic counselor, however, whether he is a medical geneticist, dentist, or physician realizes that most families with a handicapped child need more than a stark risk figure. They often need help in allaying guilt and hostility.

REFERENCES

1. Smith, D. W.: Genetic basis for clinical disorders. Southern Med. J., *64*(Suppl. 1):4, 1971.
2. Carter, C. O.: An ABC of Medical Genetics. Boston, Little, Brown and Co., 1969, p. 57.
3. Tjio, J. H., and Levan, A.: The chromosome number of man. Hereditas, *42*:1, 1956.
4. Finley, W. H.: Autosomal aberration syndromes. Southern Med. J., *64*(Suppl. 1):65, 1971.

5. Penrose, L. S., and Smith, G. F.: Down's anomaly. Boston, Little, Brown and Co., 1966, pp. 12–14.

6. Gorlin, R. J., and Prindborg, J. J.: Syndromes of the Head and Neck. New York, McGraw-Hill, 1964.

7. Edwards, J. H., and Harnden, D. G.: Cameron, A. H., Crosse, V. M., and Wolff, O. H.: A new trisomy syndrome. Lancet, *1*:7, 1960.

8. Patau, K., Smith, D. W., Therman, E., Inhorn, S. L., and Wagner, H. P.: Multiple congenital anomaly caused by an extra autosome. Lancet, *1*:790, 1960.

9. Finley, W. H., and Finley, S. C.: Triploidy in a liveborn male. J. Pediat. *81*:855, 1972.

10. Lejeune, J., Lafourcade, J., Berger, R., Vialatte, J., Boeswillwald, M., Seringe, P., and Turpin, R.: Trois cas de délétion partielle du bras court d'un chromosome 5. C. R. Acad. Sci. (Paris), *257*:3098, 1963.

11. Lejeune, J., Berger, R., and Lafourcade, J., et al.: La délétion partielle du bras long du chromosome 18. Individualisation d'un nouvel état morbide. Ann. Genet. (Paris), *9*:32, 1966.

12. de Grouchy, J., Bonnette, J., and Salmon, C.: Délétion du bras court du chromosome 18. Ann. Genet. (Paris), *9*:19, 1966.

13. Finley, S. C., Cooper, M. D., Finley, W. H., Uchida, I. A., Noto, T. A., and Roddam, R. F.: Immunological profile in a chromosome 18 deletion syndrome with I_gA deficiency. J. Med. Genet., *6*:388, 1969.

14. Caspersson, T., Zech, L., Johansson, C., and Modest, E. J.: Identification of human chromosomes by DNA-binding fluorescent agents. Chromosoma, *30*:215, 1970.

15. Federman, D. D.: Abnormal Sexual Development. Philadelphia, W. B. Saunders Co., 1967.

16. Court Brown, W. M.: Males with an XYY sex chromosome complement. J. Med. Genet., *5*:341, 1968.

29

INFECTIOUS AGENTS IN DISEASE

by JOE PRICE THOMAS

Techniques of complete diagnosis and treatment planning are described in other sections of this book. If followed systematically, these techniques insure an approach that will provide comprehensive dental care for the child patient. Longitudinal findings carefully gathered from initial and follow-up dental examination are of immense value in planning the oral care of growing children. This is especially true when a combination of influences has created an imbalance that, in turn, has altered normal patterns of growth and development. Both acute and chronic infections that commonly occur during childhood may have temporary oral manifestations, or permanent physical effects, that must be considered when the diagnostic impressions of a child are recorded. We recognize that heredity, nutrition, and hormonal balances, as well as infections, may influence the maturing process; therefore, it is seldom possible to state that an alteration has clearly resulted from a single cause. It must also be remembered that changes in a patient may have been brought on by the interrelation of two or more factors. The provision of comprehensive care for patients, with preventive dentistry as the underlying philosophy, impose a challenge on the dental profession to remember all these factors when creating a guideline for diagnosis.

Various childhood infectious disorders follow a clinical course that, to the dentist, has special significance, either because of the facial or oral symptoms present during the acute phase of the disease, or because of the long term effects on the development of the jaws and teeth.

At the onset of a disease, the child's age, sex, and stage of growth can influence his susceptibility to and the severity of an infectious attack. For example, the incidence of some infections is more prevalent at one age than at another. This relation between incidence and age may stem from one of several factors: an increased opportunity for exposure, as when starting to school; changes in patient immunity; or systemic tissue changes which are characteristic at certain ages and occasionally

646

provide conditions that are suitable for the growth of specific microorganisms. Some bacterial infections, though not restricted to a particular age bracket, may be severe and rapidly progressive in infancy, relatively innocuous between the ages of 5 to 10 years, and during adolescence may again produce severe effects.

The variation that is often evident in the clinical picture of the different age groups may be accounted for by the anatomic changes, the physiological factors, and the biochemical changes that accompany growth. The specific immunity and hypersensitivity that gradually develop as the child experiences natural infection and immunization will also affect the course of a disease.

In recent years, much of the practice and research in the field of pediatric medicine has been directed toward the prevention and treatment of infection and the management of the allergic child. Although solving these problems is primarily the responsibility of the physician, dentists can and should lend support to this effort. Being knowledgeable in the principles of epidemiology, the dentist should consider each individual who has contracted an infectious disease in relation to his background, and the extent to which the other members of his family or even larger groups may be affected.

Since it is desirable to have a health team composed of the members of the dental and medical professions, it is mandatory for these groups to coordinate their efforts in maintaining an awareness of the problems with which each is confronted, so that mutual endeavor can help them to surmount the difficulties.

The immunization of children against the common infectious diseases has produced dramatic improvements in the past 20 years. Recent live-viral vaccines against polio, measles, rubella, and mumps have become equally as effective as the smallpox vaccination and the combined immunization against diphtheria, whooping cough, and tetanus.

Infectious disease is the subject of entire texts. This chapter will touch briefly upon some of these diseases that are particularly prevalent among children, and that, because they often disturb oral health and create general physiological problems, might be the subject of a revised and more adequate approach for dental treatment.

STREPTOCOCCAL AND OTHER BACTERIAL INFECTIONS

Most human streptococcal infections are caused by beta hemolytic streptococci, of which group A is most commonly associated with infection. Penicillin has been the preferred drug for treating these infections.

Scarlet Fever (Scarlatina). An acute infection, caused by group A beta hemolytic streptococci, scarlet fever occurs mainly during the winter months and in many ways resembles acute tonsillitis. Beginning in the pharynx, this infection may cause fever, headache, delirium, tonsillitis, rapid pulse, vomiting, and rash. A bright red rash of diffuse, finely papular lesions is seen on the neck, underarms, and groin. More than half the cases also exhibit a "strawberry tongue."

The oral signs include congested mucosa, particularly in the palate, and frequently a fiery red throat. The tonsils are usually swollen and may have a grayish exudate. "Strawberry tongue," if present, occurs early in the course of the disease. This descriptive term refers to a white coated tongue with red, hyperemic, edematous, fungiform papillae. Preventive measures are not presently available for this usually mild disease. Antibiotics have been used for treatment and for prevention of complications.

Erysipelas.   An acute streptococcal infection of the skin with occasional mucous membrane involvement, erysipelas has responded to systemic penicillin treatment; local treatment is ineffective. The patient should be strictly isolated, and newborn infants should be carefully guarded against exposure since they are highly susceptible to this disease, which produces no natural immunization. Clinical manifestations may include fever, malaise, and vomiting. Skin lesions on the face, extremities, genitals, and periumbilical area are often the first signs of infection. The face, if involved, has red, tender inflammation of the cheeks and bridge of the nose ("butterfly type").

Diphtheria.   This childhood disease, caused by *Corynebacterium diphtheriae*, occurs most often during the fall and winter months. A period of incubation is followed by fever, headache, malaise, nausea, and vomiting. In the classic form of diphtheria, a local, pseudomembranous, tonsillar lesion is formed which may produce mechanical respiratory occlusion. Immunization can prevent this serious disease, and the cooperation of dentists and physicians in supporting the immunization program is of the utmost importance.

Tuberculosis.   Tuberculosis is an infectious disease caused by *Mycobacterium tuberculosis*. Although pulmonary tuberculosis is the most prevalent form of the disease, infection may occur by way of the intestines, tonsils, or skin. Oral lesions are rare, and early clinical symptoms (episodes of fever, chill, fatigability, and malaise) may be inconspicuous. A hazard of the profession is the possibility that dental personnel may contract this disease from patients with active tuberculosis. The earlier statement that age and sex are factors in resistance to infection is specifically applicable to tuberculosis. Fatality rates from tuberculosis are higher during infancy and adolescence. In late childhood and adolescence, girls exhibit higher morbidity and mortality rates than boys.

In some respects, the response of infants and small children to tuberculosis infection differs from that of older children and adults. The so-called "childhood type" of tuberculosis infection exhibits a tendency for lung lesions to localize in the lung periphery and for more regional lymph node involvement. The parenchymal and nodal lesions often heal by calcification. In the "childhood type," hematogenous dissemination of the infection is more likely to develop, and miliary tuberculosis and tuberculosis meningitis are possible complications.

Tularemia (Rabbit Fever).   This disease is brought on by *Pasteurella tularensis* after contact with infected wild rodents. In most instances, the newer antibiotics have reduced the serious nature of the disease. Ingestion of contaminated meat may be responsible for the oropharyngeal type of tularemia, in which the symptoms are necrotic ulcers in the oral mucosa and pharynx, with the possibility of a general stomatitis and cervical lymph node involvement.

Syphilis.   An infectious disease caused by *Treponema pallidum*, syphilis, if untreated, exhibits periods of activity that alternate with long periods of latency. During infancy and childhood the congenital form of syphilis is more common than the acquired form, and transplacental syphilitic infection of the fetus is possible, but infrequent, prior to the fourth gestational month. After the fourth month, this type of infection may result in spontaneous abortion or in the birth of an infant with the active disease. Children who survive congenital syphilis may have a variety of lesions, including rhinitis, choroiditis, saddle-nose, rhagades, osteochondritis, and diffuse cutaneous eruptions. Among this group of children, hypoplasia of the incisor and molar teeth (Figs. 29–1 and 29–2), eighth nerve deafness, and interstitial keratitis (Hutchinson's triad) are prevalent symptoms, though they are rarely all present in the same individual. In the last decade, the incidence of acquired syphilis has radically increased in the United States. For the protection of unborn children, all pregnant females should receive a routine serologic examination prior to the fourth month of pregnancy to lessen the possibility of transplacental infection of the developing fetus. Antibiotic treatment should be given to all persons infected with the disease.

Pertussis (Whooping Cough). This acute infection of the respiratory tract, produced by *Bordetella pertussis,* is diagnosed by a typical, severe cough. The common name derives from frequent spasmodic coughs accompanied by a forced whooping inspiration. Because this is similar in communicability to measles and chicken pox, preventive immunization is important.

Tetanus (Lockjaw). Tetanus is due to *Clostridium tetani.* During its active growing phases, it releases a potent exotoxin that causes systemic manifestations. Within two days after onset, a patient with this disease exhibits symptoms of trismus, headache, chills, and pain in the extremities. Severe spasms occur at later stages. The current mortality rate from tetanus remains high (20 to 50 per cent). Passive immunization by the injection of antitoxin has been successful if used within hours after a wound occurs, but treatment for tetanus may require weeks of constant, intensive hospital care. Active immunization effectively prevents tetanus, which like diphtheria, remains localized. Infection almost always originates from a contaminated wound, and a patient with facial or oral injuries is usually referred first to the dentist, who must be alert in singling out cases that may require treatment by a physician for tetanus prevention.

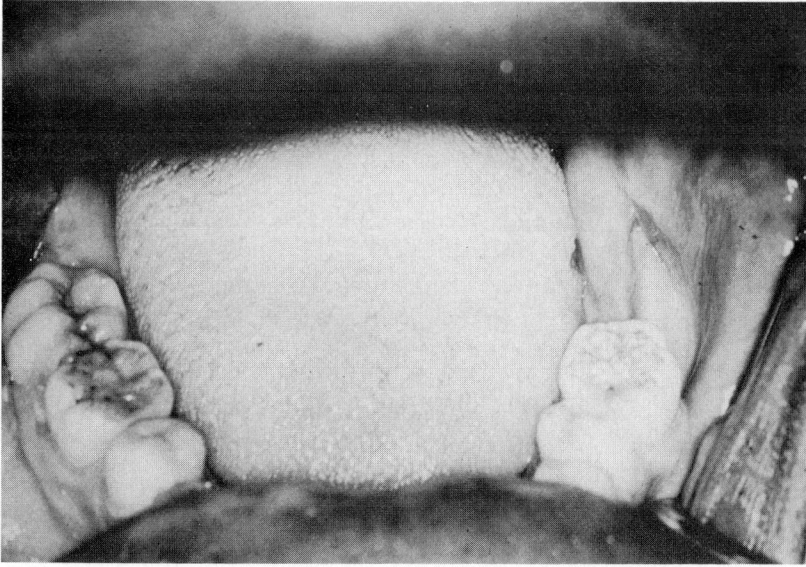

Figure 29–1 Enamel hypoplasia of congenital syphilis ("mulberry molars"). Occlusal surfaces of the mandibular first molars show many small globular malformations rather than the normal cusp and groove patterns.

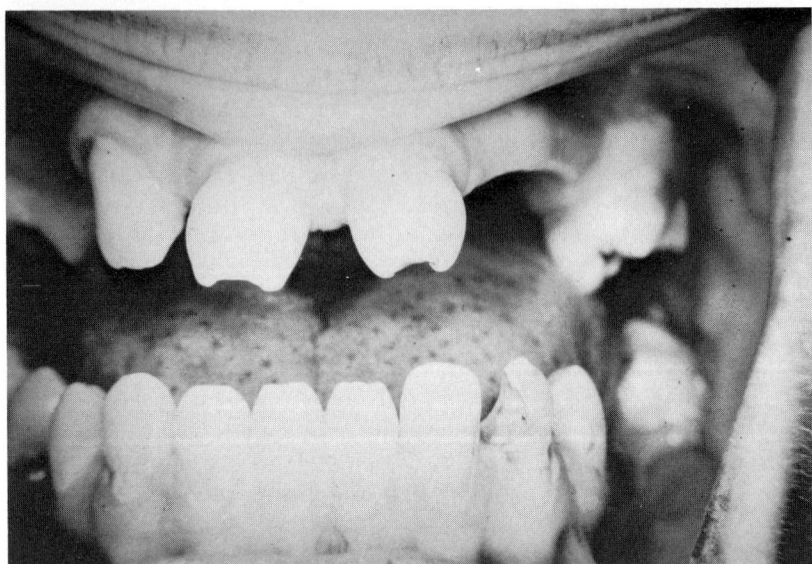

Figure 29–2   Enamel hypoplasia of congenital syphilis (Hutchinson's incisors). Notched incisal edges of the maxillary centrals and "screw-driver"-shaped incisors whose mesial and distal surfaces converge toward the incisal.

Most persons who have had a series of four tetanus toxoid injections retain a protective level of circulating antitoxin for 10 to 12 years. Therefore, routine annual boosters are now thought to be unnecessary. Boosters are injected at the time of an injury when four or more years have elapsed since the previous booster or if the wound is one of high risk. A child needing treatment of an injury to the face and teeth should be referred to his physician for a decision as to what tetanus protection is required

VIRAL INFECTIONS

Measles (Rubeola).   This is an acute, contagious, childhood disease that has a 10 to 12 day incubation period, after which an eruption called Koplik's spots is evident on the mucous membrane. This eruption is followed by malaise, fever, coughing, conjunctivitis, and photophobia. Finally, a maculopapular exanthem, or skin eruption, and high fever occur. Bed rest and treatment for relief of the symptoms is usually prescribed in uncomplicated cases.

German measles (Rubella).   German measles is a common disease with symptoms resembling those of mild scarlet fever or measles. Tender and enlarged lymph nodes in the posterior neck are a characteristic of this infection. An enanthem or mucous membrane eruption of rose-colored spots may occur on the soft palate, and 24 hours after the lymph node involvement an exanthem may occur. The high fever and photophobia experienced with measles are not present in German measles.

Only 8 to 20 per cent of the female population reaches childbearing age without acquiring immunity to German measles; unfortunately, if one of these individuals contracts the disease during the first fourteen weeks of pregnancy it is highly possible that the fetus will have some abnormality. Cleft palate and other dental anomalies are among the many possible malformations. Therefore, it is important for young girls to contract this mild disease prior to childbearing years, because the effects are seldom severe during this period. Even immune mothers may not always transfer their own immunity to the fetus. Hence, as a protective measure against the serious anomalies that are secondary to exposure to this virus, all mothers should avoid contact with this disease until after the fourth month of pregnancy.

Exanthem Subitum (Roseola Infantum). An acute viral disease, Exanthem subitum consists of a 3 to 4 day period of high fever followed by a rash, which occurs late in the infection. The principal importance of recognizing this disease is in being able to distinguish it from German measles or other infections with similar symptoms.

Erythema Infectiosum (Fifth Disease). This is a mildly infectious disease of unknown etiology, which confuses the diagnostic picture for the physician. Its first stage is marked by a rash that is similar in distribution to that in erysipelas, or lupus erythematosus. The rash spreads to the extensor surfaces of the arms, the backs of the hands, the thighs, and the buttocks. No complications from this infection have been reported and specific treatment is not indicated.

Herpesvirus. In this infection, which is almost as common in man as viral respiratory infections, oral involvement is an important clinical feature. Dentists should share the responsibility for its treatment. Since identification of the virus is an involved procedure, which occasionally requires a serologic study, the technical difficulties encountered in handling this problem are greater than those that arise from bacterial infections. Lack of therapy for viral diseases further complicates prescription of proper care for patients. Herpes simplex virus (HSV), which is responsible for a broad range of clinical diseases, is believed to become active upon the development of a primary infection that subsequently follows a course of alternate latency and activity during which transient, localized lesions tend to recur. Investigations are still in progress to determine whether a virus becomes truly latent, with a characteristic, chronic, virus multiplication, or whether exogenous reinfection occurs. One manifestation of this disease is primary acute herpetic gingivostomatitis, a systemic disease accompanied by physical signs of an acute generalized infection and distinct clinical lesions (Figs. 29–3 through 29–7).

Chicken Pox (Varicella). Caused by *Herpesvirus varicellae*, chicken pox is common in childhood and is most prevalent in the winter and spring months. An incubation period of about 14 to 21 days is followed by headache, fever, nasopharyngitis, and anorexia. Maculopapular or vesicular lesions appear first on the skin of the trunk and spread to the face and extremities. Oral lesions may occur in the buccal mucosa, palate, and pharynx. Treatment for the discomfort of symptoms is the only therapy indicated, since healing takes place in 7 to 10 days and complications are rare.

Herpes zoster This disease is thought to be due to the activation of *Herpesvirus varicellae* that has its origin from an earlier chicken pox infection. The virus remains latent in cells of the sensory ganglion and when immunity wanes, herpes zoster may occur. This disease, usually mild in children, is rarely contracted prior to age 10 (Figs. 29–8 and 29–9).

Smallpox. Smallpox is an acute, communicable viral disease with a papulo-vesicular pustular rash accompanied by severe systemic symptoms. Not a single case

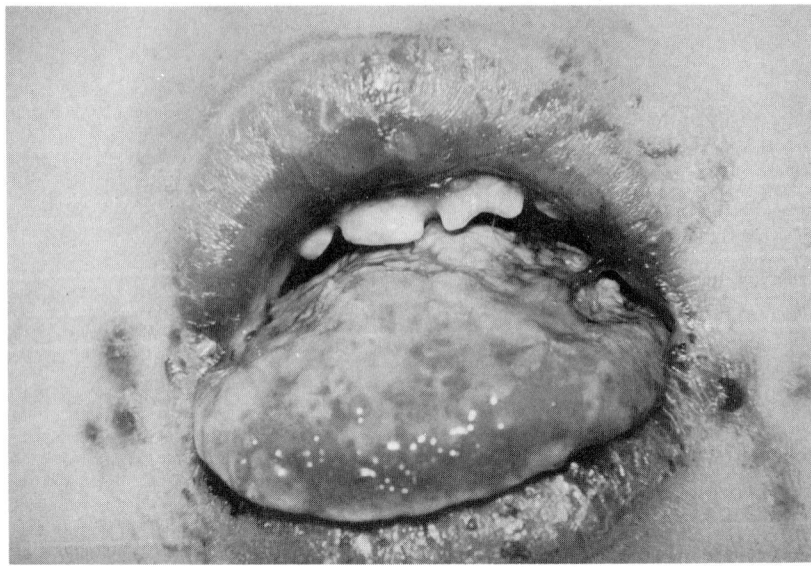

Figure 29–3 Primary herpetic gingivostomatitis. Severe involvement of the tongue, lips, skin, and mucosa. This child was dehydrated, with signs of acute generalized infection. (Courtesy of Doctors L. R. Regattieri and J. L. Parker.)

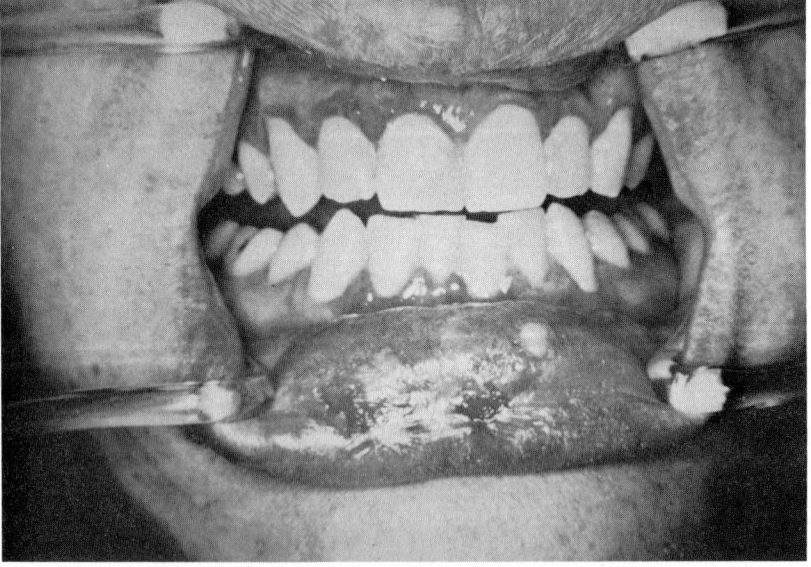

Figure 29–4 Acute herpetic gingivostomatitis. Long term factors of nutrition and oral hygiene are investigated after the acute phase. (Courtesy of Dr. T. W. Weatherford III).

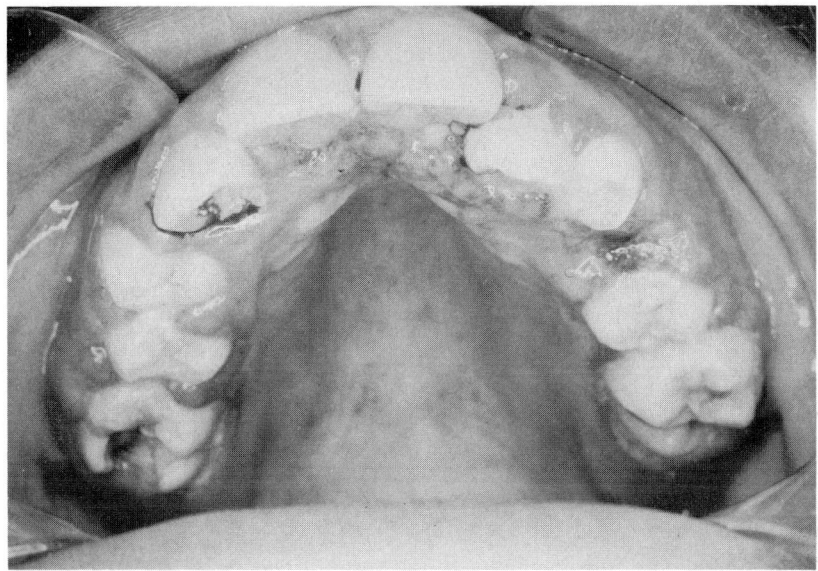

Figure 29–5   Acute herpetic gingivostomatitis. Clinical symptoms were complicated by secondary infection.

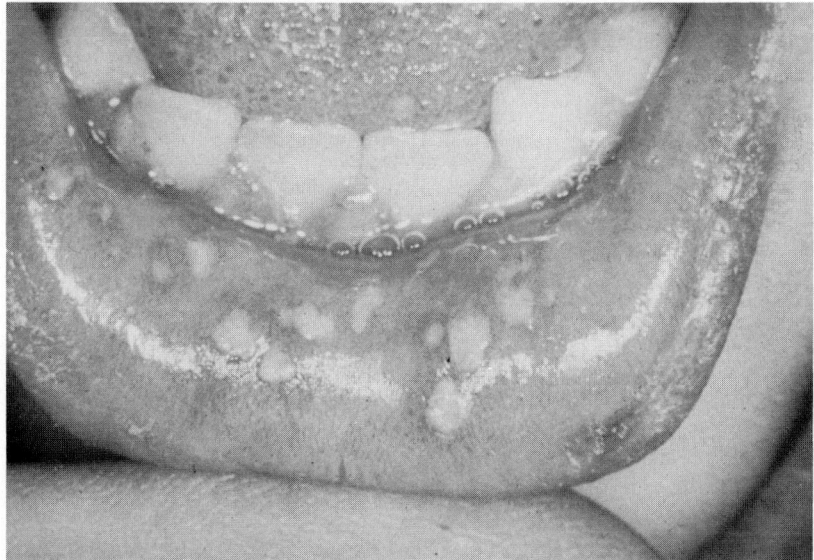

Figure 29–6   Herpetic gingivostomatitis. Moderate to severe occurrence of herpetic lesions localized on the lips. (Courtesy of Dr. T. W. Weatherford III).

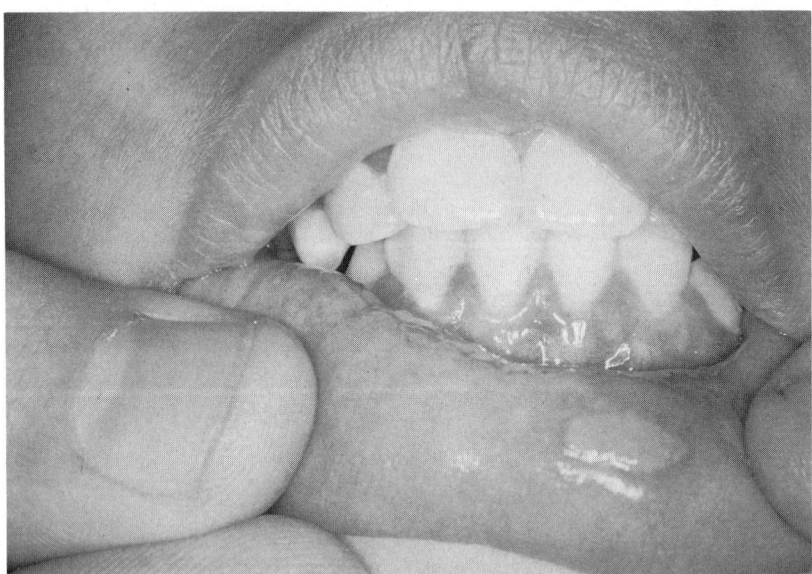

Figure 29–7 Recurrent herpetic lesion.

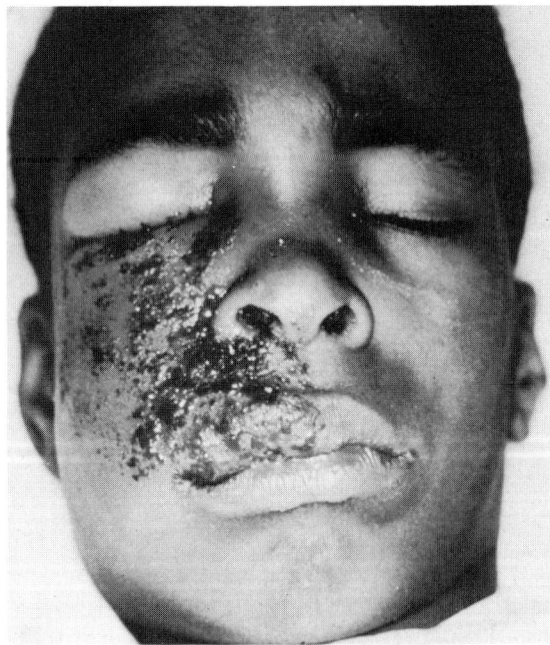

Figure 29–8 Severe herpes zoster in an adolescent patient. (Courtesy of Birmingham Children's Hospital).

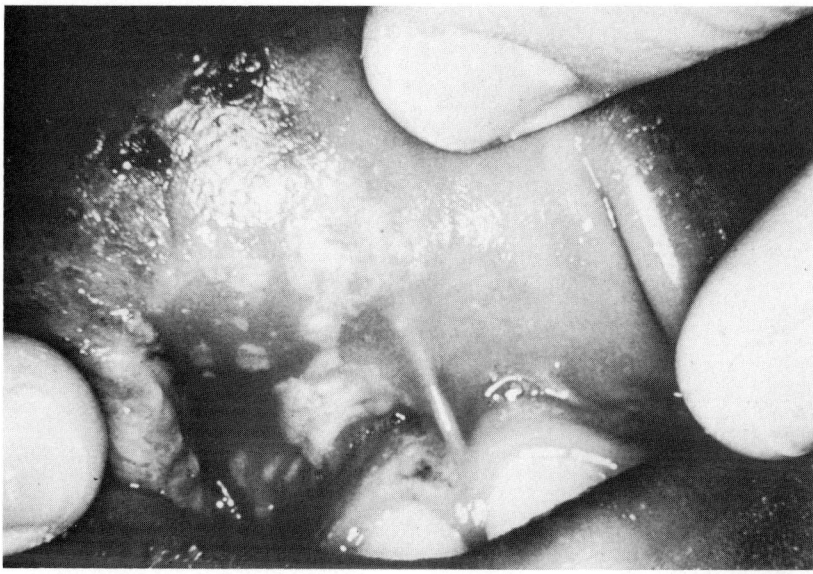

Figure 29–9　Herpes zoster. Same patient as Figure 29–8, intraoral view. (Courtesy of Birmingham Children's Hospital).

of this disease has been recorded in the United States for the past 22 years, and even in countries where endemic smallpox exists, its gradually diminishing occurrence gives a hopeful outlook for its eventual eradication. Therefore, individuals who never journey to regions where smallpox occurs may find it advisable to bypass the smallpox vaccination and avoid the risk from vaccinia sequelae. The Committee on Infectious Diseases of the American Academy of Pediatrics has recommended discontinuance of all routine smallpox vaccinations for infants. The Public Health Service advises that smallpox vaccine should be given only to persons who may be exposed; however, local health laws may experience some lag in agreeing to this new health policy. Vaccination is still required for health personnel and other individuals who travel to and from endemic areas such as Ethiopia, India, and Pakistan.

A suggested schedule for other immunizations is: diphtheria-whooping cough-tetanus (DPT)-polio to be given at ages 2, 4, and 6 months with boosters at ages 1½, 4, and 6 years; and tuberculin testing with measles-rubella vaccines, or tuberculin testing with measles-mumps-rubella, to be given at age 1.

It is probable that in the future production of a killed vaccine or a modified live vaccinia virus may improve safety levels of smallpox vaccination techniques. Until that time, it is recommended that the risk of vaccinia sequelae be reduced by gentle vaccination technique and the keeping of adequate patient histories so that vaccination can be avoided if it is deemed potentially harmful.

Mumps (Epidemic Parotitis).　A generalized, acute, contagious, viral disease, mumps is distinguished by painful enlargement of the salivary glands.(Fig. 29–10). Children under age 15 account for 85 per cent of the infections from this virus. A live attenuated strain of the virus is used for mumps immunization. This procedure is contraindicated in persons sensitive to eggs or neomycin. Though use of the virus vaccine is recommended for all prepubertal children with no history of mumps, the great number of subclinical cases renders such histories only about 50 per cent ac-

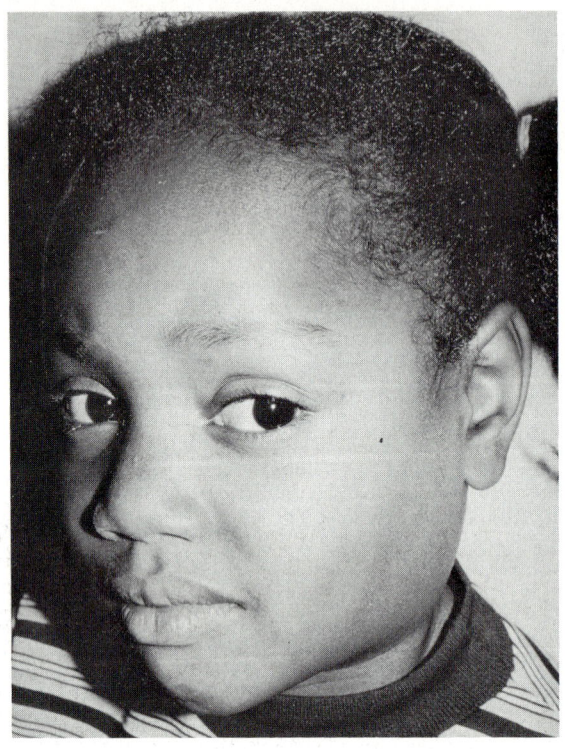

Figure 29–10 Mumps (epidemic parotitis). Firm, elastic swelling of the parotid slightly elevating the ear. (Courtesy of Doctors L. R. Regattieri and J. P. Thomas).

curate. Because of the relatively low risk of contracting mumps, The American Academy of Pediatrics has not prescribed general use of this vaccine.

Infectious Mononucleosis. Common in children from age 2 to 10 years, infectious mononucleosis is an acute disease, of unknown origin; has a variable clinical picture; and should be differentiated from throat infections, colds, influenza-like disease, and generalized rashes. The symptoms are malaise, sore throat, fever, and periorbital swelling; enlarged lymph nodes may occur and a skin rash is noted in up to 20 per cent of the cases. Diagnosis is by laboratory blood data. The prognosis is good, even in extended cases, but weakness and fatigability are occasionally prolonged.

Herpangina (Summer Disease). Herpangina is a specific viral infection caused by Coxsackie A viruses, which most frequently attack, young children. The clinical symptoms are mild sore throat, fever, and headache; small ulcers or vesicular lesions are sometimes present on the anterior faucial pillars, the hard and soft palate, and the tongue.

Hand, Foot and Mouth Disease. This infection, caused by coxsackie A16 virus, occurs in childhood and is usually mild and of short duration. Oral lesions are found on the buccal mucosa, the palate, and the tongue (Figs. 29–11 and 29–12). This disease, which frequently has distinctive clinical features, usually occurs in epidemic form among children, during the summer, and should be distinguished from other exanthems. Diagnosis is usually serologic in association with the discrete foci of the eruptions.

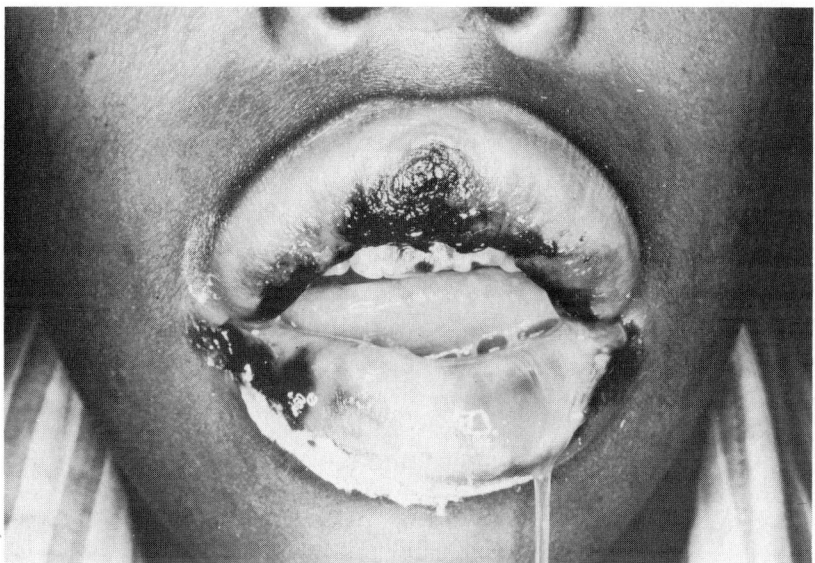

Figure 29–11 Hand, foot and mouth disease. This case demonstrated hypersalivation and dysphagia as well as severe oral lesions. (Courtesy of Doctors L. R. Regattieri and J. L. Parker).

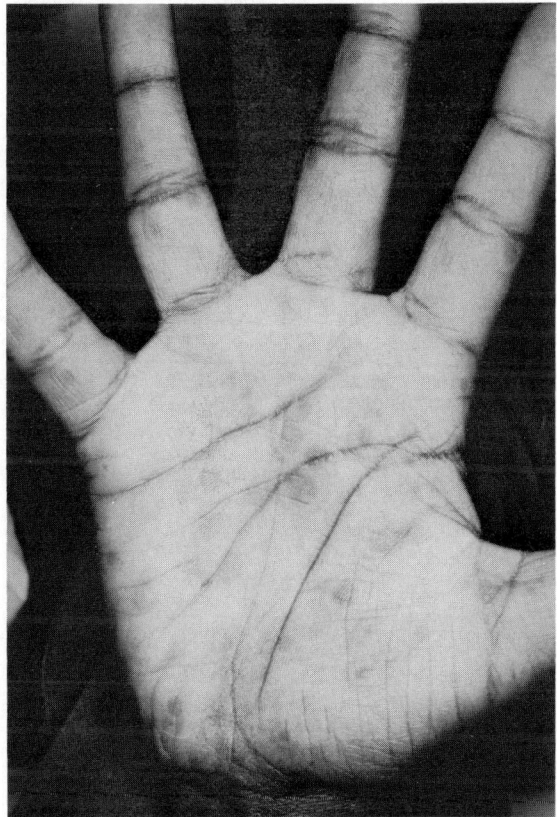

Figure 29–12 Hand, foot, and mouth disease. Hand lesion photograph taken at the same time as Figure 29–11. (Courtesy of Doctors L. R. Regattieri and J. L. Parker).

Cat Scratch Fever.   Cat scratch fever is thought to be viral (Rickettsial) in origin. Symptoms of this disease are malaise, headache, low fever, and lymphadenitis. It develops after a bite or scratch by a cat. Since the patient sometimes experiences pain in the cervical lymph nodes with inflammation of the skin that covers them, he may consult the dentist about treatment. The lesions heal spontaneously in one to three months.

FUNGUS INFECTIONS

Fungus infections are now considered more common than was previously suspected. Two of these infections, actinomycosis and blastomycosis, are more prevalent in adults than in children and will therefore not be discussed.

Moniliasis (Thrush, Candidiasis).   A disease caused by *Candida albicans*, moniliasis is most common in infants and debilitated persons who have some chronic disease, such as diabetes or avitaminosis. It is possible that in recent years, the overenthusiastic use of oral antibiotics may have been responsible for an increased incidence of moniliasis, since these drugs suppress the growth of other oral flora, which normally retard or check growth of moniliasis. Moniliasis creates soft, white, elevated plaques that usually appear on the buccal mucosa and the tongue. If the surface of these white lesions is removed, the area becomes raw and bleeding. Specific antifungal agents, such as nystatin, have been beneficial but not completely successful in treating moniliasis. When 200,000 units per ml. of nystatin is applied with cotton, and the child is allowed to swallow any of the diffusing mixture that is released, the lesions will be eliminated; however, they may recur.

REFERENCES

1. Bhaskar, S. N.: Oral lesions in infants and newborn. Dent. Clin. N. Amer. Symposium on Pedodontics, pp. 421–435, July, 1966.
2. Bhasker, S. N.: Synopsis of Oral Pathology. 2nd ed., St. Louis, The C. V. Mosby Co., 1965.
3. Bradford, W. L.: Pediat. Clin. N. Amer., Symposium on Infectious Diseases. Vol. 7, No. 4, November, 1960.
4. Cheraskin, E.. Diagnostic Stomatology; A Clinical Pathologic Approach. New York, McGraw-Hill, 1961.
5. Cooke, R. E., and Levin, S.: The Biologic Basis of Pediatric Practice. New York, McGraw-Hill, 1968.
6. Hinds, E. C.: Noninflammatory bone disease. J. Oral Surg., *28*:27–38, 1970.
7. Kempe, C. H.: Current status of immunization. Drug Therapy, *1*:45–55, 1971.
8. Meyer, I., and Shklar, G.: The oral manifestations of acquired syphilis, a study of eighty-one cases. Oral Surg., *23*:45–57, 1967.
9. Mitchell, D. F., Standish, S. M., and Fast, T. B.: Oral Diagnosis/Oral Medicine. Philadelphia, Lea and Febiger, 1971.
10. Muller, S. A.: Viral infections of the skin and mouth: A selected review. Oral Surg., *32*:752–759, 1971.
11. Nelson, W. E.: Textbook of Pediatrics. 9th ed., Philadelphia, W. B. Saunders Co., 1969.
12. Nizel, A. E.: Nutrition in Preventive Dentistry: Science and Practice. Philadelphia, W. B. Saunders Co., 1972.
13. Shafer, W. G., Hine, M. K., and Levy, B. M.: A Textbook of Oral Pathology, 2nd ed., Philadelphia, W. B. Saunders Co., 1963.
14. Zegarelli, E. V., Kutscher, A. H., and Hyman, G. A.: Diagnosis of Diseases of the Mouth and Jaws. Philadelphia, Lea and Febiger, 1969.

30

NUTRITIONAL AND HORMONAL FACTORS IN DISEASE

by JOE PRICE THOMAS

Many interrelated factors must be considered when the growth and development of a child is being evaluated in respect to his general physiology or, more specifically, to his oral condition. Nutrition, hormones, genetics, and any episodes of acute or chronic diseases that the child experiences figure prominently in the ultimate level of development and state of health he attains. The importance of these influences cannot be overemphasized because, both individually and in conjunction with each other, their effects can be far-reaching and long lasting.

After being extensively investigated for many years, the subjects of nutrition and endocrinology have come to be considered individual sciences and are recognized for the importance of their relation to disease states and abnormalities of development. Many currently published books deal exclusively with the study of these separate entities.

In this chapter the following topics will be briefly described or defined: the nutritional elements that are considered essential for growth and development or for preserving a balance in body chemistry; the principal hormones and their actions; the effects that are produced by various levels of the nutritional elements, hormones, or both, as well as the effects brought about by the interrelation that exists between the two; and the importance of recognizing imbalances in any combination of factors that may cause disease or abnormalities. It is recommended that a text concerning specific problems be consulted when there is need for extensive information on a subject.

An appraisal of a patient's physical condition at the time of his initial visit to the dentist has proved its worth as an aid in providing appropriate dental care. A continuing record of health; coordination; height; weight; the eruption sequence of the teeth; oral examinations; and hand, wrist (Fig. 30–1*A, B* and *C*), and oral roentgenograms may show that an individual deviates significantly from the normal developmental range of others of the same age and sex. A comparison of findings from the tests performed on a child over a period of time may indicate that the cause of an abnormality is a nutritional or hormonal imbalance.

Most dentists practice in communities where nutritional levels of children are

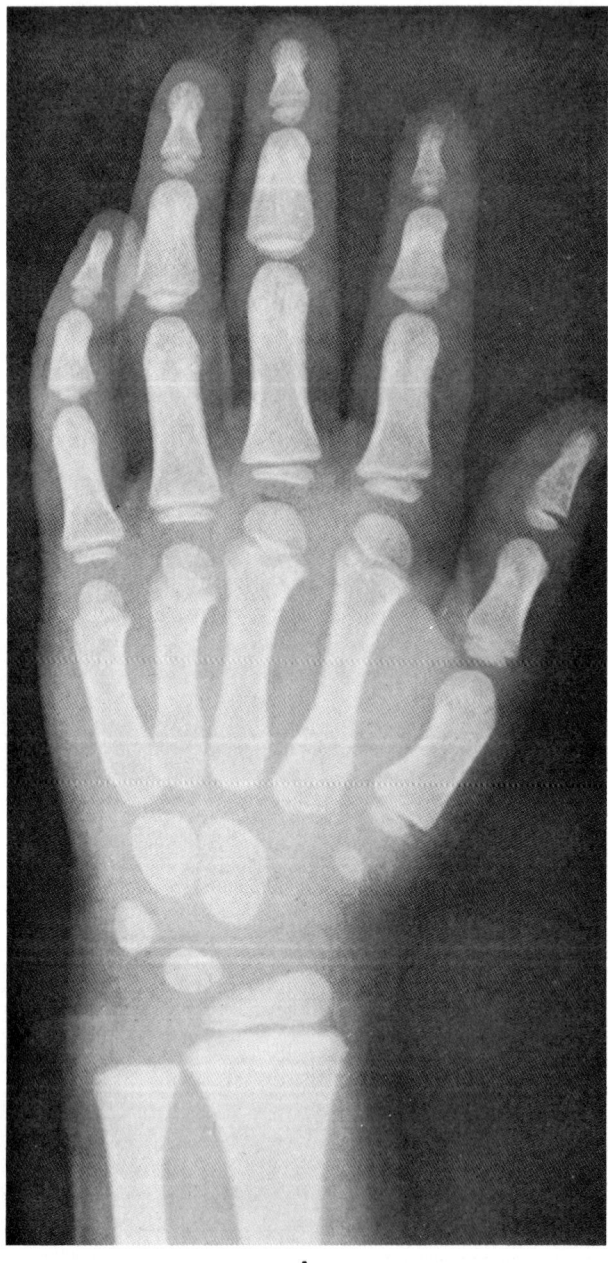

A

(Figure 30–1 continues on the following page.)

controlled by their own individual tastes or those of their parents rather than by the availability of food or the means to purchase it.

In dental practice, classic demonstrations of severe nutritional or hormonal problems are rare. Slight imbalances that cause subclinical defects, though relatively frequent, often escape detection at the time of their inception and, if untreated, may interfere with a child's general physical condition, his growth poten-

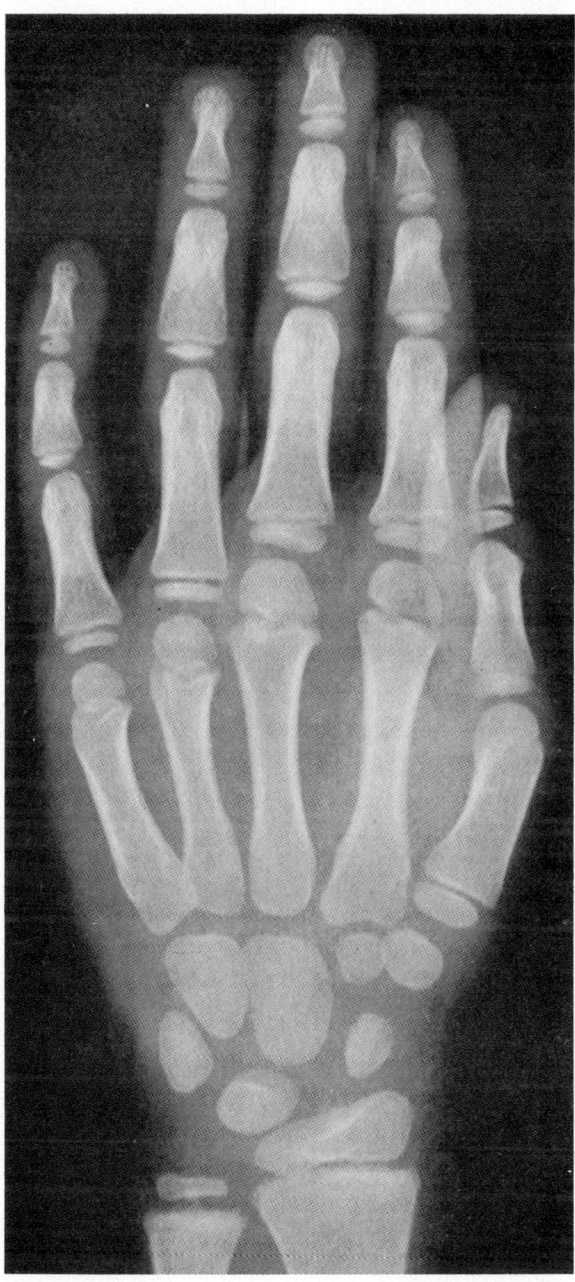

B

(Figure 30–1 continues on the following page.)

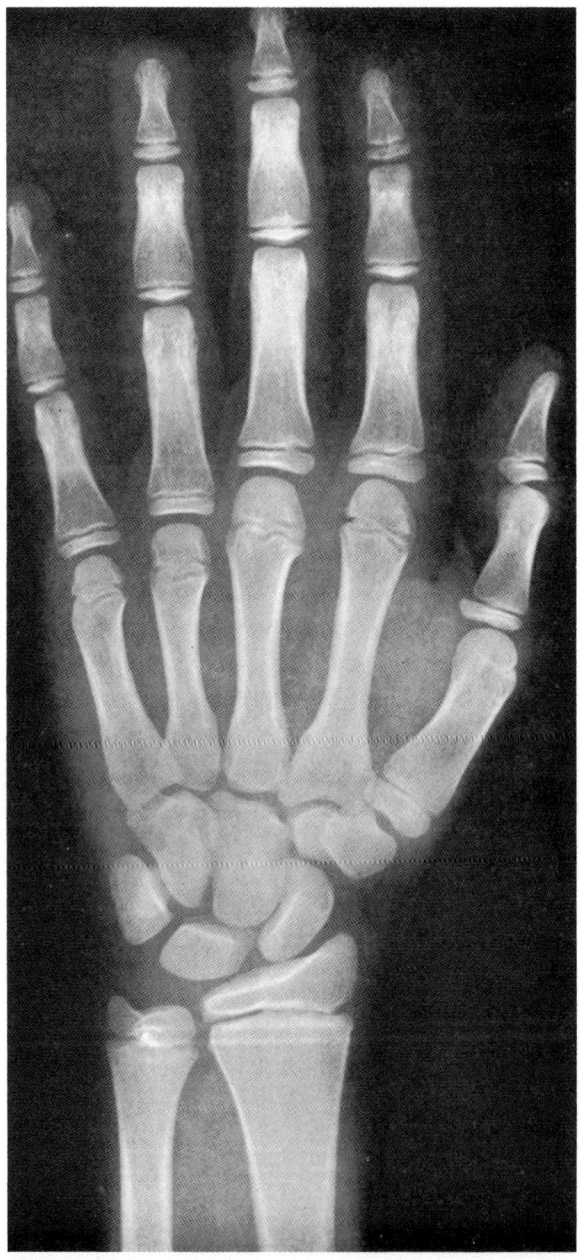

C

Figure 30–1 *A,* Male, age 5 years. *B,* Male, age 8 years. *C,* Male, age 12 years, 6 months. Radiographic standards of development of bones and wrist used to compare chronologic, dental, and bone age in diagnosis. (Reprinted from Radiographic Atlas of Skeletal Development of the Hand and Wrist. 2nd ed. by Greulich, W. W., and Pyle, S. I., Stanford University Press. Copyright © 1959, 1950).

tial, and in more extreme cases, his longevity. Experimentally, pre-eruptive nutritional influences have been shown to affect the teeth of animals in relation to histological structure, chemical composition, gross morphology, tooth size, eruption time, and caries susceptibility.

Since a child's nutritional picture is complicated by such factors as growth and development, age, sexual maturation, and exposure to childhood diseases, longitudinal nutrition studies on children are more complex to evaluate than those on adults.

Many texts on nutrition include the Table of Recommended Dietary Allowances of the Food and Nutrition Board of the National Research Council, which may be used as a guide to the levels of essential nutrients required by the average child. However, it must be remembered that children experience varying health conditions that, from time to time, dictate exceptional dietary needs. Because of these changing needs, most published tables or charts allow an intake of 50 to 100 per cent in excess of the nutrients that are needed to prevent deficiency symptoms. Complete information is not available for setting up optimal levels for some nutritional elements; therefore, levels recommended for these elements are estimates rather than established facts.

Malnutrition

This disorder, which may be caused by improper or inadequate food intake or by faulty absorption of nutrients, is influenced by stress and disease, and may be acute or chronic and either reversible or irreversible (Fig. 30–2). Clinical evidence of malnutrition can usually be traced to a deficit of more than one nutrient, but mild disturbances may escape even laboratory detection. An annual or periodic

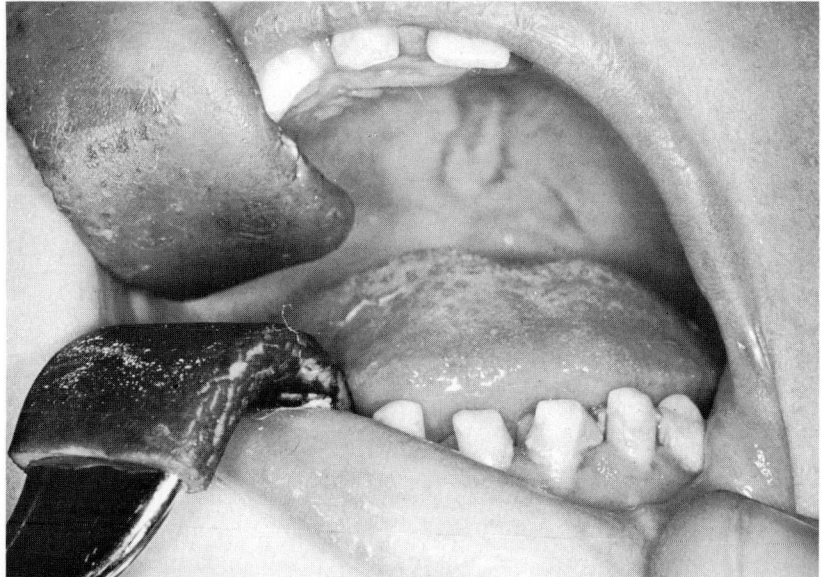

Figure 30–2 Malnutrition in a mentally retarded patient. Gingival changes, calculus and palatal ulceration noted.

record of a child's rate of growth is more reliable as an index to his nutritional status than a comparison of his size with any so-called national standard for age, weight, and height.

The dentist is in an excellent position to counsel his patients on the importance of a diet that is ample in relation to overall physical demands and as a means of preventing dental caries and periodontal disease.

GENERAL NUTRITIONAL REQUIREMENTS

Water

Water is second only to oxygen as an essential for existence. An infant's daily consumption of fluid equals 10 to 15 per cent of his body weight, whereas that of an adult equals 2 or 4 per cent of his body weight. The customary infant diet contains foods with a high water content.

Calories

The large Calorie, which represents the heat required to raise the temperature of 1 kilogram of water by 1 degree C., is used in metabolic study. The energy needs of children vary with age and difference of environmental conditions. In the first year of life the total daily energy requirement is 100 to 120 Calories per kilogram of body weight. This decreases by about 10 Calories per kilogram over each successive three year period. A child's average expenditure of Calories between the ages of 6 to 12 is approximately 50 per cent for basal metabolic rate, 12 per cent for growth, 25 per cent for physical activity, 5 per cent for specific dynamic action of food, and 8 per cent lost in feces. At puberty an accelerated rate of growth and development is accompanied by a corresponding increase in the caloric needs.

In the average balanced diet, approximately 15 per cent of the Calories consumed are derived from protein, 35 per cent from fat, and 50 per cent from carbohydrates. Heat production varies according to the oxidation rates of different foods. In general, carbohydrates and proteins provide 4 and 9 Calories per gram, respectively. The level of body fat is dependent upon the caloric intake and the daily body expenditure of energy. A consistent up or down variation of as much as 500 Calories in the daily intake will require approximately one week to effect a corresponding fluctuation of about one pound of body weight.

Protein

These compounds, which make up the predominant solid structure of the body and account for 20 percent of an adult's weight, are indispensable in the formation of cell nuclei and protoplasm. Specific proteins contain a certain type, number and arrangement of amino acids. The body can synthesize many of the 22 amino acids required for tissue protein, but eight or nine must be supplied exclusively from dietary sources. Since new tissue cannot be formed unless all essential amino acids are present in the body simultaneously and in the proper ratio, the absence of only one may create an imbalance. As with other nutritional substances, infants require larger quantities of amino acids than older children and adults. The daily protein requirement for infants is 4 to 5 grams per kilogram of body weight in contrast to the 0.9 gram per kilogram of body weight required by normal adults.

Neither the minimal nor optimal protein requirement is known. Nevertheless, the supply of this particular nutrient is most crucial, since others are available even in countries where the protein supply is limited because of underproduction, overpopulation, or lack of income.

Proteins build body tissue, furnish energy, help maintain proper water balance, and have a part in producing hormones, enzymes, and antibodies. During periods of growth the child's protein requirements are elevated; therefore, his intake must be increased to continue a positive balance for maximum growth. Adults need only keep a nitrogen equilibrium; however, a dietary lack of any essential amino acids will upset this nitrogen balance regardless of the total quantity of protein ingested. The extent of growth failure, lack of stamina, loss of muscle tissue, and increased susceptibility to infection and edema may be used to measure the degree of human protein deficiency. Severe protein deficiency, known as kwashiorkor, is a distinct clinical syndrome that most frequently appears in children from age 4 months to 5 years; marasmus, a disease common to the same age group, is caused by both protein *and* caloric malnutrition and represents a general starvation.

Carbohydrates

These nutrients, which supply the bulk in the diet as well as being the principal source of Calories, include starches, sugars, dextrins, and gums. The adult body stores carbohydrates in the liver and muscle as glycogen, which constitutes about 1 per cent of the body weight. A steady dietary supply of carbohydrates is compulsory for children because their small liver and muscle masses can store only limited glycogen reserves.

Glycolysis and the tricarboxylic acid cycle are responsible for the overall oxidation of glucose through the combined and complex activity of insulin, the pituitary and adrenal hormones, and some of the essential amino acids. The principal carbohydrate metabolic disorders are diabetes mellitus, glycogen storage disease, galactosemia, and glucose or fructose intolerance.

Fats (lipids)

Primary sources of energy from the diet, fats transport and facilitate the absorption of vitamins A, D, E, and K. Lipids help to quell hunger and prolong the sensation of satiety. Simple lipids, or esters, which develop from the reaction between fatty acids and various alcohols, are the most plentiful fats in the body and in food.

One necessary fatty acid not synthesized by humans is linoleic acid, and it must be acquired from the diet. Because of their rapid growth, infants who receive inadequate amounts of this nutrient may have dry, thickened skin with desquamation and intertrigo. These symptoms will quickly disappear if the child is fed a diet in which 1 to 2 per cent of the Calories originate from linoleic acid.

MINERALS

Minerals are inorganic nutrients that must be present in the human body in delicately balanced amounts. For the performance of their interrelated functions, bare traces of some minerals and relatively large quantities of others are needed. Of the 18 minerals required for the upkeep and regulation of the body processes, the three most important are calcium, iron, and iodine.

Before discussing the individual minerals, a review of some of their joint activities may help to clarify the overall picture. The calcium and phosphorus ratio is important in the formation of teeth and bones. The manufacture of red blood cells, as well as the synthesis of hemoglobin, requires cobalt (vitamin B_{12}), iron, and copper. Sodium, potassium, calcium, phosphorus, and chlorine function individually and in combination to keep the body fluids balanced. Zinc, molybdenum, and manganese are influential in metabolic reactions that require the enzyme catalysts in which these minerals are located. Calcium and magnesium are necessary for normal cell function in nerve and in soft tissue. Iodine is indispensable to the structure of the thyroid hormone.

The electrolytic balance between extra- and intracellular fluids is affected by calcium, magnesium, potassium, and sodium, the four most important electropositive mineral elements, and by phosphorus, sulfur, and chloride, the principal electronegative mineral elements.

Calcium

Among the most abundant minerals in the body, calcium is important for skeletal development, blood coagulation, cell permeability, muscle contractility, buffer systems, and metabolism of carbohydrates and fats. Ninety-nine per cent of the body calcium is in the bones and teeth, with 1 per cent in the other tissues. The skeletal calcium is in dynamic equilibrium with the calcium in body fluids and tissues. Normal blood contains from 9 to 11 mg. of calcium per 100 ml. of blood. Very low calcium levels may cause a characteristic tetany accompanied by convulsions.

In the small intestine, the absorption of calcium is facilitated by a low pH and by the presence of vitamin D. The parathyroid hormone regulates the amount of calcium in the blood; if the diet fails to supply enough calcium, this hormone creates a chemical action that transfers calcium from the bone to the blood. Though the lack of vitamin D is the major cause of rickets, the disease may also result from an insufficient intake of calcium and phosphorus or an imbalance in this combination.

The adult intake of calcium should be adequate to sustain body stores, since some calcium is incorporated into bone throughout the life span. A pregnant female must maintain calcium levels that will supply the combined needs of herself and the developing fetal skeleton; therefore, her intake must exceed that amount specified for the average adult or calcium will be withdrawn from the maternal skeleton to supply the fetus. Children and adolescents must also have a higher intake of calcium than adults because of their additional expenditure for growth and development (Figs. 30–3 and 30–4).

Calcium sources include dairy products, shellfish, egg yolk, and green vegetables.

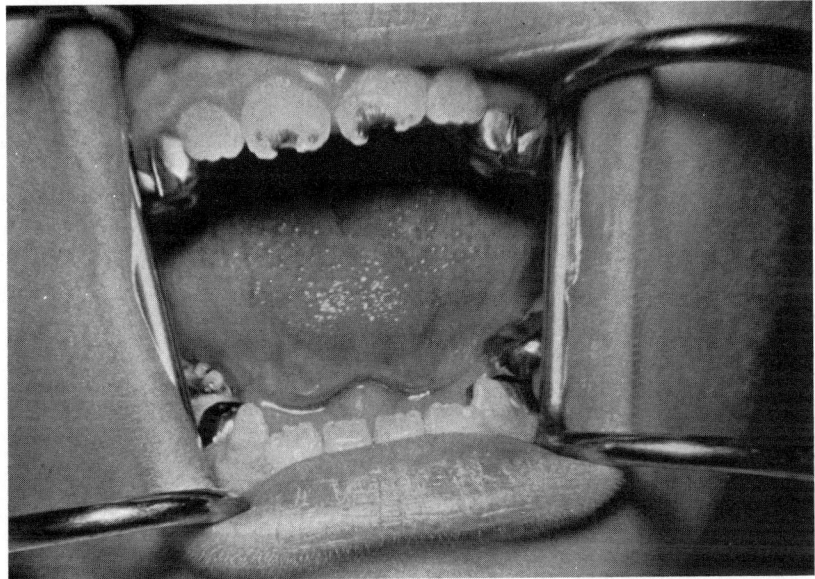

Figure 30–3 Defective enamel formation associated with a medical history of calcium deficiency. (Courtesy of Dr. R. L. Roebuck).

Phosphorus

This mineral plays a many-faceted role in the body functions; it aids in the metabolism of carbohydrates, proteins, and fats; it provides quick release of energy for muscle contraction; it helps to stabilize blood chemistry; it supports growth and

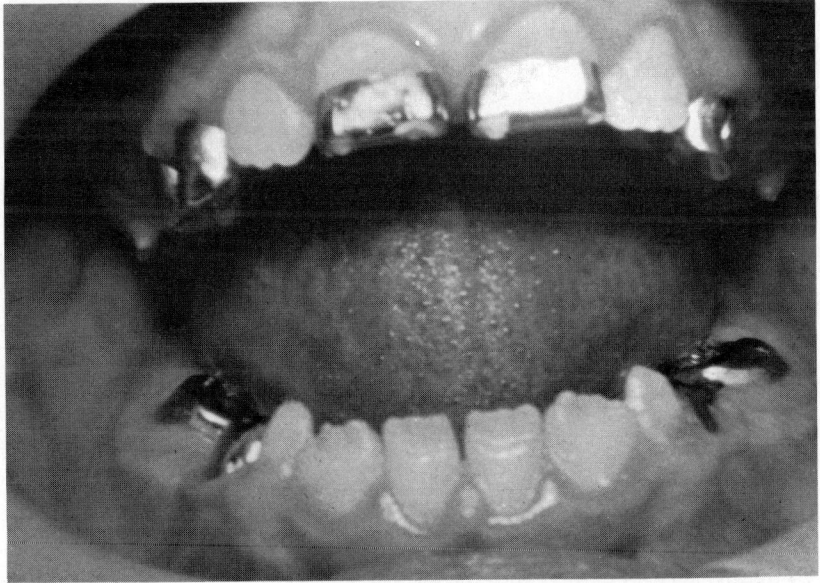

Figure 30–4 Same patient seen in Figure 30–2. Note hypoplasia of incisal thirds of the mandibular incisors. (Courtesy of Dr. R. L. Roebuck).

development of teeth and bones; and it is a medium in the transport of fatty acids. A component of many enzyme systems, phosphorus is involved in storage and transfer of energy in phosphorylated complexes such as ADP and ATP.

In the human body, 80 per cent of this important mineral is deposited in the skeletal tissue and 20 per cent in the cellular and extracellular fluids. Each 100 ml. of human blood has 35 to 45 mg. of phosphorus, of which 3 to 5 mg. is inorganic and thus readily available for chemical reaction. Normally, there is an inverse relation between serum calcium and serum inorganic phosphate. As with calcium, phosphorus absorption is favored by an acid pH in the intestine, and equal amounts of calcium and phosphate in a diet should give optimal absorption. Phosphorus is available from food sources similar to those that supply calcium.

Iron

Iron is vital to tissue respiration and the proper functioning of enzyme systems. Though only comparatively small amounts of iron are required, its function is of tremendous importance as a component of hemoglobin, which performs the indispensable task of oxygen transport in cell respiration.

Iron absorption, like that of calcium and phosphorus, is enhanced by an acid pH, and ferrous iron is more readily absorbed than ferric. It is not amiss to reiterate that the stability of the proper body chemistry depends on delicate balances. For example, an excess of phosphates may impair iron absorption.

Iron deficiency paves the way for hypochromic anemia, a disease that requires confirmation of clinical diagnosis by laboratory data concerning the hemoglobin concentration and the number of erythrocytes per unit volume in the circulating blood. Clinical signs of this deficiency may include pallor of skin and tissues, weakness, fatigability, and dyspnea upon exertion. Oral manifestations are angular cheilosis, loss of tongue papillae, and mucosal pallor (Fig. 30–5). An iron deficiency may be brought on by improper diet or poor absorption. Liver, lean meat, shellfish, dried beans, and green leafy vegetables are the best dietary sources of iron. Since milk is a poor source of iron, a wide variety of foods has been introduced in the prescribed diet for infants.

Copper

A component of the enzyme tyrosinase, which has a part in melanin pigment formation, copper also facilitates the synthesis of iron into hemoglobin and is probably involved with other oxidation-reduction enzymes in the body. No deficiency of copper in the diet has been reported.

Iodine

Iodine is necessary solely for its role in the formation of the thyroid hormone, which regulates energy metabolism of the body. Without iodine the gland forms no hormone, and this lack causes cellular hyperplasia and an increased production of colloidal material, which, together, induce excessive activity of the gland with a resultant enlargement or goiter (Fig. 30–6). During puberty and pregnancy the iodine requirement is elevated. The most critical reason for prevention of hypothy-

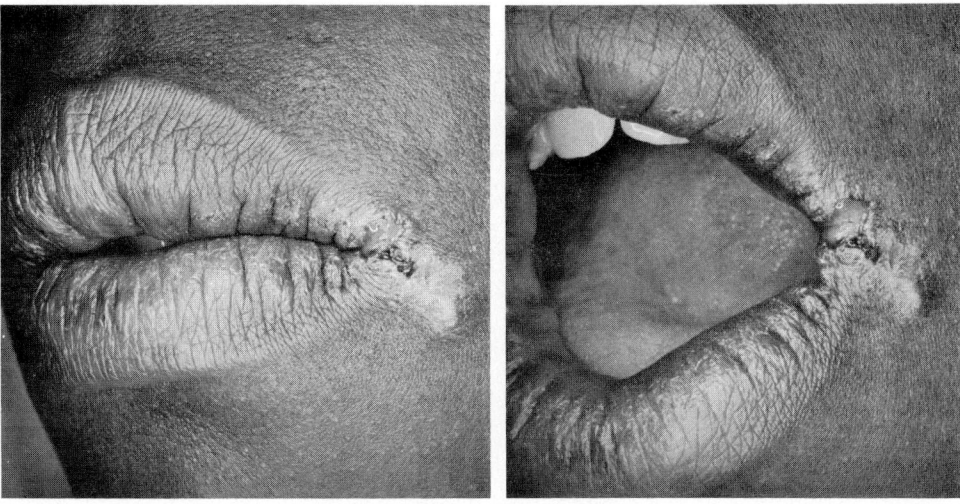

Figure 30–5 Angular cheilosis.

roidism in children is its influence in the development of cretinism and its attendant physical and mental retardation.

Vegetables grown in iodine rich soils, as well as seafoods, are good sources of iodine. Iodized salt in the United States contains 0.01 per cent of potassium iodide. In the average diet that includes iodized salt, twice the normal requirement per day would be available. If salt is restricted in a diet, use of an iodine supplement should be considered.

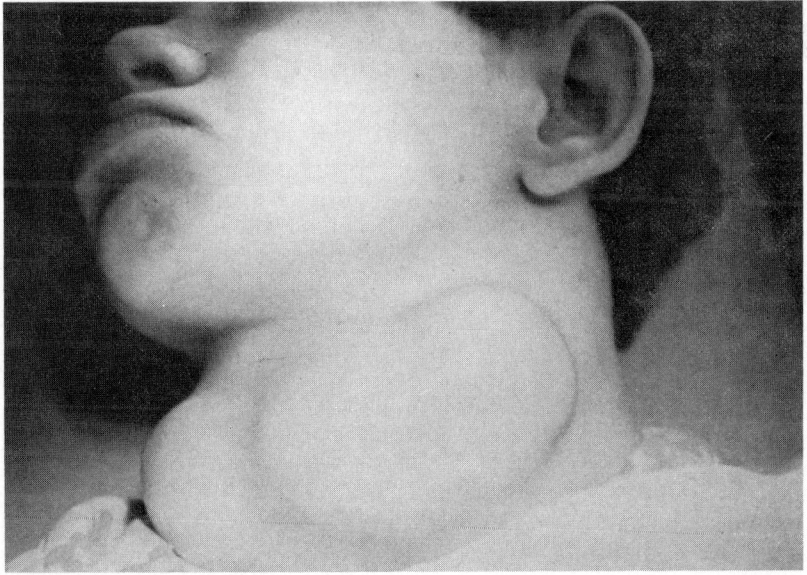

Figure 30–6 Goiter. This large untreated goiter is associated with many other problems in this patient. (Courtesy Birmingham Children's Hospital).

Cobalt

A component of vitamin B_{12}, cobalt is found in numerous common foods. The human requirement is unknown, but there are no records of any cases of cobalt deficiency.

Zinc

This mineral is present in several enzymes that serve as catalysts in metabolic reactions. For example, it is in carbonic anhydrase, which is important in the carbon dioxide exchange in red blood cells. Zinc, like cobalt, has not been indicated as a dietary requisite, and no deficiencies have been noted.

Manganese

An activator of several enzymes that are included in the Krebs cycle, manganese is part of the molecule arginase that is itself necessary for the formation of urea.

Magnesium

Magnesium is a component of both soft tissue and bone. The normal functioning of skeletal and cardiac muscles and of the nerve tissue requires a balance between magnesium and calcium ions. Magnesium is also an activator of such coenzymes as cocarboxylase and coenzyme A, and is involved in energy production, utilization of fats, and the metabolism of protein and carbohydrates. Since most vegetables and cereals contain this mineral, a deficiency in man is rare.

Molybdenum

This mineral is contained in two enzymes and probably has some influence in fatty acid oxidation. Its possible activity as a cariostatic agent has not been confirmed.

Fluoride

Present in bones and teeth fluoride has played a significant role in the achievement of maximum resistance to dental caries. The amount of fluoride present in blood is 0.10 to 0.15 ppm and in saliva 0.1 ppm. Nearly all ingested fluoride is excreted; however, prolonged excessive intake may adversely affect the calcification of the teeth and bones.

Sodium

Sodium is essential and is rarely lacking in the human diet. The principal ions of the interstitial fluid are sodium, and the basic ions of the blood are 93 per cent sodium; therefore, this element is primarily responsible for regulating the osmotic pressure of the extracellular fluids.

Potassium

A plentiful dietary requirement, potassium is mostly restricted to the intracellular areas, and its major influences are on the contractility of muscles and excitability of nerve tissue. A deficiency of potassium may cause diarrhea, abnormal kidney function, diabetic acidosis, muscular weakness, nervous irritability, and disorientation.

VITAMINS

The term "vitamin" refers to organic compounds that are required in minute amounts for energy or cellular metabolism and for promoting an individual's growth. These accessory food factors must be supplied wholly or partially from dietary intake. The exact modes of action of vitamins A, C, D, and K are still obscure, but the effects produced by their absence are well known. Vitamins are classified as fat soluble (A, D, E, K) and water soluble (B complex and vitamin C).

Vitamin A Deficiency

This disorder rarely occurs among healthy children under normal living conditions. Vitamin A has a role in the formation of visual purple, in the maintenance of epithelial tissue, and probably in the formation of mucopolysaccharides. Symptoms of deficiency include retardation of mental and physical growth, apathy, anemia, night blindness, xerophthalmia, and dry, scaly skin. During tooth formation in the rat, vitamin A deficiency produces unfavorable changes in enamel, dentin, pulp, and alveolar bone formation. Under similar conditions, these same changes might be duplicated in human beings. Ingestion of excess vitamin A may induce a serious physiological reaction accompanied by symptoms of nausea and drowsiness; however, even over an extended period, it has no effects of a dental nature.

Vitamin B Deficiencies

The components of the vitamin B complex vary greatly in function and chemical composition; several are important as coenzymes in biochemical reactions. A deficit in a single B vitamin could disrupt a chain of chemical processes and create adverse clinical manifestations. Foods poor in one B vitamin usually lack others in the complex; therefore, a sharp differential determination of a deficiency may be impossible and would, in any event, require determination through biochemical tests rather than by clinical diagnosis.

Thiamin, Vitamin B₁, Deficiency. Besides causing beriberi, this deficiency promotes the accumulation of lactic and pyruvic acids in the tissues, impairs nerve function, and increases the sensitivity of oral tissue. A vitamin B_1 deficiency is rarely seen in the United States, and most infant diets are adequate in this water-soluble vitamin.

Riboflavin, Vitamin B₂, Deficiency. This is usually encountered in conjunction with other B complex deficiencies. A diet that does not include adequate amounts of liver, milk, cheese, eggs, and leafy vegetables may occasion a deficiency of this water-soluble vitamin, and the patient will display symptoms of angular cheilosis, glossitis, eye lesions, and seborrheic dermatitis around the nose.

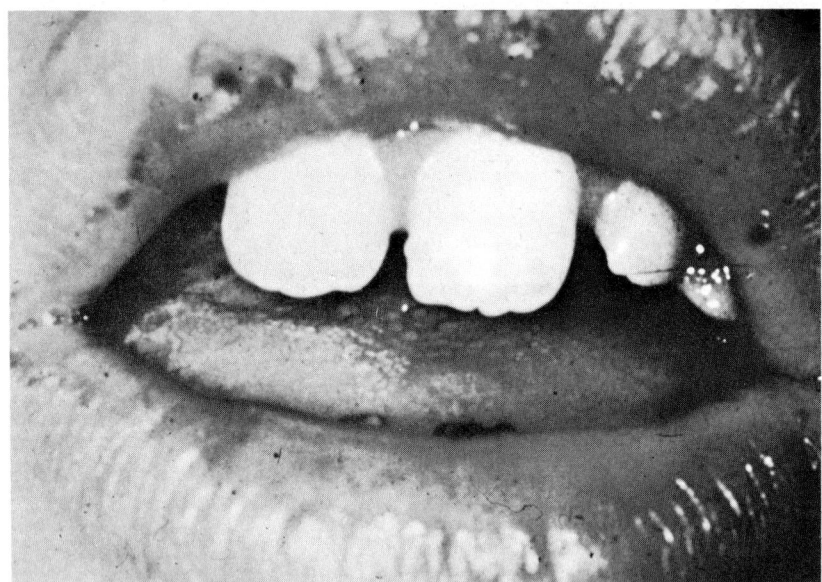

Figure 30–7   Oral view of a patient with pellagra. Painful gingivitis and glossodynia are present. (Courtesy of Dr. T. M. Weatherford, III).

Niacin Deficiency.   Niacin is a component of coenzymes I, II, and III, which are agents in glycolysis and in respiration of cells and serve as catalysts in hydrogen transfers. The niacin deficiency disease, pellagra (Fig. 30–7), is characterized by large, symmetrically developed patches of erythema on the forearms, face, neck, and backs of the hands. In the more severe cases, the patient suffers from glossitis and redness of the lateral margins and tip of the tongue, and the skin becomes dry, scaly, and pigmented. Though the clinical signs cannot be attributed to a single vitamin deficiency, the lack of niacin is probably responsible for most of the symptoms of pellagra. The best food sources for niacin are liver, yeast, meat, peanuts, and enriched cereals.

Vitamin B₆ (Pyridoxine) Deficiency.   Vitamin B_6 is composed of a group of metabolically interrelated pyridines that function mainly as coenzymes in protein and fat metabolism and in the activity of the nervous system. A deficiency of this vitamin has been associated with, though not definitely determined as the single causative of, magenta glossitis. Clinical disturbances that are due to this deficiency include infantile convulsions, peripheral neuritis, dermatitis, anemia, cheilosis, glossitis, and seborrhea around the eyes, nose, and mouth.

Pantothenic Acid Deficiency.   An important component of coenzyme A, pantothenic acid assists in the metabolic release of energy from carbohydrates and also helps in the synthesis and degradation of steroid hormones and fatty acids. A lack of this nutrient might cause fatigue, headaches, malaise, nausea, abdominal pain, and cramping of leg muscles. The production of antibodies might also be inhibited or eliminated. It is improbable that humans would be deficient in pantothenic acid because it is present in most foods.

Folic Acid Deficiency.   Folic acid (pterylglutamic acid, folacin) plays a role in the synthesis of the purine and pyrimidine compounds that are used in the formation of nucleoproteins. In man, a folic acid deficiency may induce a macrocytic anemia with the glossitis, gastrointestinal lesions, diarrhea, and malabsorption characteristic of pernicious anemia, but without its involvement of the nervous system. Folic acid is effective in treating sprue and other malabsorption syndromes.

Glandular meats, yeast, and green leafy vegetables provide the best dietary sources for folic acid.

Vitamin B$_{12}$ (Cyanocobalamin) Deficiency. Vitamin B$_{12}$ is the first compound, necessary to life, that has cobalt as a component. Thought to play a role in the transfer of single carbon intermediates (principally methyl groups), vitamin B$_{12}$ also participates in the formation of pyrimidine bases and in the metabolism of purine. Stated simply, B$_{12}$ is involved in the synthesis of red blood cells, and a deficiency of this vitamin would cause pernicious anemia. The principal dietary sources for B$_{12}$ are liver, meat, eggs, milk, cheese, and fish.

Biotin Deficiency. Biotin, an essential in many enzyme systems in bacteria, in animals, and presumably in man, is related metabolically to folacin and pantothenic acid. The richest sources of biotin are liver, kidney, egg yolk, milk, and yeast.

Ascorbic Acid (Vitamin C) Deficiency

Ascorbic acid is necessary for the normal functioning of the cellular elements of all tissues and all subcellular structures, as well as for the formation and upkeep of intercellular substances in connective tissue. Humans do not synthesize this vitamin; therefore, scurvy, one manifestation of vitamin C deficiency, may develop at any age but is rarely seen in infants and newborns. Disease states, particularly infectious and diarrheal diseases, apparently increase the need for vitamin C. A deficiency of this vitamin produces defects in formation and maintenance of intercellular substances in the supportive tissues (collagen, matrix of bone, cartilage, dentin, and vascular endothelium); early symptoms are irritability, digestive disturbance, loss of appetite, and gingivitis (Figs. 30–8 and 30–9). With a prolonged deficiency of vitamin C, growth of the endochondral bone is retarded, and recurring low grade fever and moderate secondary anemia may be among the symptoms. In this debilitated condition acute necrotizing ulcerative gingivitis caused by anaerobic organisms may destroy the periodontal membrane support so that the teeth are loosened to the point of exfoliation.

Vitamin D Deficiency

The effect of the sun's rays on the skin are instrumental in the synthesis of this vitamin, and a deficiency may occur if an individual experiences limited exposure to sunlight. Regulation of calcium and phosphorus metabolism is the principal activity of vitamin D. Therefore, prompt recognition of a deficiency of the vitamin is important to circumvent the malformations such a lack may induce in the bone and tooth structures. The difficulty of evaluating early clinical signs makes it safer to rely on dietary history for confirmation of the deficiency.

The vitamin D syndrome is rickets. Listed below are several predisposing factors that determine the extent and clinical pattern of rickets:
1. Rapid growth
2. Age of patient
3. Race (Negro children are particularly susceptible)

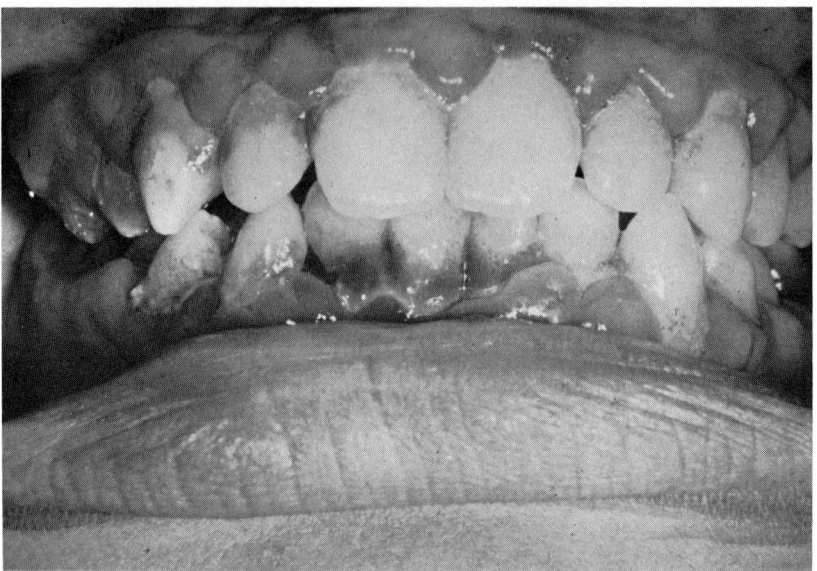

Figure 30–8   Generally debilitated oral condition of a patient with Vitamin C deficiency.

4. Genetic influences (vitamin D resistant)
5. Absorption problems (vitamin D, calcium, or both)

An excessive intake of vitamin D over a period of 1 to 3 months may cause the following symptoms: hypotonia, anorexia, irritability, constipation, polydipsia, polyuria, and pallor. The physician may also detect dehydration, hypercalcemia, and hypercalciuria in a patient who has hypervitaminosis D.

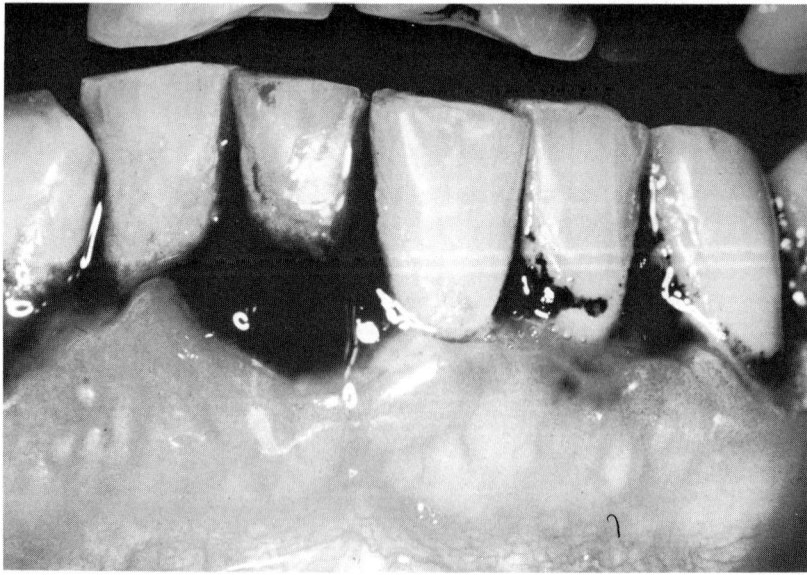

Figure 30–9   Vitamin C deficiency in an older patient who is also affected by necrotizing ulcerative gingivitis. (Courtesy of Dr. T. W. Weatherford, III)

Vitamin K Deficiency

Vitamin K is a fat-soluble substance that is essential in the formation of prothrombin. It is associated with blood clotting, and, though its exact function is uncertain, if this vitamin is not supplied or if the system fails to absorb it, hypoprothrombinemia develops. The bacterial synthesis of vitamin K that occurs in the alimentary tract may be suppressed by the use of antibiotics.

Natural sources for the vitamin are spinach, cauliflower, and cabbage.

Miscellaneous Factors

Other factors, such as roughage, digestibility, and satiety are important in the overall nutritional picture. In any population, malnutrition on a large scale is contingent on the lack of food as a result of economics or production, or both. Although the diet of low income families is apt to include little milk, fruits, and vegetables, adequately balanced, nominally priced meals can be provided for such groups if the dietary funds are expended in fifths for (1) milk (cheese), (2) meats, (3) fish and eggs, (4) bread (cereal), and (5) fats. Because of a tendency to consume local food, the geographic location assumes an important role in nutrition. For example, people living in iodine-deficient locations tend to have a higher incidence of goiter than those located where the iodine supply is adequate. In some locales the appropriate fluoride level in the water supply provides the population with a natural protection from dental caries.

HORMONES

Substances called hormones are normally produced by specialized cells in one part of the body and then transported by the bloodstream to other parts of the body where they exert an overall effect on the body responses. Brown and Barker have categorized hormones as to their three major functions: (1) integrative action, which permits the body to act as a whole in response to external and internal stimuli; (2) regulation of metabolism and growth and of the internal environmental factors such as salt and water balance; and (3) morphogenesis, or the rate and type of body growth.

Since hormones circulate in the blood and reach all cells, it is difficult to explain the selectivity with which they influence specific cells. All body tissue is subjected to hormonal influence, either in relation to the development and growth of the tissue or to the functions performed by this tissue.

As indicated earlier in this chapter, many nutritional and hormonal factors are interrelated in the child. Diverse symptoms may be encountered in a child with a health problem that issues from a hormonal imbalance, and any disturbance in growth and development may serve as a useful diagnostic factor.

Pituitary Hormones

The pituitary, master gland of the body, consists of an anterior, an intermediate, and a posterior lobe.

The anterior or more active lobe of the pituitary produces six known hormones. In addition to exercising its own specific effect upon the oral cavity and jaws, the pituitary influences the activity of most of the other so-called target glands that affect this area.

Pituitary Hormones

Anterior Lobe	Target	Activity
Thyrotrophin (TSH)	Thyroid	Producing thyroid hormone
Follicle-stimulating hormone (FSH)	Ovarian follicles	Estrogen production follicle growth
Luteinizing hormone (LH)	Corpora lutea	Estrogen production from corpora lutea
Interstitial cell stimulating hormone (ICSH)		Progesterone secretion
Leuteotrophic hormone (LTH)	Corpora lutea	Progesterone secretion
Adrenocorticotrophic hormone (ACTH)	Adrenal cortex	Growth of cortex secretion of steroid hormones
Growth hormone (STH)	Entire person	Growth
Posterior Lobe		
Antidiuretic hormone vasopressin	Kidney	Reabsorption of water
Oxytocin	Uterus	Uterine contractility
Intermediate Lobe		
Intermedin	Skin	Dispersion of pigment granules

Increased activity of the anterior pituitary occurs when the activity of the target gland is decreased (as in hypothyroidism), when there is an extra demand on the target gland (as in the corpus luteum during pregnancy), or when hypoplasia or tumors occur in the target glands or in the pituitary itself.

An overproduction of hormones is the most significant alteration induced by the hyperactivity of either the anterior pituitary gland or one of its target organs (Fig. 30–10). If hyperplasia of the anterior pituitary lobe stimulates excessive production of the growth hormone prior to age 6, hypophyseal gigantism develops. The amount of body change that ensues depends upon the age of the child at the onset of the condition. Hyperplasia between age 6 and puberty causes pituitary gigantism. If the growth phase is almost completed, the syndrome is referred to as acromegaly.

Hypophyseal infantilism is characterized by a retardation of growth and usually by a delay in sexual maturation. The body is small but proportionate, and the child's bone age lags behind his chronologic age. The primary teeth erupt and exfoliate behind schedule, and there is delayed eruption of permanent teeth. One long-term effect of this condition is an underdeveloped arch that will not accommodate the teeth, and a consequent malocclusion.

Hypofunction of the pituitary after the completion of growth will produce a hyposecretion from all target glands regulated by its anterior lobe ("panhypopituitarism").

The Thyroid Hormone

The active principle of the thyroid hormone is thyroxin, which exerts a general effect on metabolic activity and plays an essential role in cellular differentiation,

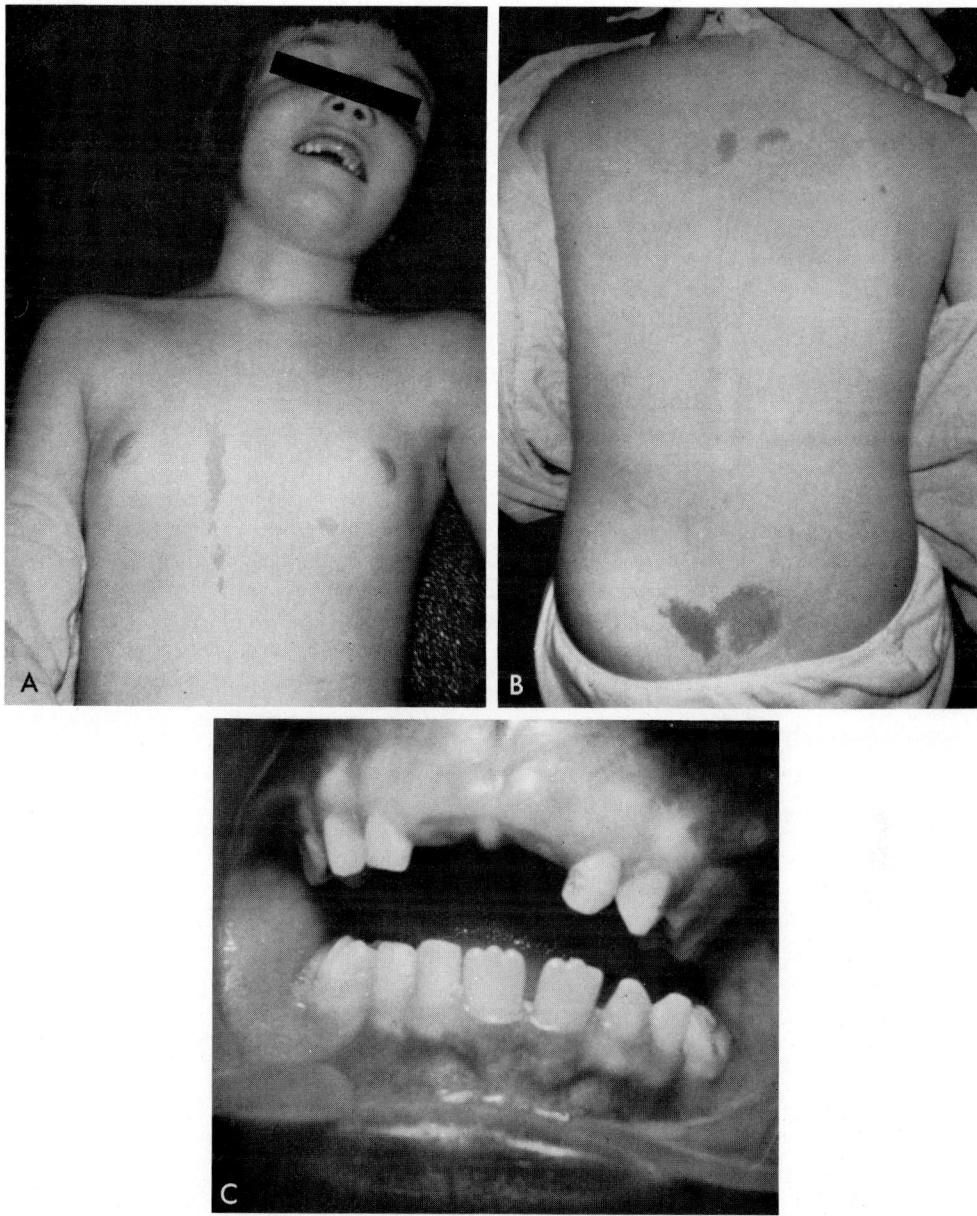

Figure 30–10 *A,* McCune-Albright syndrome. Precocious puberty associated with polyostoyic fibrous dysplasia in a six year old girl. *B,* Areas of dermal pigmentation associated with the syndrome. *C,* Oral photograph revealing erupted mandibular permanent centrals and exfoliated maxillary primary centrals. (Courtesy of Dr. R. L. Roebuck).

growth, maturation, water-electrolyte balance, metabolism of carbohydrates and lipids, protein storage, and other physiological functions.

Hypothyroidism may develop if the pituitary fails to provide enough TSH, or if the malfunction of the thyroid gland itself causes a subnormal basal metabolic rate. This failure during infancy causes cretinism, and, in an older child, juvenile myxedema.

Cretinism (Fig. 30–11) is characterized by mental retardation in conjunction with physical abnormalities such as general edema, short arms and legs, a disproportionately large head with an excessively wide face, and possibly an undersized maxilla. Hair is sparse, hair and nails are brittle, sweat glands are atrophic, and the lips and tongue are thick and enlarged. Eruption and exfoliation of primary teeth are delayed, and roots that are incompletely formed because of the lag in dentin formation are radiographically detectable.

Juvenile myxedema develops from the occurrence of a hypothyroid condition between the ages of 6 to 12 years. Since the skeletal growth of these patients is more advanced when the imbalance begins, the usual facial and body characteristics of cretinism are absent, but some obesity and delays in exfoliation of primary teeth and eruption of permanent teeth are typical of this condition.

Hyperthyroidism, referred to as Grave's disease or thyrotoxicosis, provokes an elevated basal metabolic rate, and affects nerves, muscles, and the cardiovascular, lymphatic, and reticuloendothelial systems. Clinical manifestations include protruding eyes (exophthalmos), weight loss, weakness, irritability, and tachycardia. Hyperthyroidism, which is uncommon in growing children, is encountered more often in girls than in boys. Accelerated dental development is its principal oral manifestation.

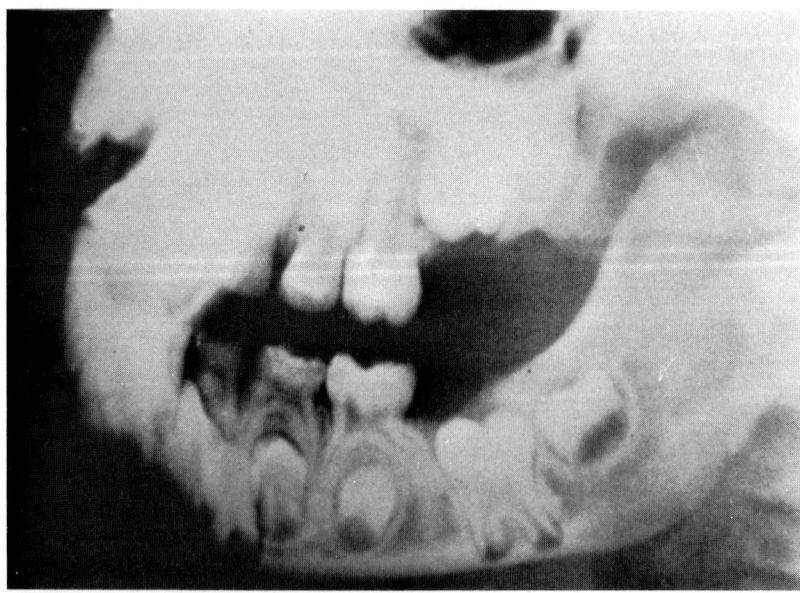

Figure 30–11   Cretinism. Note the delayed eruption pattern, particularly the mandibular first permanent molar. (Courtesy of Boston Children's Hospital).

Parathyroids

Usually four in number, the parathyroids are oval bodies located on the posterior surface of the thyroid. Two types of epithelial cells are present; those designated as chief cells produce the parathyroid hormone (PTH), which maintains the calcium-phosphorus equilibrium in the blood.

Hypoparathyroidism is characterized by low serum calcium, high serum phosphate, and low phosphate and calcium excretion in the urine. Hypocalcemia provokes increased excitability of the nerves (parathyroprivic tetany). Clinical signs of hypoparathyroidism include baldness, brittle nails, cataracts, and, if tooth development is concurrent with the imbalance, enamel and dentin disturbances.

In hyperparathyroidism poor muscle tone and a resultant decrease of neuromuscular activity are evident, as is a general radiolucency of the bones. If the disorder persists, more pronounced, oval or lobulated, radiolucent lesions are noted, which (in the jaws) may be confused with ameloblastoma, multiple myeloma, or eosinophilic granuloma. Radiographs reveal that hyperparathyroidism causes the jaw bones to have the appearance of "ground glass." This hormonal imbalance is infrequent in children. Some sources indicate that its occurrence may be related to both age and sex. Females are affected three times as often as males, and the disorder usually develops in middle age.

Adrenal Hormones

The two adrenals are small glands that are located on the upper pole of each kidney. The outer cortex of the adrenal arises from the mesoderm and has no apparent functional interrelation with the adrenal medulla, which is derived embryologically from the neural crest of the ectoderm.

Extensive research has been done on the two secretions of the adrenal medulla: epinephrine and norepinephrine; the former affects the circulatory system as a vasodilator and cardiac stimulant and the latter as a vasoconstrictor. Endocrine in nature, these secretions have metabolic effects that are not consistently correlated either with nervous activity or with their ectodermal origin.

The anterior pituitary controls the size and rate of secretion of the adrenal cortex. The hormones elaborated by the cortex, as well as the gonadal estrogens and androgens, are generally classified as steroids. The adrenals of man secrete a mixture of seven major steroids that is about 85 per cent hydrocortisone. Corticosterone and aldosterone make up the most significant proportion of the other 15 per cent of the mixture. Many steroids that are present in blood and urine have been identified during laboratory analyses. These steroids could be hormones, precursors of adrenal steroids, degradation products of metabolism, or byproducts of the chemical analytical methods. Injections of adrenal hormone may induce an elevated blood sugar that is sometimes called "steroid diabetes."

Both hypo- and hyperfunction of the adrenal cortex occur in man. The most common cause for hypofunction (Addison's disease) is destruction of the adrenal gland by tuberculosis or by a fulminating illness. When the adrenal cortex is the primary point of failure, continued secretion of ACTH by the pituitary gland fails to secrete ACTH. This disease is characterized by weight loss, weakness, increased cutaneous pigmentation, and a disturbance in mineral and carbohydrate metabolism.

Hyperfunction of the adrenal cortex assumes one of two forms. In children, a metabolic defect that provokes secretion of large amounts of androgens is referred to as the adrenogenital syndrome, and causes precocious secondary sex development in males and development of male characteristics in females. The second type of hyperfunction (Cushing's disease), though it does attack children, is primarily an adult disorder, apparently brought on by hypersecretion of the oxygenated steroids. This disease results from a defect in protein anabolism and is characterized by obesity, cessation of growth, thin skin, and asthenia.

Pancreas

The pancreas is located in the curve of the duodenum. Its endocrine cells, the islets of Langerhans, produce insulin, one of the principal hormones responsible for maintenance of a normal blood sugar level. This level is regulated by the liver, which is itself controlled by the finely balanced interaction of several hormones. Sugar uptake from the intestine is accelerated by the thyroid hormone, glycogen breakdown is stimulated by epinephrine, the blood sugar is increased through the action of the pituitary growth hormone, but the key hormone in all this activity is insulin. Glucose, a critical factor in the carbohydrate metabolic process, should be present in an approximate ratio of 100 mg. per 100 ml. of blood. Under normal circumstances, an intake of glucose, with the consequent rise in the blood sugar, stimulates the secretion of insulin which rapidly returns the blood sugar to normal.

Diabetes mellitus, a hereditary chronic metabolic disorder, is characterized by hyperglycemia and glycosuria. The long-time use of insulin to control this disease has been responsible for associating it primarily with the pancreas; however, the related and important influence of endocrine glands in the metabolism of carbohydrates lends credence to the theory that this disease may be triggered by faulty metabolism as well as by an insulin imbalance, or by a combination of the two. That the role of insulin in this disorder should not be underestimated is demonstrated by the 300 mg. per 100 ml. rise in blood sugar levels after surgical removal of the pancreas. The normal glucose level in blood is 70 to 90 mg. per 100 ml.

Diabetes, often called the poly-disease (polyphagia, polyuria, and polydipsia) is about twice as prevalent in females as in males, and in higher age brackets the incidence increases for both sexes. It has been estimated that only 4.4 per cent of all diabetics in the United States are under age 25. Hyperinsulinism may occur in a diabetic child who takes his daily insulin requirement but fails to eat his prescribed dietary allowance.

The Gonads

The male testes and the female ovaries are referred to as the gonads, and in addition to developing the cells required for reproduction, these glands produce hormones that spur the maturation of the sexual organs and develop the characteristics of masculinity and feminity.

Ovarian Hormones

Estrin is produced principally by the maturing Graafian follicle and is present after the onset of menstruation. When the female is approaching puberty the FSH of the anterior lobe of the pituitary stimulates the ovary to produce estrogen, which encourages growth of the pelvic bones, enlargement of the breasts, development and pigmentation of the nipples, and maturation of the genitalia.

Testicular Hormone

Testosterone is produced principally by the interstitial cells of Leydig. When the male nears puberty, the anterior lobe of the pituitary secrets ICSH which, in turn, causes effective amounts of testosterone to be released. This causes development of secondary sex characteristics, hastens epiphyseal maturation, and stimulates maturation of the male sex organs.

With premature or excessive production of the sex hormones, skeletal growth and sexual development are accelerated. An insufficient supply or complete absence of sex hormones will delay epiphyseal closure, which, in turn, allows a prolonged growth period that may result in disproportionately long arms and legs. Sexual maturation is also retarded by this imbalance.

REFERENCES

1. Bhaskar, S. N.: Synopsis of Oral Pathology, 2nd ed., St. Louis, C. V. Mosby Co., 1965.
2. Bernick, S.: Histochemical study of dentine in rats following hypophysectomy. Oral Surg., *23*:680–687, 1967.
3. Bernier, J. L., and Muthler, J. C.: Improving Dental Practice through Preventive Measures. 2nd ed., Philadelphia, W. B. Saunders Co., 1963.
4. Brown, J. H. V., and Barker, J. B.: Basic Endocrinology for Students of Biology and Medicine. 2nd ed. Philadelphia, F. A. Davis Co., 1962.
5. Cheraskin, E.: Diagnostic Stomatology; A Clinical Pathologic Approach. New York, McGraw-Hill, 1961.
6. Cooke, R. E., and Levin, S.: The Biologic Basis of Pediatric Practice. New York, McGraw-Hill, 1968.
7. Heinz (H.J.) Company: The Heinz Handbook of Nutrition. 2nd ed., New York, McGraw-Hill, 1965.
8. Mitchell, D. F., Standish, S. M., and Fast, T. B.: Oral Diagnosis/Oral Medicine. Philadelphia, Lea and Febiger, 1969.
9. Nelson, W. E.: Textbook of Pediatrics. 9th ed., Philadelphia, W. B. Saunders Co., 1969.
10. Nikiforuk, G.: Posteruptive effects of nutrition on teeth. J. Dent. Res., *49*:1252–1261, 1970.
11. Nizel, A. E.: Nutrition in Preventive Dentistry: Science and Practice, Philadelphia, W. B. Saunders Co., 1972.
12. Shaw, J. H.: Preeruptive effects of nutrition on teeth. J. Dent. Res., *49*:1238–1250, 1970.
13. Shafer, W. G., Hine, M. K., and Levy, B. M.: A Textbook of Oral Pathology, 2nd ed., Philadelphia, W. B. Saunders Co., 1963.
14. Zegarelli, E. V., Kutscher, A. H., and Hyman, G. A.: Diagnosis of Diseases of the Mouth and Jaws. Philadelphia, Lea and Febiger, 1969.

APPENDIX

I. THE ADHESIVENESS OF FOODSTUFFS TO TOOTH SURFACES

Foodstuff	% Moisture Content		Adhesive-ness (gm./cm.²)	Relative Adhesive-ness (0-12*)
	Before Chewing	After Chewing		
Gelatin dessert	79.0	83.0	58	0
Chocolate coated coconut bar	7.5	24.6	94	
Lima beans	71.9	71.2	97	
Raisin bran cereal	2.3	56.0	111	1
Chocolate snap cookie	4.8	29.5	160	
40% bran flakes cereal	2.0	52.0	163	
Peanut butter cookie	2.0	43.0	165	
Banana	76.5	77.0	174	
Grapenut cereal	2.0	47.0	189	
Whole wheat bread	30.6	53.7	207	2
Apple pie	44.2	34.8	224	
Deviled ham	48.1	48.7	232	
Cracker (oil sprayed)	2.0	40.0	238	
Olive	69.5	59.8	278	
Potted meat	66.3	69.0	291	
Vanilla wafer	12.2	34.7	329	3
Vienna sausage	60.8	62.0	378	
Soda cracker	1.0	52.0	384	
Liver sausage	48.0	63.0	385	
Meat ball	74.0	79.0	388	
Cheese cracker	4.4	37.3	392	
Peanut	0.8	28.5	413	4
Potato (mashed)	70.9	76.5	414	

I. THE ADHESIVENESS OF FOODSTUFFS TO TOOTH SURFACES

Foodstuff	% Moisture Content		Adhesive-ness (gm./cm.²)	Relative Adhesive-ness (0-12*)
	Before Chewing	After Chewing		
Shredded wheat cereal	3.0	50.0	424	
Raisin	13.0	30.9	427	
Cheese corn puff	0.1	47.0	432	
Peanut butter	0.6	27.2	436	
Sliced "dried" beef	51.4	71.5	438	
Rye bread	30.0	60.0	445	
Rye bread and margarine	25.0	58.0	456	
Chicken spread	58.0	73.0	477	
Sardine	49.3	62.3	480	
Peach	76.8	75.4	491	
Rice Krispie cereal	3.3	57.0	498	
Orange	88.2	83.8	502	5
Potato chip (crisp)	1.5	35.0	507	
Milk chocolate	0.5	9.2	507	
Broiled ground beef	43.9	69.4	521	
Black walnut	2.9	34.7	537	
Potato stick	1.0	47.0	551	
Doughnut	11.0	48.0	557	
Corn flake cereal	2.4	46.4	574	
White bread and margarine	32.3	58.1	595	
Black-eyed peas	72.0	77.0	606	6
White bread	26.8	64.0	610	
Date	26.0	41.8	614	
Apple (fresh)	80.5	84.7	619	
Semisweet chocolate	1.8	7.8	627	
Sandwich meat slice	61.0	73.0	646	
Cheese (American)	35.0	49.7	650	
Bologna	50.1	68.2	658	
Baked beans	66.0	70.0	672	
Canned whole kernel corn	73.0	75.0	717	7
Cherry (maraschino)	35.0	62.8	735	
Green peas	82.8	78.1	741	
Corn flakes and milk	50.3	54.2	745	
Tomato (canned)	92.0	90.0	753	
Sugar-coated corn flake cereal	2.0	50.0	754	
French bread and margarine	20.0	59.0	762	
Sweet potato	71.0	34.0	766	
Spaghetti	80.0	78.0	791	
Carrot (boiled)	91.0	92.0	804	8
French bread	18.0	63.0	811	
Chocolate cake	19.9	30.3	823	
Potato (French fried)	66.5	72.8	829	
Egg (fried)	54.1	80.0	850	
Egg (hard boiled)	70.0	71.0	948	9
Egg yolk (hard boiled)	47.0	64.0	958	
Cup cake	5.5	32.1	1006	10
Chocolate caramel	4.5	9.5	1010	
Ham (boiled)	65.0	78.0	1012	

I. THE ADHESIVENESS OF FOODSTUFFS TO TOOTH SURFACES

Foodstuff	% Moisture Content		Adhesive-ness (gm./cm.²)	Relative Adhesive-ness (0-12*)
	Before Chewing	After Chewing		
Turnip greens	90.6	90.5	1055	
Plain cake	17.0	34.1	1070	
Potato (boiled)	87.0	87.1	1100	11
Egg (scrambled)	72.2	53.4	1115	
Toffee*	4.9	9.5	2020	20
Caramel*	5.3	11.2	2630	26

*"Relative adhesiveness" is a scale (0–12) for comparing the adhesiveness of foodstuffs to teeth. Toffee and caramel are so much more adhesive than other foods that their values for relative adhesiveness are far outside the usual range.

From Caldwell, R. C.: Adhesion of foods to teeth. J. D. Res., *41*:821–832, 1962.

II. ORAL SUGAR CLEARANCE OF DIFFERENT FOODSTUFFS IN TWO PERSONS (MEAN VALUES) AND CALCULATION OF CARIES POTENTIALITY INDEX

Food Product	Sugar Content TS %	Sugar Content RS %	Ingested Quantity, Mean gm.	Max. Carbohydrate Conc., Mean TS %	Max. Carbohydrate Conc., Mean RS %	0.02% TS	0.02% RS	0.2% TS	0.2% RS	2% TS	2% RS	20% TS	20% RS	Caries Potentiality Index* TS
FLUIDS														
Light beer	1.2	0.3	32.5	0.2	0.1	0.75	0.25	0.25	—	—	—	—	—	1
Beer	1.1	0.4	27.0	0.1	0.1	1.5	1.25	—	—	—	—	—	—	2
Lemonade	9.3	8.3	20.0	0.5	0.6	1.5	1.5	0.75	0.75	—	—	—	—	2
Fruit juice	11.5	11.5	32.0	1.2	1.2	2	2.5	1	1	—	—	—	—	3
Gruel	4.5	0.3	10.5	0.6	0.2	2.5	2	1.5	—	—	—	—	—	4
Coffee + 2 sugar lumps	7.6	0.5	21.5	1.1	2.7	2.5	2.75	1.5	0.5	0.25	—	—	—	4
Tea + 2 sugar lumps	11.2	0.1	14.0	1.9	0.3	3	1.25	1	0.5	0.25	0.25	—	—	4
Chocolate (milk) + sugar	14.2	3.9	9.0	1.9	0.6	4	5.25	1	1	—	—	—	—	5
Milk	3.8	2.9	33.0	0.6	0.6	4	3	2	1.5	—	—	—	—	6
SOLIDS														
Flour, bread														
Fruit jelly	11.0	8.2	13.5	0.7	0.4	2	2.5	1.5	1.5	—	—	—	—	4
Oatmeal porridge	9.0	0.5	18.0	0.5	0.3	3.5	2.5	2	0.5	—	—	—	—	6
Cornflour pudding	7.0	2.8	24.0	0.6	0.5	4	4	2	1.5	—	—	—	—	6
Swedish hard bread, very thin + butter	3.8	0.8	4.5	1.5	0.7	4	3.5	2	1.5	0.5	—	—	—	7
Swedish hard bread, light + butter	4.4	2.7	3.0	0.9	0.5	4.5	3.5	2	1.5	—	—	—	—	7
White bread + butter	1.5	0.9	5.5	0.8	0.5	4.5	4.5	2	1	—	—	—	—	7
Rye bread, coarse + butter	2.3	1.1	6.0	1.3	0.7	5	6.25	2	2	—	—	—	—	7
Swedish hard bread, dark + butter	1.3	0	4.5	1.2	0.5	6.25	5.75	2	2	—	—	—	—	8
Special bread + butter	12.0	5.0	7.5	2.2	1.7	6.25	5	4	3	0.5	0.5	—	—	11
Wheaten bread	12.3	9.3	8.0	2.8	2.0	7.5	6.25	4	3	1	0.5	—	—	13
Danish pastry	30.0	13.5	11.0	2.4	0.7	10	5	2.5	1.5	0.5	—	—	—	13
Rye bread, fine + butter	12.0	3.5	7.5	2.6	0.9	10	6.25	4	3	1	—	—	—	15
Biscuits, sugar-containing	9.0	1.3	3.5	1.9	2.4	11.25	11.25	5	1.5	1.5	—	—	—	18

Average Clearance Time (Min.) Above Conc. Levels: 0.02%, 0.2%, 2%, 20%

II. ORAL SUGAR CLEARANCE OF DIFFERENT FOODSTUFFS IN TWO PERSONS (MEAN VALUES) AND CALCULATION OF CARIES POTENTIALITY INDEX *(Continued)*

Fruit, berries													
Strawberries	9.4	8.6	18.5	0.3	0.3	2	2.5	1	1	—	—	—	3
Orange	6.5	3.1	14.5	0.3	0.2	2	2	1	1	—	—	—	3
Apple	7.5	7.5	9.0	0.4	0.3	3.5	2.5	1	1	—	—	—	5
Banana	13.9	11.2	18.5	0.4	0.2	3.5	2.5	2	0.5	—	—	—	6
Pear	9.0	7.0	12.5	0.7	0.4	4	3.5	2	1	—	—	—	6
Marmalade + bread + butter	16.3	2.0	8.5	1.8	0.6	6.25	4	2.5	1.5	0.5	—	—	9
Marmalade	65.3	23.8	10.5	3.5	1.5	5.75	5.75	3.5	3	1	—	—	10
Red whortleberry jam	46.5	46.8	13.0	1.9	0.9	6.25	5.75	3	3	0.5	—	—	10
Vegetables													
White cabbage soup	0.1	0.1	18.0	0.1	0.1	0.5	0.5	—	—	—	—	—	1
Cauliflower, boiled	1.0	0.9	21.0	0.1	0.04	1	0.5	—	—	—	—	—	1
Carrots, boiled	2.4	0.9	10.0	0.1	0.1	1	1	1	—	—	—	—	1
Peas, boiled	0.9	0.1	13.0	0.3	0.1	3.5	3	2	1	—	—	—	5
Beans, brown	8.8	4.1	31.5	1.5	0.8	4.5	4	2	2	0.5	—	—	7
Potatoes, boiled	0.8	0.7	11.8	1.6	0.7	4.5	4	2	2	0.5	—	—	7
Potatoes, fried	3.9	1.2	13.5	0.4	0.5	4.5	3.5	2.5	1.5	—	—	—	7
Honey													
Honey	72.8	69.3	12.3	5.6	5.8	11.25	11.25	5	5	1.5	2	—	18
Honey + bread + butter	19.0	18.3	8.0	4.6	3.4	15	15	7.5	4.5	1.5	1.5	—	24
Candy													
Dragées (one)	66.6	1.4	1.0	2.3	0.1	5.75	3.5	3	—	0.5	—	—	9
Dragées (two)	66.6	1.4	6.5	6.0	0.3	6.25	4	3.5	0.5	1	—	—	11
Lozenges, white (one)	51.6	11.4	1.0	9.5	3.2	6.25	6.25	4	3	2	1	—	12
Chocolate, dark	33.7	0.1	10.0	12.8	0.04	7.5	2	3.5	1.5	1.5	—	1	13
Lozenges, black (one)	44.2	10.2	1.0	4.7	1.2	6.25	4.5	4.5	3.5	3	2	—	14
Lozenges, white (two)	51.6	11.4	2.0	13.4	3.7	7.5	7.5	5	4.5	3.5	2	—	16
Lozenges, black (two)	44.2	10.2	2.0	9.9	2.6	10	6.25	6.25	4.5	3.5	2.5	—	20
Chocolate, light	47.5	5.8	11.0	10.1	0.7	11.25	11.25	6.25	2	3	2.5	—	21
Sweets	80.0	6.0	6.0	30.6	3.5	11.25	11.25	7.25	3	3	1.5	1.5	22
Caramel	64.0	15.4	6.9	18.8	6.4	18.75	7.5	5	4	2.5	2	0.5	27
Toffee	78.0	20.0	7.0	21.7	8.1	11.25	7.5	11.25	7.5	5	3.5	2	30

II. ORAL SUGAR CLEARANCE OF DIFFERENT FOODSTUFFS IN TWO PERSONS (MEAN VALUES) AND CALCULATION OF CARIES POTENTIALITY INDEX (Concluded)

Food Product	Sugar Content TS %	Sugar Content RS %	Ingested Quantity, Mean gm.	Max. Carbohydrate Conc., Mean TS %	Max. Carbohydrate Conc., Mean RS %	0.02% TS	0.02% RS	0.2% TS	0.2% RS	2% TS	2% RS	20% TS	20% RS	Caries Potentiality Index* TS
Milk products, eggs														
Cheese	0.2	0	7.0	0.02	0.02	—	—	—	—	—	—	—	—	0
Egg, boiled	0.1	0.1	12.0	0.01	0.01	—	—	0.5	—	—	—	—	—	0
Omelette	1.3	0.9	21.0	0.3	0.2	2.5	2	1.5	1	—	—	—	—	3
Pancake	10.9	2.2	20.0	1.1	0.9	4	3	2.5	1	1	—	—	—	6
Ice cream	2.4	1.2	10.0	3.2	0.3	5	4	4	3.5	1	1	—	—	9
Whey cheese	82.0	53.5	9.0	6.8	4.6	7.5	7.5	4	3.5	1	1	—	1	13
Meat products														
Ham, boiled	0.5	0.2	8.0	0.02	0.02	0.5	1	—	—	—	—	—	—	1
Beef, boiled	0.2	0.1	10.0	0.2	0.05	1	1	—	—	—	—	—	—	1
Pork chop	0.1	0.1	13.5	0.1	0.04	1	0.5	—	—	—	—	—	—	1
Liver sausage	1.7	0.3	14.5	0.1	0.02	1.5	0.5	—	—	—	—	—	—	2
Swedish sausage, roast	0.5	0.4	8.0	0.3	0.2	2.5	2	0.5	0.5	—	—	—	—	3
Meat balls	5.3	2.8	22.5	0.6	0.2	2.5	2.5	1	0.5	—	—	—	—	4
Liver paste	3.8	1.6	13.0	0.4	0.2	3	2	1	1	—	—	—	—	4
Fish products														
Herring, salted	0	0	6.5	0.01	0	—	—	—	—	—	—	—	—	0
Cod, boiled	0.1	0.1	22.0	0.01	0	—	—	—	—	—	—	—	—	0
Herring, fried	0.5	0.3	13.0	0.1	0.1	1.5	1.5	—	—	—	—	—	—	2

From Lundqvist, C.: Oral sugar clearance: its influence on dental caries activity. Odont. Revy, 3:Supp. 1, 1952.

*Low number indicates limited caries potential. High number indicates high caries potential. For calculation of caries potentiality index see the text, Chapter 28. TS = total sugar; RS = reducing sugar.

INDEX

Page numbers in *italics* refer to illustrations; those followed by t refer to tables.

689